# THE YEARBOOK

## OF THE ROYAL COLLEGE
## OF OBSTETRICIANS
## AND GYNAECOLOGISTS

1 9 9 6

# THE YEARBOOK

## OF THE ROYAL COLLEGE
## OF OBSTETRICIANS
## AND GYNAECOLOGISTS

Edited by John Studd

*1 9 9 6*

Published,
in association with
The Parthenon Publishing Group,
by

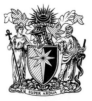

RCOG PRESS

*The Royal College of
Obstetricians and Gynaecologists*
London

A catalogue record is available
from the British Library.

ISBN 0-902331-91-4

Published in the UK and Europe in association with
The Parthenon Publishing Group Limited
by the RCOG Press

RCOG Press
Royal College of Obstetricians and Gynaecologists
27 Sussex Place, Regent's Park
London NW1 4RG

The Parthenon Publishing Group Limited
Casterton Hall, Casterton
Carnforth, Lancashire LA6 2LA

Typesetting by AMA Graphics Ltd, Preston
Printed and bound by Bookcraft (Bath) Ltd.,
Midsomer Norton, UK

# Contents

# List of contributors

**Aly Alaily PhD FRCOG**
Consultant Gynaecologist
Buchanan Hospital
St Leonards on Sea
East Sussex TN38 OTX

**Richard A. Anderson MD PhD MRCOG**
Lecturer
Department of Obstetrics and Gynaecology
Centre for Reproductive Biology
University of Edinburgh
37 Chalmers Street
Edinburgh EH3 9EW

**Janet R. Ashworth BM BS**
Specialist Registrar
University of Nottingham
Department of Obstetrics and Gynaecology
City Hospital
Huchnall Road
Nottingham NG5 1PB

**Robert D. Atlay FRCOG**
Medical Director
Consultant Obstetrician and Gynaecologist
Liverpool Women's Hospital
Crown Street
Liverpool L8 7SS

**Philip N. Baker BS MD MRCOG**
Senior Lecturer/Honorary Consultant
    Obstetrician and Gynaecologist
University of Nottingham
Department of Obstetrics and Gynaecology
City Hospital
Hucknall Road
Nottingham NG5 1PB

**Amar S. Bdesha FRCS**
Senior Registar
Charing Cross Hospital
Fulham Palace Road
London W6 8RF

**Tony Blakeborough FRCR MRCP**
Senior Registrar in Radiology
Ultrasound Department
St James's University Hospital
Beckett Street
Leeds LS9 7TF

**Sarah Bower MRCOG**
Senior Registrar
University College Obstetric Hospital
Huntley Street
London WC1E 6AU

**Timothy J. Christmas MD FRCS**
Consultant Urological Surgeon
Charing Cross Hospital
Fulham Palace Road
London W6 8RF

**Roger V. Clements FRCS(Ed) FRCOG FAE**
111 Harley Street
London
W1N 1DG

**Ian D. Cooke MB BS DGO FRCOG**
Professor
University Department of Obstetrics and
    Gynaecology
Jessop Hospital for Women
Leavygreave Road
Sheffield S3 7RE

**Peter J. Danielian MD MRCOG**
Consultant Obstetrician and Gynaecologist
Aberdeen Maternity Hospital
Cornhill Road
Aberdeen AB9 2ZA

**Anthony Davies MA MB BChir MRCOG**
Clinical Research Fellow
Minimally Invasive Therapy Unit and
    Endoscopy Training Centre
University Department of Obstetrics and
    Gynaecology
The Royal Free Hospital
Pond Street
Hampstead
London NW3 2QG

**Melanie C. Davies MA MRCP MRCOG**
Consultant
Reproductive Medicine Unit
University College Hospital
Huntley Street
London WC1E 6AU

**Anne C. Deans DCH MRCGP MRCOG**
Senior Registrar in Obstetrics and Gynaecology
Frimley Park Hospital
Portsmouth Road
Frimley
Camberley
Surrey GU16 5UJ

**Paul Devroey**
Professor
Clinical Director
Centre for Reproductive Medicine
Academisch Ziekenhuis-Vrije
Universiteit Brussel
Laarbeeklaan 101 B1090
Brussels
Belgium

**Murdoch G. Elder DSc MD FRCS FRCOG**
Professor
Department of Obstetrics and Gynaecology
Hammersmith Hospital
Du Cane Road
London W12 OHS

**Sarah Flint MB BS MRCOG**
Clinical Reasearch Fellow
Department of Obstetrics and Gynaecology
King's College Hospital
Denmark Hill
London SE5 9RS

**Donald Gibb MD MRCP FRCOG**
Consultant Obstetrician, Care Group Director
    Women's Services
Department of Obstetrics and Gynaecology
King's College Hospital
Denmark Hill
London SE5 9RS

**Abha Govind MRCOG**
Senior Registrar
Department of Obstetrics and Gynaecology
North Staffordshire Hospital Trust
Stoke-on-Trent ST4 6QG

**Alessandra Graziottin MD**
Specialist in Gynaecology, Obstetrics and
    Oncology
Docente di Sessuologia
Universita di Gonova
Via S. Secondo 19
10128 Torino
Milan
Italy

**Peter A. Greenwood MA FRCS(Ed) MRCOG**
Consultant Obstetrician and Gynaecologist
Great Yarmouth and Waveney Health Authority
James Paget Hospital
Lowestoft Road
Gorleston
Great Yarmouth
Norfolk NR31 6LA

**John Hare MA MD FRCOG**
Consultant Obstetrician
Hinchingbrooke Hospital NHS Trust
Huntingdon Park
Huntingdon
Cambridgeshire PE18 8NT

**Kelsey A. Harrison MD DSc FRCOG**
Professor of Obstetrics and Gynaecology
University of Port Harcourt
Port Harcourt
Nigeria

**Peter S. Haughton BD MA DipTh(Cantab)**
Adviser in Medical Law and Ethics
Education Development Unit
Medical School Building
Guy's Hospital
London Bridge
London SE1 9RT

**Brian Hopkinson ChM FRCS**
Head of University Department of Vascular
    Surgery
Department of Vascular Endovascular Surgery
Queens Medical Centre
University Hospital
Nottingham NG7 2UH

**Henry C. Irving FRCR**
Consultant Radiologist
Ultrasound Department
St James's University Hospital
Beckett Street
Leeds LS9 7TF

**Changulanda M. Joshi MRCOG**
Clinical Research Fellow
Department of Obstetrics and Gynaecology
North Staffordshire Hospital Trust
Stoke-on-Trent ST4 6QG

**Sean Kehoe MRCOG DCH**
Lecturer, Subspecialty Trainee in
    Gynaecological Oncology
Department of Obstetrics and Gynaecology
Division of Gynaecological Oncology
City Hospital Trust
Dudley Road
Birmingham B18 7QH

**Ronald F. Lamont BSc MB ChB DM FRCOG**
Consultant in Obstetrics and Gynaecology
Department of Obstetrics, Gynaecology and
    Genetics
Northwick Park Hospital
Watford Road
Harrow
Middlesex HA1 3UJ

**Sheila Macphail BM PhD MRCOG**
Senior Lecturer in Obstetrics and Gynaecology
    and Honorary Consultant Obstetrician and
    Gynaecologist
Department of Obstetrics and Gynaecology
4th Floor, Leazes Wing
Royal Victoria Infirmary
Newcastle-upon-Tyne
NE1 4LP

**Adam L. Magos BSc MD MRCOG**
Consultant Gynaecologist
Minimally Invasive Therapy Unit and
    Endoscopy Training Centre
University Department of Obstetrics and
    Gynaecology
The Royal Free Hospital
London NW3 2QG

**Peter J. Milton MD FRCOG**
Consultant Obstetrician and Gynaecologist
Department of Obstetrics and Gynaecology
Addenbrookes Hospital
Cambridge CB2 2SW

**Gary J. Mires MD MRCOG**
Senior Lecturer
Ninewells Hospital and Medical School
Dundee DD1 9SY

**John J. Morrison BSc DCH MD MRCOG**
Lecturer/Senior Registrar in Fetal Medicine
Department of Obstetrics and Gynaecology
University College Hospital
86-96 Chenies Mews
London WC1E 6HX

**John B. Murdoch MD MRCOG**
Consultant Gynaecologist
Directorate of Obstetrics, Gynaecology and ENT
St Michael's Hospital
Southwell Street
Bristol BS2 8EG

**P. M. Shaughn O'Brien MD FRCOG**
Professor
Keele University School of Postgraduate
    Medicine
Academic Department of Obstetrics and
    Gynaecology
North Staffordshire Hospital Trust
Stoke-on-Trent ST4 6QG

**Olusegun A. Odukoya MD FWACS MRCOG**
Clinical Lecturer
University Department of Obstetrics and
    Gynaecology
Jessop Hospital for Women
Leavygreave Road
Sheffield S3 7RE

**Pranav P. Pandya BSc MB BS**
Registrar
University College Obstetric Hospital
Huntley Street
London WC1E 6AU

**Roger J. Pepperell MGO MD FRCOG FRACOG**
Dunbar Hooper Professor of Obstetrics and
    Gynaecology
Department of Obstetrics and Gynaecology
The Royal Women's Hospital
132 Gratton Street
Carlton
Victoria 3053
Australia

**Fran Reader FRCOG BASMT MFFP**
Consultant in Reproductive and Sexual Health
    Care
Ipswich Hospital
Heath Road
Ipswich
Suffolk IP4 5PD

**Philip W. Reginald MD FRCOG**
Consultant Obstetrician and Gynaecologist
Department of Obstetrics and Gynaecology
Wexham Park Hospital
Wexham
Slough
Berkshire SL2 4HL

**Raine E. I. Roberts MBE MB ChB DCH FRCGP
    DMJ (Clin)**
Clinical Director
The St Mary's Centre
Sexual Assault Referral Centre at St Mary's
    Hospital
Oxford Road
Manchester M13 OJH

**James R. Scott MD**
Professor
Department of Obstetrics and Gynaecology
University of Utah Medical Center
50 North Medical Drive
Salt Lake City
Utah 84132
USA

**Mahmood I. Shafi MB Mch DA MRCOG**
Senior Lecturer in Obstetrics and Gynaecology
Department of Obstetrics and Gynaecology
Division of Gynaecological Oncology
City Hospital Trust
Dudley Road
Birmingham B18 7QH

**Edward J. Shaxted DM FRCOG**
Consultant Obstetrician and Gynaecologist
Northampton Medical Consultancy Unit
Three Shires Hospital
The Avenue
Cliftonville
Northampton NN1 5DR

**Anthony R. B. Smith BSc MB ChB FRCOG**
Consultant Gynaecologist
Department of Urological Gynaecology
St Mary's Hospital for Women and Children
Whitworth Park
Manchester M13 OJH

**Kevin M. Smith MB BS BSc DGM**
Registrar
Women's Centre
John Radcliffe Hospital
Headington
Oxford OX3 9DU

**Herman Tournaye**
Centre for Reproductive Medicine
Academisch Ziekenhuis-Vrije
Universiteit Brussel
Laarbecklaan 101 B1090
Brussels
Belgium

**Mark Vandervorst**
Centre for Reproductive Medicine
Academisch Ziekenhuis-Vrije
Universiteit Brussel
Laarbeeklaan 101 B1090
Brussels
Belgium

**Kathleen G. Waller MB ChB MRCOG**
Senior Registrar
Department of Obstetrics and Gynaecology
Hammersmith Hospital
Du Cane Road
London W6 OHS

**Lynne Webster MB ChB MSc FRCPsych**
Consultant Psychiatrist with a Special Interest in
    Psychosexual Medicine
Department of Psychiatry
Rawnsley Building
Manchester Royal Infirmary
Oxford Road
Manchester M13 9WL

**Andrea J. Wilkinson**
Formerly Clinical Research Fellow
University of Nottingham
Department of Obstetrics and Gynaecology
City Hospital
Hucknall Road
Nottingham NG5 1PB

# Foreword

It is a huge pleasure to see the proofs of the *Yearbook* on the desk ready for printing and publication. This volume consists entirely of printed accounts of lectures given at various College postgraduate meetings and reflects the quality and the range of subjects covered over the year to an extent that the Royal College of Obstetricians and Gynaecologists can be very proud of its contribution to postgraduate education.

Since creating the *Yearbook* four years ago I have always desired a mixture of the scientific/clinical, historical, as well as the political aspects of our specialty, enabling the *Yearbook* to be the home of the many eponymous lectures which otherwise would not find their way into print. It is important that we continue documenting the progress in subspecialty training, continuing medical education and any despair for the future of the consultant grade that we may fear. Perhaps in the next edition Shaughn O'Brien, the incoming Publications Officer and Editor, will be fortunate enough to find somebody eccentric enough to justify the Calman changes. If only one of the Colleges had had the good sense and courage to state that the Calman proposals were not workable without a huge increase in senior posts. We are heading for severe problems.

It is good that each year we include the Royal College's Historical Lecture, this time in the form of an account of the parturition chair. But there is always a danger of failing to recognise where history ends and the contemporary shame of 'poverty, deprivation and maternal health' (described by Kelsey Harrison) begins.

In addition, it is important that we carry the medico-legal advice, information on forensic medicine, as well as a chapter on the minefield of ethics in the developing areas of assisted reproduction and gynaecology. We have honoured our promise to Professor Sir Malcolm Macnaughton not to neglect ethics. Those of us who see patients dare not ignore the lawyers who are doing so much damage to our profession. This assault on doctors is merely for commercial reasons, although it masquerades as altruistic concern for patients. For my part, I am one of the increasing number of doctors who would be happy to reach retirement age without being stabbed in the back by patients who they have helped and to make sure that none of our children ever do medicine.

The remaining chapters deal with valuable updates on a wide variety of clinical problems that are frequently encountered in busy practice. In my view they are a fascinating range of subjects, well written and, although I am keen not to write my own book review, I do not see how any aspiring or current members of the Royal College of Obstetricians and Gynaecologists can fail to benefit from the information contained in this volume.

This is an excellent volume and I am very grateful to all the contributors for their time and skills, as well as to Samantha Oliver (the Scientific Editor at Parthenon Publishing) and Sandra Wegerif (of the Royal College) who pull it all together.

John Studd
*Publications Officer 1992–96*

# 1

# Subspecialty training

*Melanie C. Davies and Sheila Macphail*

## SUBSPECIALTY TRAINING ON A FLEXIBLE BASIS

Flexible training is in demand. In a Royal College of Obstetricians and Gynaecologists' survey during 1991 (Saunders 1991) no less than 59% of female trainees and 18% of their male colleagues expressed an interest in part-time training. Demand is greater among women because of the undeniable fact that women have babies. Most women doctors have children and for many of them motherhood is a decisive factor in their subsequent career choices and pathways (Allen 1988). Up to one-third of trainees passing the MRCOG are subsequently lost to the specialty (Royal College of Obstetricians and Gynaecologists 1990) and most of these are women. To reduce this wastage we need to attract and retain new graduates, more than 50% of whom are now women (Harvey 1996). The number of women consultants in obstetrics and gynaecology, after remaining static for years, is now rising steadily (Figure 1). *Opportunity 2000* (Department of Health 1992) set goals for increasing the number of women consultants; the current aim is 25% of consultants by the year 2000. Certainly, there is evidence of preference for a female physician in gynaecological consultations (reviewed by Cockburn and Bewley 1996) and there is consumer pressure to meet this target. Of the new consultants appointed in our specialty in 1995, 45% were women.

Flexible training is on the increase. Nationally, no fewer than 26% of all female senior registrars in 1994 were flexible trainees. The Royal College of Obstetricians and Gynaecologists, which obviously recognises that women have babies, has been well ahead of most other colleges in addressing the wastage of female trainees and encouraging flexible training (Francis 1987). It was the first College to appoint a specific careers adviser for flexible training. In the last five years there has been an explosion in numbers of such trainees in our specialty (Figure 2). However, subspecialty training on a part-time basis is very unusual and, to date, only one flexible trainee has completed subspecialty accreditation.

### Flexible training for senior registrars

Before the introduction of the specialist registrar grade in April 1996 (Department of Health 1996), the entry criteria for flexible training at senior registrar level required applicants to

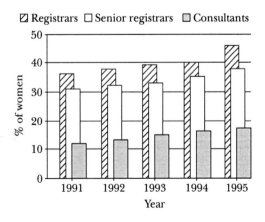

**Figure 1** *The percentage of women obstetricians and gynaecologists*

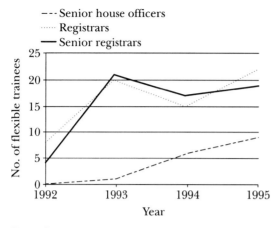

**Figure 2** *The number of flexible trainees in obstetrics and gynaecology*

be unable to work full time for 'well founded reasons'; combining part-time medicine with a second career was not encouraged. In practice, almost all those in part-time employment were women with childcare responsibilities (so, for convenience, 'she' will be used in the remainder of this article). It was possible to convert from a full-time post after appointment, but most trainees applied for and set up a part-time post which was tailor-made. Job sharing was rare because of the difficulties of finding a suitable sharer at the same career stage and in the same geographical area at the right time.

The mechanism of setting up a flexible post at senior registrar level has been described aptly by one postgraduate dean as 'a nightmare of red tape, conflicting information and delay'. Under the old regulations (Department of Health circulars PM[79]3 and EL[93]49), each specialty had a manpower quota (*sic*), set centrally, which restricted the number of posts available. The scheme was advertised once a year nationally for all specialties and competitive interviews were held to ensure that entry to part-time training was no easier or harder than to a full-time post. There was a waiting list of successful candidates awaiting a manpower slot. Having obtained manpower approval the candidate then had to set up a supernumerary post with the help of her local obstetrics and gynaecology department. She would usually be well received, because she

provided an additional pair of hands to ease the workload at little extra cost. Her basic salary came entirely from the regional (or special) health authority from a budget 'top sliced' for part-time trainees, but there was considerable regional variation in the availability of these funds, with some regions being recognised as favourable to part-time training, while others were viewed as unhelpful. However, since 1995 the budget has been held by the postgraduate dean.

After setting up a post, the timetable had to be submitted to the Higher Training Committee of the Royal College of Obstetricians and Gynaecologists for approval to ensure that the candidate would be accredited. Accreditation was achieved 'pro rata' (i.e. according to the number of sessions worked), so that for most candidates their training time was nearly doubled.

## Subspecialty training

The development of subspecialty training was proposed as long ago as 1982 (Royal College of Obstetricians and Gynaecologists 1982) in recognition of the pace of progress in obstetrics and gynaecology which made mastery of all fields an impossible task. Subspecialists are defined as '. . . having undertaken appropriate additional higher training, are recognised to have developed special expertise in the relevant field and devote a least half their working time to it'. The role of the subspecialist is envisaged as providing a service for consultation, special facilities for investigation and management of referrals (probably on a regional basis), and vital involvement in teaching, training and research.

Subspecialty training requires a two-year full-time clinical programme and one year of full-time research in the subspecialty. In practice, most trainees have undertaken research (usually for two years leading to an MD thesis) prior to entry to the clinical programme. Subspecialists are exempted from one year of general higher training. Thus, pre-Calman trainees spent a minimum of three years at the senior registrar grade.

Subspecialty training remains limited in that only 15 trainees are currently in post. Within my own field of reproductive medicine, 21 individuals have entered training programmes in 12 centres and, to date, 11 have reached accreditation. Several approved training centres have vacant positions. A major reason for these unfilled posts is lack of funding, as no designated budget is available for subspecialty trainees.

## Flexible subspecialty training

Subspecialty training is easily adapted for a flexible trainee. There are some obvious similarities. Subspecialty trainees are supernumerary to the department, like flexible senior registrars, and their posts are individually created and inspected by the Royal College of Obstetricians and Gynaecologists. The emphasis of the post is on training not service commitment and the timetable is individualised to the trainee's needs.

My personal experience of setting up both a flexible training post and subsequently a new subspecialty post showed many similarities. I found the local postgraduate dean most receptive to the idea of part-time subspecialty training and the continued provision of funding from the flexible training budget was the crucial factor in enabling me to enter the programme. The Department of Health was very supportive and extended the duration of my manpower approval to enable me to complete subspecialty accreditation.

A disadvantage is that subspecialty training cannot be undertaken on a fixed timetable, unlike general training where six sessions can be conveniently arranged as three fixed days a week. To cover the extensive curriculum, some subspecialty training programmes utilise a rotation through 'modules' of experience so that the timetable changes every few weeks or months; other programmes maintain 'core' sessions throughout the two clinical years and vary the special interest sessions, again with frequent changes of timetable. The trainee may need to attend clinic with consultant A for

3 months on Wednesday afternoon and then join consultant B for 3 months on Friday morning. This makes childcare arrangements complicated and, unless the carer is extremely adaptable, the simplest solution may be a full-time nanny — thus rather negating the point of flexible training.

On the positive side, the subspecialty trainee has a large measure of independence and flexibility. This is a great benefit in organising both work and home commitments. However, it needs considerable forward planning. Special events can be fitted in without too much difficulty — after all, consultant A's clinic will run next week, and by spending the morning in his lab this week, the trainee can get to the children's end-of-term concert in the afternoon. The rewards of these negotiations are the development of a new role as a parent who can be found at the school gates and new friendships with other parents who are delighted that she can take part in the rota for playgroups, Brownies, etc. (the full-time working mother is forever indebted to others).

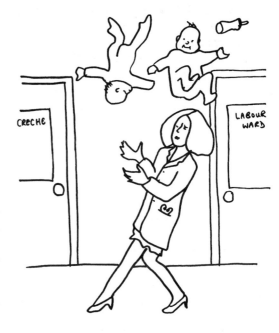

## Outcome of flexible training

The experience of flexible senior registrar training was examined by Alison Fiander, herself a flexible trainee in Wales (Fiander 1995). She surveyed all past and present trainees known to the Royal College of Obstetricians and Gynaecologists (a total of 37, all female). This demonstrated that part-time training was an excellent investment since almost one-half of the respondents would otherwise have left the specialty. Many trainees felt that part-time training could actually be better quality than full-time, because flexible posts were designed for the individual with the emphasis on training rather than service. In freeing time for family roles, the reduction in on-call commitments was particularly important to them. Many women doctors find that daytime work does not pose a problem, but covering for nights spent on call away from home is difficult with young children, particularly when the partner is also a doctor and on call. No nanny wants to work long weekends, certainly not at on-call rates of pay.

The disadvantages of flexible training are the poor salary, which may barely cover the cost of childcare, and the prolonged training period. This is extended still further by subspecialty training which may add up to two years to part-time higher training. It can be galling to be overtaken by younger colleagues who take up consultant posts and reap the material rewards, or climb the academic ladder to a Professorship before the impoverished part-timer has even reached accreditation. Flexible training has been described as full-time work for half the pay, and all those surveyed by Fiander worked more than their contracted sessions — although this is, of course, inevitable in medicine. Worryingly, no less than 80% of the trainees in the survey thought there was still prejudice against part-time workers.

Nevertheless, those who have undertaken flexible senior registrar training in general obstetrics and gynaecology are virtually all now consultants (Susan Blunt, personal communication). Most have reverted to full-time work as consultants. A small number of part-time (six session) consultant posts have recently been nationally funded, 10 of these in obstetrics and gynaecology (Royal College of Obstetricians and Gynaecologists 1996). This initiative should encourage trusts to support flexible working in the career grades.

## The future of subspecialty training

During 1996 there have been enormous changes in training in hospital medicine. The specialist registrar (SpR) grade was introduced in obstetrics and gynaecology in April 1996. An SpR appointment will provide continuity of training from senior house officer level through a five-year programme up to the award of the Certificate of Completion of Specialist Training (CCST). The details of the new arrangements for subspecialty training are still unclear. The Calman report itself (Department of Health 1993) contained ambiguities as to whether subspecialty training would be undertaken before or after the achievement of CCST. It now appears that subspecialty training will usually occur within the SpR grade (Department of Health 1996). It is likely that subspecialty trainees will enter during their fifth year and undertake the additional years of research and clinical training (years six and seven) before receiving CCST and subspecialty accreditation. Subspecialty trainees will be eligible for funding by the postgraduate dean, but the Department of Health (1996) admits 'opportunities ... may be restricted because of resource constraints'.

It is unclear how many subspecialty posts will be required. The demand for these posts may increase. After completing the SpR programme and gaining the CCST, candidates are expected to move rapidly through 'the gap' into consultant posts. Trainees fear they will have little choice but to take the first advertised post. Many may choose to develop their special interest into a subspecialty programme in the hope of achieving a better career post. In fact, very few subspecialist consultant appointments exist, and the creation of new posts at regional centres will be finite, so it is likely that in the future most subspecialty-trained candidates will become generalists with a special interest.

## Future of flexible training

The flexible training scheme at senior registrar level described above has now been wound up. In future all SpR trainees are eligible for flexible training. Equality of opportunity in the appointments procedure should be assured, because the declaration of intention to work part time is made after appointment to the SpR grade. The trainee still has to 'show that training on a full-time basis would not be practicable for well-founded individual reasons', but it is encouraging to hear that 'the deans will do all they can to ensure a smooth passage for those seeking to train flexibly' (Department of Health 1996). The deans in England and Wales hold 100% of the budget for flexible trainees. The appointment of a flexible trainee to a substantive post should bring greater professional recognition and overcome criticisms of 'favouritism' inherent in supernumerary posts. However, it may cause chaos to carefully planned SpR rotations unless specific posts are allocated for part-time training. These might have to lie vacant if there is no trainee in the right geographical location or, conversely, a waiting list may develop if there are too many flexible trainees.

More optimistically, the increasing separation of the service load from training which is emphasised by the Calman reforms will benefit part-time trainees, and the input of the postgraduate deans will be even stronger. Owing to the reductions in junior doctors' hours that are taking place (Department of Health 1991), and the shortened SpR training programme now being introduced, it is likely that the need for part-time training will lessen. This should not be taken as an excuse for lack of provision! The situation will be monitored by the powerful Flexible Training Working Group of the Conference of Postgraduate Medical Deans (COPMED). The future for part-time training may be even rosier if the recommendations of the Junior Doctors Committee (1996) are implemented. They state that training relates to knowledge acquired rather than time served, and that there is a poor association between hours worked and quality of training. As a result it should not be necessary to increase the duration of flexible training on a strict pro rata basis. They also propose that remuneration should be at the standard rate for the first 40 hours of duty; this would remove one of the greatest disadvantages of flexible training.

## Conclusions

Subspecialty training provides an opportunity for a small number of motivated trainees to develop expertise in a specialised field. Flexible training is of proven value in retaining able doctors within the specialty. Subspecialty training can easily be undertaken on a part-time basis and, following the Calman reforms, it should be easier to set up and complete.

# SUBSPECIALTY TRAINING OVERSEAS

The introduction of subspecialty training by the Royal College of Obstetricians and Gynaecologists and recognition of specific training posts within the United Kingdom has been closely followed by an increase in the number of posts recognised for subspecialty training overseas. This provides the trainee with a unique opportunity to train to some depth in a subject of personal interest, while broadening his or her education by participating in an alternative system of both health care and education. At present the Royal College will recognise one year overseas in a recognised centre towards subspecialty accreditation if the training requirements are completed in a United Kingdom centre. There are presently six trainees who have completed, or are currently undergoing, part of their training in a centre overseas. I was fortunate to be one of these and I would like to review some of the practical issues which need to be considered when contemplating a period of time overseas. Many of the issues are, however, specific to the country or unit concerned and the best solution is to talk directly with the previous trainee or the programme director.

## Availability worldwide

The number of accredited posts has increased and there are now seven recognised centres (two in fetal medicine, one in reproductive medicine and four in gynaecological oncology) distributed around the world, although they are all in countries where the predominant spoken language is English as this allows the trainee to participate fully in the work of the unit without any language barriers (Table 1). The names and addresses of the training directors of these programmes can be obtained from the subspecialty committee secretary at the Royal College. Many of these programmes are very popular and may be booked up for some years in advance, so the decision to work overseas cannot be made in haste. Furthermore, there are often lengthy administrative hurdles to be overcome, the exact nature of which varies between centres.

## Why train overseas?

Training in another country provides an added awareness of how health care is managed in countries other than the United Kingdom. It also gives an insight into different types of postgraduate training programmes, all of which are intended to prepare the medical graduates for a career as a specialist of some form. Involvement in undergraduate education may be an optional part of a subspecialty training programme, but is to be recommended to those with a passion for teaching and a desire to see how other systems operate, particularly at a time of curriculum change in the United Kingdom. Canadian medical schools have been in the vanguard of challenging traditional aspects of medical education and it is fascinating to participate in these teaching programmes at first hand.

Simply being away from home is a challenge on both a personal and professional level, and encourages the development of independent and critical opinions. It is, of course, important to be clear about which particular aspect of the host unit is attractive (other than the weather!) and to try to ascertain whether the training programme offered is compatible with your ex-

**Table 1** *Recognised centres offering subspecialty training*

*Reproductive medicine:*
  Monash University, Melbourne, Australia

*Fetal medicine:*
  Ottawa General Hospital, Ottawa, Canada
  The Perinatal Complex, University of Toronto, Canada

*Gynaecological oncology:*
  Queen Mary Hospital, Hong Kong
  Groote Schuur Hospital, Cape Town, South Africa
  Royal Hospital for Women, Sydney, Australia
  Sunnybrook Hospital, Toronto, Canada

pectations and abilities. Any programme recognised by the Royal College should provide a training menu which fulfils the syllabus requirements for each of the subspecialty areas. Even so, it is important to consider which parts of the syllabus are best covered in the home unit and which ones may be most gainfully studied overseas. While in Toronto I chose to concentrate on diagnostic ultrasound and invasive procedures and turned my attention to aspects of anaesthesia and neonatology on my return to the United Kingdom.

## Organising overseas training

Having decided that a period of subspecialty training overseas is appropriate for you and your family, and having decided the centre(s) in which you would like to work, the initial approach should be to the programme's training director. This will determine what vacancies are available, when they will occur and whether there are any local funding opportunities. Some units offer funded posts, while others expect the trainee to be funded entirely from the United Kingdom. The latter situation will require the agreement of a paid sabbatical by the regional authorities and this may become increasingly difficult to obtain when there are equally good and satisfactory programmes in the United Kingdom. However, acceptance onto a Royal College approved subspecialty training programme should enhance the chances of having the time funded from the United Kingdom, although this often results in a circular argument — with acceptance onto the programme being dependent on the availability of funding. Agreement to an unpaid leave is often easier to negotiate but, even so, it is important to clarify the temporary nature of your absence and to obtain written confirmation that employment will be available on your return. Some regions operate a limited competitive system which permits trainee staff a period of time overseas while covering the costs of locum cover in the United Kingdom.

It is also important to ensure that the Royal College of Obstetricians and Gynaecologists will recognise your training period and accepts your application to become a subspecialty trainee. This application needs to be made in conjunction with the programme director and will need to involve both the United Kingdom and overseas units. For those contemplating a period of training overseas with the subspecialty programme, it should not be assumed that the Royal College will give recognition to the training. Indeed, in all cases this should be discussed with the relevant committee in advance to avoid confusion and disappointment when recognition is not given.

## Timing and duration

Often this is not optional and it will simply be a case of undertaking the training when a space becomes available. However, if there is an element of choice, then it is sensible to think through the merits of whether the first or second year of subspecialty training is spent overseas. This will depend to some extent on the prior experience and expertise of the trainee. Clearly, it would not be prudent or personally fulfilling to spend the year learning the rudiments of the subspecialty. It would therefore be sensible for the aspiring fetal medicine specialist to be familiar with ultrasound imaging of the normal fetus, the oncologist to be surgically competent and comfortable with more complex surgical procedures and the reproductive medicine specialist to be familiar with the common procedures used regularly in assisted reproduc-

tion units. Often it is best to acquire these skills in the base unit in the United Kingdom so that your aptitude can be strengthened among familiar faces. In addition, you will then have some skills to contribute to the host unit. This will help to preserve your sense of professional identity while working in a strange and unfamiliar situation, which can be an unsettling experience when encountered for the first time (especially if it is at a relatively late stage in your professional career).

Usually, one year in an overseas centre is recognised by the Royal College as long as one of the two years of training is undertaken in a recognised United Kingdom centre. It is important to determine which centre will be the United Kingdom base and to ensure that an overseas training year will be available at the appropriate time and with the necessary funding. The introduction of Calman training schemes has led to some lack of clarity as to how and when trainees will be eligible for subspecialty training and who will fund the cost of such training. In any such negotiations it is important to clarify the nature and funding of the agreed post in writing and to have the clear support of both the programme training director and the postgraduate dean of the relevant regional authority.

To date, many of the individuals embarking upon subspecialty training had already undertaken a period of research in the relevant field. As long as this work was agreed to be suitable in terms of subject and quality by the subspecialty committee, then exemption was usually granted from a further period of full-time research, although a further short period of research is encouraged by many training programmes. However, it may be possible to undertake this research period in the overseas unit, but this will depend on many factors, the most critical being the availability of funds to cover the trainee's salary costs and the running costs of the project. If a rapport has already been established between the unit in the United Kingdom and the overseas centre, then there may already be collaborative research projects in which the trainee can become involved and which can be continued after the return to the United Kingdom.

Direct personal contact with the host unit or one of the key members is recommended and can usually be achieved by arranging to meet at a scientific meeting in the host country or elsewhere. If this is not possible, then telephone contact is worth while to obtain a sense of the unit's atmosphere and the people involved. It is helpful to contact a previous trainee to find out more about the practical aspects of the training and how it would meet your individual needs.

## Administrative details

### Immigration details

After acceptance onto a training programme there will then be the prolonged task of gaining a visa and work permit (Table 2). Rules will vary between countries, but will involve many months of form filling and several of the applications may require payment in the host currency. These details can take time and may involve a medical examination by a doctor nominated from the relevant High Commission. You should not assume that your application will be fast-tracked and so should allow the minimum recommended time to obtain the relevant document. If travelling with your family, ensure that all children are included in the application. Application for the work permit is usually initiated from the host country, but it may need further information from yourself. Departments with previous experience of overseas trainees usually have the application process streamlined and can given valuable practical advice.

### Professional registration

Just as the General Medical Council regulates the profession in the United Kingdom, there are similar bodies overseas who need to grant a licence or registration for practice. This will also vary enormously between countries and even within countries as, for example, in Canada, in which each province has a different regulating body (Table 3). A licence in one province does

**Table 2** *Administrative details*

| |
|---|
| May vary from country to country |
| May take several months to complete (6–8 months) |
| Need work visa/work permit |
| May require medical |
| All usually require payment |

**Table 3** *Factors involved in professional registration. As there is so much variation between countries, the situation in Canada is provided as an example*

| |
|---|
| Professional regulatory body |
| Professional recognition body |
| Not all medical schools recognised |
| May need to provide transcripts of grades and courses at Medical School |
| Need evidence of postgraduate education |
| Need support from host unit |
| Certificate of good standing from General Medical Council |

not grant the right to practise in another. In addition, you may also need to obtain approval from the national examining body to ensure that the training you have received is appropriate for the grade of post for which you are applying. In Canada this role is fulfilled by the Royal College of Physicians and Surgeons of Canada. These institutions will require evidence of graduation from medical school, including evidence of the grades awarded and courses undertaken (transcript of medical school progress). It is important to be aware that not all medical schools are recognised by the Canadian authorities. Any postgraduate qualifications will need to be verified by the appropriate College in the United Kingdom and original documents often need to be presented or photocopies signed by a legal authority. In addition, you will need to provide a certificate of good standing from the General Medical Council, for which there is again a fee.

## Potential problems

In the recognised overseas centres language is unlikely to be a problem, although an ability to speak French is an added bonus in Canada. In many of the centres work practices may be quite different to those in the United Kingdom and this may affect the clinical access of the trainee and opportunities to see and manage patients without direct supervision. The ultimate responsibility for the patient will lie with a senior member of staff and the degree of clinical autonomy will be dependent on the health care system as well as the personal relationship between trainee and senior staff. Again, this is an area which trainees who have reached senior registrar status or equivalent may find tricky. One of the advantages of United Kingdom training is the opportunity, even if only when on call, also to be involved in the care of women with benign conditions, or who have a normal ongoing pregnancy, and this can be an invaluable reminder that in the subspecialty arena we are dealing with only a small proportion of the population.

The question of on-call responsibility will vary between units and should be clarified in advance. Often this will depend to some extent on who is funding the post and its seniority. United Kingdom authorities are unlikely to continue out-of-hours payments and there may be no funding from the host unit to cover on-call services. However, the need to undertake on call may, to some extent, depend on the training requirements of the trainee. The lack of payment for on call may well result in a reduction in salary which should be taken into consideration when planning the trip.

Medical indemnity will vary from country to country. Indeed, cover from the United Kingdom may be available in Australia, but is not available in Canada (where cover through the Canadian Medical Protection Association [CMPA] is required). Preferential rates are usually available to those in training posts and in some instances the host unit may agree to provide cover. While you are out of the United Kingdom you may discontinue any additional personal cover, but should remember you are not then covered for providing emergency assistance out of National Health Service facilities, such as on a trans-Atlantic flight (it happened to me!).

In addition to medical indemnity, you need to ascertain who will provide health insurance for you and your family. It may be provided by the host unit and, in some countries, you may need to obtain a social security number. In order to avoid any problems, especially when travelling with young children, it is usually a good idea to take out travel insurance to cover the first couple of weeks overseas until the administrative problems are resolved. Not all schemes cover dental care and you should enquire specifically about this.

## Financial implications

You should expect a probable drop in salary due to the lack of on-call payments. It may be possible to boost your income with additional work, but be wary about the legal situation and what your work licence permits. For example, in Canada an educational licence is issued which does not allow the practitioner to work without supervision and this eliminates the chance of working as a locum. The cost of transporting yourself and your family, together with any belongings you wish to take, will need to be explored. Sea freight is often the cheapest method, but takes a long time which may not be viable if the period of time overseas is a year or less.

While you are working overseas you have the option of *not* being classed as a United Kingdom resident and this may have some tax advantages. However, it will depend on the time at which you depart from the United Kingdom and the length of time spent overseas. It is sensible to get professional advice on taxation before leaving the United Kingdom. Those who are National Health Service employees should consider continuing their superannuation contributions or making up the shortfall after they have returned. Payment will continue automatically if salary continues to be paid from the United Kingdom but, again, it is wise to discuss the details with your employing authority and the local tax office who will issue the appropriate lilac forms.

Accommodation, which may be either furnished or unfurnished, may be provided by the host institution. Taking electrical items overseas is often not helpful because of the different voltage supply. In busy university centres with many visiting staff there is often a thriving second-hand business in which items are passed from visitor to visitor with the minimum of capital outlay.

Families usually become quickly involved in the activities organised by others in a similar situation. Advice on schools is usually available from members of the host department or from other expatriates with children. There are usually many areas and aspects of the host nation to be explored and appreciated and full use should be made of these opportunities.

## Conclusions

A period of time training overseas is an invaluable experience which has many advantages in addition to those of subspecialty training. There does need to be careful planning which should

commence several months in advance of the trip and, in particular, care should be taken to ensure that employment will be available on your return. The most valuable information can usually be obtained by talking to someone who has previously worked in the unit and the Royal College of Obstetricians and Gynaecologists has a record of all these individuals and where they are currently working. The salient points of the advice I would give to somebody wishing to be involved in subspecialty training overseas are shown in Table 4.

**Table 4**  *Advice to a prospective trainee who wishes to study overseas*

| |
|---|
| It is very worth while |
| Contact host individuals, personally if possible |
| Start on recognition of qualifications early |
| Do *not* assume that the Royal College of Obstetricians and Gynaecologists will recognise the course without prior discussion |

# References

Allen, I. (1988) *Doctors and Their Careers.* London: Policy Studies Institute

Cockburn, J. and Bewley, S. (1996) Commentary: do patients prefer women doctors? *Br J Obstet Gynaecol* **103**, 2–3

Department of Health (1991) *The New Deal on Junior Doctors' Hours,* circular EL(91)82. London: Department of Health

Department of Health (1992) *Women in the NHS; an Implementation Guide to Opportunity 2000.* London: Department of Health

Department of Health (1993) *Hospital Doctors: Training for the Future. The Report of the Working group on Specialist Medical Training* (the Calman Report), circular MISC(93)31. London: Department of Health

Department of Health (1996) *A Guide to Specialist Registrar Training.* London: Department of Health

Fiander, A. (1995) Evaluation of flexible senior registrar training in obstetrics and gynaecology. *Br J Obstet Gynaecol* **102**, 461–6

Francis, W. (1987) *Memorandum of Council on the Role of Women Doctors in Obstetrics and Gynaecology.* London: RCOG

Harvey, J. (1996) Strategies for flexible training. *Med Woman* **15** (1), 11

Junior Doctors Committee (1996) *Annual Report.* London: British Medical Association

Royal College of Obstetricians and Gynaecologists (1982) *Report of the Working Party on Further*

*Specialisation within Obstetrics and Gynaecology.* London: RCOG

Royal College of Obstetricians and Gynaecologists (1990) *Manpower in Obstetrics and Gynaecology.* London: RCOG

Royal College of Obstetricians and Gynaecologists (1996) *Annual Report 1995.* London: RCOG

Saunders, P. (1991) *Recruitment in Obstetrics and Gynaecology: Report to Council.* London: RCOG

# 2

# The future of the consultant grade

*Brian Hopkinson*

Right from the earliest times some medical practitioners have had cases referred to them by their colleagues, undoubtedly because of their special interest or expertise in a particular area of medical practice. Slowly over the years, as the practice of medicine became more scientific and more specialised, medical practitioners were generally well advised to consult others in the interests of their patients. On 12 June 1886, the *British Medical Journal* stated:

> *'that a need has arisen for a class of men who will act as consultants in the strictest sense of the term.'*

During the following year, the *British Medical Journal*, on 9 February, gave the following working definition of a consultant:

> *'a gentleman, no doubt as a rule of superior culture and knowledge of his profession, who sees patients at his own house at stated hours, who is quite willing to visit them at home if requested to do so; it being understood that he confines his practice to medicine or surgery as the case may be; and that the rate of his remuneration is higher than that usually accorded to the practitioner. He is, in fact, a practitioner (though exclusively medical, surgical or obstetrical) among the rich, or among those willing to pay a guinea or more for each consultation or visit. As a point of fact, the ordinary general practitioner so called, finds the bulk of his work in medicine or obstetrics, the difference between him and the consultant really resolves into a difference of fees. We are not objecting to this. The difference of remuneration generally corresponds with a superior value of the opinion of the consultant.'*

From 1878 until the institution of the National Health Service in 1948, this superior being, the consultant, flourished in larger teaching hospitals, particularly in London, but also to a certain extent in the provinces. At this time the consultant generally made his money in private practice and donated his services free as an honorary physician or surgeon to the local voluntary hospital or poor law institute. There was a relatively small number of consultants before the Health Service. Many of them would practise on a 'hub-and-spoke' principle (i.e. they had their main session at the larger teaching hospital, but would visit smaller surrounding hospitals for sessions). Indeed, there are records of many of them travelling regularly from London to the provinces to undertake consultations and operating sessions either in the local hospitals or in the houses of the richer patients. At that time, the position of the consultant was very exalted and the spirit of the age is probably caught best by scenes in the television series *Dr Finlay's Case Book* — the consultant from Edinburgh comes to visit Tannach Brae in his Rolls Royce! In his teaching hospital the great man would be surrounded by trainees and students who counted it a privilege to associate with him and many of them were not paid wages for their services; in fact, some of them actually paid to be taught by him.

## ESTABLISHMENT OF THE HEALTH SERVICE

With the advent of the National Health Service in 1948 came the concept that every town, district and area should have its own hospital staffed by its own consultants. Many of these early consultants were part-time general practitioners who took a particular interest in medicine, surgery or obstetrics, and held consulting sessions at the local hospitals. A smaller number of registrars, housemen and students were generally associated with these provincial units. In the 1950s it became clear that trainees were having to wait until their 40s before becoming consultants and, as a result, the number of consultant posts increased to ensure that more became appointed; this led to the inevitable lowering of the consultant's status in terms of his social position, his income and his influence within the hospital environment where he worked. However, many young practitioners still aspired to become consultants and found the long hours and hard work of the apprenticeship were made tolerable by the prospects of greater freedom of action when they became consultants. Most wanted to practise independently, to be responsible for their own actions and to provide continuing care for all patients nominally under their charge. They took on the extra responsibilities happily, because they had well-trained junior staff to support them and would only be disturbed out of hours for serious and important matters which required their skill.

## CONDITIONS FOR JUNIOR HOSPITAL DOCTORS

During the 1960s and 1970s the population at large was slowly having their hours of work reduced and their hours of leisure increased, probably as a result of various technological changes in industry. Junior doctors were affected by this trend and, in the late 1960s, we saw the first move to acknowledge the heavy workload and large number of hours that juniors were undertaking. The introduction of extra duty payments, units of medical time and other devices enabled junior doctors to be paid more for excessive hours. At that time junior doctors accepted this as a form of pay rise, but did not expect to have their hours actually reduced. Through the 1970s and 1980s pressures were increasingly applied to reduce the number of hours that junior doctors worked from over 100 per week to the present 60–70 hours per week; indeed, the ultimate aim of most junior doctors'

leaders is to reduce the number of hours even further. Dr Borman, who was the chairman of the 'Junior Doctors' Committee' of the British Medical Association from 1991 to 1994, said he would like to see hours coming down even further so that nobody has to work for more than 56 hours a week. Consultants generally have a great amount of sympathy for the junior doctors in their desire to reduce the number of hours that they actually work. Unfortunately, nobody has found a way either of reducing the number of patients that need to be looked after, or increasing the number of junior doctors who are available to provide that cover. As a consequence, junior doctors increasingly cross-cover for one another. Currently, instead of looking after a small number of patients, all of whom were known to their junior doctor, they are now expected to cover an enormous number, many of whom are strangers. There is no doubt that the reduction of hours has led to some intolerable pressures due to the increased intensity of work. After all, it is much more difficult to be called in an emergency to see a patient about whom you know nothing than it is to see a patient with whom you are already familiar and whose plan of management will have been discussed at the team's ward rounds.

One of the greatest casualties of the reduction of junior doctors' hours has been the loss of team or firm identity and, in 1996, as a result of the 'new deal', consultants often find that they are managing an emergency with juniors with whom they are unfamiliar. This makes it far more difficult to delegate clinical responsibilities with confidence. As a result the consultant often sees the patient and deals with the problems him- or herself.

In my experience as a vascular surgeon, I have seen the situation change dramatically from my first appointment as a consultant surgeon in 1973. Up to 1990, I was able to train the senior registrar associated with our firm to manage virtually all the vascular surgical emergencies that could arise by spending most of the day and night with him or her during the first month of their appointment. It would then be unusual for me, personally, to have to go in to the hospital to deal with an emergency situation. Mutual trust and training had enabled this to take place between one consultant and one senior registrar. Currently, in 1996, as the registrars are only on call on one day in four, or less, they are not available for training when the emergency situations arise. As a result, I now find it very hard to provide the necessary clinical exposure to enable them to practise relatively independently in a year!

In the May 1996 issue of the British Medical Association's *News Review* there was an interesting interview with Stephen Vallely, who was the Junior Doctors' Committee Negotiating Sub-committee chairman when the 'new deal' was signed in 1991. He now feels that juniors' training is worse rather than better and is happy to call himself a dinosaur, feeling that juniors are not what they used to be. He says:

> *'I have now been a consultant radiologist for more than two years and I would have to say that on the issue of maintaining adequate training we have failed miserably ... Perhaps I am getting old, but the juniors I encounter in my day-to-day practice no longer know the patients they are treating, which will only be exacerbated by the specialist registrar grade and will not produce the calibre of the doctor we used to know. Consultants, myself included, are increasingly being expected to be first on, which is unacceptable, particularly when this is not being combined with the expected increase in consultant numbers since the new deal.'*

## SPECIALIST REGISTRAR GRADE

New training schemes for specialist registrars are designed to produce consultant candidates at an earlier age than are presently being achieved. To do this, the registrars are on rotations between different hospitals getting appropriate experience for their training and educational needs, but are only providing limited numbers of hours of service. The object is that they receive training and tuition in theoretical classes and seminars, as well as by conducting audit and, possibly, a certain amount of research. The basic concept of the 'new deal' is that refreshed and alert juniors will learn much more than if they are fainting through lack of

sleep. This may well be true for theoretical knowledge and training. Personally, I have always believed that the most valuable contribution a consultant can make to a junior's training is to be present with him at the time a difficult decision is being made or a difficult procedure undertaken. If the junior is not there when these arise, he or she will miss out. Most consultants fear that the result of the specialist registrar training programmes will be very highly educated people who are experts at the theory, but will not be competent in the management of more difficult cases. It may well be that these new-style trainees will only be exposed to more taxing situations on their own when they become consultants.

There is no question that as a result of the 'new deal' and the introduction of the specialist registrar grade, a much larger workload has been placed upon the consultants who are expected to be involved in formal teaching, audit, to take part in management affairs and to take the ultimate responsibility for patients under their charge. There are increasing pressures for consultants to become the first on call and even resident when they are on call. The theoretical answer to this increase in consultant workload recommended in the Calman report on specialist training is an annual 7–8% increase in consultant numbers to allow all these extra activities to be achieved. It is unfortunate that the actual increase has only been 2–2.5% per year. The government has fully supported the introduction of the Calman proposals, but has failed to produce the necessary cash to provide, in particular, the consultant expansion that is necessary to make it workable. Currently, I am a programme director for the Higher Surgical Training Scheme in Mid-Trent and the amount of paperwork and administration associated with this small organisation of only 18 trainees has escalated out of all proportion. This is just one of the many tasks that consultants have, in the past, gladly taken on voluntarily and as an extra contribution. However, in the future consultants, along with postgraduate deans and medical directors and clinical directors, will find themselves increasingly separated from clinical practice through the sheer pressure of hours. It is essential for maintenance of the service, and for the training of future consultants, that the consultant ranks are expanded. The consultant of the future, who has been used to a 56-hour week as a junior, will not be prepared to provide the amount of cover worked by their forebears. The intensity of work for consultants can only increase. Consultant expansion is essential.

## EFFECTS OF CONSULTANT EXPANSION

It is unlikely that the future consultant will be prepared to provide continuous responsibility for his patients when he is not officially on call. This could mean that his patients will have to be covered by colleagues during this time. Potentially, this can lead to the disruptive management of individual patients. In order to avoid this, it will be important to have teams of consultants who are familiar with each other and working together, preferably to agreed guidelines and protocols. Certainly, to bring together the contributions from different consultants to a common management plan will be in the interests of patients and it would be essential for the guidance of the resident junior doctors. However, it would be difficult for the individual consultant who happens to be on call to delegate responsibility to a registrar who also happens to be on call, especially if he is not familiar with him or her. Team working, team culture and team consensus, with written guidelines and protocols, is almost certainly going to be the safest way to work in the future.

How will future consultants acquire the necessary training and skills to practice their art? I think the answer to this lies in the method of training that applies in the United States, where they have residency training programmes which begin with more general exposure to a large number of specialties for short periods of time. Then, once basic training is completed, young doctors can either go into private practice as generalists, or go on to receive advanced training through special fellowships in prestigious units. There is no doubt that the experience and exposure the young American doctors acquire in these training units is superb and can be

achieved in a much shorter time than in the United Kingdom. However, this has only been achieved at the expense of extremely long hours of duty, far longer than are currently allowed in our own country. There are, of course, not only a far greater number of consultants per head of population in the United States, but vastly more doctors per head of population, so their individual workload is less.

In Scandinavia training programmes are accompanied by a very few number of hours per week and as a consequence it seems to take longer for them to become consultants. A surgical registrar I met recently from Scandinavia, who is a first-class trainee, is only just seeking a consultant post at the age of 45. It is to be hoped that our new specialist registrar scheme will be a better compromise than either the United States or the Scandinavian models.

## PATIENTS' EXPECTATIONS

There is no doubt that patients in the 1990s have the right to be treated by a named consultant, and also have greater expectations that the consultant will be more intimately involved in their care. If this is to happen, it is essential that consultant expansion is far greater than occurs at present.

## CONSULTANTS' CAREER EXPECTATIONS

Until now it has been quite common for a consultant to be appointed at the age of 35 and to expect to be doing essentially the same job for the next 25–30 years. The change of technology and management in medicine is such that it will be highly likely that the variety of work undertaken throughout the future consultant's career will change dramatically and more quickly than in the past. Periods of re-training and acquiring new skills will almost certainly be needed and future consultants will have to be more flexible in their work patterns. All will undoubtedly be involved to a greater or lesser extent in patient management, which is their core responsibility. However, some will concentrate more on either management and administration, teaching and research, professional representation or audit, etc. The degree to which consultants do these various other activities will have to be agreed with their colleagues, and the amount of clinical work that they perform will have to be adjusted appropriately. Certainly, most of the post-graduate deans are already full time, no longer participating in clinical activities, and many medical directors find they can only fulfil their management functions by reducing their clinical workload. Furthermore, as junior consultants may wish to take a greater amount of the emergency rota, while older consultants will probably wish to take less, suitable adjustments and negotiations about working patterns will have to be made.

Modern medicine and surgery are becoming increasingly more technical and specialised. In addition, there is a greater demand by patients that their particular problems be looked after by a specialist in that particular area. As a consequence more specialised teams of doctors are being formed in order to look after smaller and smaller areas of special interest. This has led to many of the individual specialist units requiring more complicated and expensive technical support that can only be afforded by larger units. However, as individual patients may initially be under the care of an inappropriate specialist there is always going to be a need for a generalist (not only as a general practitioner in primary care, but also in surgical or obstetric or gynaecological practice) who can recognise which is the most appropriate specialist colleague in each case.

The consequence of increasing specialisation is almost certainly going to be fewer, larger hospitals providing specialist care for a greater number of people, which will inevitably mean that patients have to travel further for their specialist care. There will still be a need for local community hospitals, probably run by general practitioners and visited by consulting specialists, but it is not practical or possible for every specialty to be represented in every community. Potentially the big problem will be the provision of emergency services, because patients do not present with neatly packaged special problems that easily identify to one particular special interest. The patients will need to be sorted out by the generalist medical attendants and transferred on as soon as appropriate to the large multi-specialty hospital. This may not always be possible in that certain emergency procedures may have to be performed at the local community level. If the local consultants at community hospital level are not kept up to date, they may easily become de-skilled. There is a very difficult balancing act to be performed between the vision of relatively local general services and the more specific specialty services which will only be available in the larger, but fewer, centres.

## PEER REVIEW AND MENTORING

In order to facilitate the career progress of consultants it will be important to have a peer review system in which the individual consultant can review his situation and make appropriate plans for his future. This can be done on an individual basis, ideally voluntarily, or through the professional review of the total service provision of a specialised unit, not merely the performance of its consultants, by a team from another part of the country. This system of mentoring, as it is called, has been pioneered by the British Thoracic Society and is attracting a fair amount of favourable press at the moment. It is important that such a scheme is peer-driven, positive, remedial, and is not punitive.

## WILL THE CONSULTANT SURVIVE?

I have no doubt that they will. Their roles and their working patterns will be very different from those in 1996. With the increasing cost of the provision of medical care, the providers will be seeking more and more cost-effective measures and it may well be that big business methods will have a much greater impact on the provision of medical services in the future. According to Professor Leslie Blumgardt, currently working in New York, the current ethos in the United States as far as provision is concerned is summed up by the phrase: 'it is not outcomes that count, it is incentives'. Make of that what you will.

# 3

# Continuing medical education: the first two years

*Peter J. Milton and Robert D. Atlay*

Continuing Medical Education (CME) may be defined as the maintenance of professional competence by the continuous updating of knowledge and skills. It is an individual's duty and responsibility to ensure sound professional development in the public interest.

The Council of the Royal College of Obstetricians and Gynaecologists approved the introduction of a mandatory programme of CME for its United Kingdom-based Fellows and Members from 1 January 1994, to encourage trained specialist staff to update themselves regularly on new knowledge, skills and procedures within their disciplines and so maintain the standards of clinical excellence necessary for optimal care of patients. The College's CME Committee is responsible for the co-ordination of the programme and for ensuring that the needs of its Fellows and Members in respect of CME are addressed.

## MONITORING PROGRESS

The half-way point in the first five-year cycle of the Royal College of Obstetricians and Gynaecologists CME programme is an opportune time to review the progress that has occurred.

Following publication of the Report of the Royal College of Obstetricians and Gynaecologists Working Party on Continuing Medical Education (Chairman Mr K. R. Peel) in 1991, the Council of the Royal College of Obstetricians and Gynaecologists decided to recommend the setting up of a CME programme for Fellows and Members in career posts. It was in the vanguard

of Royal Colleges and Faculties in deciding upon this initiative and the President at that time, Sir Stanley Simmons, invited Mr Robert Atlay to chair a Committee whose remit it was to establish and supervise CME.

From the outset it was decided that CME should be mandatory for Fellows and Members who wished their names to be included in a roll of specialists who had accumulated the requisite number of credits at the end of a five-year span. The CME Committee adopted 200 credits as the target and decided that each credit should be equivalent to one hour of educational activity. This equates to approximately 40 credits per year, or the very modest target of one hour of academic activity per week, allowing for leave (Table 1).

Following the decision of the other Royal Colleges and Faculties to adopt a target of 250 credits, we plan to elevate our target to bring it into line. This is still a modest amount in a five-year span and it was felt that, for the great majority of Fellows and Members, acquiring this number of credits would not represent a major change in their day-to-day activity, especially as a substantial number would be attainable either at the participant's own hospital or nearby.

The CME programme was designed to be flexible and charitable, with a wide range of activities being 'credit worthy'. The programme is restricted to participants working within the United Kingdom, which has proved to be a matter of contention with some Fellows and Members overseas but we felt we could not adequately provide or supervise CME for our

**Table 1**  *The Royal College of Obstetricians and Gynaecologists' (RCOG) credit allocation for the continuing medical education (CME) programme*

| Type of activity | Rate of accrual | Minimum credits |
| --- | --- | --- |
| *Hospital based:* | | |
| formal teaching | 1 per hour | — |
| clinical review meetings and other meetings related to the specialty | 1 per hour | 20 |
| *RCOG based:* | | |
| RCOG senior staff conferences | 1 per hour | 25 |
| RCOG meetings (including British congress) | 1 per hour | 30 |
| examining | 10 per exam sitting | — |
| setting MCQ/OSCE examination questions | 5 per meeting | — |
| *Personally arranged:* | | |
| publications | 5 per publication | — |
| formal presentations | 5 per presentation | — |
| CME meetings other than RCOG | 1 per hour | — |
| supervised learning | 1 per hour | — |
| personal learning project | 40 per project | — |
| *Distance learning:* | | |
| RCOG-approved video conferences | 1 per hour | — |
| RCOG-approved telephone conferences | 1 per hour | — |
| LOGIC | 10 per book | — |
| PACE reviews | 1 per review | 20 |

MCQ, multiple choice questions; OSCE, objective structured clinical examination; LOGIC, learning in obstetrics and gynaecology for in-service clinicians ; PACE, personal assessment in continuing education

overseas colleagues, whose needs might well differ from our own and whose CME would therefore be better provided locally. We are needless to say very keen not to educationally disenfranchise our overseas Fellows and Members in any way and are happy to advise them on CME matters and to provide educational material, such as PACE (personal assessment in continuing education) reviews, through the local representative committee structure. The method of recording credits is at present by means of a credit-slip book, with the slips being returned by the participants to the CME office at the Royal College of Obstetricians and Gynaecologists.

Monitoring has proved contentious, with views expressed ranging from those who feel that a very strict policy is necessary, to others who feel there should be none at all. Keeping a roll of specialists who have acquired the requisite number of credits has also proved contentious; some Royal Colleges do not intend to keep such a roll, whereas others have followed the Royal College of Obstetricians and Gynaecolo-

gists' pattern and style. This was based to a considerable extent on the CME programme devised by the Royal Australian College and it is a pleasure to acknowledge the help and advice given so freely by Roger Gabb and Alan Hewson.

Postgraduate medical education is expensive, sometimes it seems increasingly so, with not only a proliferation of courses, but high registration fees and expensive venues. For this reason, and others linked to staffing and the finances of some trusts, both the availability and funding of study leave have been a problem and may well continue to be so.

Despite some teething problems, it is felt that the CME programme was well thought out from the start and close to the original remit as defined by Council following the publication of the Peel report.

## MINOR REVISIONS

Like all vital educational activities the Royal College of Obstetricians and Gynaecologists' CME programme was designed to be flexible and amenable to change should this be deemed advisable in the light of comment and reaction from Fellows and Members. The object of CME is to maintain and, as time passes, to improve upon standards of patient care, and most would agree that CME must be beneficial in this regard. However, it is an extremely difficult concept to prove.

In developing the programme, the CME chairmen have been able to draw upon the experience of others through the very valuable CME Directors' meetings which take place regularly and which involve the chairmen and directors of all the other Colleges and Faculties. There has always been a full and generous exchange of ideas and information with other Colleges, who have drawn widely on the Royal College of Obstetricians and Gynaecologists' experience because (along with the Radiologists) they were the first in the field. Attendance at these meetings has confirmed our views that, although a degree of harmonisation between Colleges and Faculties is desirable, specialists in different fields have different requirements and hence a degree of individuality is also desirable.

One of the most difficult problems which has beset the CME Directors in trying to achieve harmonisation has been the concept of 'mandatory' as opposed to 'voluntary' CME and, although there is as yet no absolute agreement across the disciplines, there is a move towards CME being mandatory, even if the word is not actually used. The Royal College of Physicians, for example, regards CME as 'a matter of personal professional obligation'. This does not seem to us to be widely differing in its meaning from 'mandatory'.

## Registering credit allocation

As other Colleges have adopted CME (although some programmes are still not operational) we have learned that they in turn have devised simpler means of defining CME activity and registering credit allocation. As a consequence, the Royal College of Obstetricians and Gynaecologists is in the process of simplifying its own credit allocation system. In future, it is intended that participants will be asked to register their own activities in a small CME pocket diary and later to transfer the information to optically readable sheets which will be returned to the Royal College on an annual basis. It may even be possible to use direct computer transfer.

This new approach is in response to requests from our Fellows and Members for a less complex system, as well as the knowledge acquired from seeing how other programmes have developed. Some of our participants have found the categories acceptably diverse, while others felt they were too restrictive. Other Royal Colleges vary in their categorisation from the very simple and all embracing, with virtually any sort of educational activity being deemed worthy of CME credits, to the very strict, with even local meetings being scrutinised carefully. The Royal College of Obstetricians and Gynaecologists, as Fellows and Members would expect, has tried to adopt a flexible and charitable approach in devising a programme which would suit everyone's needs.

## Biased to Royal College activities

Our programme has, nevertheless, been criticised for being too heavily biased towards activities of the Royal College of Obstetricians and Gynaecologists and, in particular, for deeming it necessary for participants to attend a senior staff conference once every five years. As it is sometimes difficult for some subspecialists to derive much educational benefit from attending such conferences, which are designed essentially for the generalist, this obligatory requirement may be changed. This decision will be taken only after a great deal of thought and consultation with our participants and in committee, as it is believed that for the vast majority of specialists, particularly those involved in under- and postgraduate education, a wide knowledge of our still combined disciplines is a desirable aim. The quality of senior staff meetings and other meetings of the Royal College of Obstetricians and Gynaecologists is such that there is no doubt that they will continue to be well attended whatever the outcome; not only are they excellent in an educational sense, but they are very good value for money and present an ideal opportunity to meet specialist colleagues from all over the United Kingdom and overseas.

## 'Maxima' and 'minima'

When the programme started, there were a 'maxima' and 'minima', but this caused some consternation among those who wished to acquire more than the set maximum number of credits by extensive involvement in various types of activity. The 'maxima' have, therefore, been removed in the hope that very few, if any, participants will try to accumulate the majority of their credits by involvement in only one type of activity, but will go for the 'mixed diet' approach.

The 'minima' have been partly retained to encourage the concept of acquiring a substantial number of credits at or near base hospital and, by so doing, improve the quality of local educational activity. Also left in place is the minimum requirement to attend some Royal College of Obstetricians and Gynaecologists' activities. This is because we wish to ensure high quality educational content within the programme, which we believe the College meetings provide.

## Location of meetings

Devolution of meetings away from the Royal College will increase — in addition to the London-based conferences, there are now senior staff conferences outside London every other year, and an increasing number of excellent College postgraduate meetings and symposia are being held at provincial venues.

## Other developments/controversies

Over the past two and a half years developments have included the inclusion of non-consultant grade doctors in the programme, the inclusion of specialists in fields other than obstetrics and gynaecology (e.g. genitourinary medicine), and an increasing appreciation of the need for distance-learning programmes such as the PACE reviews (which have proved very popular) and CD-ROM (which is being introduced this year). These educational activities will surely increase in the future and other Colleges, both at home and overseas, are adopting similar distance-learning programmes.

There have been some controversial issues, including the CME Committee's refusal to award credits for reading medical literature. Interestingly, there is a split across the Colleges with regard to this point, but it is assumed that specialists in active practice will read appropriate journals to a greater or lesser extent and, as this activity cannot be measured, it remains excluded from the programme (in a similar manner to undergraduate teaching). For the time being, credits for postgraduate examining are allowed, but not all Colleges subscribe to this view. In this regard it is worth noting there are other 'credit earners' recognised by the Royal College of Obstetricians and Gynaecologists but not by other Colleges, and vice versa. Each January all activities set out in the CME programme are reviewed and appropriate alterations made.

## HOW BENEFICIAL IS CME?

Few would dispute that educational activity and keeping up to date must be beneficial for the women in our care, but it is difficult, if not impossible, to prove. The Royal College of Obstetricians and Gynaecologists is involved in a research exercise with Professor Janet Grant of the Research into Medical Education Institute, in an attempt to demonstrate that CME is effective and measurable and hopefully some answers will emerge from this project.

# 4

# The history of the parturition chair

*Aly Alaily*

*'One cannot practise a science unless one knows its history.'*

Auguste Comte

Although the use of the stool or parturition chair during delivery dates from a period of great antiquity, the custom still survives in some countries today. The midwife carried the chair from house to house among the poor and the wealthy regarded it as an indispensable article of furniture.

## HISTORICAL RECORDS

The Egyptians were the first to demonstrate the birthing chair. Figure 1 shows a sculptured stone relief in a birth house at Luxor (1450 BC) with the Queen seated on a chair, her arms being held by two divinities with bovine heads. Figure 2 shows the Egyptian Queen in labour, and the obstetric stool, in the temple of Kom Ombo by

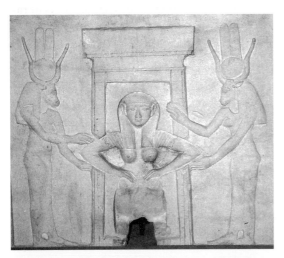

**Figure 1** *An Egyptian queen in labour helped by two divinities. (From the Cairo Museum with permission)*

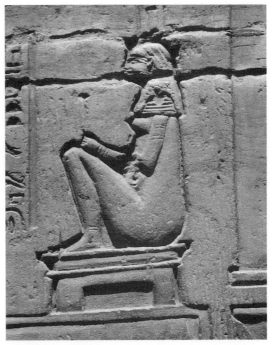

**Figure 2** *An Egyptian queen on an obstetric stool at the temple of Kom Ombo*

*This chapter is based upon the Annual Historical Lecture given at Keele University to the Royal College of Obstetricians and Gynaecologists Senior Staff Conference on 26 March 1996*

the Nile. The birth stool is perhaps the oldest parturitional posture aid.

The sitting position was practised from a very early period. The squatting position was modified slightly to form a sitting posture with the use of the birth stool depending on the custom of each tribe. The early Egyptian birthing chair consisted of three bricks on which a labouring woman sat as described in the Old Testament, in Exodus, chapter 1, verse 16. Indeed, 'to sit on stones' was synonymous in Egyptian hieroglyphics with 'to give birth'.

There is an allusion to the use of a stool in the book of Exodus, where the King of Egypt gives instructions to the Hebrew midwives; he says, '*When ye do the office of a midwife to the Hebrew women, and see them upon the stools; if it be a son then ye shall kill him: but if it be a daughter, then she shall live. But the midwives feared God, and did not as the King of Egypt commanded them, but saved the men children alive*' (Exodus, chapter 1, verses 15–16).

The Hebrew word *Ebnaim* is translated by some as 'upon the birth stool' and from the Greek text 'a bearing stool, like potter's wheel', from which one would infer it was circular in shape, rather like the potter's work table of the time (Ploss, Bartels and Bartels 1935).

Both Hippocrates (460–337 BC) and Soranus (early second century AD) recommended the use of a birth chair to the Greeks, but it was superseded by the semi-reclining position which we see depicted in Greek sculptures (Thompson 1957). There appears to be no representation of a stool or chair used by the Ancient Greeks, although in later times they are said to have employed a stool on which the assistant nurse sat on a rounded projection at the back in order to hold the patient, who sat at the front on a forked point (Ploss, Bartels and Bartels 1935). Figure 3 shows the birth stool and its correct use by Giovanni M. Savonarola (*circa* 1384–1462). An attendant sitting on the rounded projection at the apex of the stool supported the back of the parturient seated on the forked part. On the left is seen the prototype of the parturition chair (Ploss, Bartels and Bartels 1935).

The obstetric stool was used by the Romans, brought most likely by the immigrant Greek physicians, and from Rome it was taken over the Alps to be used in Germany and France throughout the Middle Ages (Thompson 1957).

The birthing stool of the earlier period appears to have developed into a chair with back and sides between the fourteenth and fifteenth centuries, although the use of a low stool still serves in some parts of Europe (Thompson 1957). The first description and representation of a chair for parturition is given by Eucharius Roeslin (the city doctor of Worms, Germany, who became physician to the Duchess of Braunschweig and Lüneburg) (Rosegarten 1513). Figure 4 shows the parturition chair described by Roeslin in 1513, with its curved back and semicircular seat which had a horseshoe-shaped piece cut out. It stood two feet in height from the ground.

The shape of the parturition chair varied in different countries because they were often constructed by carpenters who had not seen one and designed according to local ideas. Jacob Rueff in 1554 described a parturition chair similar to that of Roeslin with a semi-circular seat, but it had a curtain placed around to protect the patient and was more rounded (Rueff 1554). Indeed, Rueff, a fanatical theologian from Zürich, designed a chair that was reported to resemble more an instrument of torture, or a throne for a bow-legged monarch, than simply a birthing chair.

The peculiar custom of sitting on the lap of another person to be delivered may have led to the invention of the first parturition chair

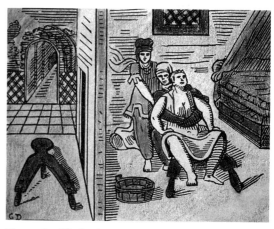

**Figure 3** *The birth stool described by G. M. Savonarola*

(Ploss, Bartels and Bartels 1935). The custom of using the lap of another during delivery, which was very widespread up to the beginning of the twentieth century, dates back to hoary antiquity. In the Bible we find allusions to the practice. For example, Rachel says to Jacob (Genesis, 23), '*Behold my maid Bilhal, go in unto her and she shall bear upon thy knees, that I also may have children by her.*' In seventeenth century Holland the so-called shott-steers were women who used to lend their laps for delivery of this kind. Sometimes it is strange men whose laps have a reputation for making easier delivery (Ploss, Bartels and Bartels 1935). Women in ancient Peru also used the lap for delivery, as was proved by Engelmann and others from Peruvian vases.

In north-western Virginia in the early nineteenth century (Engelmann 1882), as depicted in Figure 5, we find a delivery scene with the parturient sitting on her husband's lap while he is seated on a chair. This plan gives the woman complete control over the voluntary forces auxiliary to that of the uterus itself. However, it fatigues all her attendants except the doctor and, if the labour is not rapid, the husband is the greatest sufferer — but then this little tax on his affectionate nature was, in those days, considered the very least return he could make for the mischief he had occasioned (Jarcho 1934).

A crude type of obstetric chair used by negresses in Shuli village of central Africa (after Felkin) consisted of a block of wood placed against a trunk of a tree. On this the parturient sits, three and a half feet above the ground, placing her feet on the rungs of two poles resembling stilts and seizing the upper ends of the poles with her hands at the same time. Once she has taken her place, she hardly ever gives up until the child is born (Jarcho 1934).

Ambrose Paré, the renowned French surgeon who made a great contribution to obstetrics by describing the podalic version, recommended the obstetric chair in his book (Paré 1641). He believed that the obstetric chair allowed unhampered respiration and kept pressure off the sacrum, allowing the easier separation of pelvic bones.

The use of the parturition chair became common in Germany during the seventeenth cen-

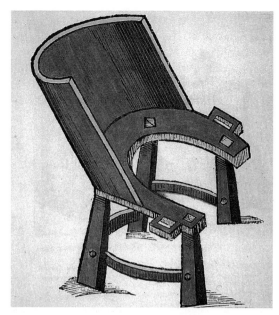

**Figure 4** *The parturition chair described by Roeslin in 1513*

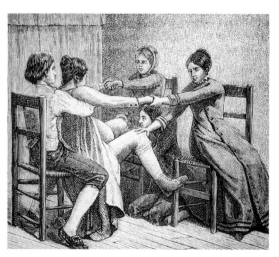

**Figure 5** *A nineteenth century delivery scene from north-western Virginia*

tury and early eighteenth century. It was modified to be higher with an open back and arms raised from the seat.

The German folding parturition chair (1701–1850) shown in Figure 6 has leg-rests and the seat tray missing. Made of wood, it has silk upholstery and leather fittings, with iron and brass studs.

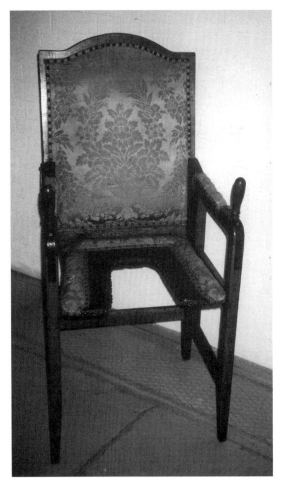

**Figure 6** *The German folding parturition chair (1701–1850). (Photo by permission of Science Museum/Science and Society Picture Library)*

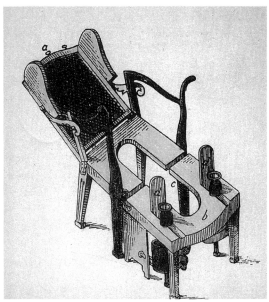

**Figure 7** *Professor Stein's chair from Germany*

Other chairs were made by Heister from Frankfurt in 1770. His chair is the first known with a moveable back which allowed the patient to take a reclining position when needed (Heister 1981).

Professor George-Wilhelm Stein of Marburg (1731–1803) designed a bed chair which he claimed could be taken to pieces; it had adjustable foot-steps which augmented the parturient's expulsive efforts. The adjustable back permitted a sitting or reclining position. An extension was added later in order that the patient could be placed in a recumbent position if desired (see Figure 7) (Stein 1805). Professor Stein's chairs were made of very expensive ma-

terial and were only available for wealthy people. Cheap standard models were eventually developed which were acquired by many communities, especially in southern Germany.

In the later eighteenth and early nineteenth centuries in Germany the obstetric chair enjoyed its greatest popularity, even with male obstetricians. Particular selling points were pillows and padding, hand-grips and foot-rests and reclining backs and ascending seats. Ease of transportation was another important feature.

Elias Von Siebold, Friedrich Benjamin Osiander and George William Stein were three of the well-known German obstetricians who engaged in this enterprise. Indeed, Elias Von Siebold designed a delivery cushion; this was a mattress containing a wedge which could be removed when required. In 1791 John Christopher Stark designed a parturition chair much lighter in construction than any previously described and which appears altogether much more comfortable (Figure 8).

François Mauriceau the leading French obstetrician, in his *Traité des Maladies des Femmes Grosses*, described a chair for delivery and a padded bed on the floor. He recommended that the best place was in the woman's own bed in a semi-recumbent position, thus saving the trouble of carrying her there after the delivery; and the woman could breath more easily and

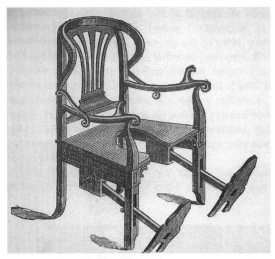

**Figure 8** *Parturition chair by John Christopher Stark (1791)*

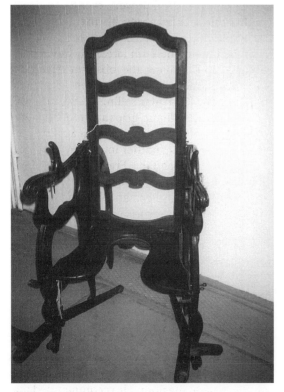

**Figure 9** *Eighteenth-century French parturition chair. (Photo by permission of Science Museum/Science and Society Picture Library)*

make better use of her pains. By this he meant the mechanical advantage of the chair.

In 1790 Herbieneux designed a chair which came into use in Flanders. It is constructed so that it can be made into a bed-chair with a mattress if necessary (Witkowski 1887).

In the latter part of the eighteenth century a further type of chair used in France was of an elaborate construction and made entirely of wood with high moveable back, arms with hand-grips and adjustable foot-rests (Figure 9).

Henrick Van Deventer, the Dutch obstetrician, in 1701, presented a new model of the parturition chair (Figure 10) with a back piece that could change position. It has two moveable hand-grips of metal which can be shortened or lengthened according to the patient's arm length. The two foot-warmers by the chair were heated through a metal jacket with hot cinders or bags of hot sand in which the patient could place her feet.

European and American chairs were designed during the eighteenth century and Figure 11 shows an American chair of elm and beech (1701–1800).

In Syria, Turkey and other parts of Asia Minor, the use of a parturition chair is still in existence (Thompson 1957).

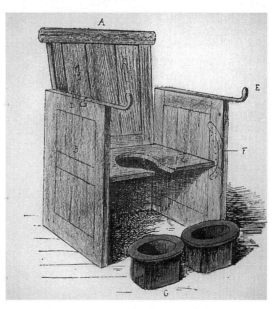

**Figure 10** *Parturition chair by Henrick Van Deventer (1701)*

A similar kind of chair is still used in Egypt (1890 and early 1900) (Simpson 1908). When transported it is usually covered with a shawl or embroidered cloth, as seen in Figure 12. Here the Aswan midwife is seen in her best attire, wearing a satin gown in which she makes a visit to her patient, taking with her a bouquet of roses at the high corner of the chair.

Figure 13 shows a type of customary confinement chair made of pine. Produced in Egypt (El Lahem, Faayum 1901–1930), it was presented by W. S. Blackmann in 1927 to the Science Museum in London. Women in Egypt gave birth in squatting position.

In old Cairo, in the Gamalieh, the 'House of El Sehimi' had been built and constructed in the sixteenth to seventeenth centuries by a wealthy merchant named Shah Bander. In this house there is a delivery room, with two delivery seats made of a large block of marble stone shaped like stools (Figure 14). The room had a window for ventilation.

Another interesting Egyptian building is the Gayer Anderson's Museum. Gayer Anderson was one of the British soldiers who became the private doctor for the family of Mohamed Ali Pasha (Viceroy of Egypt 1805–1848) and founder of the School of Medicine. He lived in this museum, which is built in Eastern style, and which included a delivery room with a number of parturition chairs, mostly made of pine (see

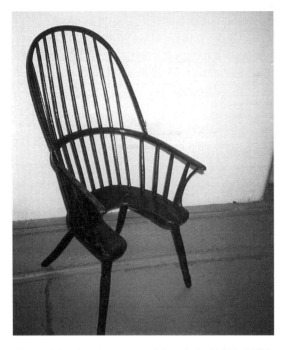

**Figure 11** *American parturition chair (1701–1800). (Photo by permission of Science Museum/Science and Society Picture Library)*

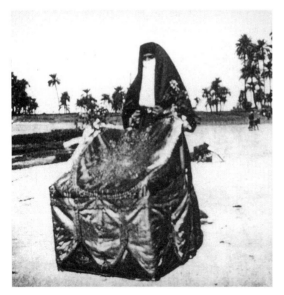

**Figure 12** *Nineteenth-century Egyptian parturition chair and Aswan midwife*

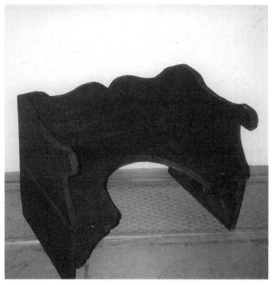

**Figure 13** *Pine chair from Egypt (1901–1930). (Photo by permission of Science Museum/Science and Society Picture Library)*

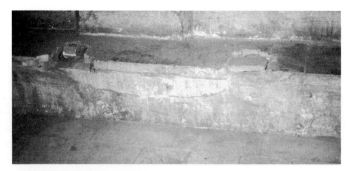

**Figure 14**    *Sixteenth- to seventeenth-century marble stone delivery stools from Cairo*

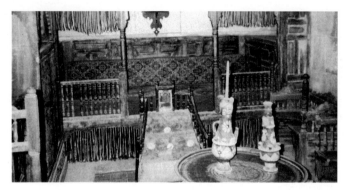

**Figure 15**    *Delivery room in Gayer Anderson's Museum, Cairo*

Figure 15). At the end of the room there is a comfortable bed for the parturient to step into after delivery. In the middle of this room there are two jars placed on a brass plate. One is green for the male child and the other red for the female child.

In Spain a vase in used for parturition. A doctor from Huelva in the south of Spain sent Alexander R. Simpson, Professor of Midwifery at the University of Edinburgh (1894), a great earthenware vessel similar to those that can still be seen in 'china shops'. It has the form of a high, steep-sided jar with a wide, flat rim. From the rim as well as from the front wall of this jar, a large piece is cut out which is two-thirds the depth of the jar. It is usually called 'bacin' by the local people. A woman in labour sits on this vessel with legs wide apart, the midwife sits in front on a low chair, examining her through the opening in the jar; the amniotic fluid and blood, etc., collect at the bottom (Ploss, Bartels and Bartels 1935).

In Japan, where the sitting position is still customary, the chair is constructed in the style of a box, the back of which is made of thin strips of wood interlaced. It is set on the floor, and the patient seated in it rests against the back in a position that would appear to be anything but comfortable (Thompson 1957).

Historically, the recumbent position was used by Mauriceau in order to apply the Chamberlen forceps more easily. The Sims position is used on the continent of Europe and to a lesser extent in other places where medical thinking has been influenced by European medical mores. As obstetricians became more skilled, access to the perineum was demanded and women were forced to accept the supine position for delivery.

The left lateral position was considered by French and German obstetricians to be the product of British prudery, preventing the parturient from looking the accoucheur in the face (Heister 1981).

Parturition chairs were abandoned because they were too simple and unstable or too heavy and complicated. This resulted in a difficult working position for the delivery assistant, operative intervention was impossible and hygiene was another problem.

## MODERN TIMES

Technology has now changed with a wide choice of materials to construct a parturition chair and several trials have been conducted to assess the outcome of delivery on the birthing chair.

Turner *et al.* (1986) at Northwick Park Hospital were the first British team to try the obstetric chair. They used an 'EZ chair' which was manufactured in Nebraska, United States. It is made of a high impact plastic material which is strong and not unattractive, but costs around £4000. In a random controlled trial, mothers were allocated to either the bed or the birthing chair for the second stage of labour. Of the 288 primigravidae and 348 multiparae, those mothers delivered on the chair were more likely to have postpartum haemorrhage and perineal tears and less likely to have an impact perineum. No evidence was found that the use of the chair was beneficial. Similar results were found by Peter Stewart and Helen Spilby in 1989 at Northwick Park Hospital using a chair manufactured by the Rocket Instrument Company in London.

Barbara Cottrell and Mary Shannahan, in Orlando in 1986, studied the effect of the birth chair on duration of the second stage of labour and maternal outcome in primigravidae (33 in the chair; 22 on the delivery table). They found the chair was an alternative delivery method which was safe in terms of maternal outcome, but it did not shorten duration of second stage of labour and perhaps increases the incidence of perineal swelling.

Elina Hemminki *et al.* (1986) from Finland studied 175 women randomly allocated to find out whether using a birth chair during the second stage of labour was more advantageous than using a delivery bed. They found mothers were more satisfied with the birth chair than they were with the delivery beds. With regard to the progress of labour and delivery and the health

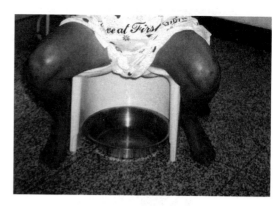

**Figure 16**   *The Birth-Mate birthing stool from Amsterdam*

of the child and mother, the groups were fairly similar.

In 1994 Kafka *et al.* from Germany studied 140 women out of a total of 1122 using the delivery chair, comparing them to a control group in the supine position. They found no increased risk to either the mother or the fetus and, therefore, concluded that the delivery chair represents an appropriate alternative to the traditional supine position for delivery.

The Birth-Mate birthing stool shown in Figure 16 was developed in 1984 by Astrid Limburg and Beatrijs Smulders, two midwives from Amsterdam, in close association with Professor Dr Kloosterman, a Dutch gynaecologist. The midwives who designed the stool have conducted over 1000 births on it since 1984 (Waldenström and Gottvall 1991). It costs about £250. The stool is moulded in plastic in the shape of a horseshoe and is 32 cm high. In our hospital (Buchanan Hospital, Hastings, United Kingdom) we found it very useful for the mothers in the first and second stages of labour, and mothers can easily stand up or move around between contractions. By tilting the mother 20° to the vertical, assisted by her partner, oedema of the peritoneum is avoided and better access allowed to the midwife for delivery. There was no evidence of postpartum haemorrhage in any of our deliveries, and better assessment of blood loss was made. Furthermore, keeping the patient out of bed prevented her from becoming unduly anxious.

The latest technology in designing parturition chairs comes from Switzerland. 'The Roma

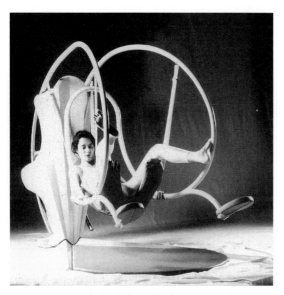

**Figure 17** *The Roma Birth Wheel from Switzerland. (Reproduced with permission of the manufacturers CH-4410 Liestal, Switzerland)*

Birth Wheel' seen in Figure 17 is made of stainless steel with powder-coated spiral and adjustable foot-rests. It has two electric 230 V motors for height adjustment and spiral adjustment with infra-red remote control. The adjustable padded seat with a horseshoe-shaped cut-out section in the base is suspended from a reinforced metal spiral frame. The mother can squat, hang or stand, using the frame as a support, or rock in the seat. It can also go into a reclining position so procedures (e.g. vaginal examinations, episiotomy or even forceps delivery) can be carried out.

## CONCLUSION

The obstetric chair, which flourished in the days of Greece and Rome, was almost forgotten in the darkness of the earlier centuries of the Christian era, although it seems to have survived in Italy (partly due to the writing of Greek and Roman authorities, and partly because the custom was handed down from generation to generation among the people). From Italy it found its way across the Alps into Germany and France. By this time, the crude stool of ancient

times had been greatly changed in shape, complicated and improved until the low stool is presented to us as the typical obstetric chair of the Middle Ages (Engelmann 1882).

In the seventeenth and early part of the eighteenth centuries the chair seems to have flourished in Germany, and also in England, and numerous modifications were introduced. Smellie says: '*In remote parts of England the patient sat upon a stool made in the form of a semi-circle.*' This was written during the decline of the chair, when the dorsal and lateral deculitis had become popular (Engelmann 1882).

It seems that the obstetric chair has had a remarkable history from antiquity to the early twentieth century. If we are to have a parturition chair in our labour ward, a delivery technique for the chair must be decided. This will obviously need the confidence of midwives before being incorporated into training courses for students.

There is certainly great popularity in the sitting or squatting position, which gives the chair a place in our current obstetric practice. If popularity of the chair increases, we may even need more than one in the delivery suite to ensure that all mothers can use it if they so wish. The parturition chair has certainly aroused enthusiasm among midwives for keeping the normal 'normal'. One of the fascinations of the history of medicine is the manner in which age-old customs are revived and this certainly seems to be the case with the parturition chair; at one stage it was perceived as an historical piece of furniture which was of interest only to museums.

It is possible today with modern techniques and materials to design a delivery chair which can satisfy the requirements of present-day obstetrics, having the advantage of giving support to the perineum, thus decreasing tissue congestion and prolapse in the future. Another important fact is that there is no one proper, or correct, delivery position. Instead, each delivery position has both its positive points and its negative points and consequently should be viewed in its cultural setting as it affects the individual (Atwood 1976). More quantitative evaluation as well as consultants' good will needs to be achieved.

## ACKNOWLEDGEMENTS

I am most grateful to librarians Mrs Jenny Turner and Mrs Margaret Ellis from the Rosewell Library at the Conquest Hospital, Hastings, and Mrs Pat Want and staff from the Royal College of Obstetricians and Gynaecologists Library, for helping me with the research and with references. I am also grateful to Mr Neil Irvine, Assistant Curator of the Science Museum, for his help with photography of the chairs from the Science Museum, to my secretary, Mrs Sue St Aubyn, for typing my literature, and to the Medical Illustration Department of the Conquest Hospital.

# References

Atwood, R. J. (1976) Parturitional posture and related birth behaviour. *Acta Obstet Gynecol Scand* 5

Cottrell, B. H. and Shannahan, M. D. (1986) Effects of the birthing chair on duration of second stage labour and maternal outcome. *Nurs Res* **35**, 364–367

Engelmann, G. J. (1882) *Labour Among Primitive Peoples*, pp. 66–73, 129. St Louis: J. H. Chambers

Hemminki, F., Virkkunen, A., Makela, A. *et al.* (1986) A trial of delivery in a birth chair. *J Obstet Gynaecol* **6**, 162–165

Mauriceau, F. (1781) *Traité des Maladies des Femmes Grosses*, pp. 238–239. Paris: L'Auteur

Jarcho, J. (1934) *Pastures and Practices During Labour Among Primitive Peoples*, pp. 41–47. New York: Paul B. Hoeber Inc.

Kafka, M., Riss, P., Von Trotsenburg, M. and Maly, Z. (1994) The birthing stool: an obstetric risk? *Geburtshilfe Frauenheilkd* **54** (9), 529–531

Paré, A. (1641) *Les Oeuvres d'Ambroise Paré*, p. 599. Lyon: Claude Prost

Ploss, H. H., Bartels, M. and Bartels, P. (1935) *Woman: An Historical Gynaecological and Anthropological Compendium* Vol. 2, pp. 722–735

Rosegarten (1513) *Der Swangern und Hebaminen.*

Rueff, J. (1554) *De Conceptu et Generatione Hominus.* Tiguri: C. Froschoverus

Simpson, A. R. (1908) 'Birth stools in Egypt' communicated to: *the Edinburgh Obstetric Society on 12.2.1908 by Emeritus Professor Sir Alexander Russell Simpson MD, DSc, LLD*

Stein, G. W. (1805) *Anleitung zur Geburtschülfe, zum Gebrauch bey Vorlesingen*, pp. 308–311. Marburg

Stewart, P. and Spilby, H. (1989) A randomised study of the sitting position for delivery using a newly designed obstetric chair. *Br J Obstet Gynaecol* **96**, 327–333

Thompson, C. J. S. (1957) 'The parturition chair, its history and use' in: Z. Cope (ed.). *Sidelights on the History of Medicine*, pp. 65–72. London: Butterworth & Co.

Turner, M. J., Romney, M. L., Webb, J. B. and Gordon, H. (1986) The birthing chair: an obstetric hazard? *J Obstet Gynaecol* **6**, 23–235.

Velpeau, A. A. L. M. (1931) *An Elementary Treatise on Midwifery* [Translated from French], p. 345. Philadelphia: John Grigg

Heister, L. (1981) *Literaturdenkmäler der Medizin und Pharmazziegeschichte*, pp. 940–941. Osnabrück: Reinhard Kuballe

Waldenström, U. and Gottvall, K. (1991) A randomised trial of birthing stool or conventional semi-recumbent position for second stage labour. *Birth* **18** (1), 5–10

Witkowski, G. J. (1887) *Historie de Accouchements chez tous les Peuples*, pp. 382–460. Paris: G. Steinheil

# 5

# Poverty, deprivation and maternal health

*Kelsey A. Harrison*

I feel very honoured by the invitation to deliver the lecture and provide a chapter for the Year-book. Of the previous William Meredith Fletcher Shaw Memorial Lectures, four were on issues related to poverty and deprivation. They discussed contracted pelvis (Kerr 1948), high maternal mortality prevention (Watson 1955), urinary fistula (Mahfouz 1957) and life in South Africa (Black 1958). In those lectures, clinical management was central, and reference to underlying social background was very peripheral. Forty years later, the times have obviously changed and my notion of progress is to discuss some topical maternal health and socio-economic issues, with particular emphasis on two major determinants of maternal mortality and morbidity; namely, unbooked emergencies and structural adjustment programmes in sub-Saharan Africa.

## INDICATORS OF POVERTY AND DEPRIVATION

On the basis of gross national product (GNP) per caput, the world's countries fall into four economic classes: the rich, the middle income, the poor and the poorest (Figure 1). Between 1950 and now, the increase in GNP is nearly threefold for the rich, 1.5-fold for the middle-income countries, marginal for poor countries and zero for the poorest countries. The gulf

between the rich and poorest, which was eight-fold in 1950, is now nearly 30-fold. The number of countries in the least developed group (24 in 1950) is currently 47, of which 29 are in sub-Saharan Africa, with all the rest being developing countries. This is real poverty to the extent that 62% of the total population of sub-Saharan Africa earn less than the equivalent of six United States dollars per week compared to 35% for Latin America and the Caribbean, 28% for North Africa and Middle East, and 25% for Asia. The stark reality is that poverty on this scale is the leading cause of premature death, especially maternal mortality. In terms of the scale in inequality between the rich and the poor, maternal mortality differentials give the widest disparity of all other health and socioeconomic indicators, including those shown in Table 1. For example, Italy with GNP per caput of US$ 20,000 has a maternal mortality rate of four per 100,000 births and a lifetime risk of dying during pregnancy and childbirth of one in 17,360; the equivalent figures for Mali in West Africa are US$ 310, 2000 per 100,000 births, and one in seven, respectively. Hence, a 66-fold difference in GNP per caput shows up as a 500-fold gap in maternal mortality rate and a 2500-fold gap in the lifetime risk of dying in pregnancy and childbirth. Gaps of similar magnitude occur within individual countries, causing increasing suffering and declining reproductive health standards which the World Health Organisation rightly wants to see checked. The challenge is to translate the idea into action.

*The 1995 William Meredith Fletcher Shaw Memorial Lecture*

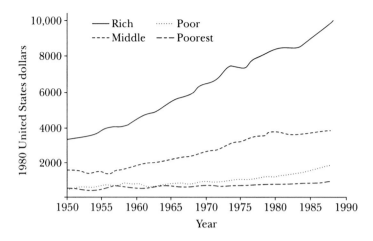

**Figure 1** *The adjusted income per person in four economic classes of nations between 1950 and 1988. (Reproduced from Bergstrom, S. (1994) 'The pathology of poverty' in: K. S. Lankinen, S. Bergstrom, P. H. Makela and M. Peltomaa (Eds.).* Health and Diseases in Developing Countries, *with permission of Macmillan Press Ltd)*

**Table 1** *Major indicators of impoverishment and deprivation*

Illiteracy
Low gross national product and wages
Poor nutrition
Unemployment
Damaging gender relations: through cultural,
  religious, social and economic barriers
High fertility rates
Low contraceptive use

## POOR NUTRITION AND MATERNAL HEALTH

### Acute undernutrition

Poor nutrition, whether in acute or chronic form, impairs reproduction. In acute undernutrition, often the results of wars or conflicts and sometimes drought, the resulting starvation causes menstrual cycles to become irregular, ovulation may cease, but those who get pregnant produce babies of low birth weight, as occurred during the Dutch famine in the 1940s and as I personally witnessed during the Nigerian civil war in the 1960s.

### Chronic undernutrition

Chronic undernutrition results from low food productivity or lack of money with which to purchase food, and it is aggravated by hard physical work coupled with food taboos imposed during pregnancy in some cultures. Energy and nutrient inadequacy become marked. They combine with rampant infections from poor housing, unsafe water supplies and poor sanitation to produce growth failure and, hence, short stature. Under these conditions, maternal height becomes a marker for difficult labour and operative delivery. The critical height below which these risks increase varies between 145 and 152 cm, depending on the genetic and socioeconomic characteristics of the population. Like acute undernutrition, chronic maternal undernutrition also impairs fetal growth. In the process much depends on the size of maternal energy available for transfer to the fetus. Prepregnancy weight, weight for height and mid-upper arm circumference are useful indicators for energy reserve. Where these anthropometric measurements are low, energy transfer to the fetus is inadequate and low fetal birth weight results. Various cut-off points for selection of those at risk in developing countries are discussed elsewhere (J. A. Kusin and F. E. Hytten, personal communication)

### Anaemia

Another important result of poor nutrition is anaemia in pregnancy. Although easily detected, the issues of its prevention, rational treatment, and the huge mortality and morbidity caused, persist because of failure to address the root problems of mass poverty and deprivation. Death is from heart failure from myocardiac oxygen lack, hypoxic and hypovolaemic shock, and from cerebral hypoxia, and it occurs when the anaemia is profound (haemoglobin 40 g/l or less). But even less severe anaemia exacerbates infections and increases various perioperative and peripartal risks. In terms of its aetiology, the contributions from iron and folic acid deficiencies, and from heavy hookworm infestation and haemoglobinopathies, are well understood. The importance of *Plasmodium falciparum* malaria is less publicised, yet this is immense. Two billion (or 40%) of the world's population are constantly exposed to this infection, and 90% of the world's malaria is concentrated in sub-Saharan Africa, the poorest region, an obvious indication of the strength of the link between poverty and malaria.

## MATERNAL AGE/PARITY AND POVERTY/PREGNANCY OUTCOME

In many areas of Africa, Asia and Latin America, a mixture of traditional customs, religious beliefs, and a background of poverty and poor educational standards, with the powerlessness the latter causes, contributes towards early marriage, early teenage pregnancy and high parity. Elsewhere, pregnancy in unmarried adolescent girls is increasing. The belief everywhere is that adolescent girls aged 16 years and under, and highly parous women with five or more previous births are at a high risk from maternal mortality and morbidity. However, detailed considerations have revealed that this is only true up to a point (Harrison 1985).

### Effect of very young maternal age

In healthy early teenage girls, it is normal for pelvic growth to lag behind linear growth so that, while growth in height stops at 16 years, pelvic growth ceases 2–3 years later. For the girl who lives in good circumstances and gets pregnant before the cessation of growth height, her pelvis is still immature, but the deficit is not sufficient to cause dystocia in most cases. Good nutrition and proper obstetric care exert a powerful protective influence against most pregnancy complications, except for pregnancy-induced hypertension, which is very common at this age.

The position is very different in young teenagers brought up in poor circumstances. Anaemia, pregnancy-induced hypertension, eclampsia and malaria (in endemic areas) are all very common. Moreover, growth stunting from poor nutrition compounds pelvic immaturity causing extreme degrees of pelvic contraction, leading to high rates of cephalopelvic disproportion and operative deliveries, and to obstructed labour, vesicovaginal fistula (VVF) and fetal death in neglected cases.

Fortunately, the worst of these disadvantages can be overcome by appropriate nutritional intervention in pregnancy. Throughout the tropics, during pregnancy, iron and folic acid supplementation combined with malaria chemoprophylaxis (in endemic areas) prevents anaemia. In Zaria, Northern Nigeria, the same regimen caused growth spurts in height with a drastic reduction of the incidence of difficult labour and operative delivery. Its application could have a great impact on the VVF situation among vulnerable populations in Africa and elsewhere. Meanwhile, in adolescents in both rich and poor countries, sexually transmitted diseases are spreading fast, and resort to induced abortion is increasing — especially in places with low contraceptive use and lacking good medical care (Brabin *et al.* 1994).

### Effect of high parity

The protective influence of good living standards is also evident in high parity. During pregnancy, highly parous women in rich countries, and highly parous women in poor countries who live in conditions close to those prevailing in rich countries, have very low death rates, their major obstetric problem being an increased risk of hypertension, probably due to the confounding effects of advanced maternal age. By contrast, under very unfavourable conditions, highly parous women experience a huge excess of deaths chiefly from anaemia and conditions requiring operative deliveries, especially obstetric haemorrhage, mechanical problems and their complications. The result is that high parity is linked with high maternal mortality rates. In addition, high maternal mortality parallels high childhood mortality, and those whose children from previous births all survived run a much lower risk of maternal death than those with poor record of child survival. Simply put, poverty and lack of knowledge are the real killers, not high parity (Harrison, Rossiter and Tan 1986; Bergstrom 1994).

## HIGH-RISK FACTORS FOR MATERNAL MORTALITY AND MORBIDITY

### Unbooked emergencies

The term 'unbooked emergencies' refers to pregnant women who, through neglect, ignorance, poverty, or especially illiteracy, fail to receive antenatal care and report for the first time when pre-existing disease worsens and the obstetric complications become life threatening. Unbooked emergencies hardly feature in rich countries, yet they make up over 80% of hospital maternal deaths and morbidities in developing countries. Anaemia, puerperal infections and obstetric conditions requiring operative delivery or treatment (i.e. eclampsia, obstructed labour, obstetric haemorrhage and complicated abortions) are the main direct causes. Haemorrhage, puerperal infection and eclampsia are important in all regions in developing countries. Obstructed labour is particularly common in Africa, where its treatment involves far more than Caesarean section. Emergency fluid, blood and antibiotic resuscitation as well as symphysiotomy, embryotomy and even hysterectomy have their place. Both vesicovaginal fistula (VVF) and obstetric palsy are important long-term sequelae for the treatment of which surgery, physiotherapy and social rehabilitation are all involved.

Besides late diagnosis, delay in getting effective treatment is always marked in unbooked emergencies (Harrison 1985; Thaddeus and Maine 1994). These delays, as well as increasing deaths and morbidities, produce other important consequences. Seldom is death in the one woman caused by a single direct obstetric complication: instead, there are two or more, so that allocation of cause to death becomes problematic. A typical example is that of a woman who dies shortly after reaching hospital with the placenta still retained three days after a home birth, with gross anaemia and septicaemia from advanced puerperal sepsis. In this case, to ascribe the death to one principal cause and classify the rest as merely contributory is misleading. Besides, treatment costs (including blood transfusion) increase when disease is very advanced and two or more maternal complications are present instead of one. For example, in the 1970s we found that in Zaria, Northern Nigeria, where nearly 30% of deliveries were unbooked emergencies, 60 units of blood per bed per year were used compared to only eight units per bed per year in the United Kingdom. Moreover, throughout West Africa and elsewhere in the entire region, patients may refuse a life-saving operation or blood transfusion for religious and cultural reasons. In developing countries' hospitals that face the problem of high rates of unbooked emergencies, the situation is compounded by a disproportionately large fraction of scarce resources and human effort being concentrated on attempts to salvage moribund women, leaving little for the care of the rest. This shift in the use of resources is one reason why pregnancy outcome among women free from major pregnancy complications is not as good as it ought to be. Indeed, during labour in hospital, they risk being neglected as attention and available resources are diverted towards dangerously ill, unbooked emergencies.

As expected, the babies of unbooked emergencies fare very badly. Birth trauma, asphyxia and intrapartum and neonatal infection do most of the damage.

There are other problems that are less obvious, but perhaps even more damaging. The risks that follow the enormous amounts of stress imposed on the maternal health care staff involved have never been assessed. The extent of the curtailment of the advancement of the society by such disease burden is not fully known. The following analysis, although crude, gives some useful indication. We examined the fetal outcomes in cases of VVF from neglected obstructed labour in Zaria, Northern Nigeria. The mean birth weights were 2.7 kg for the few survivors, and 3.14 kg for the perinatal deaths, implying that the best babies die. It has been shown that in severe anaemia (common in poor countries) fetal loss is high, the surviving babies have low body stores of iron and folic acid, their immune systems are immature (Fleming 1989) and they readily enter the cycle of malnutrition–infection which leads to stunted growth. The result is that in disadvantaged societies with high prevalence of pelvic contraction and unsupervised deliveries, the surviving babies may not necessarily be the best babies. The damaged babies grow up to become damaged adults who in turn produce damaged infants and children. The result is a nasty cycle. If it is to be broken, merely saving mothers and babies from death is not enough. What is required is to produce a generation of well-grown fetuses and infants who will then pass on the advantage to succeeding generations. Political intervention and social change will be the deciding factors, not fire brigade action in hospital.

It is clear that the unbooked emergencies are created by adverse socioeconomic, political, cultural factors and by illiteracy, and that antenatal care of good quality avoids most of the disadvantages. In moving towards this goal, several viewpoints emerge. To take but one example, antenatal care itself is under increasing scrutiny (Rooney 1992), and there are powerful advocates for fewer visits but increased efficiency at reduced costs. This is all very well in rich countries and privileged societies, but I believe that in other areas of the world, such innovations may prove counterproductive. In some Islamic societies in sub-Saharan Africa, a combination of traditional and religious beliefs cause women of reproductive age to be kept in semi-seclusion. For such women, every attendance at an antenatal clinic is eagerly awaited. It is as much a social outing as it is of health monitoring. The atmosphere is relaxed, the women talk to each other and increase their awareness of the area's obstetric and socioeconomic problems so that, with time a bond of trust between the maternity services and the local community develops, an essential step towards mortality and morbidity prevention. This is an enormous advantage: nothing must be done to disrupt it. My fear is that if the concept of 'efficiency' is applied to antenatal care in some places, this is exactly what is going to happen.

Poverty on a lesser scale, but sufficiently bad to lead to homelessness, is a growing problem in rich countries. The difference is that the health resources and infrastructure needed to deal with all the life-threatening obstetric emergencies are in place, and their efficient use keeps maternal mortality and morbidity rates very low. Nevertheless, rates of low birth weight and infant mortality remain moderately raised since they reflect bad socioeconomic conditions, whose effect emergency obstetric care of good quality cannot entirely overcome. This explains the social class differentials in perinatal and infant mortality rates that exist in nearly all rich countries. However, the gap between social classes is least in the Nordic countries (e.g. Sweden, Finland, Denmark, Norway and Iceland) where enlightened social policies have largely eliminated the grosser forms of deprivation.

## Structural adjustment programmes (SAP)

The extent and depth of the misery sub-Saharan Africa is currently experiencing through SAP has to be seen to be believed. With its prejudices against social welfare, SAP has helped to precipitate a major catastrophe in which virtually all economic, social, educational and public health gains made in the 1960s and 1970s have been lost. According to an editorial appearing in *The Lancet* (Anonymous 1994), the story began in the 1970s when prices of crude oil in the international market suddenly rose and this precipitated a world economic recession. Banking institutions, full of petrodollars on which interest had to be paid, made huge loans to developing countries. The developing countries needed new loans to make up for the fall in revenue

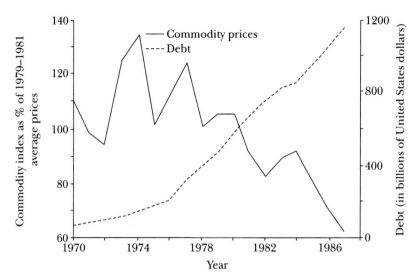

**Figure 2** *Commodity prices and debt between 1970 and 1986 in the Third World. (Reproduced from Bergstrom, S. (1994) 'The pathology of poverty' in: K. S. Lankinen, S. Bergstrom, P. H. Makela and M. Peltomaa (Eds.).* Health and Disease in Developing Countries, *with permission of Macmillan Press Ltd)*

from the decline in prices in raw materials (see Figure 2).

Significantly, the developing countries had already incurred huge losses from financial mismanagement through extreme corruption and misappropriation. Their economies became static. The World Bank and the International Monetary Fund (IMF) devised SAP as the remedy, confident in the belief that the stringent insistence on its strategies would, in the short term, check the rapid economic decline and ensure debt recovery, and, in the long term, reduce poverty through economic growth. Structural adjustment programme conditions may work in places with good administrative infrastructure and high literacy levels, but not in regions lacking these essential elements. So under SAP, East Asia advances and sub-Saharan Africa sinks (Logie and Woodroffe 1993; Wakhweya 1995; Watkins 1995). With reference to sub-Saharan Africa, expert predictions are that if the present social and economic policies continue, it will take another 330 years for the region to reach the living standards achieved 25 years ago.

Structural adjustment programmes insist on huge job losses in government posts to reduce costs, and in the private sector to maximise profits. Unemployment has therefore risen but wage settlements are lower than the rates of inflation. Without effective social welfare safety nets, dependent families of the new unemployed are driven into deeper poverty. At the same time, through removal of food and transport subsidy (another SAP condition) food prices rise. There is, therefore, simply not enough money to buy food, so that nutritional standards deteriorate. An extreme example was in Peru when food prices rose by 2500% in one year (1990), and the number of people living in poverty, already high, doubled.

Cuts in spending on public education is another of SAP's conditions. It has led to a fall in educational standards and to an increase in fees as government spending decreases drastically. Most parents cannot afford the fees charged, so school enrolment that showed a spectacular rise in the 1970s has, since the mid-1980s, fallen (see Figure 3), and drop out rates have increased.

In accordance with SAP philosophy, private schools supposedly providing better education have proliferated. Sadly, this state of affairs increasingly condemns many African children to illiteracy, with women forming two-thirds of the 900 million illiterate people in the world.

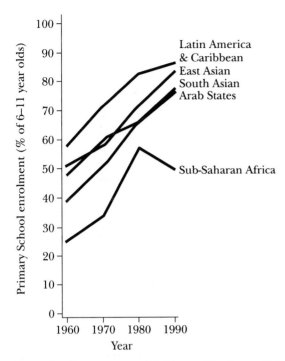

**Figure 3** *The percentage of 6–11-year olds who enrolled in primary school between 1960 and 1990. (Reproduced Grant, J. (1995) The State of the World's Children, with permission of Oxford University Press. Data acquired from the United Nations International Children's Emergency Fund [UNICEF] )*

As already stated, salary increases are much lower than the inflation rates. Thus, virtually all employees in the public sector and in most private firms, except the multinationals, are no longer paid living wages if they are paid at all. They still have to support their extended family, secure their children's future through expensive private education, pay for the high cost of very basic local food items and transport. Attempts to make ends meet result in corruption and a rise in criminal activity.

Poor resource allocation to health predates SAP, but SAP conditions make the situation worse by devaluing local currencies and further cutting financial allocations. The effects are immediate. Supply of health resources (e.g. vaccines, dressings, drugs, surgical gloves, diagnostic sets and needles, etc.) dwindle, running costs of ambulance and hospital transport increase, the services deteriorate and the distribution of all forms of supplies (including vaccines and blood for transfusion) become truncated, with very negative effects on curative and preventive care. The introduction of user fees has failed to check the decline. Most people cannot afford the fees charged, the result is increase in self-treatment (very bad news for sexually transmitted diseases), quackery and recourse to harmful traditional medicines. It is very disheartening to see the trust in orthodox maternity care, painstakingly built up over several decades, being undermined. Furthermore, this problem is compounded by the activities of rapidly growing, but controversial, evangelistic Protestant churches. While these churches help people cope with the terrific stresses of everyday life, they increasingly divert women away from orthodox maternity care with disastrous consequences: these include decline in the number of institutional deliveries, increase in unbooked emergencies with major complications, sharp increases in maternal mortality, in the number of babies admitted born before arrival, and in the incidence of neonatal deaths from sepsis (including tetanus). In Port Harcourt in Nigeria, an uncomplicated Caesarean section costs the equivalent of US$ 247, which represents 9 months' average salary. Thus, many who need the procedure for good obstetric reasons and cannot afford to pay die. While elsewhere, since the 'Safe Motherhood Initiative' was launched in 1987, maternal mortality is falling, in sub-Saharan Africa it is rising. The following experience from the University of Port Harcourt in Nigeria is fairly typical. In 1987, there were five maternal deaths among 2128 deliveries in booked women compared to 13 deaths out of 213 deliveries in unbooked emergencies. In 1994, one year after further steep increases in user fees, the equivalent figures for maternal outcome became one death out of 1068 deliveries for the booked women and 21 deaths out of 116 deliveries in unbooked emergencies. The truth is that in sub-Saharan Africa, SAP-aggravated poverty has become a major deterrent to the proper use of even the few maternity services that are available.

Women have been badly affected by cuts in education, in health (including family planning services), by lack of food for the family, and by the increase in family illness episodes these adversities cause. They find great difficulty in coping with their commitments, often being forced into prostitution, which offers one explanation for the rapid spread of the human immunodeficiency virus (HIV) among the heterosexual population in the region. Effective treatment of coincidental sexually transmitted diseases could help check the spread of HIV (Grosskuria et al. 1995), but the essential facilities for proper prevention and treatment are lacking because of poverty.

Moreover, senior medical, technical and managerial staff suffer terribly. Due to lack of funds, professional journals are not acquired, relevant medical information becomes very difficult to get, professional conferences are reduced, knowledge dissemination is curtailed, the sense of isolation engendered grows and job dissatisfaction deepens. When recently in Nigeria, withdrawal of fuel subsidy was imposed and transport cost increased abruptly, health workers found that they could not afford transport costs for more than 3 days in a 5-day working week. The forced absenteeism virtually paralysed the public services and aggravated discipline problems.

While SAP did not create the 'brain drain', it certainly has made the situation worse. Over 2100 Nigerian medical specialists now work in the United States, and an unknown number left for other countries, leaving 800 still working in the country. It is clear that many more specialists have left Nigeria than remain. Moreover, all forms of medical education have deteriorated.

Through privatisation, another SAP condition, a small number of people have become very rich, so that social inequality has widened, government authority is eroded, the number of the deprived, the hungry and the angry is growing, civil unrest is escalating, and social fragmentation is increasing. The demoralisation of the population is total except for temporary residents (e.g. international aid workers). The spirit has been knocked out of the middle classes on whom so much depends. In short, the environment in sub-Saharan Africa has become too hostile for work towards high maternal mortality reduction which is what the entire region badly needs.

## MATERNAL HEALTH 'IMPROVEMENT' INITIATIVES

The timing of SAP is most unfortunate for maternal health. Through the 'Safe Motherhood Initiative' launched in 1987, the world is much better informed about maternal mortality and morbidity. Between 1970 and 1994, the number of articles on the subject listed each year in MEDLINE from developing countries has nearly tripled, so that information on proper reduction measures for the high maternal mortality and morbidity rates is widely available (e.g. total antenatal care coverage and the establishment and use of first referral hospitals). However, due to the SAP-induced economic difficulties, permanent solutions to maternal health problems are guided by expediency rather than need. Traditional birth attendants (TBAs), retraining programmes and moves to institutionalise Caesarean sections and laparotomies by non-physicians are examples of activities whose promotion goes on despite their shortcomings.

### Traditional birth attendants

In the case of retraining programmes for traditional birth attendants (TBAs), the reasons for their failure in reducing high maternal mortality rates are very obvious (Harrison 1989a). Traditional birth attendants are handicapped by their advancing age, by their lack of requisite skill and knowledge, and by their illiteracy. Record keeping in the conventional manner is impossible, and without reliable records and periodic audit, progress is impossible. Coping effectively with life-saving management of obstetric complications and emergencies is beyond their capabilities. Furthermore, as they are female and illiterate, they are of inferior status, so that despite the high esteem in which they are held at local tribal level, they lack the political clout at the national level where the decisions affecting national development (including maternal health) are made.

**Table 2** *Female education, childbirth and maternal mortality in selected countries during 1990. (Data provided by UNICEF)*

| Country | Female literacy (%) | Births conducted by untrained birth attendants (%) | Maternal deaths per 100,000 live births |
|---|---|---|---|
| Bangladesh | 22 | 95 | 600 |
| Egypt | 34 | 59 | 270 |
| Brazil | 80 | 5 | 200 |
| Sri Lanka | 84 | 6 | 80 |

Worldwide, the trend is for births attended by TBAs to fall as literacy spreads (Table 2) leading to reduction in maternal mortality. Therefore, if moves to reduce high maternal mortality are to succeed, they must at the same time reduce illiteracy within the society. Strengthening the position of illiterate TBAs gives the wrong signals to a society wanting to increase female literacy. Indeed, if care is not taken, support for TBA activities can have the unacceptable effect of blocking female literacy. As has already been stated, progress in reducing the high maternal mortality rates requires the elimination of the unbooked emergencies, the principal high-risk group. To achieve this, tough decisions involving the underlying political, socioeconomic, cultural, religious and health causes must be taken and implemented. Traditional birth attendants are hopelessly ill-suited for any part of this mammoth task. They are too old and too set in their ways to adapt successfully to new challenges. Their replacement by midwives must be given the top priority in any safe motherhood programme.

that can have negative impacts on future health, as well as administrative and educational development (Harrison 1989a). Diagnosis and decisions for and against operative delivery must be made, and immediate and remote prognosis for future reproductive outcomes correctly assessed; clearly, non-physicians are not equipped to do this. Besides, where codes of regulation of medical practice are weak and enforcement is non-existent, quackery is bound to increase, bringing orthodox maternity care into disrepute. Disputes over career structure and payment systems for physicians as compared with non-physicians who operate will surface, with damaging consequences on the health services if they are allowed to get out of control. The creation of this class of non-physicians who operate blocks the progress of those of them who might otherwise have become physicians and then trained to become specialists. The worry is that if care is not taken, this approach can delay the emergence of top-quality indigenous medical leadership.

## Abdominal deliveries and laparotomy by non-physicians

In a desperate attempt to reduce maternal mortality in places in sub-Saharan Africa where doctors are scarce, non-physicians that are available are being encouraged to perform Caesarean sections and laparotomies in unbooked emergencies. The obvious problem with this concept is that it takes too narrow a view of the obstacles to better maternal health. Short-term outcomes of Caesarean sections by non-physicians may be favourable, but there are several consequences

## POSSIBLE SOLUTIONS

It is possible to achieve respectable levels of perinatal statistics even in poor countries, as the experience of the state of Kerala in India has shown. The gross domestic product per caput in United States dollars is 200 for Kerala and 225 for India, average births per woman are 1.9 for Kerala and four for India, the infant mortality rates are 17 per 1000 live births for Kerala and 83 per 1000 live births for India. Kerala's success comes from its strong commitment to progressive social policies, basic professional health care and female education. The percentages of literate women are 87% for Kerala and 34% for India. Girls in Kerala remain at school once they enrol, 50% drop out in India.

As for poverty alleviation, there is no need to wait for decades to achieve it, as East Asia has shown. According to United Nations Development Programme (UNDP), United Nations Fund for Population Activities (UNFPA) and United Nations International Children's Emergency Fund (UNICEF):

> '*the total cost of providing basic social services in the developing countries including health, education, family planning, clean water and all other basic social goals would be in the region of an additional 30 to 40 billion United States dollars a year. The world spends more than this in playing golf.*' (Grant 1995)

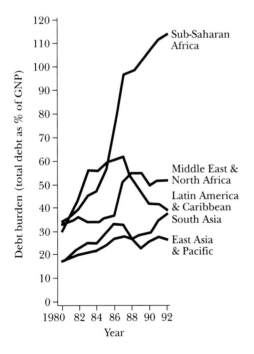

**Figure 4**  *The debt burden as shown by the total percentage of gross national product (GNP) between 1980 and 1992. (Reproduced from Grant, J. (1995)* The State of the World's Children, *with permission of Oxford University Press. Data acquired from the United Nations International Children's Emergency Fund [UNICEF])*

Between 1980 and 1990, sub-Saharan Africa's total debt as a percentage of GNP exceeded 110%, compared to 50% for the Middle East and North Africa, 35% for Latin America and the Caribbean, 33% for South Asia, and 25% for East Asia and the Pacific (see Figure 4).

It is noteworthy that the nearer the region is to Brussels, Europe's capital, the greater the debt burden. It would be unfair to blame Europe alone for the misery. However, Europe can help reduce the pain by paying fairer prices for the primary commodities from developing countries, and also through education and training, as well as by establishing and improving their infrastructure. The idea of a Marshall plan with debt cancellation has been mooted for Africa. However, as has been argued elsewhere:

> '*Even if all debts are written off, it is doubtful if sub-Saharan Africa could cope with greater economic wealth without first improving the general level of education.*' (Harrison 1989b)

The greatest strength of mass education is in raising the low status of women for socio-economic, political and health advancement and modernisation. In the process, total population census (actual counts not estimates) is essential for progress, because it registers in the minds of political and policy leadership that everybody is important, including girls and women. The case for commitment to, and investment in, education for the attainment of general development, beneficial to maternal health, is well stated by one Nigerian who said that:

> '*If you think education is expensive, try illiteracy.*'

Galbraith (1994), an economist, is in full support of these words when he wrote:

> '*There is, in our time, no well-educated, literate population that is poor; there is no illiterate population that is other than poor.*'

Research issues, the scourge of HIV infection, family planning, female infanticide and other forms of sexually dependent abuses have not been discussed, not because they are unimportant, but because other matters of life and death are at stake. In any case, they are the issues that have attracted extensive media coverage over many years and they continue to do so (Craft 1995).

## CONCLUSIONS

This chapter has tried to look at maternal mortality and morbidity, not so much from a clinical context, but from the socioeconomic and public health perspective. The inescapable conclusion is that both globally and locally, it is the exclusion of the poor from the benefits that exist that does the greatest damage and that addressing this issue will have the greatest impact. The World Health Organisation (1995) now agrees. Nigerian newspapers when carrying obituary notices sometimes display the following caption, especially in cases of maternal deaths: '*the wicked have done their worst*'. A possible rejoinder applicable not just to Nigeria or Africa, but the world at large is: '*But have the good done their best?*'

## ACKNOWLEDGEMENTS

The help received from the following during the preparation of this lecture is gratefully acknowledged: J. B. Lawson (Newcastle upon Tyne), Irma Seppanen (Tuusula, Finland), Paivi Pekkarinen and Aino Leena Nagy (National Library of Health Sciences, Helsinki, Finland), Professor J. P. Neilson, Mr Paul Nickson and Mrs Janet Storey (Liverpool, United Kingdom), Miss P. Want (Librarian, Royal College of Obstetricians and Gynaecologists) and Professor N. D. Briggs (Acting Vice Chancellor, University of Port Harcourt, Nigeria). Support over the years has also been provided by many friends and associates, in particular Frank Hytten, Robin Fox, Charles Rossiter, Adetokunbo Lucas and Staffan Bergstrom.

# References

Anonymous (1994) Structural adjustment too painful [editorial]? *Lancet* **344**, 1377–8

Bergstrom, S. (1994) 'The pathology of poverty' in: K. S. Lankinen, S. Bergstrom, P. H. Makela and M. Peltomaa (Eds.). *Health and Disease in Developing Countries*, pp. 3–120. London: Macmillan Press Ltd

Black, J. (1958) Reminiscences of fifty years of medical practice, forty seven of them spent in South Africa. *J. Obstet Gynaecol Br Emp* **65**, 933–43

Brabin, L., Kemp, J., Obunge, O. K. *et al.* (1994) Reproductive tract infections and abortions among adolescent girls in rural Nigeria. *Lancet* **344**, 300–4

Craft, N. (1995) Beijing and the future of women. *BMJ* **311**, 580–1

Fleming, A. F. (1989) Anaemia in pregnancy in tropical Africa. *Trans R Soc Trop Med Hyg* **83**, 441–8

Galbraith, J. K. (1994) The good society considered: the economic dimension [Cardiff annual lecture]. *J Law Soc*

Grant, J. (1995) *The State of the World's Children*, pp. 1–87. Oxford: Oxford University Press

Grosskuria, H., Mosha, F., Todd, J. *et al.* (1995) Impact of improved treatment of STDs on HIV infection in rural Tanzania: randomised control trial. *Lancet* **346**, 530–6.

Harrison, K. A. (1985) Childbearing, health and social priorities: a survey of 22,774 consecutive hospital births in Zaria, Northern Nigeria. *Br J Obstet Gynaecol* **92** (Suppl. 5), 14–22, 23–31, 32–9, 40–8, 72–80, 87–99, 100–115, 116

Harrison, K. A. (1989a) Maternal mortality in developing countries [correspondence, author's reply]. *Br J Obstet Gynaecol* **96**, 1121–3

Harrison, K. A. (1989b) 'Social and health factors contributing to high maternal mortality' in: C. H. W. Bullough, C. E. Lennox and J. B.

Lawson (Eds.). *Maternity Care in Developing Countries: Proceedings of a Meeting at the Royal College of Obstetricians and Gynaecologists, 30th June and 1st July, 1989*, pp 3–5. London: RCOG Press

Harrison, K. A., Rossiter, C. E. and Tan, H. (1986) Family planning and maternal mortality in the third world. *Lancet* **i**, 1441

Logie, D. E., and Woodroffe, J. (1993) Structural adjustment: the wrong prescription for Africa? *BMJ* **307**, 41–4

Kerr, M. J. M. (1948) Contracted pelvis. *J Obstet Gynaecol Br Emp* **55**, 401–17

Mahfouz, N. (1957) Urinary fistula in women. *J Obstet Gynaecol Br Emp* **64**, 23–34

Rooney, C. (1992) *Antenatal Care and Maternal Health: How Effective is it?* pp. 6–37. Geneva: World Health Organisation

Thaddeus, S. and Maine, D. (1994) Too far to walk: maternal mortality in context. *Soc Sci Med* **38**, 1091–10

Wakhweya, A. M. (1995) Structural adjustment and health. *BMJ* **311**, 71–2

Watkins, K. (1995) *Oxfam Poverty Report*, pp. 1–226. Oxford: Oxfam (UK and Ireland)

Watson, B. P. (1955) The factors responsible for the lowering of maternal mortality in the past 50 years. *J Obstet Gynaecol Br Emp* **62**, 838–52

World Health Organisation (1995) 'Bridging the gap' in: *The World Health Report 1995*, pp. 1–113. Geneva: World Health Organisation

# 6

# Physiology and pharmacology of uterine contractility

*John J. Morrison*

The factors regulating uterine contractility during pregnancy, and the precise order of events leading to the initiation of parturition in the human, are poorly understood. The question of what mediates the transformation from relative quiescence to the expulsive contractions of labour is of considerable importance, since an answer may provide insight into clinical problems such as preterm labour (Morrison 1996) and induction of labour. However, the state of excitability of the myometrium is controlled, to our knowledge, by a complex network of physiological mechanisms involving hormones, peptides, cell membrane receptors, intracellular signalling systems, calcium, neuronal and metabolic factors, gap junctions and ion channels. These various mechanisms are depicted in Figure 1 and will be dealt with separately in this chapter. Clarification of these pathways in recent years has resulted in an expansion in the number and type of pharmacological compounds with a primary action on the myometrium.

## ORGANISATION OF MYOMETRIAL SMOOTH MUSCLE

The myometrial smooth muscle cells are embedded in extracellular material composed mainly of collagen fibres, fibroblasts, macrophages and mast cells and do not form a homogeneous tissue like skeletal muscle. This

arrangement facilitates the transmission of contractile forces generated by individual muscle cells. The myometrium is composed of interlacing bundles of long, spindle-shaped smooth muscle fibres arranged in ill-defined layers. During pregnancy the myometrium grows dramatically due to hypertrophy and an increase in the number of smooth muscle cells by division (Carsten 1968). The myometrial cells communicate with one another through connections called gap junctions. No specific pacemaker cells have been identified in the uterus and the issue of pacemaker activity in the myometrium is unresolved at present.

At the subcellular level, the actin and myosin filaments of myometrium are not organised into fibres and fibrils, as is the case in striated muscle, but instead occur in random bundles throughout the myocyte (Somlyo 1980; Garfield 1984). Furthermore, unlike striated muscle, in the myometrium the continuity of these filaments is not interrupted by Z-lines. Like other smooth muscle systems, however, myometrium contains a third filament, intermediate filaments, which form a network linking protein structures known as dense bodies. The intermediate filaments and dense bodies are not actively involved in the contractile process, but are distributed throughout the entire cell forming attachments, between the cytoplasm and cell membrane. They are analogous in function to the Z-lines of striated muscle. This organised, but highly flexible, arrangement enables the uterus to adapt to many shapes and to generate force in different directions which is necessary for labour.

*Based on the William Blair-Bell Memorial Lecture delivered on 4 December 1995*

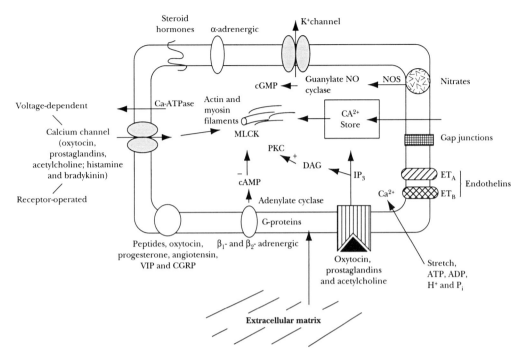

**Figure 1**  *Cellular mechanisms of modulation of myometrial contractibility. ADP, adenosine diphosphate; ATP, adenosine triphosphate; cAMP, cyclic adenosine monophosphate; cGMP, cyclic guanosine monophosphate; CGRP, calcitonin gene related peptide; DAG, diacyglycerol; $ET_A$, endothelin A receptor; $ET_B$, endothelin B receptor; G-protein, guanine nucleotide binding protein; $H^+$, hydrogen ions; $IP_3$, inositol triphosphate; $K^+$, potassium; MLCK, myosin light chain kinase; NO, nitric oxide; NOS, nitric oxide synthase; PKC, protein kinase C; and VIP, vasoactive intestinal polypeptide*

## MECHANISM OF MYOMETRIAL CONTRACTIONS

The actual contraction is based on a sliding of actin and myosin filaments, without any change in the length of either filament, in a similar manner to skeletal muscle (Huxley 1971). Contraction is preceded by a rise in intracellular calcium ($[Ca^{2+}]_i$) which results in the formation of an active complex between calcium, calmodulin and myosin light chain kinase (MLCK). It appears that MLCK is phosphorylated by agents that cause contraction and that relaxation can occur without phosphorylation of MLCK (Stull *et al.* 1990). The MLCK phosphorylates myosin light chains, which results in an increase in the actin-activated magnesium-adenosine triphosphate (ATP)ase leads to hydrolysis of ATP and contraction.

Relaxation occurs as a result of the dephosphorylation of myosin light chains by a phosphatase. Little is known about the phosphatase but, in permeabilised myometrium, the catalytic subunit of phosphatase-2A relaxed calcium-dependent contraction (Haeberle, Hathaway and De-Paoli-Roach 1985). Also, cell repolarisation results in a lowering of $[Ca^{2+}]_i$, by extrusion across the sarcolemma and uptake into the internal stores, thus inactivating the calcium–calmodulin–MLCK complex.

### Role of calcium

An increase in intracellular calcium is essential for uterine contractility, but its importance in regulation of this activity is not quite clear. As outlined earlier in this chapter, calcium binds to calmodulin and removes the inhibitory effects of proteins on both the myosin head (myosin light chain) and on actin. In the resting state, intracellular calcium is maintained at a concentration of about $10^{-7}$ M which increases to $10^{-6}$ M during contraction (Thornton and Gillespie 1992). The extracellular calcium concentration is $10^{-3}$ M. The required increase in intracellular calcium is derived from either the extracellular compartment or intracellular stores. Under normal physiological conditions extracellular calcium can enter the myometrial sarcolemma in a variety of ways. Voltage-dependent and receptor-operated calcium channels are two important means (Hurwitz 1986). These calcium channels are membrane-bound glycoproteins which are thought to exist in an open or activated state, or a closed or deactivated state. When the membrane is depolarised to an appropriate level, voltage-dependent calcium channels convert to the activated state, thus allowing a substantial calcium influx into the cell. Voltage-dependent calcium channels have been divided into long, transient and neuronal types according to their conductance properties (Ducsay 1990). The long and transient types are important in smooth muscle activation. Receptor-operated calcium channels are opened in response to activating ligands, such as hormones or neuro-transmitters, which bind to specific receptors associated with the channel. Despite their central role there is currently no information regarding the possibility of an alteration in calcium channel expression or function in association with human parturition.

Another method of calcium entry from outside the cell is the low passive resting lead that occurs with a concentration gradient. Calcium can be removed from the cytoplasm by the sarcolemmal calcium-ATPase pump. These pumps are ubiquitous single-polypeptide enzymes of molecular weight of approximately 13,000 to 15,000 (Strehler 1991). *In vitro*, the myometrial plasma membrane calcium-ATPase has been shown to be able to extrude large amounts of calcium under physiological conditions, and thus it may be, quantitatively, the most important way of removing calcium from the myometrial cell (Grover, Kwan and Daniel 1982).

The sarcoplasmic reticulum represents the major intracellular store for calcium and in the myometrium it is well developed (Garfield and Somlyo 1985; Somlyo *et al.* 1985). This calcium store is sensitive to inositol 1,4,5-triphosphate ($IP_3$) (Carsten and Miller 1985). Another potential internal source of calcium is sarcolemmal-bound calcium (Grover, Kwan and Daniel 1982), which may contribute to the rise in $[Ca^{2+}]_i$ necessary for contraction, but there is currently no evidence to support this mechanism.

## The phosphoinositide system

There is mounting evidence that binding of agonists to receptors hydrolyses phosphoinositides in the cell membrane, which in turn leads to calcium mobilisation (Berridge 1984; Carsten and Miller 1990). Although not universal, it seems to be a common system involved in the release of calcium to the cytoplasm by agonist activation. For example, the cell membrane oxytocin receptor is probably coupled to the enzyme phosphoinositidase C (phospholipase C) by guanine nucleotide binding proteins (G-proteins) (Berridge and Irvine 1984).

On binding of the agonist to the receptor, phospholipase C (a phosphodiesterase) is activated and hydrolyses phosphatidylinositol-4,5-biphosphate ($PIP_2$) to diacylglycerol (DAG) and $IP_3$. The $IP_3$ releases calcium from the sarcoplasmic reticulum, as mentioned above, possibly by opening calcium channels. It then diffuses into the cytoplasm and is broken down in turn to inositol-biphosphate ($IP_2$), inositol-monophosphate ($IP_1$) and free inositol (Carsten and Miller 1990). These inositol phosphates may have separate intracellular functions and the degradation products are used for re-formation of $PIP_2$. The DAG formed may be converted to phosphatidic acid (PA), which potentiates the effects of $IP_3$ on calcium release, or may release arachidonic acid and therefore stimulate intracellular prostaglandin formation. Diacylglycerol also increases the activity of protein kinase C (PKC). The role of PKC, and other kinases such as tyrosine kinase, in this system is less well characterised. However, it has been shown that blockade of these pathways results in a marked inhibition of contractions in isolated human pregnant myometrium, suggesting an important regulatory role (Morrison *et al.* 1996a). Further analysis of these findings is currently under way.

## Oxytocin

Oxytocin is a powerful stimulator of uterine activity and can enhance the force, the frequency and the duration of contractions. It has classically been described as being produced in, and released from the posterior lobe of the pituitary gland, but recent results indicate that it is also expressed in amnion, chorion and decidua (Chibbar, Miller and Mitchell 1993). There is a marked gestational difference in the pharmacological ability of oxytocin to cause uterine contractions, being most effective in the last trimester. This is due to the presence of more oxytocin receptors, which occurs when the ratio of oestrogen to progesterone is high (Nissenson, Flouret and Hechter 1978). The effects of oxytocin appear to be mediated mainly by resulting in increased $[Ca^{2+}]_i$ by different mechanisms (Tasaka *et al.* 1991; Thornton *et al.* 1992). The rise in $[Ca^{2+}]_i$ produced by oxytocin depends on external calcium entry through L-type calcium channels. Oxytocin also causes $IP_3$ formation, by activation of phospholipase C through a G-protein in human gestational myometrium and decidua, which can release calcium from intracellular stores (Schrey, Read and Steer 1986; Marc, Leiber and Harbon 1986). Another possible mechanism by which oxytocin may increase $[Ca^{2+}]_i$ is by inhibiting the sarcolemmal or sarcoplasmic reticulum calcium-ATPase (Magocsi and Penniston 1991). Oxytocin may also give rise to calcium- independent uterine contractility, which is probably due to phosphorylation of a cytosolic or contractile protein (Matsuo *et al.* 1989). The role that oxytocin plays in the physiology of human labour is, however, unclear and somewhat controversial. Plasma levels of oxytocin are not elevated in labour (Leake 1990). However, oxytocin may be involved in the initiation or facilitation of parturition by alteration in the number or properties of its receptors, or by potential effects on other components of the regulatory network (e.g. gap junctions or ion channels).

## Prostaglandins

The prostaglandins $PGE_2$ and $PGF_{2\alpha}$ increase uterine contractile activity in association with a rise in free $[Ca^{2+}]_i$, which appears to be due primarily to an influx of extracellular calcium (Coleman, McShane and Parkington 1988; Morrison and Smith 1994). It is not clear what changes in membrane potential occur with prostaglandin stimulation and, hence, the relative importance of voltage and receptor-operated calcium channels is unknown. In contrast to oxytocin, prostaglandins do not increase $IP_3$ production in human myometrium or release intracellular calcium stores in cultured myometrial cells (Thornton and Gillespie 1992). Oxytocin interacts with the prostaglandin pathway by phosphoinositide hydrolysis, leading to formation of diacylglycerol (DAG) which, in turn, stimulates arachidonate release and prostaglandin synthesis.

There is no doubt about the intimate involvement of prostaglandins in human labour (Morrison and Smith 1994). Their levels are markedly elevated in amniotic fluid and blood during labour and spontaneous abortion (Niebyl 1981). In addition, induction of abortion, or labour at term, can be successfully achieved with prostaglandin treatment. Colonisation of the amniotic cavity with micro-organisms is known to activate phospholipases, resulting in prostaglandin release and preterm labour (Ledger 1989). In isolated myometrial preparations, indomethacin abolished spontaneous contractions (Garrioch 1978) and prostaglandin synthetase inhibitors have been used in the treatment of preterm labour (Niebyl 1981).

## Steroid hormones

It appears that progesterone is essential to the maintenance of pregnancy, as was first outlined in 1956 by Csapo. Treatment with mifepristone, a steroid acting as an antiprogesterone at the receptor level, results in increased uterine activity as well as an increased sensitivity to prostaglandins (Swahn and Bygdeman 1988). However, the importance of progesterone in the onset of human parturition, term or preterm, is unknown. Progesterone has been traditionally described as having a relaxing effect of human myometrium and many theories have been forwarded for this, including diminished permeability for calcium, increased adenosine monophosphate (cAMP) synthesis and inhibited decidual prostaglandin formation (Egarter and Husslein 1992). However, entirely contradictory to all this, progesterone independently increases the frequency and tonus of contractions in isolated human pregnant myometrial strips (Fu *et al.* 1993). It also enhances sensitivity to, and diminishes tachyphylaxis with, oxytocin. Resolution of these issues requires further investigation.

Human pregnancy is characterised by a state of markedly increased oestrogen levels (mainly 17β-oestradiol and oestriol). Oestrogens stimulate prostaglandin production in the decidua, promote formation of gap junctions and increase the synthesis of oxytocin receptors, all of which are events that may be temporally related to the onset of labour. However, evidence for a causal role is lacking.

### Endothelins

The endothelin (ET) peptides (ET-1, ET-2 and ET-3) cause contraction in the pregnant and non-pregnant rat (Calixto and Rae 1991) uterus and in the human uterus *in vitro* (Word *et al.* 1990). In rats this ET-induced contraction of the uterus was judged to be, on a molar basis, similar to that produced by angiotensin and greater than those due to bradykinin, oxytocin, $PGF_{2\alpha}$, 5-hydroxytryptamine and acetylcholine, with the pregnant uterus being more sensitive than the non-pregnant. The increase in force appears to be related to a dose-dependent rise in $[Ca^{2+}]_i$ due to its release from stores and increased influx, producing increased myosin phosphorylation (Word *et al.* 1990).

The author and co-workers have demonstrated that $ET_A$ endothelin receptors and a smaller population of $ET_B$ endothelin receptors are found in human myometrium (Bacon *et al.* 1995). Although $ET_A$ is known to mediate myometrial contractility, the role of $ET_B$ remains to be elucidated. This group has also shown that messenger RNA for one of the endothelin peptides (ET-2) is present in amnion, chorion and placenta in pregnancy at term (O'Reilly *et al.* 1993). The implications of these findings for human labour *in vivo* are, as yet, speculative.

### Neuronal modulation

The uterus has autonomic innervation which has been known for over 300 years (Krantz 1959). Its contribution to parturition has been less well characterised than the hormonal factors involved. Myometrial cells possess all four main types of adrenergic receptors (i.e. $\alpha_1$, $\alpha_2$, $\beta_1$ and $\beta_2$ (Bottari *et al.* 1985). It has been postulated that $\alpha_1$-receptors mediate contraction and that $\beta_2$-receptors are predominantly responsible for relaxation (Bulbring and Tomito 1987). Both $\beta_1$- and $\beta_2$-receptors are coupled to adenylate cyclase via an intermediate G-protein ($G_S$). The increased cAMP that results from activation of adenylate cyclase activates cAMP-dependent kinase, which ultimately leads to a reduction of phosphorylation of myosin light chains, and relaxation, as discussed previously. Cyclic AMP has other effects which result in relaxation, such as calcium sequestration and efflux of calcium through the cell membrane (Diamond 1990; Thornton and Gillespie 1992). The α-adrenergic receptor is coupled to adenylate cyclase by an inhibitory G-protein ($G_I$). This $G_i$ may directly reduce adenylate cyclase activity or may prevent stimulation of the enzyme by $G_S$. Finally, α- and β-adrenergic agents may have effects which appear to be independent of cAMP.

Cholinergic stimulation causes uterine contractions and this appears to occur by increasing $IP_3$ and elevating $[Ca^{2+}]_i$ (Marc, Leiber and Harbon 1986). However, the uterine parasympathetic system receives more attention for its role in pain perception than effects on motor activity.

## Ion channels and excitation–contraction coupling

The resting membrane potential that exists across a cell membrane arises as a consequence of an unequal distribution of ions on either side of the membrane. The resting membrane potential of human myometrium is approximately –50 mV (Inoue *et al.* 1990). Changes in the myometrial membrane potential, as a result of a flow of ions across the membrane, are fundamental to the control of uterine activity. Spontaneous contractions are preceded by action potentials, which can be altered in frequency and duration by agonists. The ion channels involved in the generation of electrical signals can be described in relation to their ionic selectivity (i.e. calcium [discussed above], potassium, chloride and sodium). In myometrium, as in other smooth muscle tissues, each action potential consists of a rapid depolarisation phase followed by a slower return to baseline. The inward current of the depolarisation phase is mediated via calcium and sodium ions (Young and Herndon Smith 1991; Young, Herndon Smith and Anderson 1991). Activation of a chloride conductance in smooth muscle would also tend to depolarise the cell membrane towards the threshold for an action potential (Shoemaker, Naftel and Farley 1985). The number of channels in the open state at any one time determines the permeability of the membrane to these ions. Each channel can exist in an open, closed or inactivated state. The repolarisation phase, which returns the membrane potential to its resting level, is associated with inactivation of the calcium current and efflux of potassium ions through potassium channels (Jmari, Mironneau and Mironneau 1986; Toro, Stefani and Erulkar 1990).

The author's group has demonstrated that potassium channels play a role in the excitability of human myometrium during pregnancy and labour. There are many types of these channels, but the predominant one in electrophysiological recordings of human myometrial cells was a large conductance, calcium-activated potassium-channel (Khan *et al.* 1993). The physiological and pharmacological properties of this channel were markedly altered by the onset of labour.

As well as voltage activation, the activity of many channels can be influenced by neurotransmitters and hormones. Ligands may also influence channels indirectly by inducing production in the cell of enzymes or second messengers (e.g. cAMP, cGMP, protein kinases, inositol phosphates and G-proteins) which in turn regulate channel activity (Parkington and Coleman 1990). The potential for interaction of biochemical and electrical processes to modulate uterine contractility is vast and a considerable amount of work is still required to elucidate these mechanisms in human labour.

## Gap junctions

Gap junctions are composed of membrane spanning proteins of the connexin family and it is thought that they provide a low-resistance pathway between individual myometrial cells, allowing easy spread of action potentials, as in a syncytium (Garfield, Sims and Daniel 1977; Cole, Garfield and Kirkaldy 1988). Garfield and co-workers (1977) first observed the sudden appearance of gap junctions conjoining myometrial cells in rats just prior to and during parturition. There is a marked increase in levels of connexin-43 messenger RNA and protein, and in the density and size of gap junctions, towards parturition in successful labour, whether this occurs at term or preterm (Garfield and Somlyo 1985; Chow and Lye 1994). It appears that expression of gap junction proteins is a necessary component of term and preterm labour (Balducci *et al.* 1993). More work is necessary in defining the mechanism of action of gap junctions and their role in promoting labour.

## Extracellular matrix

Uterine growth during pregnancy, and cervical ripening and dilatation in parturition, involve major changes in the extracellular matrix. Collagen is the main structural molecule in the uterine extracellular matrix and is involved in the maintenance of its three-dimensional integrity (Danforth and Buckingham 1973). The other components of this connective tissue include fibronectin, laminin, proteoglycans, glycoaminoglycans, oligosaccharides and other macromolecules. The synthesis and metabolism of collagen are altered during pregnancy and labour (Danforth and Buckingham 1973; Rajabi, Dean and Woessner 1990). The mechanism and regulation of this altered collagen metabolism, and its relationship with the onset of labour at term and preterm, have been studied.

The enzymes that degrade extracellular matrix are known as the matrix metalloproteinases of which there are three major subclasses; the collagenases, the gelatinases and the stromelysins. The activity of the metalloproteinases is regulated by a potent glycoprotein of 28,000 molecular weight, tissue inhibitor of metalloproteinases (Matrisian 1990). Altered collagenase activity in preterm labour has been reported with associated changes in serum levels (Rajabi, Dean and Woessner 1987). Interestingly, the author's group has found that the tissue inhibitor of metalloproteinases levels are similarly altered in term and preterm labour, suggesting that the enzyme and inhibitor come from the same source and are co-ordinately regulated (Clark et al. 1994). The group has also reported that the altered collagenase activity in term and preterm labour does not appear to be due to tissue collagenase (matrix metalloproteinase-1), confirming suggestions that neutrophil collagenase may be primarily involved (Morrision et al. 1994). Further studies to investigate the expression of these enzymes in reproductive tissues may provide valuable information on the mechanisms regulating parturition.

## Metabolic modulation

Hypoxia, as may occur during prolonged uterine contractions, reduces contractions in isolated rat and rabbit myometrial strips (Wray et al. 1992). Acidification, with the lowering of pH that may occur with hypoxia, can depress uterine contractions (Wray et al. 1992; Parratt, Taggart and Wray 1994). A rise in intracellular

pH can increase the frequency, and to a lesser extent the amplitude, of contractions in rat and human uterine strips (Heaton, Taggart and Wray 1992). Little is known about intracellular pH regulation in the myometrium. There is no knowledge on the potential *in vivo* role of these factors in human term or preterm labour.

## Nitric oxide

Recent reports from different animal species, including humans, have suggested that the L-arginine–nitric oxide (NO) system is important in inhibition of uterine activity during pregnancy. Nitric oxide synthase activity in rabbit decidua and in the gravid rat uterus is reduced towards the end of gestation (Natuzzi et al. 1993; Sladek et al. 1993). L-arginine at high concentrations (millimolar) has been shown to relax contractions of rat myometrium (Yallampalli, Garfield and Byam-Smith 1993). The NO synthase inhibitor, NG-nitro-L-arginine methyl ester, again at millimolar concentrations, caused an increase in the contractile activity of the pregnant rat uterus *in vitro* (Yallampalli, Garfield and Byam-Smith 1993). The author's group has reported that NO donor compounds are affective relaxants of isolated human pregnant myometrium, but did not observe a relaxant effect with NO substrate or a stimulatory effect with NO synthase inhibitor (Morrison et al. 1996b).

## Oxidoreductases

The physiological importance of oxidation–reduction reactions in cellular regulation has long been recognised (Holmgren 1985). In addition, it is now known that oxidative damage is a form of tissue injury involved in the pathophysiology of many disease processes (Haliwell 1994). The author and co-workers have shown that the regulation of such interconversion between the oxidised and reduced states of proteins is an ongoing process in amnion, chorion and placenta during pregnancy and labour, and that increased levels of one such oxidoreductase (thiol protein disulphide isomerase) occurs in preterm labour before 30 weeks' gestation (Morrison et al. 1996c). These findings add a new dimension to our understanding of the molecular mechanisms regulating parturition at term, and the lack of regulation that occurs preterm.

## Stretch

Stretch (distension) is a contractile stimulus to smooth muscle. Thus, in the uterus the role of stretch in parturition has been considered. Preterm labour is more common in multiple pregnancies where, for gestation, relative uterine distension is a feature. Stretch may cause an increase in intracellular calcium (Himpens *et al.* 1988) and it has been demonstrated that stretch can result in an increase in phosphorylation of myosin in the uterus (Csabina, Barany and Barany 1986). Its contribution to the network of interactions resulting in labour, at term or preterm, is not known.

## PHARMACOLOGICAL INHIBITION OF PRETERM LABOUR

Through the years a variety of drugs with different pharmacological principles have been used to suppress unwanted uterine activity. Tocolytic treatment should fulfil certain preconditions:

(1) There should be no maternal or fetal reason for which delivery might confer some benefit;

(2) The fetus should be at a gestational age (generally less than 32 weeks' gestation) at which it is expected to benefit from the treatment in excess of the potential risks imposed; and

(3) Contraindications to a particular tocolytic must be lacking and the fetal membranes should generally be intact.

In the properly selected patient, it is hoped that intervention with an effective means of tocolysis may decrease morbidity and mortality. Using these basic guidelines most obstetricians will use a drug with a sound pharmacological principle to postpone preterm labour.

The tocolytics currently in use, or under consideration for benefit in recent years, are β-adrenergic agonists, prostaglandin synthetase inhibitors, calcium channel blockers, magnesium sulphate, oxytocin antagonists, potassium channel openers, NO donor compounds, ethanol and miscellaneous agents such as diazoxide and progesterone derivatives.

## β-adrenergic agonists

The smooth muscle relaxing properties of the β-adrenergic agonists is derived from their interaction with $\beta_2$-adrenergic receptor sites on the myometrial cell membrane leading to activation of adenylate cyclase and an increase in intracellular concentrations of cAMP. This in turn activates protein kinase and phosphorylation of intracellular proteins, including membrane proteins in the sarcoplasmic reticulum, leading ultimately to decreased availability of free intracellular calcium to actin and myosin (Roberts 1984). Myosin light chain kinase is also phosphorylated, which decreases its affinity for calmodulin (Scheid, Honeyman and Fay 1979; Roberts 1984). The cumulative results of these actions is that uterine smooth muscle is relaxed.

Isoxsuprine was the first such agent demonstrated to relax uterine smooth muscle and has $\beta_1$- and $\beta_2$- adrenergic effects (Lish, Hillyard and Dungan 1960). The second generation of β-adrenergic agonists, with selectivity for $\beta_2$-adrenergic receptors, are the agents now most used. These include ritodrine, terbutaline, salbutamol, fenoterol and hexoprenaline. Ritodrine is currently the only tocolytic agent licensed for this use in Britain and was the first such agent approved by the Food and Drug Administration in the United States in 1980 (Merkatz, Peter and Bardon 1980).

Unfortunately, in terms of clinical effectiveness, the inhibition of contractions by β-adrenergic agonists is often short lived. Escape from their tocolytic effect is well described both *in vitro* and *in vivo* (Casper and Lye 1986; Caritis, Chiao and Kridgen 1991). In their meta-analysis, King *et al.* (1988) reviewed 16 controlled trials in which tocolytic agents, chiefly ritodrine, were evaluated. The β-adrenergic agonists were found to be effective in reducing the proportion of women who delivered within

24 hours and within 48 hours of treatment. However, this treatment did not decrease the likelihood of preterm delivery and had no effect on perinatal mortality or neonatal morbidity. A more recent randomised, controlled, multicentre Canadian trial, which involved 708 women receiving either ritodrine or placebo, concluded that the use of ritodrine in the treatment of preterm labour had no significant beneficial effect on perinatal morality, the frequency of prolongation of pregnancy to term, or birth weight (Canadian Preterm Labor Investigators Group 1992). The accumulated evidence, therefore, shows that treatment with a β-adrenergic agonist reduces the rate of delivery within 48 hours, but that this immediate effect has not led to clinically significant reductions in the rates of preterm birth or low birth weight and, most importantly, has not resulted in an improvement in outcome in terms of severe neonatal respiratory distress syndrome or perinatal death.

Maternal side effects of the β-adrenergic agonists can be unpleasant and occasionally life threatening (Alger and Crenshaw 1989). The potentially fatal ones are cardiac arrythmias, myocardial ischaemia and pulmonary oedema. The mechanism of development of pulmonary oedema with their use is unknown, but its incidence has been reported as being as high as 3–9% (Leveno and Cunningham 1992), and the debate concerning the safety of β-adrenergic agonists has intensified in the United Kingdom in recent times (Lamont 1993). Their use requires close clinical monitoring. The dilemma is that the failure of properly supervised use of β-adrenergic agonists, and equally, but conversely, the failure to use such drugs, can have far-reaching cost and medico-legal implications (Lamont 1993). In addition, their reported fetal and neonatal side effects include hypoglycaemia, hypocalcaemia, ileus, hypotension and death (Alger and Crenshaw 1989). Despite these problems, β-adrenergic agonists remain as the primary, and most commonly used, method of tocolysis in the developed world. Until more effective and safer tocolytic agents are available, appreciation of these cautions and limitations is mandatory for obstetric practice.

## Prostaglandin synthetase inhibitors

There is a large amount of evidence that supports intimate involvement of prostaglandins in the uterine contractions of labour (this has been discussed earlier in the chapter). Furthermore, indomethacin is the most commonly used prostaglandin-synthetase inhibitor for treatment of preterm labour. Some of the early studies, in the 1970s, reported good results for inhibition of preterm contractions, but a review of these studies reveals that many were uncontrolled (Niebyl 1981). One prospective, randomised, double-blinded study suggested that indomethacin was more effective than placebo in the first 24 hours of treatment, but there was no difference between the groups with respect to gestational age at delivery, birth weight, neonatal morbidity and perinatal mortality. In other studies, the success rates with indomethacin have been comparable to those achieved with β-agonists (Morales et al. 1989; Besinger et al. 1991).

As the use of prostaglandin-synthetase inhibitors for preterm labour has increased, questions have arisen about their safety for both mother and fetus (Niebyl 1981). However, more recently, it has been demonstrated that the incidence of serious neonatal complications associated with antenatal indomethacin treatment (e.g. necrotising enterocolitis, patent ductus arteriosus, intracranial haemorrhage and renal dysfunction), is significantly increased in infants born at or before 30 weeks' gestation (Norton et al. 1993). This had not previously been appreciated due to a preponderance of more mature infants in earlier studies concerning safety of indomethacin. This introduces a dilemma for the future use of indomethacin, because the fetuses most in need of tocolysis are those at most risk of serious complications from the treatment.

## Calcium channel blockers

As discussed earlier in the chapter, myometrial contractility is intrinsically dependent on the availability of free intracellular calcium and, as a consequence, blockade of sarcolemmal calcium channels would lead to relaxation. Dihydro-pyridine derivatives, such as nifedipine, bind to the inside of the myometrial L-type voltage-dependent calcium channels, causing them to remain in the closed state (Triggle and Janis 1987). They are potent inhibitors of tension development in uterine smooth muscle (Parkington and Coleman 1990).

Published experience with these agents is limited to small series and successful treatment of preterm labour has been reported in limited numbers of patients (Leonardi and Hankins 1992). Attempts to combine their use with that of β-agonists, in order to modify the side effects of the latter agents, have not been successful. Of concern is the finding of reduced uterine blood flow, in parallel with decreased fetal oxygen saturation and a trend towards fetal acidosis, caused by these agents in sheep (Harake *et al.* 1987). Nifedipine also affects placental vascularisation and there is the unresolved question of embryotoxicity (Richichi and Vasilenko 1992). Their place and safety in preterm labour requires further evaluation.

## Magnesium sulphate

For many years it has been recognised that magnesium sulphate inhibits myometrial contractility, since clinical use of magnesium for the treatment of pre-eclampsia frequently resulted in decreased uterine activity as a side effect. Its exact mechanism of action is unknown, but it is believed that magnesium alters nerve transmission by affecting acetylcholine release and sensitivity at the motor endplate, and that it may displace calcium in the transmission of a nerve impulse (Petrie 1981). The reports concerning its tocolytic efficacy have been either observational or comparisons with various β-adrenergic agents. Its success in the treatment of preterm labour appears, in general, to be comparable to that of β-adrenergic agonists (Beall *et al.* 1985; Hollander, Nagey and Pupkin 1987). It has been reported that the combination of the two treatments may be more effective, but this approach requires great caution regarding the potential for cumulative side effects (Hatjis *et al.* 1987). The maternal side effects include nausea, dizzi-

ness and pulmonary oedema. Indeed, hypermagnesaemia which results from impaired renal function can lead to respiratory and cardiac compromise (Petrie 1981). Respiratory and motor depression have been observed in infants with elevated cord magnesium concentrations.

## Oxytocin antagonists

As previously discussed, the role of oxytocin in labour, at term and preterm, is controversial, but its mechanisms of action in promoting myometrial contractions are well documented. For this reason, agents that can interfere with these mechanisms have been investigated as potential tocolytic agents. A series of oxytocin antagonists were synthesised and screened in both *in vitro* and *in vivo* animal pharmacology experiments in the early and mid 1980s (Melin 1993). Åkerlund *et al.* (1987) reported successful inhibition of contractions in an uncontrolled pilot study in which 13 patients used [mpa$^1$D-Tyr(Et)$^2$Thr$^4$Orn$^8$]OT (atosiban). The initial results from a multicentre study in the United States have revealed that atosiban diminished the frequency of contractions by 70.8% and completely stopped contractions in 61% (Melin 1993). However, no overall relationship between the effect of the drug and the length of gestation was apparent. Of concern was the fact that umbilical vein plasma levels were 12% of the maternal uterine vein plasma levels, indicating the importance of follow-up studies on infants born to women receiving oxytocin antagonists. Further evaluation of these agents is currently required.

## Potassium channel openers

It has been demonstrated that potassium channel openers are effective relaxants of isolated human pregnant myometrium (Cheuk *et al.* 1993; Morrison *et al.* 1993) and that this inhibitory effect is of equal potency before and after the onset of labour (Morrison *et al.* 1993). This method of uterine inhibition is physiologically appealing because the outward current of potassium offsets depolarising stimuli and so suppresses regenerative electrical activity, thereby rendering the myometrial cell quiescent. In addition, the nature and diversity of potassium channels and the increasing number of compounds available for their modulation introduces the concept of uterine selectivity, as it is being developed in other clinical applications in a way not possible with previous methods of tocolysis. There is currently no information available from clinical studies with these compounds.

## Nitric oxide donor compounds

As discussed earlier in the chapter, it has been shown that NO donor compounds are relaxants of rat and human pregnant myometrium *in vitro* (Morrison *et al.* 1996b). Provisional clinical results, as yet uncontrolled and derived from small numbers, point to the possibility that NO donor compounds in the form of topically applied glyceryl trinitrate patches may have a role in the treatment of preterm labour (Lees *et al.* 1994). There are currently two prospective randomised trials under way in the United Kingdom to further investigate this hypothesis and the results are awaited with interest.

## Ethanol

Ethanol acts both centrally (inhibiting neuro-hypophyseal secretion of oxytocin and vasopressin) and peripherally (interfering with calcium mobilisation, and stimulating cAMP production) to inhibit uterine activity (Fuchs and Fuchs 1981). It was the first widely used tocolytic agent in the late 1960s and early 1970s. Its administration requires constant supervision because of its many associated side effects which include intoxication, vomiting, restlessness, disorientation, hangover, lactic acidosis, dehydration and neonatal depression. The most serious of all is the risk of vomit aspiration by a sleepy, intoxicated woman. For all these reasons its use is no longer justified.

## Miscellaneous

Diazoxide, a benzothiazide derivative which has been discussed earlier in the chapter, has

uterine-relaxant activity and has been used successfully to inhibit labour in humans (Landesman and Wilson 1968; Landesman *et al.* 1969). However, as it is a chemical derivative of the thiazide drugs, it results in unacceptable side effects, including hyperglycaemia, hyperuricaemia, stimulation of the renin–angiotensin system, abnormal hair growth and fluid retention (it does not have diuretic properties). For these reasons its use was discontinued (Alger and Crenshaw 1989). Pregnenolone sulphate, an immediate precursor of placental progesterone, has been reported in small trials to inhibit uterine activity (Alger and Crenshaw 1989). The tocolytic effect of oral micronised progesterone was not as intense, or as rapid, as that of β-mimetics in a double-blind study of 57 women, of whom 29 received a single oral dose of 400 mg progesterone (Emy, Pigne and Provost 1986). Progesterone is not routinely used in current obstetric practice.

## CONCLUSION

In conclusion, it is apparent that many factors are involved in the regulation of myometrial contractility in pregnancy and labour. Many of these processes interact, and agents that cause uterine contraction or relaxation often have multiple sites of action. It appears that these processes are similar in normal labour at term and in preterm labour, and the latter may simply be the consequence of an early, often unknown, triggering event. Despite the fact that great advances have been made in the characterisation of mechanism of action of contracting and relaxing agents on myometrial cells, our understanding of these issues is still incomplete. Disorders of this process, such as preterm labour and delivery, continue to have a significant impact on perinatal outcome in the 1990s and the standard perinatal mortality statistic is a poor yardstick of this situation (Morrison and Rennie 1995). There is, of course, no one simple answer to these problems, as there will undoubtedly be interplay between the various modulatory factors outlined in this chapter. The pursuit of a solution to this problem demands sound scientific investigation followed by rigorous clinical appraisal. Clarification of these issues should open pathways for the development of new therapeutic agents which are highly effective and selective.

# References

Åkerlund, M., Stromberg, P. Hauksson, A. *et al.* (1987) Inhibition of uterine contractions of premature labour with an oxytocin analogue. Results from a pilot study. *Br J Obstet Gynaecol* **94**, 1040–4

Alger, L. S. and Crenshaw, M C. (1989) 'Preterm labour and delivery' in: A. Turnbull and G. Chamberlain (Eds.). *Obstetrics*, pp. 49–70. Edinburgh: Churchill Livingstone

Bacon, C. R., Morrison, J. J., O'Reilly, G., Cameron, I. T. and Davenport, A. P. (1995) $ET_A$ and $ET_B$ endothelin receptors in human myometrium characterised by the subtype elective ligands BQ123, BQ3020, FR139317 and PD151242. *J Endocrinol* **144**, 127–34

Balducci, J., Risek, B., Gilula, N. B. *et al.* (1993) Gap junction formation in human myometrium: a key to preterm labour? *Am J Obstet Gynecol* **168**, 1609–15

Beall, M. H., Edgar, B. W., Paul, R. H. and Smith-Wallace, T. (1985) A comparison of ritodrine, terbutaline and magnesium sulfate for the suppression of preterm labour. *Am J Obstet Gynecol* **153**, 854–9

Berridge, M. J. (1984) Inositol triphosphate and diacylglycerol as second messengers. *Biochem J* **220**, 345–60

Berridge, M. J. and Irvine, R. F. (1984) Inositol triphosphate, a novel second messenger in cellular signal transduction. *Nature* **312**, 315–21

Besinger, R. E., Niebyl J. R., Keyes, W. G. and Johnson, T. R. (1991) Randomized comparative trial of indomethacin and ritodrine for the long-term treatment of preterm labor. *Am J Obstet Gynecol* **164**, 981–8

Bottari, S. P., Vokaer, A., Kaivez, E., Lescrainier, J. P. and Vauquelin, G. (1985) Regulation of α- and β-adrenergic receptor subclasses by gonadal steroids in human myometrium. *Acta Physiol Hung* **65**, 335–46

Bulbring, E. and Tomito, T. (1987) Catecholamine action on smooth muscle. *Pharmacol Rev* **39**, 49–96

Calixto, J. B. and Rae, G. A. (1991) Effects of endothelin, Bay K8644 and other oxytocics in non-pregnant and late pregnant rat isolated uterus. *Eur J Pharmacol* **192**, 109–16

Canadian Preterm Labor Investigators Group (1992) Treatment of preterm labor with the beta-adrenergic agonist ritodrine. *N Engl J Med* **327**, 308–12

Caritis, S. N., Chiao, J. P. and Kridgen, P. (1991) Comparison of pulsatile and continuous ritodrine administration. Effects on uterine contractility and β-adrenergic cascade. *Am J Obstet Gynecol* **164**, 1005–12

Carsten, M. E. (1968) 'Regulation of myometrial composition, growth and activity' in: *The Maternal Organism*, Vol 1 of the Biology of Gestation Series, pp. 355–425. New York: Academic Press

Carsten, M. E. and Miller J. D. (1985) $Ca^{2+}$ release by inositol triphosphate from $Ca^{2+}$-transporting microsomes derived from uterine sarcoplasmic reticulum. *Biochem Biophys Res Commun* **130**, 1027–31

Carsten, M. E. and Miller, J. D. (1990) 'Calcium control mechanisms in the myometrial cell and the role of the phosphoinositide cycle' in: M. E. Carsten and J. D. Miller (Eds.). *Uterine Function: Molecular and Cellular Aspects*, pp. 121–67. New York: Plenum Press

Casper, R. F. and Lye, S. J. (1986) Myometrial desensitization to continuous but not to intermittent β-adrenergic agonist infusion in the sheep. *Am J Obstet Gynecol* **154**, 301–5

Cheuk, J. M. S., Hollingsworth, M., Hughes, S. J., Piper, I. T. and Maresh, M. J. A. (1993) Inhibition of contractions of the isolated human myometrium by potassium channel openers. *Am J Obstet Gynecol* **169**, 953–60

Chibbar, R., Miller, F. D. and Mitchell, B. F. (1993) Synthesis of oxytocin in amnion, chorion and decidua may influence the timing of human parturition. *J Clin Invest* **91**, 185–92

Chow, L. and Lye, S. J. (1994) Expression of the gap junction protein connexin-43 is increased in the human myometrium toward term and with the onset of labour. *Am J Obstet Gynecol* **170**, 788–95

Clark, I. M., Morrison, J. J., Hackett, G. A. *et al.* (1994) Tissue inhibitor of metalloproteinases: serum levels during pregnancy and labor, term and preterm. *Obstet Gynecol* **83**, 532–7

Cole, W C., Garfield, R. E. and Kirkaldy, J. S. (1988) Gap junctions and direct intercellular communication between rat uterine smooth muscle cells. *Am J Physiol* **249**, C20–31

Coleman, H. A., McShane, P. G. and Parkington, H. C. (1988) Gestational changes in the utilization of intracellularly stored calcium in the myometrium of guinea pigs. *J Physiol (Lond)* **399**, 13–32

Csabina, S., Barany, M. and Barany, K. (1986) Stretch-induced myosin light chain phosphorylation in rat uterus. *Arch Biochem Biophys* **249**, 374–81

Csapo, A. L. (1956) Progesterone 'block'. *Am J Anat* **98**, 273–91

Danforth, D. N. and Buckingham, J. J. (1973) 'The effects of pregnancy and labor on the amino acid composition of the human cervix' in: R. J. Blandau and K. Moghissi (Eds.). *The Biology of the Human Cervix*, pp. 351–5. Chicago: University of Chicago Press

Diamond, J. (1990) 'β-Adrenoreceptors, cyclic AMP, and cyclic GMP in control of uterine motility' in: M. E. Carsten and J. D. Miller

(Eds.). *Uterine Function: Molecular and Cellular Aspects,* pp. 249–75. New York: Plenum Press

Ducsay, C. A. (1990) 'Calcium channels: role in myometrial contractility and pharmacological applications of calcium entry blockers' in: M. E. Carsten and J. D. Miller (Eds.). *Uterine Function: Molecular and Cellular Aspects,* pp. 169–94. New York: Plenum Press

Egarter, C. H. and Husslein, P. (1992) Biochemistry of myometrial contractility. *Clin Obstet Gynecol* **6**, 755–69

Emy, R., Pigne, A. and Provost, J. (1986) The effects of oral administration of progesterone for premature labor. *Am J Obstet Gynecol* **154**, 525–9

Fu, X., Masoumeh, R., Löfgren, M., Ulmsten, U. and Bäckström, T. (1993) Antitachyphylactic effects of progesterone and oxytocin on term human myometrial contractile activity *in vitro*. *Obstet Gynecol* **82**, 532–8

Fuchs, A.-R. and Fuchs, F. (1981) Ethanol for prevention of preterm birth. *Semin Perinatol* **5**, 236–51

Garfield, R. E., (1984) 'Myometrial ultrastructure and uterine contractility' in: S. Bottari, J. P. Thomas and A. Vokaer (Eds.). *Uterine Contractility*, pp. 81–109. New York: Mason

Garfield, R. E., Sims, S. M. and Daniel, E. E. (1977) Gap junctions: their presence and necessity in myometrium during parturition. *Science* **198**, 958–60

Garfield, R. E. and Somlyo, A. P. (1985) 'Structure of smooth muscle' in: *Calcium and Contractility*, pp. 1–36. Clifton, NJ: Humana

Garrioch, D. B. (1978) The effect of indomethacin on spontaneous activity in the isolated human myometrium and on the response to oxytocin and prostaglandin. *Br J Obstet Gynaecol* **85**, 47–52

Grover, A. K., Kwan, E. Y. and Daniel, E. E. (1982) $Ca^{2+}$ dependence of calcium uptake by rat myometrium plasma membrane-enriched fraction. *Am J Physiol* **242**, C278–82

Haeberle, J. R., Hathaway, D. R. and De-Paoli-Roach, A. A. (1985) Dephosphorylation of myosin by the catalytic subunit of a type-2 phosphatase produces relaxation of chemically skinned uterine smooth muscle. *J Biol Chem* **260**, 9965–8

Haliwell, B. (1994) Free radicals, antioxidants, and human disease: curiosity, cause or consequence? *Lancet* **344**, 721–4

Harake, B., Gilbert, R. D., Ashwal, S. and Power, G. G. (1987) Nifedipine: effects on fetal and maternal hemodynamics in pregnant sheep. *Am J Obstet Gynecol* **157**, 1003–8

Hatjis, C. G., Swain, M., Nelson, L. H., Meis, P. J. and Ernest, J. M. (1987) Efficacy of combined administration of magnesium sulfate and ritodrine in the treatment of preterm labor. *Obstet Gynecol* **69**, 317–22

Heaton, R. C., Taggart, M. J. and Wray, S. (1992) The effects of intracellular and extracellular alkalinization on contractions of the isolated uterus. *Pfuegers Arch* **422**, 24–30

Himpens, B., Matthijs, G., Somlyo, A. V., Butler, T. M. and Somlyo, A. P. (1988) Cytoplasmic free calcium, myosin light chain phosphorylation, and force in phasic and tonic smooth muscle. *J Gen Physiol* **92**, 713–29

Hollander, D. I., Nagey, D. A. and Pupkin, M. J. (1987) Magnesium sulfate and ritodrine hydrochloride: a randomized comparison. *Am J Obstet Gynecol* **156**, 631–7

Holmgren, A. (1985) Thioredoxins. *Annu Rev Biochem* **54**, 237–71

Hurwitz, L. (1986) Pharmacology of calcium channels and smooth muscle. *Ann Rev Pharmacol Toxicol* **26**, 225–58

Huxley, H. E. (1971) The structural basis of muscular contraction. *Proc R Soc Lond [Series B]* **178**, 131–49

Inoue, Y., Nakao, K., Obabi, K. *et al.* (1990) Some electrical properties of human pregnant myometrium. *Am J Obstet Gynecol* **162**, 1090–8

Jmari, K., Mironneau, C. and Mironneau, J. (1986) Inactivation of calcium channels current in rat uterine smooth muscle: evidence for calcium- and voltage-mediated mechanisms. *J Physiol (Lond)* **380**, 111–26

Khan, R. N., Smith, S. K., Morrison, J. J. and Ashford, M. L. J. (1993) Modification of large-conductance $Ca^{2+}$-activated $K^+$-channel properties of human myometrium during pregnancy and labour. *Proc R Soc Lond [Biol]* **251**, 9–15

King, J. F., Grant, A., Keirse, M. J. N. C. and Chalmers, I. (1988) β-Mimetics in preterm labour: an overview of the randomised controlled trials. *Br J Obstet Gynaecol* **95**, 211–22

Krantz, K. E. (1959) Innervation of the human uterus. *Ann NY Acad Sci* **75**, 770–84

Lamont, R. F. (1993) The contemporary use of β-agonists. *Br J Obstet Gynaecol* **100**, 890–2

Landesman, R. DeSouza, J. A., Coutinko, E. M., Wilson, K. H. and de Sousa, M. B. (1969) The inhibiting effect of diazoxide in normal term labour. *Am J Obstet Gynecol* **103**, 430–3

Landesman, R. and Wilson, K. H. (1968) The relaxant effect of diazoxide on isolated gravid and nongravid human myometrium. *Am J Obstet Gynecol* **101**, 120–5

Leake, R. D. (1990) 'Oxytocin in the initiation of labour' in: M. E. Carsten and J. D. Miller (Eds.). *Uterine Function: Molecular and Cellular Aspects*, pp. 361–71. New York: Plenum Press

Ledger, W. J. (1989) Infection and premature labour. *Am J Perinatol* **6**, 234–6

Lees, C., Campbell, S., Jauniaux, E. *et al.* (1994) Arrest of preterm labour and prolongation of gestation with glyceryl trinitrate, a nitric oxide donor. *Lancet* **343**, 1325–6

Leonardi, M. R. and Hankins, G. D. V. (1992) What's new in tocolytics. *Clin Perinatol* **19**, 367–84

Leveno, K. J. and Cunningham, F. G. (1992) β-Adrenergic agents for preterm labour. *N Engl J Med* **327**, 349–51

Lish, P. M., Hillyard, I. W. and Dungan, K. W. (1960) The uterine relaxant properties of isoxsuprine. *J Pharmacol Exp Ther* **129**, 438–43

Magocsi, M. and Penniston, J. T. (1991) Oxytocin pretreatment of pregnant rat uterus inhibits $Ca^{2+}$ uptake in plasma membrane and sarcoplasmic reticulum. *Biochem Biophys Acta* **1063**, 7–14

Marc, S., Leiber, D. and Harbon, S. (1986) Carbachol and oxytocin stimulate the generation of inositol phosphates in the guinea pig myometrium. *FEBS Lett* **201**, 9–14

Matrisian, L. M. (1990) Metalloproteinases and their inhibitors in matrix remodelling. *Trends Genet* **6**, 121–5

Matsuo, K., Gokita, T., Karibe, H. and Uchida, M. K. (1989) $Ca^{2+}$-independent contraction of uterine smooth muscle. *Biochem Biophys Res Commun* **155**, 722–7

Melin, P. (1993) Oxytocin antagonists in preterm labour and delivery. *Clin Obstet Gynecol* **7**, 577–600

Merkatz, I. R., Peter, J. B. and Barden, T. P. (1980) Ritodrine hydrochloride: a β-mimetic agent for use in preterm labor: II. Evidence of efficacy. *Obstet Gynecol* **56**, 7–11

Morales, W. J., Smith, S. G., Angel, J. L., O'Brien, W. F. and Knuppel, R. A. (1989) Efficacy and safety of indomethacin versus ritodrine in the management of preterm labour: a randomized study. *Obstet Gynecol* **74**, 567–72

Morrison, J. J. (1996) 'Prediction and prevention of preterm labour' in: J. Studd (Ed.). *Progress in Obstetrics and Gynaecology*, Vol. 12, pp. 65–83. Edinburgh: Churchill Livingstone

Morrison, J. J., Ashford, M. L. J., Khan, R. N. and Smith, S. K. (1993) The effects of potassium channel openers on the isolated human pregnant myometrium before and after the onset of labour: potential for tocolysis. *Am J Obstet Gynecol* **169**, 1277–85

Morrison, J. J., Charnock-Jones, D. S. and Smith, S. K. (1996c) Messenger RNA encoding thiol protein disulphide isomerase in amnion, chorion and placenta in human term and preterm labour. *Br J Obstet Gynaecol* **103**, 873–8

Morrison, J. J., Clark, I. M., Powell, E. K. *et al.* (1994) Tissue collagenase: serum levels during pregnancy and parturition. *Eur J Obstet Gynaecol Reprod Biol* **54**, 71–5

Morrison, J. J., Dearn, S. R., Smith, S. K. and Ahmed, A. (1996a) Activation of protein kinase C, tyrosine kinase and phospholipase are involved in oxytocin-induced contractility in human pregnant myometrium. *Hum Reprod* (in press)

Morrison, J. J., Perera, D., O'Brien, P., Marshall, I. and Rodeck, C. H. (1996b) Effects of nitric oxide (NO) substrate, NO donors and NO synthase inhibitors on contractions of isolated human myometrium. *Br J Obstet Gynaecol* **103**, 483–4

Morrison, J. J. and Rennie, J. M. (1995) Changing the definition of perinatal mortality. *Lancet* **346**, 1038

Morrison, J. J. and Smith, S. K. (1994) 'Prostaglandins and uterine activity' in: J. G. Grudinskas and J. L. Yovich (Eds.). *Cambridge Reviews in Human Reproduction: Uterine Physiology*, pp. 230–51. Cambridge: Cambridge University Press

Natuzzi, E. S., Usrell, P. C., Harrison, M., Buscher, C. and Riemer, R. K. (1993) Nitric oxide synthase activity in the pregnant uterus decreases at parturition. *Biochem Biophys Res Commun* **194**, 1–8

Niebyl, J. R. (1981) Prostaglandin synthetase inhibitors. *Semin Perinatol* **5**, 274–87

Nissenson, R., Flouret, G. and Hechter, O. (1978) Opposing effects of estradiol and progesterone on oxytocin receptors in rabbit uterus. *Proc Nat Acad Sci USa* **75**, 2044–8

Norton, M. E., Merrill, J. O., Cooper, B. A. B., Kuller, J. A. and Clyman, R. I. (1993) Neonatal complications after the administration of indomethacin for preterm labor. *N Engl J Med* **329**, 1602–7

O'Reilly, G., Charnock-Jones, D. S., Morrison, J. J. *et al.* (1993) Alternatively spliced mRNAs for human endothelin-2 and their tissue distribution. *Biochem Biophys Res Commun* **193**, 834–40

Parkington, H. C. and Coleman, H. A. (1990) 'The role of membrane potential in the control of uterine motility' in: M. E. Carsten and J. D. Miller (Eds.). *Uterine Function: Molecular and Cellular Aspects,* pp. 195–248. New York: Plenum Press

Parratt, J., Taggart, M. and Wray, S. (1994) Abolition of contractions in the myometrium by acidification *in vitro. Lancet* **344**, 717–18

Petrie, R. H. (1981) Tocolysis using magnesium sulfate. *Semin Perinatol* **5**, 256–73

Rajabi, M. R., Dean, D. D. and Woessner, J. F. (1987) High levels of serum collagenase in premature labor — a potential biochemical marker. *Obstet Gynecol* **69**, 179–86

Rajabi, M. R., Dean, D. D. and Woessner, J. F. (1990) Changes in active and latent collagenase in human placenta around the time of parturition. *Am J Obstet Gynecol* **163**, 499–505

Richichi, J. and Vasilenko, P. (1992) The effects of nifedipine on pregnancy outcome and morphology of the placenta, uterus, and cervix during late pregnancy in the rat. *Am J Obstet Gynecol.* **167**, 797–803

Roberts, J. M. (1984) Current understanding of pharmacologic mechanisms in the prevention of preterm birth. *Clin Obstet Gynecol* **27**, 592–605

Scheid, C. R., Honeyman, T. W. and Fay, F. S. (1979) Mechanism of β-adrenergic relaxation of smooth muscle. *Nature* **277**, 32–6

Schrey, M. P., Read, A. M. and Steer, P. J. (1986) Oxytocin and vasopressin stimulate inositol phosphate production in human gestational myometrium and decidua cells. *Biosci Rep* **6**, 613–19

Shoemaker, R., Naftel, J. and Farley, J. (1985) Measurement of $K^+$ and $Cl^-$ channels in rat cultured vascular smooth muscle cells. *Biophys J* **47**, 465a

Sladek, S. M., Regenstein, C. C., Lykins, D. and Roberts, J. M. (1993) Nitric oxide synthase activity in pregnant rabbit uterus decreases on the last day of pregnancy. *Am J Obstet Gynecol* **169**, 1285–91

Somlyo, A. V. (1980) 'Ultrastructure of vascular smooth muscle' in: D. F. Bohr, A. P. Somlyo and H. P. Sparks (Eds.). *Handbook of Physiology. The Cardiovascular System,* Vol. 2, pp. 33–70. Bethesda: American Physiological Society

Somlyo, A. V., Bond, M., Somlyo, A. P. and Scarpa, A. (1985) Inositol triphosphate induced calcium release and contraction in vascular smooth muscle. *Proc Natl Acad Sci USA* **82**, 5231–5

Strehler, E. E. (1991) Recent advances in the molecular characterization of plasma membrane $Ca^{2+}$ pumps. *J Membr Biol* **120**, 1–15

Stull, J. T., Hsu, L.-C., Tansey, M. G. and Kamm, K. E. (1990) Myosin light chain kinase phosphorylation in tracheal smooth muscle. *J Biol Chem* **265**, 16683–90

Swahn, M. L. and Bygdeman, M. (1988) The effect on the antiprogestin RU-486 on uterine contractility and sensitivity to prostaglandin and oxytocin. *Br J Obstet Gynaecol* **95**, 126–34

Tasaka, K., Masumoto, N., Miyake, A. and Tanizawa, O. (1991) Direct measurement of intracellular free calcium in cultured human puerperal myometrial cells stimulated by oxytocin: effects of extracellular calcium and calcium channel blockers. *Obstet Gynecol* **77**, 101–6

Thornton, S. and Gillespie, J. I. (1992) Biochemistry of uterine contractions. *Contemp Rev Obstet Gynaecol* **4**, 121–6

Thornton, S., Gillespie, J. I., Greenwell, J. R. and Dunlop, W. (1992) Mobilization of calcium by the brief application of oxytocin and prostaglandin $E_2$ in single cultured human myometrial cells. *Exp Physiol* **77**, 293–305

Toro, L., Stefani, E. and Erulkar, S. (1990) Hormonal regulation of potassium currents in single myometrial cells. *Proc Natl Acad Sci USA* **87**, 2892–5

Triggle, D. J. and Janis, R. A. (1987) Calcium channel ligands. *Ann Rev Pharmacol Toxicol* **27**, 369–74

Word, R. A., Kamm, K. E., Stull, J. T. and Casey, M. L. (1990) Endothelin increases cytoplasmic calcium and myosin phosphorylation in human myometrium. *Am J Obstet Gynecol* **162**, 1103–8

Wray, S., Duggins, K., Iles, R., Nyman, L. and Osman, V. A. (1992) The effects of metabolic inhibition and intracellular pH on rat uterine force production. *Exp Physiol* **77**, 307–19

Yallampalli, C., Garfield, R. E. and Byam-Smith, M. (1993) Nitric oxide inhibits uterine contractility during pregnancy but not during delivery. *Endocrinology* **133**, 1899–1902

Young, R. C. and Herndon Smith, L. (1991) Characterization of sodium channels in cultured human uterine smooth muscle cells. *Am J Obstet Gynecol* **164**, 175–81

Young, R. C., Herndon Smith, L. and Anderson, N. C. (1991) Passive membrane properties and inward calcium current of human uterine smooth muscle cells. *Am J Obstet Gynecol* **164**, 1132–9

# 7

# The gynaecologist as defendant and expert witness

*Roger V. Clements*

Gynaecologists, like all other citizens, are subject to the law and need to understand the legal framework within which they operate (Clements and Puxon 1992).

## THE LEGAL FRAMEWORK

Some of the more important areas of law affecting the practice of the gynaecologist are illustrated in Table 1. While the law on female circumcision and on abortion (Paintin 1994) is enshrined in statute law, manslaughter is a matter of common law (Puxon 1995a). Assault and battery may be crimes or civil offences. 'The doctor, while liable to prosecution like any other citizen for criminal assault and battery in his ordinary life, is unlikely to be prosecuted in the criminal courts for acts within his professional activity, however gross his neglect of the patient's wishes in respect of treatment' (Puxon 1995b). Nevertheless, *civil* actions for battery *do* occur within the context of the gynaecologist's professional activities.

## Standard of care

In civil law the doctor is in the same position before the law as any other person offering professional skills. The level of skill required is that which other members of that particular profession regard as fair and reasonable at the time of the alleged act of negligence. Thus, the standard imposed is that of his or her peers — not of the public, nor of the judge, although it will be the judge's decision, after hearing all the evidence, to decide what was in fact the accepted standard of care at the time. This has been clearly described by Lord Edmund-Davies in *Whitehouse v. Jordan* (1980):

'*Doctors and surgeons fall into no special category and ... I would have it accepted that the true doctrine was enunciated by McNair J in* Bolam *v.* Friern Hospital Management Committee *(1957) in the following words*

"*When you get a situation which involves the use of some special skill or competence, then the test as to whether there has been negligence or not is not the test of the man on the top of a Clapham omnibus because he has not got this special skill. The test is the standard of the ordinary skilled man exercising and professing to have that special skill.*"

*If a surgeon fails to measure up to that standard in **any** respect ("clinical judgement" or otherwise) he has been negligent and should be so adjudged.*'

**Table 1**  *The framework of the law*

*Criminal law:*
  abortion
  manslaughter
  female circumcision

*Civil law:*
  breach of contract
  negligence*/breach of duty
  assault and battery

*Negligence is a tort, a wrongful act at common law for which the law provides a remedy

## Burden of proof

To succeed with an action the plaintiff must prove on the balance of probabilities that the defendant was negligent. The defendant does not have to prove that he was *not* negligent. Even if negligence is proved, there can be no finding of liability against the doctor unless the plaintiff can also prove, again on the balance of probabilities, that the injuries and loss complained of were directly caused by that particular negligence.

## The expert witness

In deciding whether the defendant has been negligent the judge will have to hear expert evidence called by both the plaintiff and the defendant.

It is important, both from the public's point of view and that of the medical profession, that experts of high calibre should be readily available to give their independent and disinterested opinions in such cases. Good opinions, given at an early stage, will often avert litigation or produce a reasonable settlement without a court hearing.

## Consent

### What is it?

No one may lay hands on another against their will without running the risk of criminal prosecution for assault and, if injury results, a civil action for damages for trespass or negligence. In the case of a doctor, consent is often implied, but if there is doubt it must be explicit and the limits of that consent must be respected (Clements 1995a; Clements 1995b).

The term 'informed consent' is often used, but there is no such concept in English law (Barton 1995). Consent must be real, that is, there must be:

(1) Competence;

(2) Voluntariness; and

(3) Knowledge.

### The consent form

The signing of a consent form provides some evidence that the patient has been given an opportunity to decide whether or not to undergo the operation (or procedures) after full information has been given. However, in a court of law it is not as important as the evidence of the surgeon as to what he or she said to the patient and whether or not the patient understood it (National Health Service Management Executive 1990). The surgeon needs no consent for any urgent emergency procedures (Francis 1995).

### Consent by third parties

Except in the case of minors, no person may consent to any surgical procedure on the body of another.

### Consent for the mentally handicapped

No person may give consent to gynaecological or obstetric treatment on another adult. Even the courts do not have the jurisdiction to give or withhold consent for an operation on an adult, but a court can make a declaration that the proposed operation is lawful 'in the circumstances in the best interests of the woman'. For operations such as sterilisation where the benefits to the patient are questionable, a court's jurisdiction should be invoked beforehand. Where there is no doubt about the benefit of the operation, the doctor has a common law duty to operate in the best interests of the patient.

## THE GYNAECOLOGIST AS DEFENDANT

The doctor's first duty is always to his or her patient; any duty to peers comes second. After a medical accident the doctor is naturally concerned about his own responsibility, criticism by his peers, the possibility of litigation, fear of appearing in court and, ultimately, a finding of negligence. However, the clinician's first concern should be the consequences of the accident to the patient. His or her duty is to establish what went wrong, find out why, explain to the patient, seek to rectify the damage and see that she is properly advised about her legal rights. Only after these duties have been discharged should peer loyalties arise. There is often a suspicion that after an accident occurs, the caring stops.

## Avoidance of litigation

The maintenance of a reasonable standard of care will ultimately avoid a finding of negligence. A proper standard of note keeping will make it easier for an independent assessor to understand the care given. In the last resort, while the maintenance of a reasonable standard of care and meticulous note keeping will defeat litigation, good communication will often obviate it.

## Risk management

The aims of clinical risk management (Vincent 1995) are summarised in Table 2. Adverse outcome reporting is a key element in any system of risk management (Roberts 1995). It should allow:

(1) Identification;

(2) Analysis; and

(3) Control.

Following assessment the response to the injured patient can be swift and appropriate. A good risk-management system does not operate to the detriment of the patient because, while a

**Table 2**  *The aims of clinical risk management*

The reduction, and as far as possible the
  elimination, of harm to the patient

Improvement in the quality of care

*Dealing with the injured patient:*
  continuity of care
  swift compensation for the justified claimant

*Safeguarding the assets of the organisation:*
  financial
  reputation
  staff morale

defensible case may be better defended, those in which there is clear evidence of liability may be rapidly settled.

## Letter before action

Without a good risk-management system the first intimation of a claim is the letter from the plaintiff's legal adviser many months, often many years, after the event. At this point the notes should be disclosed, once a *prima facie* case has been made out.

## Documents to be disclosed

Only communications between solicitor and client are privileged — and even then only in certain circumstances. Risk-management reports and other accident investigations are *not* privileged. Witness statements taken early in the investigation of an adverse outcome are thus vulnerable to discovery and should confine themselves to *facts only.*

## Conduct of the defence

Except in private practice, the defence of an action is now the responsibility of the provider unit. The *claims manager* and *medical executive director* have a vital role in this process. The merits of the case should be tested internally but, at some stage, if the matter is to be defended, legal advisers will need to be instructed. In many small claims the trust may decide to settle the case without instructing lawyers.

At an early stage in the proceedings the defendant doctor should give a full account of his part in the case, the reasons for acting as he or she did and an assessment of his or her own (and others') responsibilities. The doctor should have some say in the choice of expert and should try to ensure that the expert chosen to help the defence is the right one, with appropriate experience; ideally, this should be recent and in circumstances similar to those of the defendant doctor.

It is essential that the defendant doctor should understand the expert evidence which is to be given on his behalf. He should read the expert's report and make sure he or she either agrees with it or provides appropriate comments. The defendant should read all of the authorities on which the expert seeks to rely.

When the case is to be defended, the doctor must ensure that he or she attends a conference with counsel at which the experts are also present, so that it is certain that due weight is given to the doctor's own experience and it corresponds with the expert's view.

## Appearing in court

Before appearing in court the defendant doctor will have the opportunity to read the expert evidence from the plaintiff. This will indicate where the main thrust of cross-examination will lie. The doctor should become familiar with the authorities upon which the plaintiff's experts rely and make sure that his or her own experts fully understand the case. Although a witness of fact, the defendant doctor is inevitably an expert in their own field; nevertheless, they should be encouraged to concentrate upon facts. In giving evidence the defendant doctor must be modest, succinct and intelligible.

## THE GYNAECOLOGIST AS EXPERT WITNESS

### Definition

A salient feature of an expert witness is that he or she is unconnected with the case in question and can give an independent opinion about the standards of care provided by the defendant. The expert must have specialised knowledge and experience in the particular field relevant to the facts under investigation.

It is desirable that the expert should have current practical contact with the specialty; he or she should not be tempted to stray outside his or her own particular field of expertise.

### Role of the expert

When first asked for an opinion, the expert should approach the analysis of the case in an objective fashion, forming an opinion without

fear or favour. He or she must give a clear indication of an assessment of the standards of care, but once that opinion has been formed he or she cannot be disinterested — although at all times remaining balanced. In an adversarial system the expert who gives evidence on behalf of either plaintiff or defendant becomes part of a team assembled to conduct the litigation and will have a responsibility to assemble evidence and advise the lawyers on the best ways of presenting it. The expert will be expected not only to justify his or her own opinion, but also to deal with contrary arguments advanced by the other side.

When giving evidence in court the expert will be subjected to cross-examination in which his or her views will be challenged and contrary views advanced; he or she must be able to marshall the evidence in such a way that the independent opinions advanced can be justified. The expert should be able to support those views from textbooks current at the time of the incident.

### The medical report

For the plaintiff's expert, it is an essential prerequisite to interview the plaintiff before compiling a report. It is unrealistic to expect a defence expert to fulfil his or her role without the opportunity of discussing management with the doctors concerned; unfortunately, they are frequently asked to do so.

It is seldom that an expert, whether acting for plaintiff or defendant, will find it possible to produce only one report in a medical negligence case which comes to trial. The purpose of the initial report is to guide the counsel and provide help in drafting or rebutting the statement of claim. The first report will often need to deal with contrary arguments and discuss controversial issues (Clements 1994). It will usually be in three parts:

(1) The *first* part of the report is a careful analysis of all the hospital records;

(2) The *second* part explains the technical matters involved; and

(3) The *third* part relates the case in point to this technical explanation.

Finally, the expert should give an unequivocal assessment of standards of care and, if he or she believes these to be defective, should list the areas in which care fell short of the reasonable standard to be expected.

In this discussion the expert should avoid the use of the term 'negligence', since this is a question of law and may be misunderstood by doctors; in any event, it is for the court to decide after hearing evidence what is acceptable to the profession and, hence, whether the care has been negligent.

## Conference

The earlier the expert is involved in a meeting with solicitors and counsel the better.

## The pleadings

The pleadings are the formal statements of each party's case. They set out the case on each side, defining the allegations and limiting the area of dispute. No evidence can be given that does not relate to allegations in the pleadings. It is essential that no pleadings should be served without the expert's approval.

## Disclosure of reports

With the particulars of claim, the plaintiff will be required to serve a report which describes the damages that she has suffered. No report on liability should be disclosed until *after*:

(1) Close of pleadings;

(2) The exchange of lay witness statements; and

(3) A conference has occurred with the counsel.

Only then can the expert know the facts upon which he or she is asked to advise. Only then is it safe to make the report public. The final report for exchange will form the basis for the

expert's evidence in court, upon which he or she may be cross-examined.

The court also has the power to order a 'without prejudice' meeting between experts, but in medical negligence cases this rarely happens.

## Giving evidence in court

This may be a daunting experience, but some simple rules may help:

(1) The judge, especially in the High Court, will have a basic scientific knowledge enabling him to understand complex explanations.

(2) The judge will take down in longhand all the germane points of the evidence, often word for word.

(3) The expert should face the judge and watch his pencil, giving evidence no faster than the judge can write it.

(4) In cross-examination the expert's views will be attacked. Sometimes it is necessary to concede a point; it should be done gracefully.

(5) The expert should bear in mind the 'bottom line' beyond which he is not prepared to retreat. This needs to be carefully rehearsed beforehand.

It is essential that the expert should hear the evidence given by the expert acting for the 'other side' and should be readily available to his or her own counsel during cross-examination; without expert advice, the counsel may be unable to cross-examine effectively.

## Responsibilities of the expert witness

In *National Justice Compania Naviera S. A.* v. *Prudential Assurance Co. Ltd*, Cresswell J. recently summarised the responsibilities of the expert witness in the civil courts. Although the judgment concerned marine insurance, the principles are no less applicable to medical negligence litigation.

'(1) *Expert evidence presented to the Court should be, and should be seen to be, the independent product of the expert uninfluenced as to form or content by the exigencies of litigation.*

(2) *Independent assistance should be provided by the court by way of objective unbiased opinion regarding matters within the expertise of the expert witness. An expert witness in the High Court should never assume the role of advocate.*

(3) *Facts or assumptions upon which the opinion was based should be stated together with material facts which could detract from the concluded opinion.*

(4) *An expert witness should make it clear when a question or issue fell outside his expertise.*

(5) *If the opinion was not properly researched because it was considered that insufficient data were available then that had to be stated with an indication that the opinion was provisional. If the witness could not assert that the report contained the truth, the whole truth and nothing but the truth, then the qualification should be stated on the report.*

(6) *If, after exchange of reports, an expert witness changed his mind on a material matter, then the change of view should be communicated to the other side through legal representatives without delay, and, when appropriate, to the Court.*

(7) *Documents referred to in the expert evidence had to be provided to the other side at the same time as the exchange of reports.'*

# References

Barton, A. (1995) Who decides? The prudent patient or the reasonable doctor? *Clin Risk* **1**, 86–8

Bolam v. Friern Hospital Management Committee [1957] 1 WLR 582

Clements, R. V. (Ed.) (1994) 'The role of the expert for plaintiff and defendant' in: *Safe Practice in Obstetrics and Gynaecology: A Medico-legal Handbook*, pp. 89–94. Edinburgh: Churchill Livingstone

Clements, R. V. (1995a) 'Law and the clinician' in: D. K. Hirst and R. V. Clements (Eds.). *Clinical Director's Handbook 1995/96*, pp. 171–96. Edinburgh: Churchill Livingstone

Clements, R. V. (1995b) Consent 1: the consultant's view. *Diplomate* **2** (2), 139–43

Clements, R. V. and Puxon, M. (1992) 'The gynaecologist as defendant and expert witness' in: R. W. Shaw, W. P. Soutter and S. L. Stanton (Eds.). *Gynaecology*, pp. 791–802. Edinburgh: Churchill Livingstone

Whitehouse v. Jordan [1981] A11 ER 267

Francis, R. (1995) Consent; treatment of the unconscious patient. *Clin Risk* **1**, 160–4

National Justice Compania Naviera S. A. v. Prudential Assurance Co. Ltd (Ikarian Reefer) [1993] *The Times* **5 March**

National Health Service Management Executive (1990) *A Guide to Consent for Examination or Treatment,* HC(90)22. London: Department of Health

Paintin, D. B. (1994) 'Induced abortion' in: R. V. Clements (Ed.). *Safe Practice in Obstetrics and Gynaecology: A Medico-legal Handbook*, pp. 345–63. Edinburgh: Churchill Livingstone

Puxon, M. (1995a) Manslaughter and the doctor. *Clin Risk* **1**, 129–31

Puxon, M. (1995b) Assault and battery. *Clin Risk* **1**, 189–91

Roberts, G. (1995) Untoward incident reporting: quality improvement and control. *Clin Risk* **1**, 168–70

Vincent, C. A. (Ed.) (1995) Clinical risk management. *Quality Health Care* **4** (2), June 1995

Watt, J. (1995) Leading cases in medical negligence: Whitehouse v. Jordan. *Clin Risk* **1**, 157–9

# Further reading

Clements, R. V. (Ed.) (1994) *Safe Practice in Obstetrics and Gynaecology: A Medico-Legal Handbook.* Edinburgh: Churchill Livingstone

Jones, M. A. (1995) *Medical Negligence,* 2nd edn. London: Sweet & Maxwell

Powers, M. J. and Harris, N. H. (Eds.). (1994) *Medical Negligence,* 2nd edn. Butterworths

Vincent, C. (Ed.) (1995) *Clinical Risk Management.* London: BMJ Publishing Group

# 8

# A suggested framework for obstetric risk limitation

*John Hare*

The cost of litigation to the National Health Service is rising dramatically. It is estimated by the Department of Health that this cost will have more than doubled from £80 million to £175 million between 1992 and 1996. At the individual unit level liability accrues at a frightening rate; for example, it is estimated that each of the 49 first-wave trusts have built up liability of £10 million over a four-year period, a rate of £2.5 million a year (Anonymous 1996). Moreover, large claims predominate. Actuaries acting for the new Clinical Negligence Scheme for Trusts have indicated that 80% of the total number of claims for clinical negligence will represent only 20% of the total liability, whereas just 3% of claims represent 60% of the total cost. Obstetric claims dominate that 3%. Symonds, writing in 1993, stated that:

> '*It seems likely that in 1992 total payments for obstetric claims alone were in excess of £60 million. At this rate it has been estimated that within five years settlements for claims on brain damaged babies will exceed the total budget for the maternity services. A major part of the liability is related to claims for cerebral palsy and mental retardation.*'
> (Symonds 1993a)

This author wrote in the same year that, on a national scale, known liabilities for brain-damaged babies were valued at between £600 million and £1 billion (Symonds 1993b).

Risk management and prevention are, therefore, of paramount priority in obstetric practice. In attempting to suggest a framework for tackling this problem, the author proposes adopting the principles of risk management as laid down in the National Health Service Management Executive document *Risk Management in the NHS*, published in 1993. They suggest the approach should be:

(1) To identify the risk;

(2) To analyse and evaluate; and

(3) To attempt to control by avoidance, prevention or in some cases acceptance, and, if the risk is accepted, make available funding to meet the liability.

How can the risks in obstetric practice be identified? The author would suggest a three-step approach. First, the study of national and regional reports which comment on adverse outcomes and poor standards of practice. Second, by audit of legal claims; such audits have been published by individuals and organisations. Third, for each individual unit to undertake a local audit of perinatal and maternal morbidity and mortality from adverse incident reports by staff, patient complaints, letters before action and cases proceeding to litigation.

## NATIONAL AND REGIONAL AUDIT

National audit provides details of mortality but not morbidity. Two publications need to be considered: the trienniel *Reports on Confidential Enquiries into Maternal Deaths in the United Kingdom* and the *Confidential Enquiry into Stillbirths and Deaths in Infancy Report (CESDI)*, which is published annually.

### Report on Confidential Enquiries into Maternal Deaths in the United Kingdom

This collates all deaths related to pregnancy and categorises them as either:

(1) *Direct*, that is, related directly to the pregnancy itself;

(2) *Indirect*, where for example pregnancy modifies pre-existing disease;

(3) *Fortuitous*, where the death happens to occur in a pregnant woman but is not related to her pregnancy; or

(4) *Late*, where deaths occur outside the 42-day follow-up period after delivery, but, nevertheless, are thought to have been due to the effects of pregnancy.

The numbers of maternal deaths in all categories rose between 1985–1987 and 1988–1990: Direct deaths rose from 139 to 145; indirect deaths were 86, 93 and 100; fortuitous deaths were 26, 65 and 46 and late deaths from 16, 48 and 46 (Department of Health 1991; 1994; 1996).

In each section of the report the deaths are assessed and a decision made as to whether substandard care (which may include lack of co-operation by the patient herself) has contributed to the adverse outcome. In some categories, for example deaths from thromboembolic disease and deaths from amniotic fluid embolus, care is usually held to be satisfactory and there is very little that the assessors consider could have been done to alter the course of disease. However, in other major causes of maternal death (including hypertensive disease, haemorrhage and ruptured uterus) the assessors have decided that in the majority of cases care has been substandard. Direct and clear guidance is given by the panel of assessors and examples of recommendations in the 1994 report (Department of Health 1994) include:

'*(1) New medical and midwifery staff should have an induction course when they take up an appointment before taking clinical responsibility.*

*(2) Continuing education programmes should include regular rehearsals of emergency procedures,*
especially practice in cardiopulmonary resuscitation.

*(3) There is a need for continuing review of the staffing structure in obstetric units, with increased consultant involvement in acute obstetric care.*

*(4) The number of deaths from haemorrhage increased in this triennium (1988–1990) and substandard care was a major feature. The need for a team approach to the management of severe haemorrhage is apparently not adequately recognised.*

*(5) With regard to sepsis, microbiological investigation was often incomplete and initiated too late. Full details of antibiotic therapy were rarely available to assessors, but in several cases it was evident that therapy was not sufficiently aggressive. The importance of seeking advice from a microbiologist at an early stage in the treatment of sepsis is emphasised.*'

This last recommendation highlights the common finding that poor note keeping and poor practice go together; indeed, it is highly disturbing that after the death of some maternity patients due to infection, the assessors cannot even work out the timing and nature of her antibiotic therapy!

### Confidential Enquiry into Stillbirths and Deaths in Infancy

The 1993 programme for CESDI was on normally formed babies weighing 2.5 kg or more, and reported on deaths up to the end of six completed days after birth possibly related to problems during labour (National Advisory Body 1995). Among its findings were that:

(1) Thirty per cent of babies studied were born at weekends, when senior cover was scanty or absent;

(2) Twenty-one per cent of stillbirths occurred on a Saturday; and

(3) In total, 42.3% of the 387 cases studied had suboptimal care that influenced outcome.

The assessors' most common criticism of obstetricians was failure to act appropriately and the most common criticism of midwives and general practitioners, failure to recognise a problem. Failure to act appropriately was the most common adverse criticism, and was thought to have been a significant factor in the loss of the baby in 34% of cases. Failure to recognise a problem (29%) and communication failures (17%) were also frequent criticisms. Interestingly, lack of staff and/or lack of equipment were only thought relevant in a total of 7.5% of cases. Among their conclusions the CESDI authors criticised:

'(1) Inadequate account taken of complications, for example, hypertension, diabetes and infection;

(2) Poor techniques of induction of labour, including overdosage of Syntocinon and prostaglandins;

(3) Poor monitoring and lack of involvement with senior staff;

(4) Inappropriate counselling if mothers' wishes were contrary to safety;

(5) Poor recognition of cardiotocographic (CTG) abnormalities and poor response to these; and

(6) Hyperstimulation with Syntocinon or prostaglandins of a uterus with a scar from a previous Caesarean section with consequent rupture.'

Major issues that the CESDI authors felt should be tackled were:

'(1) Weekend and out-of-hours cover;

(2) Staffing and availability of senior staff;

(3) Risk assessment; and

(4) Neonatal resuscitation.'

For a number of years each National Health Service Region has also produced its own CESDI report.

## AUDIT OF CLAIMS

A number of studies have been published on the legal claims made within the specialty; Brown (1985) in the *Annual Report and Accounts of the Medical Protection Society* analysed 257 claims. Forty-four per cent of these related to stillbirth, neonatal death and cerebral palsy and the most common adverse features were forceps delivery and breech delivery. Ennis and Vincent (1990) reviewed 64 cases which were also taken from the files of the Medical Protection Society. They highlighted:

'(1) Inadequate fetal monitoring (not done in 11 cases, unsatisfactory in six and disregarded in 14);

(2) Mismanagement of forceps delivery, often with multiple attempts; and

(3) Inadequate supervision by senior staff. Seniors should have attended but did not in 20 of these 64 cases; in a further 20 the notes were unclear as to whether the senior had attended or not.'

In the same year (1990) Capstick and Edwards, from a firm of defence solicitors, looked at trends in their obstetric malpractice claims. In 100 cases the causes were said to be:

'(1) Disregarding meconium liquor (32 cases);

(2) Inadequate fetal monitoring (58 cases);

(3) Prolonged labour (40 cases); and

(4) The use of Kielland's forceps (20 cases).'

The following year Symonds and Senior (1991) analysed 110 cases that had gone to litigation. Seventy per cent involved CTG abnormalities; 24% involved forceps delivery; in 52% of cases the most senior staff involved were registrars; 11% had the senior house officer as the most experienced person present and 15%, the midwife. The importance of monitoring and correct interpretation of the CTG was also emphasised by Symonds in 1993, who stated:

'In reviewing 100 cases of "brain damage" claims I formed the opinion that 53 of the claims would be indefensible in court mainly because no action was taken or there has been a considerable delay before action was taken.' (Symonds 1993b)

The author has undertaken an audit of a group of 134 obstetric cases on which he prepared reports for medico-legal use. His instructions were from solicitors acting for plaintiffs or defendants in a ratio of 2 : 1, and the author has excluded cases which involve allegations of wrongful birth which make up to about 10% of the total.

Out of the 134, there were allegations of negligence before 24 weeks' gestation in 12 cases, of which 10 have now been settled in some manner. There were 24 cases of between 24 and 36 weeks' gestation, of which 11 are now completed and 13 are still (in mid-1996) waiting for a decision. By far the majority of cases (98 of 134) related to events after 36 weeks' gestation, of which 56 are now completed cases and 42 are still awaiting decision. The author's experience therefore supports Symonds and Senior (1991), who wrote:

> 'Although prematurity is related to a large number of cases in handicap, litigation does not seem to be prompted by this.'

Of the 56 completed cases after 36 weeks' gestation, 34 settlements were made broadly in favour of the plaintiff, although liability was admitted or found in court in only a minority. The same themes were found that had been obvious in earlier work, namely:

(1) The use of prostin to induce labour, including after previous delivery by Caesarean section;

(2) The use of Syntocinon;

(3) Failure to recognise and act upon abnormal CTG patterns; and

(4) Attempts at instrumental delivery, not always successful. This occurred in five cases where Kielland's forceps were used, in eight cases with other forceps, in three cases with Ventouse and in four cases where there were multiple attempts.

A subgroup of special concern are mature babies with cerebral palsy, not least because of the very high cost of settlements made in their favour. In this audit there was a group of 21 cases, all of whom had the following characteristics:

(1) All were over 36 weeks' gestation.

(2) All were agreed to be in good condition at the start of labour.

(3) All were either stillborn or developed hypoxic ischaemic encephalopathy (HIE) soon after birth; if they developed HIE they either died or developed severe cerebral palsy agreed to be typical of the pattern thought consequential to hypoxia in labour and delivery.

(4) All settled in favour of the plaintiff, either in court or by out-of-court settlement very close to the amount claimed.

In these 21 cases there was misreading of the CTG or failure to act on the CTG findings in 16 cases. Prostin induction had been used in nine cases. Syntocinon had been used in 16 cases, in 14 of which it had been used to a degree which would be described as aggressive.

There were two cases involving breech delivery, and in three cases the baby was one of twins. Delivery with Kielland's forceps was attempted in four cases, and multiple attempts at vaginal delivery (three or more) were made in three cases. In four cases signs of umbilical cord entanglement, including CTG traces, were neglected.

## LOCAL AUDIT AND REVIEW

Each unit should discover its own pattern of obstetric risk, based on audit of mortality and morbidity for both mother and baby, patient complaints, solicitors' letters before action and cases proceeding to litigation. A confidential system of adverse incident report must be set up, and time, money and human resources dedicated to this work. Assessment and advice from professionals from outside the unit may be of great benefit, although involvement of staff from a neighbouring trust may be difficult if there is local competition for contracts and referrals. In some situations, a short but comprehensive review from experienced risk assessors and managers may set a unit on the path for improvement.

## RISK PREVENTION STRATEGY

National information, together with that obtained locally, should enable a unit to design a risk prevention strategy. The author suggests that this be conducted on three levels, namely:

(1) *Level 1 prevention strategy*: this is the attainment of good standards of practice as judged by present standards and conventions.

(2) *Level 2 prevention strategy*: which is slightly more controversial, and is the rearrangement of use of resources to base resource allocation on risk profile.

(3) *Level 3 prevention strategy*: which is much more controversial, and is the reappraisal of the usefulness of high-risk procedures and strategies.

### How are good standards determined?

At the present time two relatively new factors are having a great influence on the way obstetrics is practised; these are the concept of research-based or evidence-based medicine and the perception of the wishes of the consumer. Evidence-based medicine made a great impact with the publication of *Effective Care in Pregnancy and Childbirth* (Chalmers *et al.* 1989) and the subsequent development of the Cochrane Database (Enkin *et al.* 1995). For many aspects of obstetrics, evidence-based medicine leads to better, safer, more humane and more economical, although not necessarily cheaper, medicine. However, evidence-based medicine does not, will not and cannot provide a blueprint for the whole of obstetric practice, and to rely on this source alone is a recipe for disaster. Material from all sources of medical knowledge must be considered in decision making, including that from the study of adverse outcome. This was summarised by Sackett and others in their editorial from the *British Medical Journal* on 13 January 1996:

'*External clinical evidence can inform, but cannot replace, individual clinical expertise, and it is this expertise that decides whether the external evidence applies to the individual patient at all, and, if so, how it should be integrated into the clinical decision.*

*The practice of evidence-based medicine means integrating individual clinical expertise with the best available external clinical evidence from systematic research.*

*Increased expertise is reflected ... especially in more effective and efficient diagnosis, and in more thoughtful identification and compassionate use of individual patients' predicaments, rights and preferences in making clinical decisions about their case.*'

The Cochrane Database and CESDI should not be seen as in conflict, but as complementing each other!

The perceived wishes of the patient are often used as a stick with which to beat the obstetrician, with high intervention rates being considered undesirable, in particular high rates for Caesarean section. Yet, Thornton and Lilford (1989) found that the average pregnant woman wanted intervention by Caesarean section if there was a risk of 1 in 15,000 of her baby being otherwise lost during the course of labour and delivery. Such a level of risk is, of course, totally impossible for the obstetrician to prevent and this unreal impression of our skills and ability may well be a factor in causing dissatisfaction when things go wrong. In contrast, the same authors found that the average woman booked for home confinement was content to accept a risk to her baby of 1 in 100. If those who lead consumer pressure groups that lobby over the provision of maternity care have different concepts of risk from the majority of those they seek to represent, then more rather than less dissatisfaction will result.

### Level 1 prevention strategies

Most of the level 1 prevention strategies are common sense, and were summarised by James in 1993 as '*medicolegal pitfalls in the labour ward*'. She highlights:

'*(1) Lack of continuity between teams to include failure to define a chain of responsibility;*

*(2) Failure to recognise high-risk patients because clinical notes are either not available or not read; and*

*(3) Lack of consultant supervision or inability to contact a consultant in an emergency.'*

The author of this chapter would add that chains of responsibility should reflect increasing experience; for example, a senior house officer should not be able to override an experienced midwife. When chains of responsibility are long, for teaching purposes an effective bypass system must be available for emergencies; this must include the stated permission for a senior midwife to telephone a consultant if a problem becomes acute. James continues:

*'(4) Lack of clear guidelines about interpretation of CTG traces;*

*(5) Failure to date and time CTG traces;*

*(6) Failure to report deficient equipment or failure to maintain equipment; and*

*(7) Vaginal examinations recorded in insufficient detail or not at all.'*

The CTG issue is absolutely crucial. Every doctor or midwife in a position of responsibility on the labour ward must understand the significance of CTG patterns. Regular tutorials, assessments and discussions should be held, and each unit should agree on the standards they will use for CTG interpretation. Most published schemes are satisfactory, and the guidelines set down by the International Federation of Gynecology and Obstetrics (FIGO) in 1987 are a good starting point (FIGO Subcommittee on Standards in Perinatal Medicine 1987). James (1993) continues;

*'(8) Protocols not reviewed regularly and dates of introduction and withdrawal not recorded.'*

The issue of guidelines and protocols, their comprehensiveness and how strictly they are to be followed is difficult, but guidelines are needed whatever grade of staff work on the labour ward. Tight protocols are needed if juniors are allowed to make decisions and carry out actions unsupervised. Particular points needing attention include the use of Syntocinon and rules for junior doctors undertaking instrumental deliveries without direct supervision. James (1993) concludes with:

*'(9) Unavailability of trained obstetric anaesthetists or paediatric staff;*

*(10) Lack of efficient call systems;*

*(11) Failure to make full records in the case notes;*

*(12) Undue delay between the decision to carry out emergency Caesarean section and its implementation; and*

*(13) Inadequate monitoring of oxytocin infusions and other methods of stimulating labour.'*

The relative importance of these and other points will be determined by local audit.

## Level 2 prevention strategies

Level 2 prevention strategies concern the allocation of resources, of which the most important in health care is human resource. If risk and liability are generated to a great degree in one particular area, it seems logical to direct more resource into that area to lessen the risk and liability. At present the highest risk area, the labour ward, is often under the control of junior and inexperienced doctors. Experienced midwives will often allow themselves to be overruled and permit junior doctors to make decisions and take actions that they know are wrong. Senior midwives must be given, and must take, greater responsibility. Consultants must spend more hours on the labour ward, not just visit it for nominal ward rounds. They must show both interest and ability. The daily presence of a consultant should be accepted as important, and consultants should expect to work during unsocial hours. The probationary period during which junior doctors' or midwives' practice is physically supervised should be much longer than at present.

The concept of a 24 hours a day, 7 days a week visible commitment by consultants which is proven by regular rounds and attendance at a high proportion of Caesarean sections and complicated vaginal deliveries is considered unacceptable by many working in this grade in the United Kingdom. Yet elsewhere in the world this commitment is a reality. Since 1993, the Accreditation Council for Graduate Medical Education in the United States has insisted:

*'On an obstetrics and gynecology service, adequate supervision requires the 24-hour presence of faculty in the hospital. Faculty must be immediately available to the resident if clinical activity is taking place in the operating rooms and/or labor and delivery areas. Faculty must be within easy walking distance of patient care units.'*

There is also some evidence that the traditional view that out-of-hours labour ward work is left to juniors is not held by younger obstetricians. In the *Survey of Training* conducted by the Royal College of Obstetricians and Gynaecologists National Trainees Committee in 1995, 28% of doctors preparing for a career in obstetrics and gynaecology stated that consultant posts should have a resident on-call consultant and 51% agreed that, in future, consultants would be required to be resident while on call.

### Level 3 prevention strategies

Similar views are held in most Northern European countries. What this author has designated as level 3 prevention strategies are the most controversial of all. When looking at the data concerning complaints, adverse outcomes and litigation, certain obstetric managements, procedures and strategies are over-represented. Some of these, for example the use of Syntocinon, simply need to be revised to sensible protocols and safeguards. Others may carry a high risk of adverse outcome, and in the author's own legal practice this group would include:

(1) The use of Kielland's forceps with the risk of damage to mother and baby; and

(2) The use of prostaglandin pessaries to induce labour after previous Caesarean section with the risk of uterine rupture.

Each unit should decide if these and some other procedures are a necessary part of obstetric practice, or whether they could be replaced with some alternative management which might be associated with less risk of an adverse outcome.

## CONCLUSION

There is a long way to go. We must depart from the idea that obstetric litigation presents unwarranted victimisation of our specialty. Honesty is required about our shortcomings. Niswander and colleagues (1984) considered that, even with satisfactory perinatal outcomes, a significant number of women were cared for in a suboptimal fashion (the figures for substandard care being 4.5% in pregnancy and 14% in labour).

Gaffney and colleagues (1994) looked at 339 babies developing cerebral palsy who were born in the Oxford region between 1984 and 1987. Using figures derived from the Office of Population Censuses and Surveys (OPCS) there were about 132,000 babies born in that region during that period, giving a rate for cerebral palsy of 2.6 per thousand. Forty-one of these 339 were born at term, had no other cause for cerebral palsy and developed HIE in the perinatal period. Almost all of these 41 had adverse features in labour which could have been better managed; such management is likely to have led to a better outcome. 'Preventable' cerebral palsy may therefore represent one in eight of all cases, and occur once in every 3000 births. The reduction in the number of these cases, together with avoidable stillbirths and maternal death and damage, must be the target for the future. With proper action and resource it is likely that this reduction can be achieved for, as Sir Stanley Simmons, past President of the Royal College of Obstetricians and Gynaecologists, wrote in 1993:

*'Most of the claims that are against us are due to bad obstetric practice, not because of obscure interpretations of the CTG.'*

# References

Accreditation Council for Graduate Medical Education, USA (1993) 'Special requirements for residency accreditation in obstetrics and gynecology' in: *Graduate Medical Education Directory*, p. 91.

Anonymous (1996) Medical litigation faces British revolution [news]. *BMJ* **312**, 330

Brown, A. G. D. (1985) 'Medicolegal problems in obstetric practice' in: *Annual Report and Accounts of the Medical Protection Society*, pp. 25–9. London: Medical Protection Society

Capstick, J. B. and Edwards, P. J. (1990). Trends in obstetric malpractice claims. *Lancet* **336**, 931–2

Chalmers, I., Enkin, M., Kierse, M. J. N. C. (1989) *Effective Care in Pregnancy and Childbirth*, Vols 1 and 2. Oxford: Oxford University Press

Department of Health (1991) *Reports on Confidential Enquiries into Maternal Deaths in the United Kingdom 1985–1987*. London: HMSO

Department of Health (1994) *Report on Confidential Enquiries into Maternal Deaths in the United Kingdom 1988–1990*. London: HMSO

Department of Health (1996) *Report on Confidential Enquiries into Maternal Deaths in the United Kingdom 1991–1993*. London: HMSO

Enkin, M. W., Kierse, M. J., Renfrew, M. J. and Neilson, J. P. (Eds.) (1995) *Pregnancy and Childbirth Module*, Cochrane Database of Systemic Reviews, Issue 1. Available from BMJ Publishing, London

Ennis, M. and Vincent, C. A. (1990). Obstetric accidents: a review of 64 cases. *BMJ* **336**, 931–2

FIGO Subcommittee on Standards in Perinatal Medicine (1987) Guidelines for the use of fetal monitoring. *Int J Gynecol Obstet* **25**, 159–67

Gaffney, G., Flavell, V., Johnson, A. *et al.* (1994) Cerebral palsy and neonatal encephalopathy. *Arch Dis Child* **70**, F195–200

James, C. E. (1993). 'The consequences of legal issues that face the obstetrician' in: J. A. D. Spencer and R. H. T. Ward (Eds.). *Intrapartum Fetal Surveillance*, pp. 347–57. London: RCOG Press

National Advisory Body (1995). *The Confidential Enquiry into Stillbirths and Deaths in Infancy Report (CESDI)*, report for 1 January–31 December 1993, parts 1 and 2, F51/036 2382 20k March 95. London: Department of Health

National Health Service Management Executive (1993) *Risk Management in the NHS*, 10M. London: Department of Health

Niswander, K., Henson, G., Elbourne, D. *et al.* (1984) Adverse outcome of pregnancy and the quality of obstetric care. *Lancet* **ii**, 827–30

Royal College of Obstetricians and Gynaecologists National Trainees Committee (1995) *Survey of Training*. London: RCOG

Sackett, D. L., Rosenberg, W. M. C., Muir-Gray, J. A., Haynes, R. B. and Richardson, W. S. (1996) Evidence based medicine, what it is and what it isn't. *BMJ* **312**, 71–2

Simmons, S. C. (1993) 'Introduction' in: J. A. D. Spencer and R. H. T. Ward (Eds.). *Intrapartum Fetal Surveillance*, pp. xvii–xviii. London: RCOG Press

Symonds, E. M. (1993a) 'Legal issues of fetal monitoring' in: J. A. D. Spencer and R. H. T. Ward (Eds.). *Intrapartum Fetal Surveillance*, pp. 359–69. London: RCOG Press

Symonds, E. M. (1993b) Litigation and the cardiotocogram. *Br J Obstet Gynaecol* **100** (Suppl. 9), 8–9

Symonds, E. M. and Senior, O. E. (1991) The anatomy of obstetric litigation. *Curr Obstet Gynaecol* **1**, 241–3

Thornton, J. G. and Lilford, R. J. (1989) The Caesarean section; patients' choices are not determined by immediate emotional reactions. *J Obstet Gynaecol* **9**, 283–8

# 9

# Forensic gynaecology and sexual assault

*Raine E. I. Roberts*

*Forensic: 'pertaining to, connected with, or used in courts of law'*

*Shorter Oxford Dictionary*

Doctors are increasingly involved with courts for a number of reasons. Patients are increasingly litigation minded and very much more ready to sue their doctors than they were a few years ago.

Women are much more willing to report rape and other sexual assaults and to go through the trauma of giving evidence in court.

Child sexual abuse is now well recognised as a major problem for society, but there is continuing difficulty about how best to present medical evidence to courts and continuing controversy and lack of knowledge about the significance of various findings.

Lawyers are now very well aware that medical testimony can often be successfully challenged and are much more willing to do just that. Events such as the Cleveland controversy have highlighted the fact that medical testimony in court can be unsound. Doctors giving evidence in court are commonly perceived by lawyers as tending to be biased in favour of the prosecution if they have examined the complainant.

## RECORD KEEPING

Any consultation may contain matters which could at a later date become the subject of court proceedings and it is important to make good (but not necessarily long) notes, bearing in mind that any such notes may be ordered to be disclosed to the court. Following recent decisions in the Court of Appeal, notably in the Guinness and Judith Ward cases (*R.* v. *Ward*), requests or orders for disclosure of all notes have become commonplace. If the doctor considers that the notes contain matters which are not material to the case, or the disclosure of which may harm the patient or be against the public interest, he should take the notes to court to be evaluated by the judge who will decide whether all or part of them should be disclosed. The advice of a doctor's defence organisation and the legal department of the hospital should be sought in such cases.

Good note keeping is particularly important with regard to any genital complaint in a child where the possibility of sexual abuse may need to be considered.

In the past many children have attended gynaecologists and other doctors with symptoms and signs which were due to sexual abuse and this has not been recognised. In future, such patients may disclose abuse and may be prepared to sue their doctors for negligence if he or she did not consider this possibility. What would have been acceptable practice in 1976 might well be criticised in 1996 and be the subject of an action for damages in 2016!

## CONSENT AND CONFIDENTIALITY

If any forensic matters arise, issues of consent and confidentiality are different from those in an ordinary medical consultation. In the usual doctor–patient relationship consent is usually implied and confidentiality expected, although it is never absolute. Consent to any examination where court proceedings may possibly follow, whether this is of an adult or a child, should ideally be obtained in writing, although oral consent is no less valid. Furthermore, both the doctor and the patient should be clear that any information gathered in such an examination may be disclosed to the court and be seen by lawyers and other doctors, including those acting for other parties such as the alleged abuser or rapist.

In cases of suspected child abuse, confidentiality cannot be offered and local child protection procedures should be known by any doctor who becomes involved in what might prove to be a sexual abuse case. These procedures require information about such matters to be shared. No doctor should keep information about possible child abuse to him or herself. Usually, it is best to discuss the problem with senior colleagues within the department before making a decision to inform social services departments or the police.

The General Medical Council has recently issued new guidance on confidentiality. Generally, confidentiality must not be broken, but:

> '*if you believe a patient to be a victim of neglect or physical or sexual abuse and unable to give or withhold consent to disclosure you should usually give information to an appropriate responsible person or statutory agency in order to prevent further harm to the patient. In these and similar circumstances you may release information without the patient's consent, but only if you consider that the patient is unable to give consent and that the disclosure is in the patient's best medical interests.*'
> (General Medical Council 1995)

## RAPE

While there is increasing readiness by women to report rape to the police, and the national incidence of reported rapes continues to rise, this represents probably only a very small proportion of those women who are raped.

Well over 5000 rapes and 32,000 other sexual offences are reported to the police each year in the United Kingdom (Home Office 1996), but surveys such as the 'No' Means 'No' Survey carried out by university students a few years ago, suggested that only one in 50 cases was reported. Dr Tim Jordan of Oxford Brookes University reported at the British Psychology Conference in 1994 that one in three women students had been sexually assaulted and one-half of them had previously been assaulted. Twelve per cent of his study reported the offence to the police. Reasons for not reporting included a fear of not being believed, guilt and self-blame and, in a minority of cases, fear of retaliation by the attacker.

Jill Saward, who was raped by two assailants who broke into her home, wrote a book about her experiences (Saward 1990). She was worried for three years about acquired immunodeficiency syndrome (AIDS) and felt that every minor symptom was the beginning of the end. She suffered from flashbacks and nightmares for years and felt that it was important for well-being and recovery that the complainant should know that she was believed.

In some parts of the country, including West Yorkshire (the Star Project) and Northumbria (the Reach Project), as well as the St Mary's Centre in Manchester, there are now services which include forensic, medical and counselling aspects, but provision is still very patchy. Indeed, Temkin showed in a questionnaire survey (of only 22 women) in the Sussex area (Temkin 1995) that women were often dissatisfied with some aspect of the care which they received. They regarded the positive points as being seen by a woman doctor and a doctor who was kind and sympathetic and who explained what was happening, but often found the examination humiliating and stressful. In some cases the attitude of trained police officers was more helpful than that of the doctors.

### The St Mary's Centre

At St Mary's Hospital in Manchester, a comprehensive service is offered to women (and now to men) who report a serious sexual offence to the police and those who self-refer (self-referring includes those referred by general practitioners, gynaecologists, accident and emergency departments, and community and voluntary services). The centre is staffed by a team of forensically trained doctors, with the complainant choosing whether he or she sees a male or female doctor. Furthermore, there is also a team of trained counsellors, many of whom have a background in nursing, including gynaecology and midwifery.

The centre opened in Manchester in December 1986 as a unique collaborative venture between the Central Manchester Healthcare Trust and the Greater Manchester Police Authority. It is funded jointly, with the police authority contributing approximately £150,000 and the trust approximately £30,000. Its objectives are:

(1) To provide forensic investigation of the highest standard in order to facilitate the collection and collation of objective and impartial evidence;

(2) To provide non-judgemental emotional and psychological support for individuals, their partners and their families;

(3) To provide medical investigation and treatment when necessary;

(4) To safeguard and promote the right of individuals to make informed decisions consistent with their own wishes; and

(5) To provide information and advice about the work of the centre and issues related to it, for the benefit of interested professionals, other organisations and the community in general.

The centre is open from 9.00 a.m. to 8.00 p.m. Monday to Friday and operates an emergency 'on-call' system at all other times, enabling an immediate response to be provided 24 hours a day. Services include:

(1) A telephone counselling/advice line staffed by trained personnel;

(2) Emotional and practical response to victims of assault consistent with their wishes in a safe and supportive atmosphere;

(3) Immediate access to police personnel and forensic physicians;

(4) Postcoital contraception and pregnancy testing service;

(5) Fortnightly sexually transmitted disease screening clinic, together with HIV pre- and post-test counselling;

(6) One-to-one counselling for individuals and their supporters with fully trained counsellors; and

(7) Support through criminal proceedings and compensation claims.

The St Mary's Centre has, since its opening almost 10 years ago, seen over 3700 attenders.

The total number of attenders has risen from 301 in 1987 to 456 in 1995, with the rise being due to the number of police referrals (Figures 1 and 2). This is presumably mainly due to the increased readiness to report rape to the police because of public perception that services have improved, rather than an increase in incidence.

There has been a marked rise in the numbers of young women, those under 18 and, most worryingly, those under 16, presenting with an allegation of rape (Figures 3–5). Many of these cases are alcohol related and in a number of them the young woman cannot even remember what has happened.

In one genitourinary medicine clinic (Dr Williams, Clwyd, personal communication) 5% of the attenders were under the age of 16 and 49% of them were self-referrals. Fifty per cent of the *Chlamydia* cases seen in this clinic were under the age of 19. This clearly poses a serious medical problem. It seems likely that the risk of pelvic inflammatory disease from *Chlamydia* is greater during the adolescent years.

Furthermore, sexual assault of those with learning difficulties is increasingly being recognised as people are more prepared to listen to what these women say (Brown, Stein and Tark 1995). At St Mary's we are aware of an increasing number of young adult women with learning difficulties who are alleging rape. It can be extremely difficult to assess these people. Issues

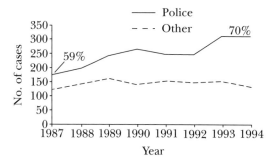

**Figure 1** *The source of referrals in 3131 sexual assault cases to the St Mary's Centre, Manchester, between 1986 and 1995*

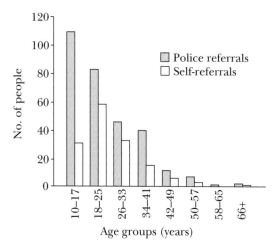

**Figure 2** *The type of referral of sexual assault victims to the St Mary's Centre, Manchester in 1995 related to age*

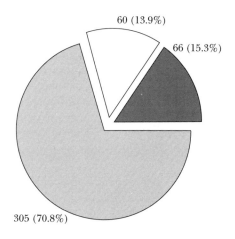

**Figure 3** *The number of sexual assault victims attending the St Mary's Centre, Manchester, in 1995 who were under 18 years of age*

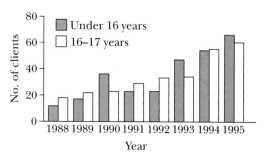

**Figure 4** *The number of sexual assault victims attending the St Mary's Centre, Manchester, between 1988 and 1995 who were under 18 years of age*

of consent and their capacity to give reliable evidence in court are major problems.

If a woman feels that she does not fit the perceived stereotype of the rape victim (i.e. that she was *not* attacked by a stranger [Figures 6 and 7], the incident occurred at home and she was not injured), she is less likely to be able to report to the police. In many cases rape is about degradation and control and a woman may find it impossible to tell anybody that, for instance, she actually took her own blouse off; indeed, she may even allege that it was forcibly removed and may damage it afterwards to substantiate her story because she cannot admit, perhaps even to herself, that she was so controlled that she did what the rapist ordered. The rapist defines the behaviour of the victim in his terms (Wyre

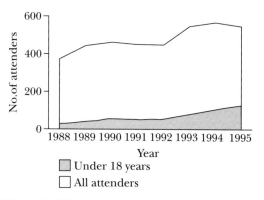

**Figure 5** *The proportion of sexual assault victims attending the St Mary's Centre, Manchester, who were under 18 years of age between 1988 and 1995. They are compared with the overall number of attenders*

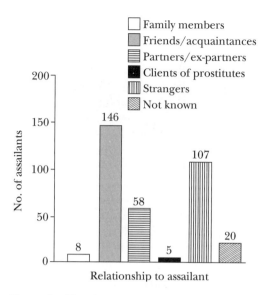

**Figure 6** *The relationship of the assailant to the victim of sexual assault in 1995*

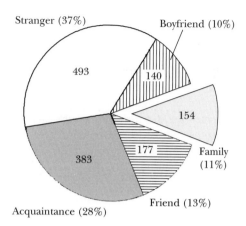

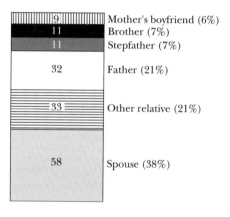

**Figure 7** *The relationship of the assailant to the victim of sexual assault in 1347 cases recorded from 1500 incidents*

1990). Those women subjected to degrading practices and made to take an active part in the sexual activity, and those who have no injuries, may find it impossible to report it to anybody, let alone the police. When they do report to the police they may well subsequently withdrew the allegation.

Of the attenders at St Mary's, approximately one-third of women withdraw the allegation and decide not to pursue the matter through the court. Some of these are false allegations and in a small proportion of cases the woman will admit that the story was false. However, in many cases a rape has occurred, but the woman decides that she cannot go through the further trauma of a court appearance and wishes to put the episode behind her. Such women may present to gynaecologists with a number of complaints. It is common for women to feel that they have been damaged because they experience pain or bleeding during the unwanted sexual activity. They may then present with a variety of symptoms, but are not able to tell the doctor the nature of the real problem. Sympathetic and understanding doctors who have the time and empathy to allow the patient to talk will sometimes find out more, and in some cases the patient will tell the nurse what she is unable to tell the doctor.

Several of our crisis counsellors at St Mary's also work in the gynaecology and midwifery departments of the hospital and their experience of both aspects of their work brings increased understanding to each part. Women do tell the nurses that they have been sexually abused as children or have been raped when they have not mentioned this to the doctors.

Chronic atypical pelvic pain is common in women who have been raped, as are psychosexual problems (Walker 1993). Urinary retention and unusual or bizarre complaints in a young woman should alert the gynaecologist to the possibility that sexual abuse played a part in the aetiology of the woman's problems. An example is shown in the following case history:

> A 27-year-old woman had been admitted to hospital on numerous occasions with acute retention of urine requiring catheterisation. Hospital investigations revealed no bladder disease. She did not disclose sexual abuse to those caring for her in hospital, but went to see a therapist elsewhere and during sessions with her began to describe grotesque acts of satanic abuse which were alleged to have involved her family and others. The police investigated and could find no evidence to corroborate the story, which bore striking resemblance to accounts of abuse in various paperback books being published at that time, including the presence of a 'Master' and ritual abortion and child sacrifice.
>
> It is very unlikely that these allegations were true, but there may well have been sexual abuse within the family which might have played a major part in the aetiology of her disturbed mental state and physical problems.
>
> If those caring for her gynaecological problems had considered the possibility that child sexual abuse accounted for some symptoms and enabled her to talk, it *might* have saved much morbidity, not to mention use of expensive hospital resources.

Adults are increasingly claiming that they have been sexually abused and those in therapy, sometimes with untrained counsellors and therapists, are sometimes encouraged to ascribe all their symptoms to repressed memories of abuse. There is considerable concern as to whether some or all of such memories are false (Pople and Hudson 1995), but many people in the 'caring professions' are convinced that they are usually true. There is, however, no firm evidence that people forget traumatic events occurring after infancy.

## Genital injuries

In our attenders at St Mary's who are examined by doctors within five days of the alleged assault,

the incidence of genital injuries is about 22%. Similar findings have been observed in cases seen in London where 21% of 217 women had genital injuries (F. Lewington, Metropolitan Police Forensic Science Service, personal communication). Other studies have shown a similar incidence (Solola *et al.* 1983). The most common injury is fresh splitting or abrasion of the fourchette, followed by bruising or abrasion of the labia minora (Figure 8). For many of those presenting at St Mary's, their first sexual intercourse is the subject of the allegation. In a series of the author's own cases, 17% of 480 women alleging rape were virgins prior to the alleged offence. Findings in them varied from no injury, slight tearing of the hymen, a full-width tear, multiple tears or, rarely, a tear of the hymen extending into the lower-third of the vagina necessitating stitching.

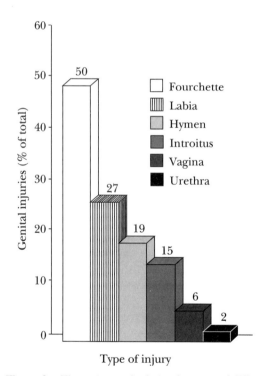

Type of injury

**Figure 8** *The variety and relative frequency of different genital injuries observed in sexual assault victims at the St Mary's Centre, Manchester, between 1986 and 1991. The injuries included two knife wounds to the vulva. It is important to note that 223 women out of a total of 946 (23.6%) victims had injuries*

Injuries to the vagina are rare and consist of a spiral tear, usually caused by the insertion of something like a bottle, or penile penetration in a young child or elderly woman. Occasionally, scratches or abrasions on the cervix are caused by fingers or other objects. What is not known is the incidence of such findings in consenting sexual activity. Doctors giving evidence in court are liable to say, or to assume, that the injuries prove rape. However, it is well known among gynaecologists that first intercourse between consenting adults can occasionally cause an injury which requires surgical treatment. It is important to understand, however, that rape commonly occurs without causing genital injury and that genital injuries may occur in consenting sexual activity, but there is a pressing need for more hard evidence.

## Forensic evidence

If a woman presents within a week of being raped and is unsure whether she wishes to report to the police, it is worth taking forensic specimens which can be stored indefinitely in a four-star freezer which, if properly labelled and sealed, can subsequently be examined and used as evidence in court. Ordinary plain hospital swabs, moistened with sterile water, should be used on dry surfaces such as skin, and the specimens should then be placed in tubes which are sealed with sticky tape and frozen immediately.

The laboratory investigation is based on Locard's principle that 'every contact leaves a trace' and seeks to establish links between the suspect, the victim and the scene.

Swabs should be taken from any part of the body which has been sucked or licked and any bodily orifice which has been penetrated.

The forensic medical examination is described in detail in standard texts such as *Gynaecology* (Shaw *et al.* 1992), and *Clinical Forensic Medicine* (McLay 1992). A brief outline of the possible signs of injury to the body is shown in Figure 9. Table 1 lists the different types of injury and the parameters used to describe the injury.

In most cases in the United Kingdom forensic doctors (police surgeons) are now well trained and are willing to give advice or, in some cases, as in Manchester, to attend and conduct a forensic examination without need to inform the police. The police force operations room should be contacted for advice.

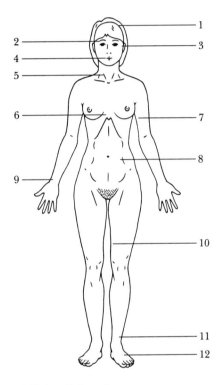

1. Hair pulled out, bumps
2. Black eye, bloodshot, pupil size (alcohol, drugs), petechiae (strangulation)
3. Bruising of ear, behind ear or side of face
4. Cuts, bruises, petechiae in mouth (fellatio)
5. Grip marks, love bites, ligature marks
6. Bruises, bite marks
7. Bruises, grip marks
8. Scratches from pulling off clothing
9. Ligature marks, handcuff marks
10. Fingertip bruises
11. Ligature marks
12. Dirt, cuts, bruises

**Figure 9** *The possible signs of injury to the body of sexual assault victims that are recorded by the examining doctor*

**Table 1** *The different types of injury to record when examining the victim of an alleged sexual assault and the parameters used to describe the injury*

*Type:*
  bruises
  abrasions (scratches)
  lacerations (tearing injuries)
  incised wound (cut)

*Parameters measured:*
  size
  shape
  colour
  distance for fixed body point (e.g. elbow crease)

## CHILD SEXUAL ABUSE

There is no doubt that sexual abuse of children is common and has frequently gone unrecognised. It is also true that in recent years it has sometimes been overdiagnosed. Where a child makes a spontaneous allegation, the management of the case is relatively straightforward, but particular problems arise where:

(1) There may be a perception, perhaps by professionals (e.g. therapists, social workers or teachers), that a child has been abused because she exhibits sexually explicit behaviour or has other psychological problems which have sometimes been found in sexually abused children;

(2) There are genital problems; and

(3) In custody disputes where, occasionally, a parent, usually the mother, will allege sexual abuse on very shaky evidence or, rarely, may herself cause genital injuries to the child.

When a child presents to a doctor with any genital problem it can be argued that it would now be negligent not to consider sexual abuse in the differential diagnosis, but it is imperative that doctors use their clinical skills in evaluating these problems. It is important to take a full history, examine the patient, carry out all the appropriate investigations consider a differential diagnosis and, if possible, reach a diagnosis.

In this field it is, unfortunately, true that doctors frequently act as an advocate for the child rather than giving unbiased, accurate information to the courts. They are too ready to ascribe findings (e.g. tramline redness of the inside of the labia majora, redness persisting for more than a few days or labial adhesions) to abuse without thoroughly considering other possibilities.

Gynaecologists who see children and perform examinations under anaesthetic would be in a good position to carry out studies of the non-abused children. Some studies have been performed in the United States (although none in the United Kingdom) and, while there might be difficulties with ethical committees, as well as with parental and child consent, the lack of hard facts means that courts are sometimes misled and decisions reached on the basis of medical evidence which will not stand up to scientific evaluation. The following findings have caused problems:

(1) Concerning *tramline redness.* How common is it? What are its causes? Is it ever significant as a sign of sexual abuse?

(2) How long does *redness persist after trauma* (e.g. after indecent rubbing without actual injury)? Claims have been made and evidence given in court that redness seen weeks or even months later is supportive of such an allegation.

(3) *Labial adhesions* are well recognised in children in nappies and are not uncommon in older girls. How common are they? What is their exact mechanism? Are they always caused by slight trauma whether indecent or not?

(4) *Atrophic vulvitis* is associated with fourchette friability and is well known to be associated with low oestrogen status and respond to oestrogen cream. How common is it in children who have been indecently touched? Is it sometimes a chance, incidental finding?

(5) Does *scarring of the fourchette* occur after single or only after repeated injury? Can atrophic vulvitis cause scarring of the fourchette?

(6) Is a *hymenal orifice which is open* on first inspection a sign of abuse? Some doctors refer to this as 'gaping' (Hobbs *et al.* 1995).

(7) Does the *hymen ever repair* after a tear without leaving a defect or any sign that it has been torn? Does the hymen develop true scars?

(8) Do *tampons ever damage the hymen* in ordinary use? (Emans *et al.* 1994). Emans found no difference in genital anatomy between tampon users and non-users.

Evidence continues to be given in court by doctors, and is commonly unchallenged, which asserts with equal, but unscientific, certainty all aspects of the above points.

A major problem which has caused controversy in court is where doctors have testified that tears of the hymen caused prepubertal damage to the membrane, so that it does not respond to the influence of oestrogen and grow normally during puberty. It has been claimed that a thin, wispy, hymenal remnant seen in a teenage girl indicates that the hymen was damaged before puberty and that large hymenal defects support allegations of prepubertal penetration. Is this a reasonable hypothesis? Is it evidence which should be put before a court? Many doctors aware of this claim have looked in vain for such signs and there is no published work on the subject. In the author's experience, the only finding which is a significant pointer to abuse before puberty is where there is a full 'U'-shaped posterior tear of the hymen which extends into the posterior fourchette, because there had been a very large tear due to disproportion between the penis and vagina.

## HEALING OF INJURIES

There is some anecdotal evidence about the healing of injuries following sexual assault, both in adults and children, but there is little published work on this matter. Gynaecologists are, however, uniquely placed to carry out studies of healing in the genital area which would be of enormous value.

## THE LEGAL CASE

When a doctor is called to court, either as a professional or expert witness, it is important to understand the differences between the medical and legal mind. According to Gee and Mason (1990):

'*The scientist is accustomed to the rules of scientific enquiry, to making observations, forming hypotheses from them, conducting experiments to check the hypotheses and thus formulating theories. The object is to establish the truth; there are no compromises. The court on the other hand is there to resolve a dispute between two parties either between two persons in a civil action or between an individual and the State in a criminal action.*'

Mr Justice Cazalet (Cazalet 1988) set down the criteria which experts should use in preparing reports and giving opinions. These are that the expert should:

(1) Provide a straightforward and not a misleading opinion;

(2) Be objective and not omit factors which do not support their opinion; and

(3) Be properly researched.

## CONCLUSIONS

Forensic gynaecology is of increasing importance. The needs of victims call for understanding and professional skill. Much evidence given in court is of dubious scientific worth. There is a pressing need for good research on genital findings, patterns of injury and progress of healing in both adults and children.

# References

Brown, H., Stein, J. and Tark, V. (1995) Report of a second two year incidence survey on the reported sexual abuse of adults with learning disabilities. *Ment Handicap Res* **8**(1), 1–22

Cazalet, J. [1988] Family Law Reports (FLR) 607 at 612

Emans, S. J., Woods, E. R., Allred, E. N. and Grace, E. (1994) Hymenal findings in adolescent women: impact of tampon use and sexual activity. *J Pediatr* **125**(1), 153–60

Gee D. J. and Mason, J. K. (1990) *The Courts and the Doctor.* Oxford: Oxford University Press

General Medical Council (1995) *Duties of a Doctor. Guidance from the General Medical Council*

Hobbs, C. J., Wynne, J. M. and Thomas, A. J. (1995) Colposcopic findings in prepubertal girls assessed for sexual abuse. *Arch Dis Child* **73**, 465–71

Home Office (1996) *Home Office Criminal Statistics 1995.* London: HMSO

McLay, W. D. S. (Ed.) (1992) *Clinical Forensic Medicine.* Pinter Publishers Ltd for the Association of Police Surgeons

Pople, H. G. and Hudson, J. I. (1995) Can memories of childhood sexual abuse be repressed. *Psychol Med* **25**, 121–6

*R. v Ward* [1993] 96 Cr. App R1

Saward, J. (1990) *Rape — My Story.* London: Pan Books

Shaw, R. W., Stanton, S. and Soutter, P. (Eds.) (1992) *Gynaecology.* Edinburgh: Churchill Livingstone

Solola, A., Scott, C., Severs, H. and Howell, J. (1983) Rape: management in an institutional setting. *Obstet Gynecol* **61** (3), 373–7

Temkin, J. (1995) 'A questionnaire in the Sussex area' in: *Proceedings of the Conference on Care of Survivors of Sexual Assault,* London, September

Walker, E. A. (1993) Sexual victimisation and chronic pelvic pain. *Obstet Gynecol Clin North Am* Dec. **20** (4), 795–807

Wyre, R. and Swift, A. (1990) *Women, Men and Rape.* London: Headway

# 10

# Ethics, the law and the fetus

*Peter S. Haughton*

'*More than a body part but less than a person, where it is, is largely what it is.
From the standpoint of the pregnant woman, it is both me and not me. It "is"
the pregnant woman in the sense that it is in her and of her and is hers more
than anyone's. It "is not" her in the sense that she is not all that is there.*'

MacKinnon (1991)

This is an enormous topic of book-length proportions. In this chapter there is the need to be selective, since the whole ground cannot possibly be covered. What it does cover is the examination of the ambivalence that society has over the moral status of the human fetus, with a critical appraisal of the general position of bioethicists, and how society's ambivalence is pragmatically worked out in the law.

## THE ARGUMENTS

My starting point is to make two assumptions. The first is that all who read this were once human fetuses and the second is that none of the readers can remember what it was like when they were a fetus. If we can accept that these two assumptions are true, it may become evident why so much ethical and legal controversy continues to surround the fetus. It may also help in bringing a fresh perspective to this ongoing controversial area.

The recognition that, in order to be who we are today, it was necessary for each and every one of us to have successfully completed the fetal stage of development, at first seems a powerful argument for affording protection to the fetal stage, both legally and morally. The potentiality that we had then has been realised

in who we are now. Yet, such an argument, as it stands, is in need of considerable buttressing in order for it to have any strength, for it makes a number of assumptions and further questions need to be raised. These are:

(1) When does someone/something become morally valuable and how is this determined?

(2) Is it when a new life begins and, if so, can we agree when this is the case?

(3) Does the fetal stage of development have a claim to the 'right to life' and what do we mean by such a claim?

(4) How do we resolve the inevitable conflicts between the fetus' right to life and other rights, such as those of the mother and society?

### Polarisation of belief

These are all elements of the well-rehearsed arguments surrounding the fetus that are also used when discussing abortion. Initially, it seems that there is a polarisation between those who advocate the rights of the fetus and those who advocate the right of the mother-to-be to choose whether to continue with the pregnancy. Society appears to be divided into those who are 'pro-life' or 'pro-choice'. Much effort and argument has been made for both positions, to such an extent that it appears, at first sight, that a compromise can never be found. On one side, there are those who hold that a human fetus is already a moral subject, an unborn child, with corresponding moral rights, from the moment of its conception. This group would wish society to recognise the fetus' moral rights through a tightening of the law. Opposed to this are those who would argue that a recently conceived fetus is no more than a collection of cells, although these are unique, that has the potential to develop, given the right circumstances; a human fetus is no more a child than a caterpillar is a butterfly. The division of society is particularly acute in the United States of America where it is one of the key issues in current political and social debate.

## Understanding the content

To understand and to accept the arguments merely in this polarised form is to take too pessimistic a view. Furthermore, the approach of Ronald Dworkin (1993) has much to commend it, in that he steers the reader through the arguments and removes the apparent polarisation of the two positions by recasting the arguments in a new light. He writes:

'*[The polarised] understanding of the character of the abortion argument is wrong, [for] it is based on a widespread intellectual confusion we can identify and dispel ... I can describe this intellectual confusion at once in very general terms. The public argument over abortion has failed to recognise an absolutely crucial distinction. One side insists that human life begins at conception, that a fetus is a person from that moment, that abortion is murder or homicide or an assault on the sanctity of human life. But each of these phrases can be used to describe two very different ideas.*

*First, they can be used to make the claim that fetuses are creatures with interests of their own right from the start, including, prominently, the interest in remaining alive, and that therefore they have the rights that all human beings have to protect these basic interests, including a right not to be killed. Abortion is wrong in principle, according to his claim, because abortion violates someone's right not to be killed, just as killing an adult is normally wrong because it violates the adult's right not to be killed. I shall call this the* derivative *objection to abortion because it presupposes and is derived from rights and interests that it assumes all human beings, including fetuses, have. Someone who accepts this objection, and who believes that government should prohibit or regulate abortion for this reason, believes that government has a derivative responsibility to protect a fetus.*

*The second claim that the familiar rhetoric can be used to make is very different: that human life has an intrinsic, innate value; that human life is sacred just in itself; and that the sacred nature of a human life begins when its biological life begins, even before the creature whose life it is has movement or sensation or interests or rights of its own. According to this second claim, abortion is wrong in principle because it disregards and insults the intrinsic value, the sacred character, of any stage or form of human life. I shall call this the* detached *objection to abortion, because it does not depend on or presuppose any particular rights or interests. Someone who accepts this objection, and argues that abortion should be prohibited or regulated by law for this reason, believes that government has a detached responsibility for protecting the intrinsic value of life.*' (Dworkin 1993, page 10)

Dworkin advocates that almost all of us regard the abortion argument as of this second kind, the detached view, whether we be conservative or liberal, Catholic, feminist or atheist (Dworkin 1993, page 24). In other words, in spite of the rhetoric, people hold that a developing human fetus has intrinsic innate value. The argument, then, is not so much about whether or not a fetus has a right to life, but how much does society value this 'intrinsic innate value' and, further, whether it should be protected through legal sanctions.

However, since so much of the debate is conducted in terms of 'right to life' it is helpful to look at an argument advanced by the bioethicists such as Glover (1977), Harris (1985) and Singer (1993). They argue that it is the notion

ETHICS, THE LAW AND THE FETUS

of 'persons' that is morally relevant; and that it is only 'persons' who have this right to life. Their argument in deductive form can be expressed as the following three premises:

(1) Not all human beings are persons;

(2) Only persons have the right to life; and

(3) Some human beings have no right to life.

It is this type of argument that is used by bioethicists to justify, in certain cases, abortion, infanticide and some forms of euthanasia.

The argument set out above lies within the rules of deductive logic, with the conclusions following the premises. Hence, any weakness within the argument is not in the logic itself, but rather in the truth claims employed by the premises. There are three areas within the premises for which greater clarification is needed, namely:

(1) What are the differences, if any, between human beings and persons?

(2) What do we understand by the 'right to life'?

(3) It it *only* persons who have that 'right to life'?

### What are the differences, if any, between human beings and persons?

Human beings could be defined in entirely empirical terms in that a human being is a member of a particular species, namely *homo sapiens*, and as such has certain characteristics that can be measured and described. The word 'person' is not so easily defined, for although in common usage the terms person and human being are often used synonymously, much depends on the definition accepted for the word 'person' as to what the differences are between the two terms. If we accept, as most bioethicists do, a definition similar to that of the seventeenth century philosopher John Locke, who defined a person as '*a thinking intelligent being that has reason and reflection and can consider itself as itself, the same thinking being, in different times and places*', then it is clear that there are two

elements which are critical to the notion of being a person, namely:

(1) Rationality; and

(2) Self-consciousness.

It is also worth noting that these characteristics that define a person are those necessary to be a moral agent. It is equally clear that not all humans possess these characteristics, for example, infants, those with a mental handicap, the senile and, of course, fetuses. For being human, as with other forms of life, is a dynamic process of growth and decay, whereas the idea of a person, once a definition is accepted, is a static notion. Furthermore, being human is a closed concept, namely belonging to a certain species, whereas being a 'person' is open to all who exhibit such characteristics that the definition requires.

It is clear that there are differences between a human being and a 'person', given the definitions used. Therefore, we have no difficulty in accepting the first premise that 'not all human beings are persons' and that human fetuses are not 'persons', but only, at best, 'potential persons'.

### What do we understand by the 'right to life'?

The phrase 'right to life' is a short-hand phrase that could mean a number of things, but is generally understood to mean either the right to have one's own life protected and enhanced, or, alternatively, the right not to be killed. The right to life can be understood either as a positive right (i.e. the right to be saved) or as a negative right (i.e. the right not to be killed). Taken at face value, it is a positive right and it is clear that there would be a corresponding duty imposed on others that promotes life. Alternatively, it can be expressed in terms of a negative right, and this in turn imposes a negative duty on others of not killing those processing this right.

Further, the right to life can either be an absolute right or a relative right. If it is absolute, then those on whom this right is conferred, or who can claim this right, should not under any circumstances have their life taken from them (even if those beings wished for their life to be ended by others). Many of those who identify with the 'pro-life' lobby would regard the right to life to be absolute and that the human fetus has this right. If the right to life is relative, then it may be overridden by other conflicting rights.

However, whichever form is taken, the question of boundaries and scope of the right to life is raised; in other words, 'Who or what has the right to life?' For the moment, this question will be left and answered later. Instead, the answer to an easier, related question (namely, 'Who or what can uphold a right?') will be given which, in turn, provides a way of finding an answer to the scope of the right to life.

It would seem that only those who can comprehend the notion of rights and duties can uphold a right. Those without this facility cannot be morally culpable for not upholding right. In fact, it seems that it is only 'persons', in the philosophical sense of Locke's definition, or institutions that are made up by such persons, that can uphold rights. In other words, only 'persons' or institutions made up of persons can take upon themselves such duties that will uphold whatever moral right is being sought.

### Is it *only* persons who have a right to life?

We have stated as being self-evident that duties cannot be imposed on non-persons. Only persons can uphold rights; only persons, or institutions made up of persons, can have duties imposed on them. But it does not follow that only persons have rights. Anything or anyone could have rights provided that there are persons to uphold those rights and that there are persons who are prepared to act as proxy to make claim of those rights bestowed on non-persons that are incapable of exercising their rights. Now, it may be that persons decide that only persons can have the particular right to life. Alternatively, the right to life could be extended to other non-persons, but there needs to be consensus among persons as to the scope of the right to life in order that such persons can uphold that right. It is here that lies the apparent conflict between the 'pro-life' faction and their 'pro-choice' opponents. For the 'pro-life' lobby would wish to extend the right to life for all human fetuses, while the 'pro-choice' lobby recognises that there are competing rights that may take precedence over the human fetus' right to life.

It would seem that the notion of rights in general, and the right to life in particular, is fraught with complications of language and application. A more fruitful approach would be to seek consensus among persons to determine what is of moral value, and from this vantage moral objectives could be advanced by the promotion of those things deemed to have moral value or worth, rather than resorting to the language of rights.

### Summary of the bioethicists' argument

There is no difficulty accepting that 'persons' as defined earlier in the chapter and 'human beings' are two different notions in which there are beings that can belong to both, or just one, of these two categories. We, therefore, accept the initial premise that not all human beings are persons. It is the second premise that is the weak link in the argument in that, although it is true that only persons can uphold a right (and the right to life in particular), it does not follow that only persons have the right to life, as persons could confer such a right on non-persons. Given the weakness of the second premise, it follows that the conclusion that some humans do not have the right to life is itself weak in that it is dependent upon the second premise. It is perfectly possible that persons could wish to confer the right to life upon, for example, the whole of the species *Homo sapiens* and/or upon other living beings; that persons would wish to extend the notion of enhancing and promoting life to non-persons, rather than to confine it solely to the category of person.

### Consequences of accepting the argument

The consequences of accepting the argument, as it stands, are enormous and, for many, they are sinister. For, if the argument is accepted, then those beings (human or otherwise) that are not persons are denied the right to life. We have already noted that, whatever definition we use for a person, that definition will be static. Someone or something is, at any point in time, either a person or is not a person. Yet, life itself is a dynamic process so that a living thing may be considered a person at certain points in time and not a person at others. For example, at one end of the spectrum of life a being (human or otherwise) who was once a person can become afflicted by senile dementia and lose the right to life. Then, at the other end of the spectrum of life, at its beginnings, we have a situation where a being has not yet developed those attributes of self-consciousness and rationality, but in the normal course of events would go on to become a person; in other words, it is a potential person. It seems that such 'potential persons', such as fetus and infants of those species that exhibit the attributes of personhood, would also be denied the right to life. Thus, the argument implies that such potential persons may morally be killed. I suggest that such a notion would be deeply repugnant to many that are persons.

## Is the argument helpful in medical ethics?

We have examined this argument at length because it is popular among those in the field of bioethics, but I believe it to be of limited value in the field of medical ethics. That said, it does raise the issue of the scope of medicine; that is, whether medicine is for persons or for humans? Quite clearly, medical practice is not solely for persons, but for humans. This avoids the issue over whether it is morally relevant that our ethics are overtly 'specieistic'. Indeed, much of medical practice is done for those whose self-consciousness and rationality are impaired by illness and disease and the task of medicine is to restore to such beings their autonomy. In other words, as well as the duty to respect autonomy, much of health care is about the creation of autonomy within the individual.

Yet, the human fetus has no autonomy to respect, for it will never, as a fetus, have any autonomy. As the fetus grows and develops, its potential to become an autonomous being increases, but as a fetus *per se*, it will only ever have the *potential* for autonomy. Furthermore, it is also true that the fetus, in the character of the fetus, has no interests; rather it has the potential to develop interests. Many people have difficulty in accepting this idea because they project their current values onto a stage of life in which those values are not apparent. The question that faces society is what moral value we ascribe to this potentiality, both of autonomy and interests, and whether it is appropriate to use law to protect this potentiality.

## Potentiality

Arguments around the issue of the potentiality of the human fetus are often confused mainly, I suggest, because they are conducted from the point of view of those with realised potential. This can be illustrated by taking an example where potential has not been realised. I have the potential to become an old age pensioner and if I reach the age of 65, then I will be entitled to a state pension (other things being equal). If I die in my sixty-fifth year then I shall not receive a penny of my pension. In order for me to realise my pension I have to reach the required age, but if I die before pensionable age my rights have not been infringed for those rights only come into being when potential is realised. In a similar way, the so-called rights of a fetus can only come into being when the fetus ceases to be a fetus and has successfully realised its potential in becoming an independent member of the human race. This is not to say, nor has it been argued, that human society does not have interest in human fetuses realising their potential. Clearly, it does and English law reflects society's concern and interest in the fetus.

## ENGLISH LAW AND THE FETUS

English law does not treat human fetuses in the same manner as human beings. To kill the latter deliberately is usually regarded as murder. As far as the law is concerned, the fetus is not regarded as a person, but neither is it merely regarded as a chattel or a piece of property. A fetus does not have legal rights, although the destruction of the fetus and prenatal injury are both statutory matters.

The Abortion Act (1967), as amended by the Human Fertilisation and Embryology Act (1990), specifies the criteria for a legal abortion. The act is pragmatic, stating who may perform an abortion and in what circumstances an abortion may take place. The law does not seek to answer such philosophical questions posed earlier; rather its purpose, by regulating abortion and making it legal in controlled circumstances, is to do away with the horrors that many women once faced if seeking abortion, with its consequent health risks, when practised by those with dubious skills.

The Congenital Disabilities (Civil Liability) Act 1976 was enacted, following the recommendations of the Law Commission in its 1974 report (number 60) on *Injuries on Unborn Children* to deal with prenatal injury. However, it can only be brought into effect if the fetus has successfully become a human being. This is the recognition by society that detrimental events occurring prenatally are subject to compensation. This indicates that society does in fact have an interest in the welfare of the fetus although, in practical terms, it should be noted that clinicians cannot be said to have a duty of care towards the fetus, but that the duty of care is primarily with the mother-to-be. Or so it seemed.

On the whole, the law reflects the view that society values the interest of the mother-to-be when it is in conflict with the continuance of the pregnancy. It was therefore surprising and somewhat disturbing to learn of the judgement in *Re S*, in which a woman was compelled to undergo a Caesarean section despite a previously successful vaginal delivery, as the doctors had predicted that only a section would save the baby. It would seem that the former notion of 'unity of persons' representing both the mother and the fetus has been dented. Andrew Grubb writes (Grubb 1995):

'So where does this leave the law? If neither the "unity of persons" or the "separateness of persons" approach makes common sense or sensible law, what should the law do? The solution lies in an approach which is widely recognised as seeing the fetus as a de facto entity (though not a legal person) which has interests that the law must take account of when any decision is made, or action taken, affecting the fetus ... Some have termed this de jure unity but de facto separateness as a co-existence "Not-One-But-Two". Why should English law embrace this approach? There are a number of reasons. First, it is more flexible than the other two approaches and allows for a sensitive accommodation of the interests of the mother and fetus[*]. It does not dictate, merely by its description, whose interests should prevail in mother and fetus cases. It does not, for example, mean that the mother may always have her way regardless of the effect on the fetus; neither may the claims of the fetus always trump the claims of the mother. It allows both sets of interests to be taken into account. Secondly, it actually reflects how we popularly conceptualise the position of the pregnant woman. Thirdly, alien though all this may sound to the more rigid, and black or white, attitude of English law, it is in fact reflected in the law already. It is what much of English law concerned with the fetus is actually based on: for example, when an abortion may be carried out; that the contingent interests of a fetus may justify a prenatal injury action in tort or inheritance by as-yet unborn children and why courts have genuine concerns when a pregnant woman's refusal of medical treatment may harm her fetus.'

Where once the law seemed to be so clear, we now recognise that the ambivalence that is found within society is also reflected in the law that governs society. A consequence of this is the need for rigorous ethical debate to continue to take place. It is hoped that this article has made some contribution to the debate.

---

[*] *'Interest of mother and fetus' for reasons already given, I wish this phrase to be understood as shorthand for 'the interests of the mother and the interests that society has in seeing that that particular fetus is/was brought to term'.*

# References

Dworkin, R. (1993) *Life's Dominion. An Argument about Abortion and Euthanasia.* London: Harper Collins

Glover, J. (1977) *Causing Death and Saving Lives.* London: Penguin Books

Grubb, A. (1995) Commentary on unborn child (pre-natal injury); homocide and abortion. *Med Law Rev* **3**, 307

Harris, J. (1985) *The Value of Life.* London: Routledge & Kegan Paul

MacKinnon, C. A. (1991) Reflections on sex equality under law. *Yale Law J* **100**, 1316

Re S (*Adult Refusal of Medical Treatment*) [1992] 4 A11 E.R. 671

Singer, P. (1993) *Practical Ethics*, 2nd edn. Cambridge: Cambridge University Press

# 11

# The adolescent and the obstetrician/gynaecologist

*Roger J. Pepperell*

Whereas the gynaecologist may be asked to see a newborn baby with ambiguous genitalia, or see a child between the ages of three and eight years with vaginal discharge and vulval irritation, which usually is shown to be due to 'atrophic' vaginitis, by far the most common time for paediatric gynaecological opinion is during adolescence.

It is during this time that peer pressure results in sexual experimentation by both adolescent boys and girls, at a time when many seem to fail to consider the consequences of their activity in terms of pregnancy and the transmission of a variety of sexually transmitted diseases. These diseases not only adversely affect their subsequent fertility but, as is the case with acquired immunodeficiency syndrome (AIDS), can (and will) cause their premature death. It is almost as if, despite the widespread information about AIDS and the known risk of transmission during unprotected sexual activity, the adolescent believes 'this could not happen to me'. The possibility that their sexual behaviour, often with multiple partners, may also lead to an increased risk of cervical cancer is not even considered.

One of the major responsibilities of all physicians is, therefore, to ensure that information concerning the risks of unprotected sexual activity is readily available to all adolescents. Furthermore, it is important to encourage society to 'stop burying its head in the sand' and accept the need for sexual education in the latter years of primary school and throughout all secondary education. The available data clearly indicate that sexual activities in teenagers is increasing, with > 50% of 16-year-olds sexually active, and the abortion and delivery rate in teenagers still on the increase. The ready availability of both advice and methods of contraception for adolescents is an absolute priority. Unfortunately, many of them do not want to listen to this advice, nor attend the current sites where this is available such as family planning clinics, gynaecological clinics in major hospitals, adolescent clinics in children's hospitals or free-standing clinics in the community which specialise in the needs of adolescents. Some lateral thinking will probably be necessary to ensure that information and contraceptive techniques are readily available to those who need it.

It is not the intention of this chapter to dwell at length on the problems confronting both the adolescents and society due to the sexual revolution in our teenagers, despite the fact these are clearly more important than most other problems in terms of financial cost and effects on lifestyle, etc. It will, however, consider the many other problems experienced by the adolescent female which may lead them to see a gynaecologist (see Table 1).

## PROBLEMS OF BODY IMAGE

During adolescence body image assumes ever-increasing importance with the teenage magazines encouraging the excessively thin, tall physique and overemphasising the importance of 'adequate breast development'. The increasing

**Table 1** *Adolescent problems encountered by the gynaecologist*

*Disordered body image:*
  height
  weight
  breast size
  acne

*Sexuality:*
  contraception
  sexually transmitted diseases
  teenage pregnancy

*Abnormalities of menstruation:*
  primary amenorrhoea
  irregular cycles
  excessive blood loss

*Abdominopelvic pain:*
  dysmenorrhoea
  other causes

*Müllerian duct abnormalities:*
  absence
  duplication
  obstruction

*Care of the handicapped child:*
  coping with menstruation
  contraception
  complicating factors (e.g. public opinion,
    guardianship boards and Supreme/Family
    Court)

contact with boys clearly influences the clothes and swimming garments that adolescent girls wear; any problem with breast development is likely to result in the girl not being prepared to wear a swimsuit at all. The occurrence of acne at this time also produces considerable concern in the afflicted girl, who then sees herself as unattractive to her peers and the opposite sex.

## Ideal body weight

Preoccupation with ideal body weight results in many adolescents dieting to the extent that too much weight is lost, with some girls displaying all the features of anorexia nervosa. A considerate gynaecological consultant may well address part of this problem; however, assistance from a psychiatrist experienced in this area is often required. Where the anorexia is of such

degree that secondary amenorrhoea results, it should not be forgotten that a return of ovarian function often takes up to 12 months, even where weight has been gained and ideal body weight achieved. It is important that the girl is advised of this or she may not maintain her weight and may well become anorexic again.

## Disturbances of height

Abnormalities in height also upset many adolescent girls, with short stature being much more frequently identified as a problem than excessive height. Although an organic cause for excessive height (e.g. gigantism due to growth hormone excess, Marfan's syndrome, XXX chromosome complement, agonadal eunuchoidism and thyrotoxicosis) is sometimes found, the usual cause is familial. Organic causes of short stature (e.g. chromosome abnormalities [45X or 46XX/45X] and growth hormone deficiency) are much more common but other causes (e.g. previous precocious puberty, delayed menarche, a 'deprived' child or a child who was just born small) also need consideration. Assessment of the estimated mature height (EMH) by wrist radiography forms an important part of the evaluation of both short and tall girls, as this information is required to assist with treatment.

Excessive height is rarely a problem to the girl concerned, although many tall girls are brought to a paediatric endocrinologist or gynaecologist by her parents because they perceive that a problem exists. As the tallness is usually familial, the EMH result allows a rational plan of management to be advised, with hormonal treatment often being proposed if the EMH is 183 cm or more. The most extensive report of this treatment so far is that of Wettenhall *et al.* (1975), who recommended that the hormonal treatment should be commenced when the girl reached 168 cm in height and should last for two years, with the expectation that the reduced height achieved would be 3.5–7.3 cm. The therapy used was 150 μg ethinyloestradiol per day (initially commencing at a lower dose until tolerance was achieved), with norethisterone being administered in a dosage of 5 mg twice daily for the first four days of each calender month. Although the duration of progestogen therapy is clearly less than would currently be recommended when hormone replacement therapy is being given, no apparent problems were identified during treatment or in a follow-up period of more than 20 years.

Providing an organic cause for small stature can be excluded, and any 'deprivation' factor addressed, a decision can usually be made as to whether any hormonal treatment is warranted. This is particularly the case for girls shown to have a delay in their menarche, as hormonal replacement to stimulate the growth spurt usually seen at puberty will certainly achieve a significant increase in height. It should also be remembered that oxandrolone therapy has achieved considerable height increase in girls with Turner's syndrome (45X) and trials of growth hormone therapy are currently being evaluated in many countries for such individuals.

In a prepubertal girl, knowledge of the amount of height increase expected once the growth spurt commences is important, as this will often allay anxiety that 'she is always going to be the smallest in her class'. Whereas the growth velocity is usually 4–5 cm per year prior to the growth spurt, it doubles during the spurt for a period of about two years prior to the menarche, with a further 5.5 cm (average) of growth occurring after the menarche (Tanner 1962). For girls who are first seen during their growth spurt, the postmenarchal growth can be up to 10 cm, especially if the menarche occurs before the age of 11 years.

## Disturbances of breast size/symmetry

Unequal breast development during puberty is common and equalisation of growth usually takes place over time without treatment. There is no evidence that hormone treatment, such as supplemental oestrogen, is more likely to affect the smaller than the normal breast, although it may result in both breasts increasing in size.

If the breasts are not equal in size by the age of 16 years, and if the menarche has already occurred, it is unlikely the discrepancy will be resolved without either reduction mammoplasty of the larger breast, augmentation mammoplasty of the smaller breast or the use of an external prosthesis to augment the size of the smaller breast.

Surgical treatment is also indicated in the presence of a congenital abnormality of the breast (e.g. Poland's syndrome, aplasia or extreme hypoplasia) or where the breast abnormality follows damage to the breast bud by a chest wall incision used during infantile cardiac surgery. In each of these instances a most satisfactory result can be obtained by a combination of plastic surgery and the use of a tissue expander. In Poland's syndrome, where pectoralis major is missing, latissmus dorsi muscle is transposed, and a tissue expander placed deep to the transposed muscle.

Although many adolescents are reluctant to accept the use of an external prosthesis, the currently available prostheses are remarkably lifelike in both feel and appearance and can be placed in a pouch in a specially designed bra or one-piece swimsuit. Their major use currently is in girls who are either hoping for some spontaneous equalisation of size with time or those with some, but an inadequate amount of, breast tissue on one side.

## Adolescent acne

Most adolescent acne is mild and can be adequately controlled with either 2.5–10% benzoyl peroxide gel, 0.025–0.05% tretinoin gel, 0.05% isotretinoin gel or 4–10% sulphur lotion. These agents should not be used if there is a risk of pregnancy.

In moderate inflammatory acne an antibiotic should be used in addition to the above. These have included topical clindamycin (1%), or oral tetracycline, minocycline or erythromycin.

In severe cystic acne oral sulphonamides or a short course of corticosteroid therapy may be added. If six months of antibiotic therapy does not control the acne, consideration should be given to the use of the Dianette (Schering Health Care Ltd, Burgess Hill, West Sussex), the contraceptive pill containing 35 μg of ethinyloestradiol and 2 mg of cyproterone acetate, or the use of a six-month course of isotretinoin (Roaccutane; Roche Products Ltd, Welwyn Garden City, Hertfordshire). This latter agent usually produces a long-term remission, although pregnancy must be avoided during therapy and for one month after it is stopped. Dianette is generally only effective while the treatment is continued and for a short time after its cessation.

## ABNORMALITIES OF MENSTRUATION

Puberty usually commences with the growth spurt, followed sequentially by breast development, pubic and axillary hair development and finally the first period (menarche). The usual time interval between the commencement of breast development and the menarche is two years. The first few periods are often quite irregular, although regular ovulatory cycles usually occur within two years of the menarche.

### Primary amenorrhoea

Where an adolescent has not had her menarche by the age of 16 years, she is deemed to have primary amenorrhoea. As the cause of this can be at the level of the hypothalamus, pituitary, adrenal, ovary, uterus and vagina, the need for both clinical examination and a number of special tests is obvious. In general, this evaluation is delayed until the age of 16 years, but if the growth spurt and breast development have not started by 14 years, where more than three years have elapsed since the breast development commenced or where cyclical lower abdominal pain is occurring, the evaluation should occur earlier.

In the presence of apparently normal pubertal development, but where the menarche has not occurred, the possibility of Müllerian duct absence or obstruction of the vagina to the egress of blood (such as seen in the presence of an imperforate hymen) must be suspected. Müllerian duct absence is found in 5–10% of girls with primary amenorrhoea. If the vagina is found to be short, the possibility of androgen

insensitivity syndrome must also be considered, and this diagnosis confirmed by chromosome analysis. Inspection and gentle clinical examination of the vulva, with insertion of a small probe into the vagina to measure its length, and pelvic (abdominal) ultrasound examination will usually enable the correct diagnosis to be made without the need for examination under anaesthesia or laparoscopy. The presence of normally functioning ovaries in association with Müllerian agenesis can be confirmed on basal body temperature assessment or with the use of a series of weekly progesterone measurements over a four-week period. Where an imperforate hymen is identified, it should be incised; where Müllerian duct absence is confirmed, the need for creation of a vagina must be raised; where androgen insensitivity is diagnosed, removal of the gonads which are predisposed to the development of gonadoblastoma and disgerminoma, followed by long-term oestrogen administration should be advised.

If there is little or no evidence of pubertal breast development, a hypothalamic cause will ultimately be identified in approximately 50% of individuals. Hypothalamic hypogonadism with a deficiency in gonadotrophin releasing hormone (GnRH) production will be the cause in two-thirds of these, with the remainder having a delayed onset of puberty. It is not always possible to differentiate between these causes, except through observation over time, but hormone replacement therapy should be considered (initially in low doses) to promote the normal pubertal growth and breast development and to normalise the amount of calcium laid down in the skeleton during the teenage years.

The remaining individuals will generally be shown to have either a pituitary disorder (10%) or an ovarian disorder (35%) (Evans 1971). The usual pituitary disorder is an adenoma or craniopharyngioma, which will normally be associated with an elevated prolactin (PRL) level and abnormal radiography. The ovarian disorders are predominantly ovarian agenesis (10%), ovarian dysgenesis with chromosome complements of 45X or 46XY (20%), or prepubertal polycystic ovarian disease (3%). The evaluation required in these individuals should be the assessment of serum follicle stimulating hormone (FSH), luteinising hormone (LH) and PRL levels, the assessment of thyroid function, and the measurement of oestradiol levels as an indication of current ovarian activity. Where the FSH and LH levels are elevated, a chromosome analysis is required to assess the possibility of a chromosome abnormality which would necessitate the removal of the gonads (e.g. if an XY line was found).

## Irregular menstruation

As the ovarian cycles in the first one to two years after the menarche are usually anovulatory, the periods are often irregular, heavy and prolonged. In an attempt to prevent anaemia, supplemental iron should be administered and the individual observed to see if a spontaneous resolution occurs. Fortunately, this is what usually happens. Where anaemia occurs, or the individual is not prepared to put up with the abnormal periods any longer, hormone therapy can be instituted. In general, this is best achieved using a medium-dose oral contraceptive pill containing 50 µg of ethinyloestradiol. Lesser doses of oestrogen are likely to be ineffective and breakthrough bleeding will further complicate the already unacceptable bleeding problem.

## Excessive menstrual loss (metrostaxis)

In addition to the heavy periods referred to above, in a small number of adolescents extremely heavy menstrual loss occurs despite the use of a medium-dose contraceptive pill or as an isolated heavy period. Under such circumstances it is imperative that an underlying haematological cause (e.g. von Willebrand's disease, immune thrombocytopenia or acute leukaemia) should be excluded prior to commencing hormone therapy. Such a cause is found in up to 30% of individuals with pubertal metrostaxis where blood transfusion is required because of the extent of the blood loss.

As distinct from adult women, especially those over 40 years of age, it is extremely rare for dilatation and curettage to be required in an adolescent girl with metrostaxis, because the possibility of an organic cause within the uterine cavity is remote and the bleeding can usually be controlled by medical means.

When an underlying haematological cause is identified, appropriate treatment should be instituted in addition to hormonal therapy. The excessive bleeding in individuals with von Willebrand's disease can usually be controlled with an oral contraceptive pill containing 50–75 µg of oestrogen, but the pill will need to be continued throughout the reproductive life (except, of course, when a pregnancy is desired).

Where an underlying haematological cause is not identified, high-dose progestogen therapy with norethisterone (10 mg two-hourly for six doses followed by 10 mg three times daily for three weeks) will often cause the bleeding to cease. Where this does not occur, or where a medium-dose contraceptive pill has already been administered unsuccessfully, no further norethisterone should be given, but high-dose oestrogen therapy provided instead. If the progestogen is continued while the high-dose oestrogen is also administered, it will prevent the oestrogen exerting a proliferative effect on the endometrium and this is required to control the bleeding. The most effective oestrogen is Premarin, given intravenously in a dose of 20 mg twice daily for two days and then orally in a dose of 2.5 mg three times daily. If the bleeding does not stop, the response of the endometrium to the oestrogen therapy can be checked by performing an ultrasound examination; if the endometrial thickness is still < 8 mm, the unopposed oestrogen should be continued for longer. Generally, however, after about one week, 10 mg of norethisterone twice daily can be added and all hormone therapy ceased after a further two weeks to allow menstruation to occur. Thereafter, high-dose hormonal treatment (e.g. 100 µg of ethinyloestradiol per day and 10 mg of norethisterone twice daily for the last two weeks of each month's treatment) should be given for a further six months before ceasing all therapy to see if the disorder has resolved. Fortunately, this is usually the case.

## ABDOMINOPELVIC PAIN

Abdominal pain is a common symptom in adolescence, even prior to the menarche. It is often difficult to explain and a variety of different diagnoses need to be considered in a logical sequence if an appropriate assessment is to be made. Pathology within the urinary tract, genital tract, gastrointestinal system or the peritoneal cavity can all result in pain during adolescence, just as later in life. It is outside the scope of this chapter to discuss all these in detail.

Although most adolescents with pelvic pain, especially dysmenorrhoea, do not have an organic cause identified for this symptom, it is unusual for the dysmenorrhoea to commence at the menarche and, where this is the case, both unilateral Müllerian duct obstruction and a complicated ovarian cyst need to be excluded. Pelvic ultrasound examination enables these two diagnoses to be made.

Pelvic endometriosis also needs to be considered if the dysmenorrhoea fails to respond to traditional therapies (e.g. prostaglandin synthetase inhibitors, oral contraceptive pills, etc.).

## MÜLLERIAN DUCT ABNORMALITIES

Adolescents with Müllerian duct abnormalities will generally present with either primary amenorrhoea or recurrent (often cyclical) lower abdominal pain. If the duct is absent or totally obstructed, primary amenorrhoea will be present, whereas when the obstruction is incomplete, or on one side of a duplicated system, periods will occur and a Müllerian duct problem may not be suspected. Dysmenorrhoea experienced soon after the menarche, or lower abdominal pain occurring intermittently or cyclically, may be seen in total or incomplete Müllerian duct obstruction. Under such circumstances the pain is due to retention of menstrual loss within the genital tract (haematocolpos, haematometra or haematosalpinx) or the development of endometriosis consequent on the retrograde menstruation which almost inevitably occurs.

A large number of Müllerian duct abnormalities have been described, with the most common being shown in Figure 1. The first (Figure 1(A)) is not really a Müllerian duct abnormality as the Müllerian ducts themselves are normal, but the hymen is imperforate due to failure of the membrane between the Müllerian duct and the urogenital sinus to break down. A cruciate incision in this membrane quickly rectifies the problem.

Figure 1(B) indicates the findings when both the uterus and the vagina are absent. In some instances a very short vagina can be identified, but the perineum is frequently flat with no evidence of where the vaginal opening should be located. Although the only symptom is usually that of primary amenorrhoea, a decision does need to be made as to when and how a vagina should be created to allow normal sexual activity to occur. Sometimes this can be achieved using pressure alone (Frank 1955); however, an operative procedure such as that described by McIndoe (1950) or Sheares (1960) is commonly required. It is important that the adolescent with this abnormality is reassured that a vagina can be created with minimal difficulty and that, despite the fact it may be shorter in length than a normal vagina, sexual gratification for both herself and her partner should be normal.

In Figure 1(C) there is no vagina, but a functioning uterus is present. Creation of a vagina by one of the surgical techniques described above is essential and urgent, with the cervical canal then needing to be connected to the newly created vagina. Although maintaining a patent track between the uterus and the created vagina is often difficult, it is much more likely to be successful where a cervix is present than where the lower pole of the uterus is globular. Under the latter circumstances a hysterectomy is usually required (Fliegner & Pepperell 1994).

The complete duplication of the uterus and vagina shown in Figure 1(D) is not usually discovered during adolescence unless the individual concerned attempts to use vaginal tampons rather than sanitary napkins. Difficulty may be experienced inserting the tampon if the diameter of the vagina on that side is too small, or satisfactory insertion of the tampon may not

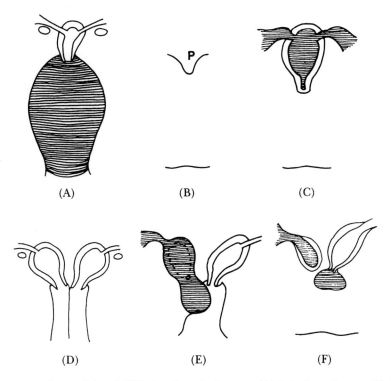

**Figure 1** *Six common abnormalities of Müllerian duct development: (A) imperforate hymen with haematocolpos (a haematometra is usually not present with this abnormality); (B) absent uterus and vagina; (C) absent vagina, obstructed uterus with cervix containing haematometra; (D) double uterus, cervix and vagina — all patent; (E) left uterine horn normal and empties into patent left vagina, but right vagina obstructed producing a haematocolpos, haematometra, haematosalpinx and often right-sided endometriosis (also has absent right kidney); (F) multiple developmental abnormalities, including absent lower two-thirds of vagina, obstructed right uterus with no cervix and containing haematometra, obstructed left upper vagina with small haematocolpos, haematometra and haematosalpinx*

result in all of the menstrual loss being absorbed as this is passing down the vagina which does not contain the tampon, thus staining her underwear.

Figure 1(E) shows the most common form of unilateral Müllerian duct obstruction encountered in clinical practice. Menstruation occurs from the left uterus, whereas the right side is obstructed at the vaginal level resulting in retention of menses in the vagina, uterus and tube on that side. The kidney on the affected side is also usually absent. Division of the vaginal septum from below, ensuring the obstructed vagina is widely opened from its most dependent point inferiorly to the level of the cervix superiorly, is a straightforward procedure and allows the retained menses to be released and subsequent menstruation to occur from the pre-

viously obstructed side. Sometimes endometriosis resulting from the retrograde menstruation also needs to be treated.

In Figure 1(F) two separate obstructed uteri are shown along with an absent vagina. The right uterus does not have a cervix and it is therefore best removed. The left uterus is functional, with its menstrual loss being collected in a small upper vagina which has become the site of a haematocolpos. Following the surgical creation of a vagina, and connection of this to the lower pole of the haematocolpos, little difficulty should be experienced in maintaining patency. This is in contrast to the problem shown in Figure 1(C), where no haematocolpos is present, and connection of the newly created vagina directly to the cervical canal would be necessary.

**Table 2** *The various therapeutic options for the gynaecologist caring for the mentally handicapped adolescent in Melbourne, Australia*

| Option | Consent required | Supervision required | Cycle control | | Contraception | Effect on premenstrual syndrome | Major side effects |
|---|---|---|---|---|---|---|---|
| | | | Timing | Loss | | | |
| Oral contraception | P | yes, daily | yes | less | yes | variable | breakthrough bleeding |
| Depo-Provera | P (< 18 years) GB (> 17 years) | doctor, 3 monthly | yes | amenorrhoea | yes | better | irregular bleeding |
| Prostaglandin antagonist | P | yes, 5 days/month | no | slightly less | no | none | gastrointestinal bleeding |
| Endometrial ablation | FC (< 18 years) GB (> 17 years) | operation | no | less or amenorrhoea | no | none | operative procedure |
| Tubal sterilisation | FC (< 18 years) GB (> 17 years) | operation | no | unchanged | yes | none | operative procedure |
| Hysterectomy | FC (< 18 years) GB (> 17 years) | operation | yes | amenorrhoea | yes | none, unless ovaries also removed | operative procedure |

P = parent or guardian, FC = Family Court, GB = Guardianship board

## MENTALLY HANDICAPPED ADOLESCENT

The gynaecologist is faced with a number of separate requirements when providing care for such an individual who may have profound physical problems in addition to being mentally handicapped. These requirements often include:

(1) The need to regulate the menstrual cycle to enable the care-givers to anticipate when menstruation will commence and thus be prepared.

(2) The need to reduce the menstrual loss, especially where this has been heavy or the normal amount is poorly managed by the girl concerned.

(3) The need to provide adequate pain relief if she is apparently disturbed by dysmenorrhoea.

(4) The need to alter the hormonal milieu in an attempt to reduce any premenstrual syndrome (PMS); this is likely to have been manifest by a change in behaviour in the premenstrual phase or a worsening in the frequency or severity of any underlying epileptic tendency at the time.

(5) The need to provide adequate contraception.

The whole matter is made even more complicated by the need to take into account the often competing views of some members of society and the parents, the fact that a sterilisation procedure or hysterectomy usually requires a court order if it is to be performed on a person under the age of 18 years, and that after the age of 18 years a guardianship board or court may be required to give approval before such an operative procedure can be performed on a mentally handicapped individual. In Melbourne, guardianship board approval is required if treatment with Depo-Provera is to be continued after the age of 18 years, even where the adolescent concerned is still living with her parents and they have been allowed to give permission for its administration prior to that age.

The various options available are listed in Table 2, along with their individual effects on the requirements needing to be addressed. Depo-Provera is often the option advised as it not only provides adequate contraception but usually renders the individual amenorrhoeic after six months of therapy. The maintenance of hormones at a constant level often results in a reduction in symptoms and abnormal behaviour previously seen in the premenstrual phase and also a decrease in any epilepsy.

The final decision for any one individual needs to be made after considering all of the options, but should generally be left until after the menarche has occurred. It is only then that the actual effect of the period on the individual will be known, including her own ability to cope with the menstrual loss.

# References

Evans, J. H. (1971) A review of 50 cases of primary amenorrhoea. *Aust NZ J Obstet Gynaecol* **34**, 467

Fliegner, J. R. H. and Pepperell, R. J. (1994) Management of vaginal agenesis with a functioning uterus. Is hysterectomy advisable? *Aust NZ J Obstet Gynaecol* **34**, 467

Frank, R. T. (1955) The formation of an artificial vagina without operation. *Am J Obstet Gynecol* **35**, 1054

McIndoe, A. (1950) Treatment of congenital absence and obliterative conditions of the vagina. *Br J Plast Surg* **2**, 254

Sheares, B. H. (1960) Congenital atresia of the vagina: a new technique for tunnelling the space between bladder and rectum and construction of the new vagina by a modified Wharton Technique. *J Obstet Gynaecol Br Emp* **67**, 24–31

Tanner, J. M. (1962) *Growth at Adolescence*, 2nd edn. Oxford: Blackwell Scientific

Wettenhall, H. N. B., Cahil, C. and Roche, A. F. (1975) Tall girls: a survey of 15 years of management and treatment. *Adolesc Med* **86**, 602

# 12

# Male contraception

*Richard A. Anderson*

The choice of contraception currently available to men is between the condom and vasectomy, and this contrasts with the wide range of hormonal, barrier and intrauterine methods (which can be active for up to five years) available to women. The two male methods, however, provide contraception for approximately 35% of couples in England and Wales (Oddens *et al.* 1994), demonstrating the demand for male methods of contraception. The readiness of men to use new methods is supported by opinion polls: in 1991, 56% of German men were willing to accept a hormonal male contraceptive, compared to 14% in 1977 (Nieschlag *et al.* 1992). In this chapter I will discuss some of the current issues in male contraception, including the methods in development.

## CONDOMS

The use of condoms has come full circle since their description in the sixteenth century as protection against syphilis, with the current resurgence of interest in condoms as protection against sexually transmitted infection including the human immunodeficiency virus (HIV). Their use as contraceptives came later, and is paralleled by the current promotion of use of a hormonal method in addition to a condom (Bromham and Cartmill 1993). This century has seen their development from linen and animal intestine, via vulcanised rubber, to the latex, multi-coloured, multi-flavoured varieties available today. Condoms are currently used for contraception by 20% of couples in the United Kingdom and by approximately 40 million couples worldwide. They are particularly popu-

lar in Japan, where they are used by 50% of couples. Two of the major issues relating to condom use are their reliability and the degree of protection against infection.

## Potential problems

The efficacy of condoms as contraceptives varies greatly between populations, with Pearl Indices of between 2% and 12% being found (Vessey *et al.* 1988). Reasons for failure include inconsistent use and problems such as breakage and slippage: user-related problems outweigh manufacturing defects. Breakage or slippage have been reported to occur in as many as 12% of intercourse acts, and are more common in the young and inexperienced (Sparrow and Lavill 1994). Others have found breakage rates of up to 12% and between 0.6% and 2% (Rinehart 1990; Cates and Stone 1992). Breakage rates also vary widely between countries, and while there is a good correlation between 'expected' breakage rates (on the basis of laboratory testing) and actual rates, in one study the best predictor of breakage rate was age of the condom (Steiner *et al.* 1992).

Other problems are caused by the expectations of the 'one size fits all' approach. The British Standards Institution specifies a flat width of 52 mm, while World Health Organisation (WHO) data suggest that 30% of men have larger penises than this (WHO 1992). While unrolled condoms can expand greatly, this is not possible when they are rolled up, as when being put on, and condom failure is significantly higher in the 19% of men who report that condoms are too tight (Tovey and Bonell 1993).

The two major United Kingdom manufacturers also supply narrower condoms, 48 mm and 49 mm flat width. The European Community has recently issued a new standard for condom manufacture, allowing condoms between 44- and 56-mm flat width, with harmonisation of manufacturing and testing procedures across Europe (Carnall 1996). Condoms also continue to be regarded as messy and inconvenient, reducing sexual pleasure and with connotations of infidelity (Stewart *et al.* 1991; Choi, Rickman and Catania 1994; Oddens *et al.* 1994).

## Reducing sexually transmitted diseases

Condoms reduce the transmission of many sexually transmitted diseases. Spermicides such as Nonoxynol-9, which are added to the lubricant during manufacture, also have anti-infective properties, although activity against HIV is less certain (Feldbum *et al.* 1995). Nonoxynol-9 also has a dose-dependent irritant effect on vaginal and cervical epithelium, possibly reducing the protection offered with frequent use. Natural membrane condoms do not provide as much protection against infection (Lytle *et al.* 1990). Worldwide, the spread of HIV infection depends on heterosexual intercourse, and there is now evidence that condom use can protect both men and women against heterosexual transmission of the virus. A large amount of government money has been spent on promoting the 'safe sex' message, and use of barrier methods in the United Kingdom by women aged 15–24 years has doubled between 1984 and 1992 (Oddens *et al.* 1994). In the United States condom sales more than doubled in 1987 following similar publicity (Moran *et al.* 1990). A meta-analysis of retrospective data from studies of partners of HIV-positive subjects suggests that consistent use of condoms may reduce the risk of transmission by 69% (Weller 1993). The importance of co-existing infection is demonstrated by a study of Zairean prostitutes, in which condom promotion was allied with sexually transmitted disease treatment. The incidence of HIV infection declined with time from 11.7 per 100 woman years in the first six months to 4.4 per 100 woman years over six months, three

years later. There was an increase in regular condom use from 11% to 68%, and seroconversion was associated with irregular condom use, gonorrhoea, trichomoniasis and genital ulcerative disease (Laga *et al.* 1994). A benefit has also been demonstrated in a prospective study of 304 heterosexual couples where one partner was HIV positive who were followed up for an average of 20 months (De Vincenti 1994). There were no seroconversions in 124 couples who used condoms consistently, compared to a rate of 4.8 per 100 person years in inconsistent users. While this study provides good evidence of a protective effect of consistent condom use, it is noteworthy that nearly half the couples studied continued to have unprotected intercourse despite counselling. Thus, a high incidence of risk-taking in the general population should not be unexpected, although the potential benefits of consistent condom use are clear. Male-to-female transmission of HIV is approximately twice as likely as female-to-male (Haverkos and Battjes 1992). Condom use has also been suggested to protect against the development of cervical intraepithelial neoplasia (CIN) II and III. An odds ratio of 0.5 for 'ever use' of condoms was found, with a greater effect in those using barrier methods for longer periods of time (Coker *et al.* 1991).

## VASECTOMY

Vasectomy is increasingly popular as a method of contraception, and is now used by more couples than female sterilisation in England and Wales (Oddens *et al.* 1994). The reasons for this include its ease, as it is performed as an outpatient under local anaesthesia, infrequency of complications and low failure rate, as well as reflecting a change in attitude in the population.

As with female sterilisation, counselling of the couple is the most important factor in reducing the incidence of regret, which is estimated to be 3%. The couple should be made aware of the possibility of failure of the method, estimated to be between zero and 2.2% (Liskin, Pike and Quillin 1983), usually due to failure to await the confirmation of azoospermia and late recanalisation. A recent survey of British urologists suggests that approximately 5% of vasectomies are repeated within six months (Benger, Swami and Gingell 1995).

## Confirming azoospermia

Azoospermia, the complete absence of spermatozoa from the ejaculate, is routinely confirmed by analysis of two ejaculates at 12 and 16 weeks postoperatively, which will allow identification of those patients in whom the surgical technique was incorrect. Motile sperm are absent from the semen after 10 ejaculates in 35% of men, but this can take up to 50 ejaculations to occur in others (Sivanesarantham 1990). It is thus essential that sexual activity is resumed after only a brief period of abstinence (approximately one week). The abstinence is to allow sufficient healing of the cut ends of the vas deferens to prevent 'blow out' by the forceful peristalsis which occurs during ejaculation. Earlier testing has been recommended, with the absence of motile spermatozoa in the ejaculate after four weeks being found to be as reliable as complete azoospermia (Edwards 1993). Further testing was required only if there were motile spermatozoa present, and this regimen was found to be independent of the number of post-vasectomy ejaculations.

Late recanalisation probably occurs more frequently than has been recognised. Cases of proven paternity (by DNA analysis) in the presence of azoospermia have been reported (O'Brien et al. 1995), and a survey of 1000 men one year after successful vasectomy demonstrated the presence of spermatozoa in six, although only intermittently and at very low density (Smith, Cranston and O'Brien 1994).

## Complications

Complications of vasectomy include haematoma formation, granulomas (either from suture material or spermatozoa), infection and the development of antisperm antibodies. In one study of 200 men in Edinburgh, 17% had reported to their general practitioner within two weeks of vasectomy with scrotal pain and swelling (Milne et al. 1986). Other studies have found postoperative complications in approximately 10%, although in one retrospective study of men four years after vasectomy, 33% complained of chronic pain, although only three of these 56 men regretted the operation as a result (McMahon et al. 1992). This may be sufficient to require further surgery (e.g. epididymectomy), which has been reported to give good results in only 50% of cases (Chen and Ball 1991). Other surveys have found less worrying results, finding chronic pain in only one in 200 men (Denniston and Kuehl 1995). Chronic pain, although severe in only a very small proportion of men, may therefore be an underestimated result of vasectomy, and counselling should cover this possibility. A reduction in sexual function is also reported by approximately 12% of men (Canter and Goldthorpe 1995), but there is an absence of good controlled studies.

The possibility that vasectomy may cause an increase in the incidence of prostatic and testicular carcinoma has attracted considerable attention, both scientifically and in the media. Initially this was based on two small studies, one from Scotland and one from Ireland, involving only eight and three cases, respectively, of testicular carcinoma (Thornhill, Butler and Fitzpatrick 1987; Cale et al. 1990). Subsequently, large studies in the United Kingdom and United States (involving over 600 men with testicular carcinoma) found no increase in cancer risk in men in whom the vasectomy had been carried out over 20 years before (Giovannucci et al. 1992). The Oxford linkage project study compared 13,246 men after vasectomy with 22,196 controls, and suggested a reduced risk of testicular carcinoma (Nienhuis et al. 1922). Little, however, is known about the long-term effects of vasectomy on the human testis (Jarow et al. 1985; McDonald 1990). The major effect on the epididymis is the development of a chronic inflammatory infiltrate, the degree of which is related to the development of antisperm antibodies (Flickinger, Howards and Herr 1995). The increase in pressure in the epididymis is not transmitted to the seminiferous tubules.

Two large studies in the United States have suggested an association between vasectomy and prostatic carcinoma, particularly after a delay of 20 years or more, with a relative risk of 1.6 (Giovannucci *et al.* 1993a; 1993b). While these two studies, one prospective the other retrospective, were very carefully performed, the opportunity for bias remains, particularly as the subjects were of above average educational and socioeconomic status, and in a population with a high and rising incidence of prostatic cancer. Prostatic cancer is much less common in other populations, varying 50-fold across the world, and risk factors for the disease are poorly understood. There is also no convincing biological explanation for a causal relationship. Thus extrapolations of the United States data may not be of relevance in countries where the prevalence is low. Both the World Health Organisation and the United States National Institute of Health have issued statements discussing these points (Farley *et al.* 1993; Healy 1993), and conclude that there is no reason to change current practice. The WHO has also concluded that large studies in developing countries where the prevalence of prostatic cancer is low and vasectomy is widely practised are a low priority (Wildschut and Monincx 1994). It would, however, appear to be prudent to discuss this continuing uncertainty during counselling for vasectomy. The increase in atherosclerosis seen in monkeys after vasectomy appears not to be of relevance in man.

## FUTURE PROSPECTS

The clearest gap in male methods of contraception is the lack of availability of a hormonal method. This area of research has a clear physiological basis in our understanding of the gonadotrophin-dependent nature of spermatogenesis, and is the area closest to becoming a reality. Other areas of research include chemical and thermal interference with testicular and epididymal function, but many avenues thus far explored have been hampered by problems of toxicity.

## Hormonal male contraception

As spermatogenesis is dependent on gonadotrophin secretion, complete suppression of gonadotrophin secretion would produce azoospermia. This has been the basis for the investigation of possible hormonal methods of male contraception for 50 years, following the demonstration that administration of testosterone (as the propionate ester) to normal men caused a reversible reduction in spermatogenesis without affecting libido or potency (McCullagh and McGurl 1939). This has subsequently been confirmed and enlarged upon in many other studies using a variety of testosterone derivatives, alone or in combination with other hormonal agents. However, the goal of complete suppression of spermatogenesis to provide the required degree of contraceptive efficacy with the maintenance of libido, without side effects and in an acceptable method of delivery, remains elusive. This approach is illustrated in Figure 1. Trials involving the use of testosterone alone currently provide the most information and illustrate the major problems.

### Androgens alone

Two recent multicentre trials organised by the WHO have given us much information about the contraceptive potential of hormonally-suppressed spermatogenesis (WHO Task Force on Methods for the Regulation of Male Fertility 1996). Both involved the administration of 200 mg testosterone oenanthate weekly intramuscularly, which results in azoospermia in the majority of men, and severe oligozoospermia in the remainder (Figure 2), although by the end of the trial (i.e. 15–18 months treatment) only two of 33 men from the Edinburgh cohort had detectable spermatozoa in the ejaculate. In the first of these studies only men who became azoospermic were allowed to use the testosterone injections as their only contraceptive. The basis for this was that demonstration of azoospermia in masturbatory samples may not equate with azoospermia during sexual intercourse. In that study, only one pregnancy was reported in a total of 1486 months of exposure,

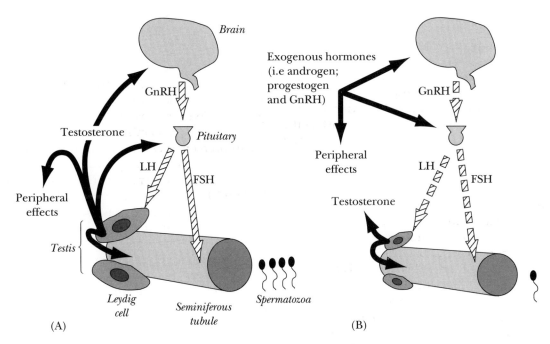

**Figure 1** *Hormone pathways involved in the control of spermatogenesis: (A) the normal situation; and (B) the environment induced by potential hormonal male contraceptives, with increased negative feedback from exogenous steroids at the hypothalamus and pituitary, reduced secretion of luteinising hormone (LH) and follicle stimulating hormone (FSH), and consequent reduction in Leydig cell activity and spermatogenesis. GnRH, gonadotrophin hormone releasing hormone*

giving a Pearl Index of 0.8 pregnancies per 100 woman years.

In the second study, men were required to use no other contraception once their sperm count had fallen to below three million/ml. Ninety-eight per cent of 349 men who entered the trial were successfully suppressed to below this level, and went on to use no other contraception for a further year. The overall pregnancy rate was only 1.4 per 100 woman years, and was related to sperm density at, or near to, the date of conception (Figure 3). These data are similar to those reported for the chance of spontaneous conception in oligozoospermic men attending an infertility clinic (Hargreave and Elton 1986). Following discontinuation of the testosterone injections, sperm density recovered to normal in all men, with a median duration of recovery to > 20 million/ml at 16 weeks.

While these large trials provide much encouragement that a hormonally-based male contraceptive method is possible, they also illustrate many of the present problems. These include incomplete suppression of spermatogenesis in a large proportion of men. Although only a very small proportion of men still maintained a rate of spermatogenesis incompatible with adequate contraception, complete and universal cessation of spermatogenesis would have clear benefits. Incomplete suppression of spermatogenesis has been a consistent finding in all studies of hormonal male contraception, whether using androgens alone or in combination with progestogens or GnRH analogues (see below), with azoospermia being achieved in 50–70% of men in most studies. This is in the absence of detectable follicle stimulating hormone (FSH) secretion, and may be the result of a low rate of ongoing steroidogenesis in the testis maintaining a sufficient intratesticular testosterone concentration to support spermatogenesis to a degree. In the studies just described, the very high peaks in peripheral testosterone concentration may have been sufficient to influence intratesticular events. The

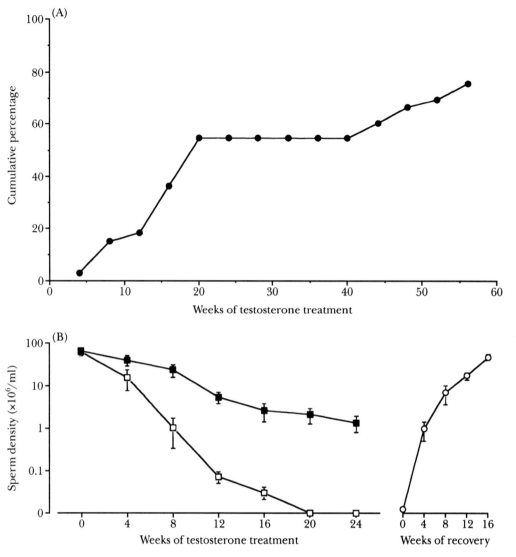

**Figure 2** *Data on suppression of spermatogenesis by testosterone oenanthate (200 mg per week intramuscularly): (A) cumulative percentage of men achieving azoospermia; and (B) sperm counts in men who became azoospermic within 20 weeks testosterone treatment (open symbols) and those remaining oligozoospermic at 20 weeks (filled symbols). Mean ± standard error of mean. Recovery data refer to all men: sperm densities had continued to decline in the oligozoospermic group with continuing testosterone oenanthate treatment. Data refer to the 33 men who comprised the Edinburgh cohort of a multicentre World Health Organisation study. (Reproduced from Anderson, R. A. and Wu, F. C. W. (1996) Comparison between testosterone enanthate-induced azoospermia and oligozoospermia in male contraceptive study. II. Pharmacokinetics and pharmacodynamics of once-weekly administration of testosterone enanthate. J Clin Endocrinol Metab **81** (3), 896–901.* © *The Endocrine Society)*

proportion of men achieving azoospermia also varied between centres in the WHO studies, with those with a predominantly white population reporting lower rates of azoospermia than those with Chinese populations, in which azoospermia was achieved in over 90% of men studied. The basis for this difference is unknown, although ethnic differences in androgen metabolism have been recognised for many years.

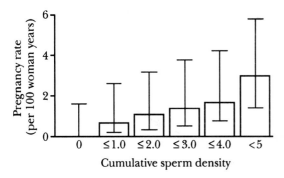

**Figure 3** *Pregnancy rate according to cumulative sperm concentration in testosterone-induced oligozoospermia. Mean ± 95% confidence interval. (From World Health Organisation Task Force on Methods for the Regulation of Male Fertility (1996) Contraceptive efficacy of testosterone-induced azoospermia and oligozoospermia in normal men. Fertil Steril 65, 821–9. Reproduced with permission of the publisher, The American Society of Reproductive Medicine [formerly The American Fertility Society])*

Side effects of testosterone treatment are a second problem, and reflect the supraphysiological dose used. Peak concentrations of bio-available testosterone were found to be tenfold higher than pretreatment, an effect amplified by the fall in sex hormone binding globulin (SHBG). Side effects include changes in haematocrit, high-density lipoprotein cholesterol, coagulation factors and prostatic size (Wallace *et al.* 1993; Anderson, Ludlam and Wu 1995; Anderson, Wallace and Wu 1995) which may indicate significant long-term risk. Other effects include a high incidence of acne and increases in lean body mass. The frequency of sexual intercourse did not change, although detailed testing revealed an increase in psychosexual stimulation, a measure related to arousability (Anderson, Bancroft and Wu 1992).

The large peaks in plasma testosterone reflect release of the testosterone ester from the site of injection, and are a characteristic of all currently available preparations with the exception of pellets of crystalline testosterone. Treatment of normal men with a dose of 1200 mg testosterone in the form of pellets resulted in a slightly quicker suppression of spermatogenesis than with injectable testosterone, but the proportion of men achieving azoospermia was similar (Handelsman, Conway and Boy-

lan 1992). A novel ester, testosterone buciclate, is being developed by the WHO, and has much more favourable pharmacokinetics. Thus, a single dose of 600 mg will provide androgen replacement in hypogonadal men for 12 weeks without initial supraphysiological levels (Behre and Nieschlag 1992). Preliminary studies in normal men demonstrated that a single dose of 1200 mg induced azoospermia in three out of eight men (Behre *et al.* 1995), but this drug may be of greater use in combination with a non-androgenic drug to suppress gonadotrophin secretion. This would then require only physiological testosterone replacement to prevent hypogonadal symptoms. Both progestogens and GnRH analogues may be used for this, and are discussed below.

A further potential problem is the relatively slow onset and offset of suppression of spermatogenesis. Median duration of suppression to reach three million/ml was 15 weeks, and recovery time was similar (although fertility is restored more quickly). This duration of suppression is likely to be similar for all hormonal methods, and is similar to the time needed for achievement of azoospermia after vasectomy. The acceptability of these aspects of hormonal male contraception still needs to be carefully explored in the general population, but is clearly important in designing a method for widespread practical use.

*Androgen–progestogen combinations*

Progestogens inhibit gonadotrophin secretion in men, with subsequent suppression of spermatogenesis. The most widely studied combination has been depot medroxyprogesterone acetate (MPA) with testosterone oenanthate, but as with testosterone administration alone, azoospermia is not uniformly achieved. The steroid 19-nortestosterone has both androgenic and progestogenic effects, and in combination with MPA causes azoospermia. In one trial in Indonesia, in which testosterone oenanthate or 19-nortestosterone were administered weekly in combination with depot-MPA every six weeks, azoospermia was achieved in 98% and very similar patterns of suppression were achieved with the two androgens (WHO Task Force on Methods for the Regulation of Male Fertility 1993).

A promising alternative is oral administration of the progestogen. Levonorgestrel plus testosterone replacement caused profound suppression of spermatogenesis (Bebb *et al.* 1996), with azoospermia achieved in 12 out of 18 men receiving 500 mg levonorgestrel daily and 100 mg testosterone oenanthate weekly, with sperm density of less than three million/ml in the remaining men. Interestingly, the combination of the potent progestogen and antiandrogen, cyproterone acetate, with testosterone caused azoospermia in all 10 men tested (Meriggiola *et al.* 1995). While this combination may seem illogical, it is possible that the antiandrogenic effect of cyproterone acting within the testis may have had a crucial effect. Further data are required to clarify the validity of this finding. There is, so far, no published data using third-generation progestogens in this context, but trials are in progress. The combination of an oral progestogen with a long-acting androgen, such as testosterone buciclate, may prove to be a major step towards an acceptable form of administration. Additional possibilities include implant preparations of progestogen, as used for female contraception.

*Analogues of gonadotrophin releasing hormone*

Analogues of gonadotrophin releasing hormone (GnRH) with both agonist and more recently antagonist properties have been developed and investigated as male contraceptive agents, both alone or in combination with androgens. The GnRH agonists are in widespread use in gynaecological practice in a variety of pharmaceutical forms, but results in men have been disappointing with azoospermia not being consistently achieved. In a trial using an implant of the long-acting GnRH agonist buserelin, the combination of buserelin with 19-nortestosterone caused less consistent suppression of spermatogenesis than when the androgen was given alone. Treatment with buserelin resulted in FSH concentrations returning towards baseline levels after nine to 15 weeks of treatment despite continuing inhibi-

tion of luteinising hormone (LH) secretion (Behre *et al.* 1992).

The more recent development of GnRH antagonists has led to a resurgence in interest in this method of male fertility regulation despite initial problems with histamine-like side effects. As with other non-androgen methods, replacement androgen is required. This has the additional advantage of having an inhibitory effect on GnRH secretion, which would otherwise increase and, thus, tend to overcome the effect of the antagonist.

As with the GnRH agonists, FSH secretion is relatively resistant to suppression, but azoospermia was achieved in seven out of eight subjects using a protocol in which the antagonist was administered followed by a low dose of testosterone oenanthate after two weeks (Pavlou *et al.* 1991). With the replacement dose used the plasma concentration of testosterone was only approximately 20% of baseline, but this appeared sufficient to prevent complaints of reduced libido or sexual activity. This finding has recently been confirmed by a further seven out of eight subjects achieving azoospermia following treatment with the same GnRH antagonist, although a more physiological replacement dose of testosterone was used (Tom *et al.* 1992). New GnRH antagonists are becoming available, but only very preliminary pharmacodynamic data are available (Behre *et al.* 1992). These results suggest that GnRH antagonists are promising agents for male fertility regulation, but there are clearly major problems with administration to be overcome, in addition to questions about the degree to which spermatogenesis is suppressed.

Therefore, it appears that inhibition of gonadotrophin secretion by progestogen or GnRH antagonists with replacement testosterone administration results in azoospermia in the majority of men, and the use of these agents rather than androgen alone avoids or reduces the incidence of side effects related to the supraphysiological doses of androgen required. This will be associated with a reduction in the possible risks of long-term androgen replacement therapy. Conversely, the use of non-androgenic gonadotrophin suppression and subphysiological testosterone replacement offers the possibility of health benefits of hormonal male contraception, analogous to the effects of the combined contraceptive pill on the risk of endometrial and ovarian cancer in women. The Contraception Development Network in Edinburgh is currently carrying out a survey of men's attitudes to contraception in general and proposed hormonal male contraceptives in particular, and perceived health benefits rate very highly as desired characteristics of a 'male pill'. A hormonal method of male contraception for widespread use therefore remains elusive for the present, although the most recent results either are considerable steps forward in themselves or suggest clear pathways for future development using existing pharmaceutical products.

## Non-hormonal methods

Non-hormonal methods of male contraception rely on the ability to interfere with specific processes in sperm maturation in the testis or epididymis, or with sperm-specific biochemical pathways. Clearly, a logical approach requires an adequate understanding of the relevant physiology and biochemistry, which is at present not available. A serendipitous approach has generally been used in the past, but more systematic and rational studies are currently been undertaken. One potential advantage over hormonal methods is the possibility of rapid onset and offset of action.

The best known non-hormonal agent is gossypol. This is an extract of cotton seed oil which has been long recognised to have an antifertility effect. The recognition that gossypol resulted in severe suppression of spermatogenesis led to large-scale clinical studies in China, in which gossypol was 99% effective in producing azoospermia or severe oligozoospermia (Qian and Wang 1984). Unfortunately, recovery is slow, and in 10% the effect is irreversible. Additional side effects include weakness, gastrointestinal upset, loss of libido and hypokalaemia, which was serious in a small proportion (Liu *et al.* 1981). While a number of potentially important biochemical effects of gossypol have been described (reviewed by Wu 1988), it is unclear which are relevant *in vivo* as the antifertility effect is specific to one steroisomer. Gossypol, therefore, may have a role in the investigation of potential sites of action of antifertility agents, but the toxicity of the natural product precludes further clinical study at present.

Extracts of a second Chinese plant may have more promise. *Tripterygium wilfordii* Hook.f. is a vine used in herbal medicine for a wide variety of complaints, and was noted to have an antifertility effect in men. Systematic experiments in rats revealed a marked effect on sperm motility, with less of an effect on density, which was reversible without apparent toxicity (Qian, Zhong and Xu 1986). Similar effects were noted in a small group of men (Qian *et al.* 1986), and subsequently a systematic approach to fractionated extracts has been undertaken (Qian, Xu and Zhong 1995). Six compounds with antifertility action were isolated, with testicular and epididymal effects. Higher doses had an immunosuppressive action. Much needs to be done to investigate the toxicity of these compounds, but this work demonstrates the potential value of a systematic approach.

While a specific epididymal action is very attractive as it avoids interference with the endocrine function of the testis, lack of understanding of epididymal function has limited this approach. Several compounds with epididymal effects have been investigated, including α-chlorohydrin and the 6-chloro-6-deoxysugars. Both groups of compounds act by inhibition of spermatozoal glucose metabolism (Ford and Waites 1978), but their clinical use is limited by toxicity.

Scrotal warming reduces spermatogenesis in experimental animals without altering testosterone levels, although higher LH levels indicate a greater drive to the testis (Galil and Setchell 1988). This approach has also been used in humans (Mieusset *et al.* 1985; Shafik 1992), azoospermia being achieved in all 14 subjects and maintained for one year. Full reversibility was indicated by recovery of sperm density in the ejaculate, and by successful pregnancy thereafter (Shafik 1992). This is an important consideration as defective embryological development has been reported following scrotal insulation in rams (Mieusset *et al.* 1992).

## CONCLUSION

Male methods make a disproportionate contribution to overall contraceptive use, despite the major deficiencies of existing methods. Two-thirds of couples who took part in a recent WHO contraceptive efficacy trial in Edinburgh gave inability to find a contraceptive method with which they were happy as the main reason for taking part, despite the experimental and uncertain contraception offered. The remaining third gave the desire to see new male methods becoming available as their main reason for participating (author's unpublished observations). It is clear that there is considerable hidden demand for safe and effective male methods, hormonal or chemical, but the current involvement of the pharmaceutical industry is minimal. Nevertheless the developments discussed above show the range of approaches being investigated and, particularly with epididymal methods, illustrate the importance of increasing our basic knowledge of male reproductive function.

# References

Anderson, R. A., Bancroft, J. and Wu, F. C. W. (1992) The effects of exogenous testosterone on sexuality and mood of normal men. *J Clin Endocrinol Metab* **75**, 1503–7

Anderson, R. A., Ludlam, C. A. and Wu, F. C. W. (1995) Haemostatic effects of supraphysiological levels of testosterone in normal men. *Thromb Haemost* **74**, 693–7

Anderson, R. A., Wallace, E. M. and Wu, F. C. W. (1995) Effect of testosterone enanthate on serum lipoproteins in man. *Contraception* **52**, 115–19

Anderson, R. A. and Wu, F. C. W. (1996) Comparison between testosterone enanthate-induced azoospermia and oligozoospermia in male contraceptive study. II. Pharmacokinetics and pharmacodynamics of once-weekly administration of testosterone enanthate. *J Clin Endocrinol Metab* **81** (3), 896–901

Bebb, R. A., Anawalt, B. D., Christensen, R. B. *et al.* (1996) Combined administration of levonorgestrel and testosterone induces more rapid and effective suppression of spermatogenesis than testosterone alone: a promising male contraceptive approach. *J Clin Endocrinol Metab* **81**, 757–62

Behre, H. M., Baus, S., Kleisch, S. *et al.* (1995) Potential of testosterone buciclate for male contraception: endocrine differences between responders and non-responders. *J Clin Endocrinol Metab* **80**, 2394–403

Behre, H. M., Klein, B., Steinmeyer, E. *et al.* (1992) Effective suppression of luteinizing hormone and testosterone by single doses of the new gonadotrophin-releasing hormone antagonist Cetrorelix (SB-75) in normal men. *J Clin Endocrinol Metab* **75**, 393–8

Behre, H. M., Nashan, D., Hubert, W. and Nieschlag, E. (1992) Depot gonadotrophin-releasing hormone agonist blunts the androgen-induced suppression of spermatogenesis in a clinical trial of male contraception. *J Clin Endocrinol Metab* **74**, 84–90

Behre, H. M. and Nieschlag, E. (1992) Testosterone buciclate (20-Aet-1) in hypogonadal men: pharmacokinetics and pharmacodynamics of the new long-acting androgen ester. *J Clin Endocrinol Metab* **75**, 1204–10

Benger, J. R., Swami, S. K. and Gingell, J. C. (1995) Persistent spermatozoa after vasectomy: a survey of British urologists. *Br J Urol* **76**, 376–9

Bromham, D. R. and Cartmill, R. S. V. (1993) Are current sources of contraceptive advice adequate to meet changes in contraceptive practice? A study of patients requesting termination of pregnancy. *Br J Fam Plann* **19**, 179–83

Cale, A. R. J., Farouk, M., Prescott, R. J. and Wallace, I. W. J. (1990) Does vasectomy accelerate testicular tumour? Importance of testicular examinations before and after vasectomy. *BMJ* **300**, 370

Canter, A. K. and Goldthorpe, S. B. (1995) Vasectomy-patient satisfaction in general practice: a follow up study. *Br J Fam Plann* **21**, 58–60

Carnall, D. (1996) Condom trade barriers come down across Europe. *BMJ* **312**, 597

Cates, W. and Stone, K. M. (1992) Family planning, sexually transmitted diseases and contraceptive choice: a literature update — part 1. *Fam Plann Perspect* **24**, 75–84

Chen, T. F. and Ball, R. Y. (1991) Epididymectomy for post-vasectomy pain: a histological review. *Br J Urol* **68**, 407–13

Choi, K.-H., Rickman, R. and Catania, J. A. (1994) What heterosexual adults believe about condoms. *N Engl J Med* **331**, 406–7

Coker, A. L., Hulka, B. S., McCann, M. F. and Walton, L. A. (1991) Barrier methods of contraception and cervical intraepithelial neoplasia. *Contraception* **45**, 1–10

Denniston, G. C. and Kuehl, L. (1995) Open-ended vasectomy: approaching the ideal technique. *J Am Board Fam Pract* **7**, 285–7

De Vincenti, I. (for the European Study Group on Heterosexual Transmission of HIV) (1994) A longitudinal study of human immunodeficiency virus transmission by heterosexual partners. *N Engl J Med* **331**, 341–6

Edwards, I. S. (1993) Earlier testing after vasectomy, based on the absence of motile sperm. *Fertil Steril* **59**, 431–6

Farley, T. M. M., Meirik, O., Mehta, S. and Waites, G. M. H. (1993) The safety of vasectomy: recent concerns. *Bull World Health Organ* **71**, 413–419

Feldblum, P. J., Morrison, C. S., Roddy, R. E. and Cates, W. Jr (1995) The effectiveness of barrier methods of contraception in preventing the spread of HIV. *AIDS* **9** (Suppl. A) 585–93

Flickinger, C. J., Howards, S. S. and Herr, J. C. (1995) Effects of vasectomy on the epididymis. *Microsc Res Tech* **30**:82–100.

Ford, W. C. L. and Waites, G. M. H. (1978) Chlorinated sugars: a biochemical approach to the control of male fertility. *Int J Androl* (Suppl. 2), 541–64

Galil, K. A. A. and Setchell, B. P. (1988) Effects of local heating of the testis on testicular blood flow and testosterone secretion in the rat. *Int J Androl* **11**, 73–85

Giovannucci, E., Ascherio, A., Rimm, E. B. *et al.* (1993a) A prospective cohort study of vasectomy and prostate cancer in US men. *J Am Med Assoc* **269**, 873–7

Giovannucci, E., Tosteson, T. D., Speizer, F. E. *et al.* (1992) A long-term study of mortality in men who have undergone vasectomy. *N Engl J Med* **326**, 1392–8

Giovannucci, E., Tosteson, T. D., Speizer, F. E. *et al.* (1993b) A retrospective cohort study of vasectomy and prostate cancer in US men. *J Am Med Assoc* **269**, 878–82

Handelsman, D. J., Conway, A. J. and Boylan, L. M. (1992) Suppression of human spermatogenesis by testosterone implants. *J Clin Endocrinol Metab* **75**, 1326–32

Hargreave, T. B. and Elton, R. A. (1986) Fecundability rates from an infertile male population. *Br J Urol* **58**, 194–7

Haverkos, H. W. and Battjes, R. J. (1992) Female-to-male transmission of HIV. *J Am Med Assoc* **268**, 1855

Healy, B. (1993) Does vasectomy cause prostate cancer? *J Am Med Assoc* **269**, 2620

Jarow, J. P., Budin, R. E., Dym, M. *et al.* (1985) Quantitative pathologic changes in the human testis after vasectomy. A controlled study. *N Engl J Med* **313**, 1252–6

Laga, M., Alary, M., Nzila, N. *et al.* (1994) Condom promotion, sexually transmitted diseases treatment, and declining incidence of HIV-1 infection in female Zairian sex workers. *Lancet* **344**, 246–8

Liskin, L., Pike, J. M. and Quillin, F. (1983) Vasectomy: safe and simple. *Popul Rep* **Series D** (4)

Liu, Z. Q., Liu, G. Z., Hei, L. S., Zhang, R. S. and Yu, C. Z. (1981) 'Clinical trial of gossypol as a male antifertility agent' in: C. F. Chang, D. Griffin and A. Wackman (Eds.). *Recent Advances in Fertility Regulation*, pp. 160–3. Geneva: Atar

Lytle, C. D., Carney, P. G., Vohra, S., Cyr, W. H. and Bockstaher, L. E. (1990) Virus leakage through natural membrane condoms. *Sex Transm Dis* **17**, 58–62

McCullagh, E. P. and McGurl, F. J. (1939) Further observations on the clinical use of testosterone propionate. *J Urol* **42**, 1265–7

McDonald, S. W. (1990) Vasectomy and the human testis. *BMJ* **301**, 618–19

McMahon, A. J., Buckley, J., Taylor, A. *et al.* (1992) Chronic testicular pain following vasectomy. *Br J Urol* **69**, 188–91

Meriggiola, M. C., Valdiserri, A., Pavani, A. *et al.* (1995) A combined regimen of cyproterone acetate (CPA) and testosterone enanthate (TE) as a potentially highly effective male contraceptive: effects on spermatogenesis and hormones. *Am Endocr Soc* OR29–5

Mieusset, R., Grandjean, H., Masat, A. and Pontonnier, F. (1985) Inhibiting effect of artificial cryptorchidism on spermatogenes. *Fertil Steril* **43**, 589–94

Mieusset, R., Quintana Casares, P., Sancheq-Partida, L. G. *et al.* (1992) Effects of heating the testes and epididymides of rams by scrotal insulation on fertility and embryonic mortality in ewes inseminated with frozen sperm. *J Reprod Fertil* **94**, 337–43

Milne, R., Munro, A., Scott, R. and Louden, N. (1986) A follow up study of 200 men after vasectomy. *Health Bull* **44**, 137–42

Moran, J. S., Janes, H. R., Peterman, T. A. and Stone, K. M. (1990) Increase in condom sales following AIDS education and publicity, United States. *Am J Public Health* **80**, 607–8

Nienhuis, H., Goldacre, M., Seagroatt, V., Gill, L. and Vessey, M. (1922). Incidence of disease after vasectomy: a record linkage retrospective study. *BMJ* **304**, 743–6

Nieschlag, E., Behre, H. M. and Weinbauer, G. F. (1992) 'Hormonal male contraception: a real chance?' in: E. Nieschlag and U.-F. Habenicht (Eds.). *Spermatogenesis–Fertilization–Contraception. Molecular, Cellular and Endocrine Events in Male Reproduction*, pp. 477–501. Berlin: Springer-Verlag

O'Brien, T. S., Cranston, D., Turner, E., MacKenzie, I. Z. and Guillebaud, J. (1995) Temporary reappearance of sperm 12 months after vasectomy clearance. *Br J Urol* **76**, 371–2

Oddens, B. J., Visser, A. Ph., Vemer, H. M., Everaerd, W. Th. A. M. and Lehart, Ph. (1994) Contraceptive use and attitudes in Great Britain. *Contraception* **49**, 73–86

Pavlou, S. N., Brewer, K., Farley, M. G. *et al.* (1991) Combined administration of a gonadotrophin-releasing hormone antagonist and testosterone in men induces reversble azoospermia without loss of libido. *J Clin Endocrinol Metab* **73**, 1360–9

Qian, S. Z. and Wang, S. G. (1984) Gossypol: a potential antifertility agent for males. *Ann Rev Pharmacol Toxicol* **24**, 329–60

Qian, S. Z., Xu, Y. and Zhong, J. W. (1995) Recent progress in research on *Tripterygium*: a male antifertility plant. *Contraception* **51**, 121–9

Qian, S. Z., Zhong, C. Q., Xu, N. and Xu, Y. (1986) Antifertility effect of *Tripterygium wilfordii* in men. *Adv Contracep* **2**, 253–4

Qian, S. Z., Zhong, C. Q. and Xu, Y. (1986) Effect of *Tripterygium wilfordii* on the fertility of rats. *Contraception* **33**, 105–10

Rinehart, W. (1990) Condoms — now more than ever. *Popul Rep* **H 8**, 10–12

Shafik, A. (1992) Contraceptive efficacy of poly-ester-induced azoospermia in normal men. *Contraception* **45**, 439–451

Sivanesarantham, V. (1990) Vasectomy — an assessment of various techniques and the immediate and long-term problems. *Br J Fam Plann* **16**, 97–100

Smith, J. C., Cranston, D. and O'Brien, T. (1994) Fatherhood without apparent spermatozoa after vasectomy. *Lancet* **334**, 30

Sparrow, M. J. and Lavill, K. (1994) Breakage and slippage of condoms in family planning clients. *Contraception* **50**, 117–29

Steiner, M., Foldesy, R., Cole, D. and Carter, E. (1992) Study to determine the correlation between condom breakage in human use and laboratory test results. *Contraception* **46**, 279–88

Stewart, D. L., DeForge, B. R., Hartmann, P., Kaminski, M. and Pecukonis, E. (1991) Attitudes towards condom use and AIDS among patients from an urban family practice center. *J Natl Med Assoc* **83**, 772–6

Thornhill, J. A., Butler, M. and Fitzpatrick, J. M. (1987) Could vasectomy accelerate testicular cancer? The importance of prevasectomy examination. *Br J Urol* **59**, 367

Tom, L., Bhasin, S., Salameh, W. *et al.* (1992) Induction of azoospermia in normal men with combined Nal-Glu gonadotrophin releasing hormone antagonist and testosterone enanthate. *J Clin Endocrinol Metab* **75**, 476–83

Tovey, S. J. and Bonell, C. P. (1993) Condoms: a wider range needed. *BMJ* **307**, 987

Vessey, M. P., Villard-Mackintosh, I., McPherson, K. and Yeates, D. (1988) Factors affecting the use–effectiveness of the condom. *Br J Fam Plann* 1988; **40**, 43

Wallace, E. M., Pye, S. D., Wild, S. R. and Wu, F. C. W. (1993) Prostatic specific antigen and prostate gland size in men receiving exogenous testosterone for male contraception. *J Androl* **16**, 35–40

Weller, S. C. (1993) A meta-analysis of condom effectiveness in reducing sexually transmitted HIV. *Soc Sci Med* **36**, 1635–44

Wildschut, H. I. and Monincx, W. (1994) Vasectomy and risk of prostatic cancer. *Bull World Health Organ* **72**, 777–8

World Health Organisation (1992) *Specifications and Guidelines for Condom Procurement.* Geneva: WHO

World Health Organisation Task Force on Methods for the Regulation of Male Fertility (1993) Comparison of two androgens plus depot-medroxyprogesterone acetate for suppression of azoospermia in Indonesian men. *Fertil Steril* **60**, 1062–8

World Health Organisation Task Force on Methods for the Regulation of Male Fertility (1996) Contraceptive efficacy of testosterone-induced azoospermia and oligozoospermia in normal men. *Fertil Steril* **65**, 821–9

Wu, F. C. W. (1988) Male contraception: current status and future prospects. *Clin Endocrinol* **29**, 443–65

# 13

# Urinary tract ultrasound

*Tony Blakeborough and Henry C. Irving*

The urinary tract was one of the first of the body systems to be investigated by ultrasound, with initial interest being focused on the kidneys. The advent of transrectal probes has improved imaging of the lower urinary tract, particularly the prostate gland, but this article will be limited to the female urinary tract.

It is not surprising, considering the close embryological relationships, that developmental anomalies of the genital tract are often associated with anomalies of the urinary tract. In addition, pathology in the urinary tract may present with symptoms that simulate pathology in the genital tract, and vice versa. Consequently, it is good practice to routinely examine the kidneys as well as the pelvic organs during gynaecological examinations. This adds little to the overall examination time, and considerable delays in diagnosis can often be pre-empted.

## TECHNIQUE

There is no specific preparation required prior to renal ultrasound, but the bladder is best assessed when fully distended, although any collecting system dilatation should be reassessed after micturition as a full bladder may be responsible. Conversely, collecting system dilatation which first appears or increases after micturition indicates vesicoureteric reflux, so it is useful to scan the kidneys before and after micturition in patients with urinary tract infections, especially children.

The right kidney can usually be examined with the patient supine, scanning in the anterior axillary line. Either an intercostal or subcostal approach can be used, and the right kidney

is usually clearly visualised using the liver as an acoustic window. In difficult cases full inspiration, raising the right side or scanning more posteriorly may help.

The left kidney is more difficult to visualise and it is best to start with the left side raised and by scanning in the posterior axillary line. The spleen can be used as an acoustic window for the upper pole, but unless it is enlarged it does not cover the lower pole.

While scanning young children the prone position may be useful to assess both kidneys, in older children and adults attenuation of the ultrasound by the paraspinal muscles reduces image quality.

Once a kidney has been located, the probe should be rotated to obtain the maximum longitudinal length from pole to pole as oblique scans will underestimate the true renal size. When the true longitudinal plane has been attained, rotation of the probe through 90° will find the transverse plane, and each kidney should be systematically scanned in both the longitudinal and transverse planes. It is important to scan through and 'off' the kidneys at both extremes in each plane to avoid missing peripheral abnormalities.

It is useful to obtain an image of the right kidney adjacent to liver and the left kidney adjacent to spleen in order to compare the relative echogenicity of the renal parenchyma. The parenchymal thickness and the presence of any hydronephrosis can usually be quickly established, and if the latter is noted an attempt should be made to trace the ureter. The lower ureters, if dilated, are best seen behind a distended bladder.

The bladder should be scanned in transverse and sagittal planes looking for intraluminal masses and irregularities or focal thickening in the bladder wall.

When a solid renal mass is discovered it is useful to look for para-aortic nodes and assess the patency of the renal vein and inferior vena cava as this may help characterise the nature and stage of the lesion.

## NORMAL APPEARANCE

### Position

The kidneys are retroperitoneal organs which lie on either side of the spine angled relatively to the coronal, sagittal and transverse anatomical planes. The upper poles are tilted posteriorly, with the lower poles lying more anteriorly. In addition, the lower poles diverge with the upper poles which are placed more medially. Finally, the hilum of each kidney is rotated about 45° so that the renal pelvis lies anterior relative to the lateral border.

### Kidney size

A reasonable estimate of renal size can be achieved by measuring the longest craniocaudal length, and this will vary according to age and size of the patient (the normal range in adults is 8.5–11.5 cm) with the left kidney often being slightly larger than the right. The kidneys are smaller on ultrasound than when measured at urography, because of the combined effects of geometric magnification of radiography and the osmotic diuresis induced by the contrast medium. Pregnancy results in an increase in renal size, while dehydration will have the opposite effect.

### Appearance

The normal kidney has a characteristic appearance with a central cluster of echoes caused by the highly reflective sinus fat around the pelvicalyceal system, surrounded by an outer zone of relatively poorly reflective renal parenchyma (Figure 1) (Amis and Hartman 1984). Within the parenchyma, the more reflective cor-

tex can be differentiated from the relatively less reflective medulla. The latter can be identified as the (medullary) pyramids with their bases against the inner cortical margin and apices pointing into the renal sinus echoes. Corticomedullary differentiation is variable in normal subjects and may be lost or enhanced due to various disease processes. The interlobar arteries run between the medullary pyramids and give rise to the arcuate arteries which run along the corticomedullary junction, where they may appear as small, highly reflective foci and should not be misdiagnosed as renal calculi. Their true nature can be confirmed with colour Doppler and, since they mark the corticomedullary junction, they allow true cortical thickness to be measured.

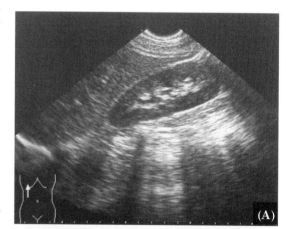

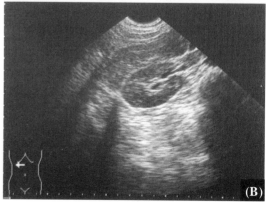

**Figure 1**  *The ultrasound scans of a normal kidney: (A) longitudinal view; and (B) transverse view*

## Renal cortex

The reflectivity of the renal cortex can be compared with the liver (right kidney) or spleen (left kidney) and should be of similar reflectivity to the adjacent organs. When the echogenicity of the renal cortex is significantly greater than that of the liver and spleen, renal parenchymal disease is highly likely.

## Renal parenchyma

The parenchymal thickness is variable in normal individuals and progressively reduces as part of the normal ageing process, when there is often an associated increase in the size of the central sinus echo as fatty replacement of the atrophic renal tissue occurs. Deciding that parenchymal thickness is pathologically reduced can be subjective and, although usually obvious when advanced, a lesser degree of thinning may only be apparent to the experienced observer. Increased cortical echogenicity usually accompanies chronic parenchymal disease. Focal areas of parenchymal scarring are easier to appreciate and are typically seen in chronic pyelonephritis, but may also be seen following cortical infarcts.

## Renal lobes

Embryologically, the kidneys develop from several lobes which normally merge during development but, occasionally, these may partially persist, giving rise to a lobulated contour to the renal outline which the unwary may interpret as either cortical scarring — due to the gaps between adjacent lobes — or the lobes themselves may simulate a tumour (Figure 2). With careful scanning the key observations are that:

(1)  There is normal cortical thickness over the medullary pyramids; and

(2)  The indentations between the lobes are between adjacent pyramids. It is the cortex overlying a pyramid that is reduced with true cortical scars.

Other examples of renal pseudotumours include splenic humps, seen as a lateral cortical

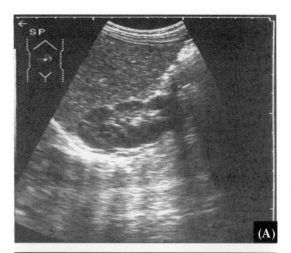

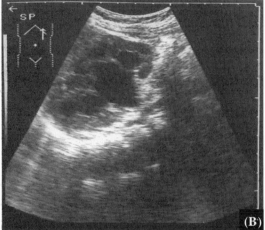

**Figure 2**   *The ultrasound scan of a three-year-old child who presented with a urinary tract infection showing: (A) a normal right kidney showing fetal lobulation; and (B) a hydronephrotic left kidney due to pelviureteric junction obstruction*

bulge in the mid-polar region of the left kidney adjacent to the lower pole of the spleen, and prominent septa of Bertin, which are simply columns of cortical tissue extending between medullary pyramids towards the sinus fat. In all these normal variants, the tissue reflectivity and echo-pattern within the pseudotumour is identical to that of the rest of the cortex, and there is no distortion of parenchymal anatomy.

## Renal vessels

The renal vessels can often be seen arising from the aorta and inferior vena cava and followed for a variable extent to the renal hila with the vein anterior to the artery. The right renal artery passes behind the inferior vena cava, while the left renal vein crosses the midline between the aorta and superior mesenteric artery. Multiple renal arteries and veins are not uncommon and may be detected with ultrasound. At the renal hilum, each vessel divides into several branches which can be seen as echo-free spaces within the highly reflective central sinus. Colour Doppler reveals their vascular nature, but they can also be distinguished from a dilated collecting system in that they do not extend to the peripheral parts of the sinus and are not connected to the renal pelvis. The renal vascular bed has a low peripheral vascular resistance and spectral Doppler waveforms show continuous flow through diastole.

*Pelvicalyceal system*

The pelvicalyceal system only becomes identifiable within the sinus when the urothelial surfaces are separated by more than the normal thin film of fluid and is thus normally not visible on ultrasound. Occasionally, an extra-renal pelvis is sufficiently 'baggy' to be visible, but the ureters are not seen unless there is obstruction or reflux.

*Bladder*

The bladder is best assessed when distended, should have a uniformly thin wall with no intraluminal masses, and should empty completely on micturition. The ureteric orifices cause small bulges in the bladder wall in the region of the trigone, and jets of urine emanating forth from the orifices can be graphically demonstrated on colour Doppler.

## CONGENITAL RENAL VARIANTS

### Duplex collecting system

Duplex collecting systems are not uncommon. They may be partial or complete, unilateral or bilateral, and are usually best demonstrated by urography. The kidney of a duplex system is usually larger and ultrasound may show separation of the central sinus fat into the upper and lower moieties. There may be an associated ureterocoele which appears as a thin membrane projecting into the bladder lumen at the site of insertion of the upper moiety ureter (Figure 3).

### Ectopic location and agenesis

When a kidney is not identified in its normal position, the possibilities include ectopic location or agenesis. A normal-sized contralateral kidney implies functioning renal tissue elsewhere and should prompt a search for an ectopic kidney as unilateral renal agenesis is associated with compensatory hypertrophy of the single kidney.

The majority of ectopic kidneys lie within the pelvis on the ipsilateral side (Figure 4), and when located on the contralateral side they are usually fused with the other kidney — crossed fused ectopia. Ectopic kidneys often have unusual shapes and may be malrotated. Some dilatation of the collecting system may be normal.

### Horseshoe kidney

Horseshoe kidneys are another variant. The lower poles converge and are linked across the spine via the isthmus, which may contain functioning renal parenchyma. Malrotation is again present, and the renal pelvis lies more anteriorly with the ureter passing over the isthmus.

## COLLECTING SYSTEM DILATATION

Ultrasound is sensitive in detecting collecting system dilatation, as even slight distension of the pelvicalyceal system is readily apparent within the central sinus echo-complex. Obstruction leads to hydronephrosis and can usually be excluded if ultrasound establishes that no pelvicalyceal dilatation is present (Lycus, Matthews and Evans 1988). Dilatation of the collecting system is recognised by multiple intrarenal fluid collections which communicate with each other and the central renal pelvis (Figure 2); this

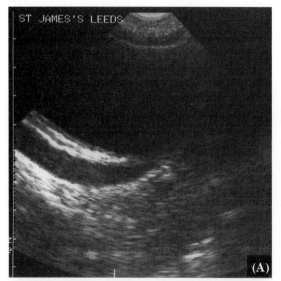

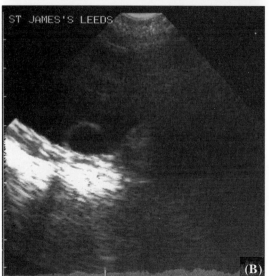

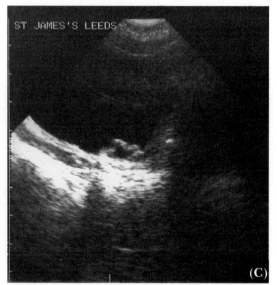

**Figure 3** *The ultrasound scan of a ureterocoele showing: (A) a dilated ureter running behind bladder towards the bladder base; (B) a ureterocoele distended with urine; and (C) a collapsed ureterocoele after expulsion of urine into bladder*

distinguishes them from multiple renal cysts which do not communicate. This has been referred to as the 'Mickey Mouse sign', where the central renal pelvis represents the head, and the dilated calyces the ears. However, not all dilatation of the renal collecting system is obstructive (Amis *et al.* 1982).

## Non-obstructive dilatation

There may be mild dilatation of the collecting system, particularly when the bladder is full during routine pelvic scans. Furthermore, the transient diuresis induced by the rapid water ingestion prior to the investigation could also contribute. In practice, mild dilatation is not uncommon and any dilatation present should, therefore, be reassessed after micturition.

During pregnancy, the majority of women will show some dilatation of the collecting system. This may increase throughout the pregnancy but, typically, disappears soon after the birth, usually within a few days (although minor dilatation of the collecting system may persist). Clearly, the mechanical effect of the enlarging uterus plays a part, but other factors have been implicated such as hormonal effects and increased renal blood flow (Peake, Roxburgh and Langlois 1983; Cietak and Newton 1985).

## Obstructive dilatation

When dilatation of the pelvicalyceal system is present an attempt should be made to trace the ureter in order to identify the level and possibly the cause of the obstruction. The upper ureter, if dilated, can be seen if the probe is angled

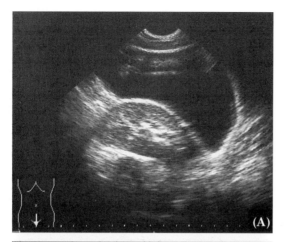

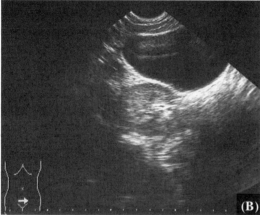

**Figure 4** *The ultrasound scans of a pelvic kidney: (A) a longitudinal view; and (B) a transverse view*

anteriorly from the renal pelvis. The mid-ureter is usually hidden by bowel loops, but the distal dilated ureter is best seen behind a full bladder (Figure 3). Marked dilatation of the pelvicalyceal system but not the ureter suggests pelviureteric junction obstruction.

Occasionally, the cause of the obstruction may be apparent. A variety of masses may appear within the dilated collecting system and be responsible for the obstruction. These include calculi, blood clots, sloughed papillae and transitional cell carcinoma. A bladder tumour may invade the ureteric orifice and cause dilatation of the ureter down to the vesicoureteric junction.

A renal calculus is seen as a highly echogenic focus with distal acoustic shadowing (Figure 5).

The larger the stone the easier it is to see, whatever the composition, as this has no effect on the ultrasound appearance. Higher frequency probes also improve detection, but they do not penetrate as far. Small stones can easily be missed and, surprisingly, large stag-horn calculi can sometimes be difficult to appreciate, so that a plain radiograph is recommended if calculus disease is suspected. Air in the collecting system (from infection or instrumentation) and vascular calcification can mimic calculi by giving rise to highly reflective foci. (These reflections result when ultrasound passes between substances of differing densities.) Finally, sloughed papillae and transitional cell tumours may calcify or become encrusted with urinary salts and present similar ultrasound appearance as calculi.

With a duplex system, there may be localised dilatation if only one moiety is obstructed, usually the upper one, which may have an ectopic ureteric insertion. This can be into the vagina or urethra, but vesical insertions are commonly associated with a ureterocoele which is a cause of obstruction itself and also predisposes to stone formation. In such an instance urography produces the classical 'drooping lily' appearance, which on an ultrasound scan looks like a fluid collection above a small, but otherwise normal looking, kidney (i.e. the lower moiety). The ureterocoele can be identified within the bladder as a 'cyst within a cyst' (Figure 3).

Low-level echoes within the dilated collecting system may form a gravity-dependent layer of debris resulting from either blood or infection, but ultrasound alone cannot distinguish between them. Clinical suspicion of infection in the presence of obstruction is an indication for urgent intervention. Treatment will depend on the exact circumstances, but the options include percutaneous nephrostomy under ultrasound guidance.

## RENAL CYSTS

One of the great strengths of ultrasound is its ability to demonstrate whether masses are solid or cystic. Simple renal cysts become increasingly common with age and are perhaps part of

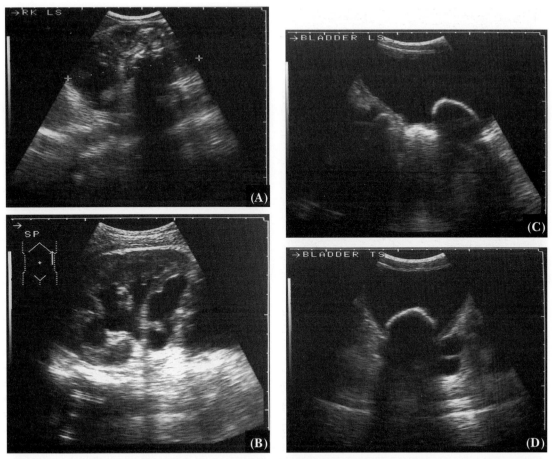

**Figure 5** *The ultrasound scans of calculi in a nine-year-old with repeated urinary tract infections: (A) the renal pelvis contains material that casts a strong acoustic shadow due to a stag-horn calculus, but there is no collecting system dilatation; (B) the collecting system of the left kidney is hydronephrotic; (C) a longitudinal scan through the bladder showing a large calculus; and (D) a transverse scan through the bladder showing dilated duplex ureters on the left side*

the normal ageing process. They are rare in children. The vast majority of renal cysts are asymptomatic, incidental findings but, occasionally, symptoms may result if they become infected or bleed, and a large cyst may rarely obstruct the collecting system. In practice, the most important distinction is between a simple renal cyst and a cystic mass (e.g. a necrotic tumour). The ultrasonic criteria for the diagnosis of a simple cyst are a spherical or oval shape with no internal echoes, and a sharply defined posterior wall with acoustic enhancement beyond it. Atypical findings include irregular shape, internal echoes, septation, solid components and calcification and, if any of

these features are present, then further investigation (e.g. computed tomographic [CT] scanning or cyst puncture/aspiration under ultrasound guidance) is indicated. If the ultrasonic criteria for a simple cyst are strictly applied and fulfilled, no further investigation is required because the diagnosis is sufficiently accurate (Bosniak 1986).

Multiple renal cysts are not uncommon in older patients, in either one or both kidneys which otherwise appear normal. This is in contrast to adult type (autosomal dominant) polycystic kidney disease in which, by the time it typically presents in early middle age, both kidneys are enlarged with complete disruption

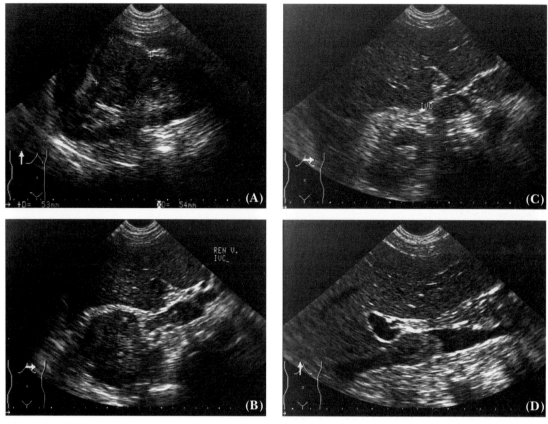

**Figure 6**  *Ultrasound scans of a renal carcinoma showing: (A) longitudinal view through a right kidney with a large solid mass; projecting anteriorly (the margins of the mass are indistinct in parts); (B) transverse scan showing tumour extending along the renal vein; (C) transverse scan showing tumour within the inferior vena cava; and (D) longitudinal scan showing tumour within the lumen of the inferior vena cava*

of the normal renal architecture by innumerable cysts of varying sizes and cysts may be present in other organs (e.g. the liver and, occasionally, in the pancreas or spleen). Relatives can be screened with ultrasound and if no cysts are present at 20 years of age it is most likely that the disease has not been inherited (Bear, McManaman and Morgan 1984). Tuberose sclerosis and von Hippel–Lindau disease are the other inherited conditions which are associated with multiple renal cysts, but other features of these conditions should allow them to be distinguished. Haemodialysis patients with end-stage renal failure develop multiple small simple cysts on their native kidneys, and patients with such acquired cystic disease have an increased risk of renal carcinoma.

## SOLID RENAL MASSES

Solid renal masses may be neoplastic or inflammatory and, although certain tumours have a typical appearance, there is sufficient variability and overlap in the ultrasonic appearances that ultrasound alone cannot distinguish between the histological types. Even the pseudotumours previously mentioned can cause diagnostic uncertainty. Therefore, while ultrasound will identify the mass, further investigation is usually required. The history may be helpful (e.g. previous trauma may suggest haematoma), which could then be followed up with repeat ultrasound. When a renal mass is discovered it is important to check the renal vein and inferior vena cava for invasion (Figure 6), para-aortic lymphadenopathy and liver metastases.

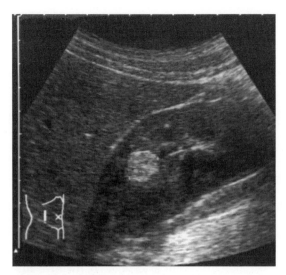

**Figure 7** *Longitudinal ultrasound scan showing a highly reflective well-demarcated angiomyolipoma mass*

Benign neoplasms include adenoma, angiomyolipoma and oncocytoma. Angiomyolipomas are typically small, well-defined, highly reflective tumours which gives them a characteristic appearance (Figure 7), but when haemorrhage has occurred the picture may be complicated. They have an association with tuberose sclerosis, when they are often multiple. Computerised tomography (CT) will confirm the fat content of these tumours which gives them that highly reflective appearance on an ultrasound scan. An oncocytoma generally shows a central stellate scar which is also shown on CT. If the diagnosis is suspected, a preoperative biopsy may allow partial nephrectomy.

Malignant neoplasms of the kidney include renal cell carcinomas, which are by far the most common in adults, Wilms' tumour (nephroblastoma) and, very rarely, sarcoma. Metastases to the kidney do occur and when lymphoma affects the kidney, this is usually by direct invasion from retroperitoneal nodes, which is almost invariably of the non-Hodgkins type.

Renal cell carcinomas are usually of similar reflectivity to normal parenchyma, but are heterogeneous in echo-texture. Cystic degeneration may occur and thus complex cysts require further investigation.

## BLADDER

The normal bladder is best examined when full, and appears as a smooth-walled, cystic structure with no intraluminal masses. Focal thickening of the wall or polypoid lesions projecting from it warrant further investigation, usually cystoscopy. Blood clots or sloughed papillae also appear as polypoid masses, but are mobile. Bladder stones are recognised by their ultrasonic appearances as with calculi elsewhere (i.e. highly reflective structures with distal acoustic shadowing, Figure 5), but are gravity dependent and will move if the patient is turned onto her side, which differentiates them from calcification on the surface of neoplasms which will be fixed in position.

## RENAL TRANSPLANTS

Ultrasound is useful for the initial assessment and subsequent follow-up of the transplanted kidney (Blakeborough and Irving 1995). Conventional ultrasound will demonstrate peri-transplant collections and hydronephrosis, and can be used for guiding subsequent percutaneous interventional techniques. Doppler sonography can assess vascular patency. Ultrasound is not specific for the diagnosis of rejection, although in biopsy-proven cases it can be useful for monitoring response to appropriate therapy. Routine surveillance will provide a baseline study and may lead to the early detection of complications before they are clinically apparent, alerting the clinician to impending transplant dysfunction.

# References

Amis, E. S., Cronan, J. J., Pfister, R. C. and Yoder, R. C. (1982) Ultrasonic inaccuracies in diagnosing renal obstruction. *Urology* **19**, 101–5

Amis, E. S. and Hartman, D. S. (1984) Renal ultrasonography: a practical overview. *Radiol Clin North Am* **22**, 315–32

Bear, J. C., McManaman, P. and Morgan, J. (1984) Age at clinical onset and at ultrasonographic detection of adult polycystic kidney disease: data for genetic counselling. *Am J Med Genet* **18**, 45–53

Blakeborough, A. and Irving, H. C. (1995) Ultrasound in the assessment of renal transplants. *Br Med Ultrasound Soc Bull* **2**, 18–24

Bosniak, M. A. (1986) The current radiological approach to renal cysts. *Radiology* **158**, 1–10

Cietak, K. A. and Newton, J. R. (1985) Serial qualitative maternal sonography in pregnancy. *Br J Radiology* **58**, 399–404

Lycus, K., Matthews, P. and Evans, C. (1988) Obstructive uropathy without dilatation: a potential diagnostic pitfall. *BMJ* **296**, 1517–18

Peake, S. C., Roxburgh, H. B. and Langlois, S. le P. (1983) Ultrasonic assessment of the hydronephrosis of pregnancy. *Radiology* **146**, 167–70

# Further reading

Cosgrove, D., Meire, H. and Dewbury K. (Eds.). *Abdominal and General Ultrasound*, Vol. 2, Chapters 28–35. Edinburgh: Churchill Livingstone

# 14

# Intractable incontinence

*Amar S. Bdesha and Timothy J. Christmas*

Although urinary incontinence can occur in any individual, the incidence increases with age. It affects 15–30% of elderly individuals in the community and up to one-half of those in institutions (Resnick 1988; Herzog and Fultz 1990). In the United States it has been estimated that the annual cost of managing incontinence is more than 10 billion dollars (Hu 1990). This is greater than the annual cost of providing renal dialysis services and coronary artery bypass grafting surgery combined. Most affected individuals respond to a variety of first-line treatments, which may include measures such as weight loss, drugs and physiotherapy. The majority of individuals who fail to respond to such measures will benefit from standard surgical treatments, including either transvaginal or transabdominal surgery, or a combination of the two. A minority of patients will not, however, respond to any of these procedures and these people are said to be suffering from intractable incontinence. In order to avoid condemning these patients to a lifetime with this condition, with its attendant risks of physical and psychological complications, it is necessary to recognise that a number of surgical treatments are available for such patients. Carefully planned and meticulously performed surgical procedures in specialised units may dramatically enhance the patients' quality of life.

## INCREASING URETHRAL RESISTANCE

The surgical options for patients with intractable incontinence can be divided into several categories. The first group of patients are those who require an increase in urethral resistance which cannot be accomplished by conventional surgery. This can be achieved in a number of ways, including periurethral injection treatment and by using an artificial urinary sphincter. These will now be discussed in turn.

## Periurethral injection treatment

An increase in urethral resistance can be achieved by the injection of bulk-enhancing agents at the bladder neck. The use of such agents is not new as the first literature reports appeared in 1938, when Murless described his experience of treating 20 women with injections of sodium morrhuate (a sclerosant). Subsequently, a variety of different agents, including polytetrafluoroethylene (Polytef), gluteraldehyde cross-linked collagen (GAX) (commercially marketed as Contigen), bioplastique and autologous fat have all been used. Polytef is an extremely thick paste that is a sterile mixture of polytetrafluoroethylene micropolymer particles (ranging in size from 4–100 μm), glycerine and polysorbate. Success and improvement rates of 70–90% have been reported with Polytef (Appell 1990).

The surgery is performed as a day-case procedure, either under general or regional anaesthesia, or under local anaesthetic augmented with sedation. Aliquots of 1–3 ml of the bulking agent are injected submucosally at two or three points around the circumference of the bladder neck. A satisfactory result is achieved when narrowing and occlusion of the proximal urethra occurs. Injection can be accomplished either transurethrally via a nephroscope or periurethrally. The procedure can be repeated in those patients with a poor or partial response.

Concern has been reported about the use of certain agents, particularly Polytef, since a number of complications may occur. These include distant emboli, migration, local granuloma formation and carcinogenesis. However, all of these data have been derived from animal experiments and it is not known whether such effects occur in humans. Furthermore, these potential problems may be circumvented by using the more inert substances such as GAX and bioplastique. GAX is a highly purified bovine dermal collagen lightly cross-linked with glutaraldehyde and dispersed in phosphate-buffered physiological saline. Appell (1990) summarised the results of a multicentre study which demonstrated an overall success rate of 95%. In patients with hypermobility type related stress incontinence the success rate was much lower. In those patients in whom GAX is employed it is essential to perform skin testing to identify the patients who would be allergic to it.

## Artificial urinary sphincter

Although the first attempt at prosthetic augmentation of urethral resistance was made by Berry in 1961, the first true attempt at placement of an artificial sphincter was in 1973 (Scott, Bradley and Timm 1973). Subsequently, the prostheses have undergone considerable modification. The modern artificial sphincter consists of three essential components: a cuff, a pump and a reservoir (see Figure 1).

This technique is best suited to incontinent individuals who have a compliant bladder which they are able to empty, but who have poor outflow resistance. Prior to placing an artificial sphincter the upper urinary tract should be assessed and, if obstruction or reflux is present, this should be corrected.

Before surgery, sterile urine should be documented and the procedure should be covered with the use of broad-spectrum antibiotics. All patients have a light bowel preparation to ensure that the rectum is empty and vaginal packs are placed to aid bladder neck and proximal urethra dissection.

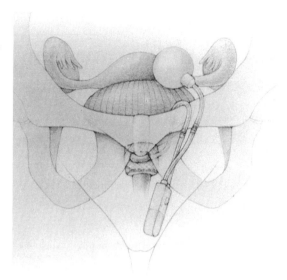

**Figure 1** *Diagrammatic representation of artificial urinary sphincter* in situ

The patient is catheterised, placed in the supine position and a lower midline or transverse abdominal incision is made. The bladder neck is identified and dissected free. This process is aided by incision of the endopelvic fascia. After the urethra has been mobilised, a sphincter sizer is placed around the urethra to ensure the correct sphincter cuff length is chosen. The cuff is then placed around the urethra but remains deflated. The tubing from the cuff is passed through the abdominal wall to the subcutaneous space anterior to the rectus fascia. The sphincter pump is placed in a dependent position in the labia, while the balloon reservoir is placed intra-abdominally (or in the paravesical space if there is adequate space) to avoid compression of the reservoir. Occasionally the reservoir must be placed intraperitoneally. Once the sphincter is in place and connected, the device is tested to ensure that it functions properly. It is then left deactivated for four to six weeks to allow healing to take place and to allow the formation of a collateral blood supply.

Urinary retention occurs in most patients for five to seven days due to oedema of the bladder neck and posterior urethra. This is best managed by either self-catheterisation with a small indwelling urethral catheter, or a suprapubic catheter situated well away from the device and tubing to minimise the risks of infection. Indwelling catheters, particularly those of a large calibre, are generally avoided to reduce the chance of cuff erosion.

Satisfactory continence is achieved in 95% of cases (Fishman, Shabsigh and Scott 1989). The incidence of mechanical dysfunction, including cuff leakage or pump malfunction, has been reduced with improvements in sphincter design. Other complications (e.g. infection, cuff erosion and cuff migration) can be minimised by following the precautions outlined earlier and by performing surgery in a specialised unit while employing a meticulous surgical technique. Many series, however, still report re-operation rates of up to 35% (Gundian, Barrett and Parulkar 1989), but this is in patients with incontinence from a variety of causes and those whose incontinence has resulted from prior surgery and for whom re-operation rates tend to be higher.

## INCREASING BLADDER CAPACITY AND COMPLIANCE

In those patients in whom the urethral resistance is adequate, but whose primary problem is a defect of the bladder storage phase, treatment is directed at the bladder rather than the outlet. Such patients would include those whose incontinence is due to detrusor instability which is refractory to drug treatment, and those whose incontinence is secondary to a diminished capacity bladder which may coexist with decreased bladder compliance. In such patients, *augmentation cystoplasty* is an appropriate and highly effective treatment. However, while this type of surgery can create a large bladder with better compliance, it may result in poorer bladder emptying. As such it is vital to ensure that the patient is adequately trained in the technique of intermittent self-catheterisation (ISC) prior to surgery. This is critical, not only to empty the bladder, but also to prevent the build up of mucus with consequent spontaneous bladder rupture in some patients. Any patient unable to perform ISC should not be a surgical candidate. Such patients would

include those who were quadriplegic, although in some cases a carer may be able to perform the catheterisation if it is required.

Careful patient selection is crucial to ensure optimal outcome. Care should be exercised in patients with renal impairment, since the use of bowel segments for augmentation may induce metabolic disturbances, particularly acidosis. Caution should also be exercised in patients with hepatic dysfunction, as the resorption of ammonia can lead to hepatic coma, and where there is poor urine output, since accumulation of mucus is more likely to occur.

Urodynamics, preferable with fluoroscopy, should be performed in all patients in order to define a bladder of insufficient volume and/or poor compliance. A leak point pressure of greater than 40 cm water is necessary for dryness in most patients.

Prior to surgery, all patients undergo standard bowel preparation and the procedure is covered with prophylactic antibiotics. Although a number of different bowel segments may be employed, the segment of bowel used for augmentation is not nearly as important as its size or configuration (Hinman 1989). The exact segment chosen is usually based on the surgeon's preference. Different bowel segments do, however, exhibit particular characteristics. For example, while the colon has a tendency to greater mucus production than stomach, the stomach can produce acid which is unbuffered and can potentially lead to painful irritation or even ulcer formation in the bladder. A number of bowel segments, including ileum, caecum and sigmoid colon, have all been used.

The technique of ileal cystoplasty is described, since this illustrates the general principles of augmentation cystoplasty and is the most widely used technique. This segment of bowel was first used experimentally by Tizzoni and Foggi in 1888.

The bladder is opened in a sagittal or coronal plane with electrocautery. It is important to divide the bladder almost to the bladder neck to prevent a subsequent 'hourglass' configuration which may lead to incomplete bladder emptying (Bramble 1982). A length of suture material is placed along the length of the opened bladder in order to determine the length of ileum required. The appropriate length of ileum (usually 20–40 cm) is then resected ensuring an adequate blood supply and bowel continuity is restored. The ileal segment is irrigated with saline and opened along the anti-mesenteric border with electrocautery. At this point the ureters are cannulated with ureteric catheters to prevent inadvertent damage during the anastomosis. The segment of bowel is then anastomosed with running Vicryl sutures to the opened bladder. Just prior to completion of the anastomosis the ureteric catheters are removed. A large-bore urethral catheter is placed and left *in situ* for 10 days. Depending on the degree of mucus production, regular bladder wash-outs may be necessary. After catheter removal the patient's voiding is assessed, renal function carefully monitored and, if necessary, ISC commenced.

## URINARY DIVERSION

In some patients increasing urethral resistance or augmentation cystoplasty will be an inadequate or inappropriate treatment. Such patients will require more radical surgery to achieve continence and this fundamentally involves either an internal diversion or a cutaneous diversion may be fashioned. The techniques include suprapubic cystostomy and bladder neck closure, cutaneous ureterostomy, ileal conduit jejunal conduit and colon conduits. These will now be discussed in turn.

### Suprapubic cystotomy and bladder neck closure

In certain patients incontinence can result from a failure in the storage phase of bladder function with a coexisting problem with the bladder neck and urethra. Such patients would include those with a variety of neurological disorders. Although some of these patients may be treated with ISC, with time, and particularly in those patients who have had indwelling urethral catheters, the urethra may demonstrate a marked increase in diameter. Even if a suprapubic catheter is placed in such cases they can still experience considerable urethral leakage of urine. Therefore, the best method of treatment involves formal closure of the bladder neck and placement of a permanent suprapubic catheter or formal suprapubic cystotomy.

The technique of bladder neck closure is of utmost importance, since simple closure has a high failure rate. Closure is achieved by dividing the urethra which is then inverted into the bladder. The inverted urethra is then closed from within the bladder, thus creating an 'ink well' closure.

### Cutaneous ureterostomy

Urinary diversion by means of cutaneous ureterostomy has the advantage of being able to achieve urinary diversion without the need for bowel surgery. The cutaneous ureterostomy can be fashioned either in a double-barrelled fashion, when both the ureters are brought to the surface, or by bringing one ureter to the surface and fashioning a transuretero-ureteric anastomosis. The major disadvantage of cutaneous ureterostomy relates to the condition of the ureters themselves. If normal calibre ureters are used, then, even with a V-flap technique designed to widen the ureters, there is a high incidence of stomal stenosis (Chute and Sallade 1961). In addition, due to the long length of ureter that must be freed of its blood supply in order for it to reach the anterior abdominal wall, an adequate collateral blood supply is necessary. Moderately dilated ureters are therefore of greatest use in creating a cutaneous ureterostomy, because they allow a double-barrelled stoma to be created, minimising the risk of stomal stenosis. If only one ureter is dilated this is best brought to the surface while the other ureter is used to fashion a transuretero-ureterostomy.

This technique is generally only feasible in children in whom cutaneous stenosis is much less likely to occur.

### Ileal conduit

The first reported construction of an ileal conduit appeared in 1935. However, this description by Seiffert suffered from the lack of an effective external collecting device (Seiffert 1935). Thus, it was not until 1950, when the procedure technique was described by Bricker, that an appropriate collecting device was included and the technique gained popular acceptance.

Prior to surgery the patient must be carefully assessed to ensure that they will be able to care for their stoma. In addition, the site of the stoma should be marked with extreme care. Skin creases and the belt or skirt line should be avoided, and the site should not be too close to previous scars which might interfere with proper adherence of the appliance. The site should be easily visible to the patient and the stoma sited as far away from the midline as possible, while still allowing the bowel to traverse the rectus muscle to minimise the risk of parastomal herniae. To ensure these criteria are met, the services of a skilled stoma nurse are invaluable.

Before the operation starts a full-bowel preparation is administered and perioperative prophylactic antibiotics are given. Surgery involves division of the ureters and their direction, usually to the right iliac fossa. An appropriate length of ileum is mobilised on its blood supply and the bowel transected, ensuring a good blood supply to the conduit. Bowel continuity is restored and the proximal end of the conduit is closed in two layers with Vicryl sutures. The ureters are anastomosed separately to the proximal part of the conduit using interrupted Vicryl sutures. This anastomosis is completed over ureteric stents or catheters. No attempt is made to create an anti-reflux mechanism, since this increases the incidence of anastomotic stricture. The overall incidence of anastomotic stricture is 6% if this particular ureteroileal anastomotic technique is employed. It is important to maintain the ileal loop in an isoperistaltic direction to ensure optimal drainage. The mesenteric defect is then closed to prevent internal hernias and the loop brought through the rectus sheath to the previously marked stoma site. A standard ileal stoma is fashioned with an adequate spout to prevent skin irritation. The ureteric stents are removed after 10 days.

## Jejunal conduit

The use of jejunum as a bowel segment to divert urine allows areas of pelvic irradiation to be avoided. However, metabolic consequences (including hyponatraemia and hyperchloraemic acidosis) are sufficiently common and severe to ensure that jejunal conduits are only used where no other suitable alternative exists (Golimbu and Morales 1975).

## Colon conduits

These conduits employ either the sigmoid or transverse colon. The ureters are anastomosed to the colon using a tunnelled approach in order to create an anti-reflux anastomosis to avoid upper tract deterioration. This technique is, however, unsuitable for patients with dilated ureters, since any hydronephrosis will be accentuated. A sigmoid conduit should also be avoided in the heavily irradiated pelvis.

## INTERNAL URINARY DIVERSION

The use of conduits, particularly the ileal conduit, has been proven over time as a safe and effective treatment for patients with intractable incontinence. The ileal conduit remains the 'gold standard' against which other forms of urinary diversion must be compared. However, conduits are not suitable for all patients and a number of problems may occur; for example, in some countries suitable external collecting devices are not available and the psychological effects of external stomas (their perceived social unacceptability and effects on sexual function) should not be underestimated. In an attempt to overcome these problems, a number of internal urinary diversion techniques have been developed. These include ureterosigmoidostomy, ileocaecal sigmoidostomy and rectal bladder urinary diversions. They will now be discussed in turn.

## Ureterosigmoidostomy

Ureterosigmoidostomy can be regarded as the original internal urinary diversion. Reports of this procedure can be found in the medical literature dating back to the 1870s (Smith 1879). Careful patient selection and preparation is essential to minimise the risks which can arise from connecting the ureters to the intact faecal stream. These potential complications include hyperchloraemic acidosis, hypokalaemia, pyelonephritis, renal failure and colonic malignancy as well as deterioration of upper tract function (Figure 2). The operation is usually reserved for older patients in view of the incidence of long-term complications. Contraindications include patients with neurogenic bladder dysfunction (as there may be coexisting anal sphincter dysfunction), patients with hepatic dysfunction, dilated ureters, impaired renal function or a history of previous pelvic irradiation.

Preoperatively the colon is evaluated to exclude any coexisting pathology and the integrity of the anal sphincter confirmed. This is done by instilling 400–500 ml of a semi-solid substance

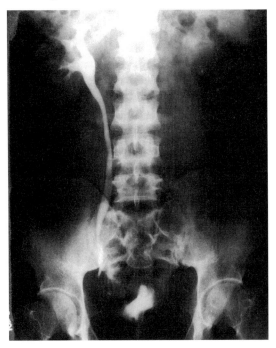

**Figure 2** *Loss of function of the left kidney following ureterosigmoidostomy*

(e.g. porridge) into the rectum and asking the patient to retain this for an hour while ambulant. If the patient is able to remain continent then the integrity of the anal sphincter is confirmed.

The surgical technique involves division of the ureters and the formation of ureterosigmoid anastomoses within submucosal tunnels to minimise the incidence of reflux. Stenting of the anastomoses is essential to reduce the incidence of anastomotic leaks. Although several studies have demonstrated the benefits of performing non-refluxing anastomoses to preserve renal function (Elder, Moisey and Rees 1979; Husmann, McLorie and Churchill 1989), other studies have shown none from such anastomoses (Shapiro, Lebowitz and Colodny 1975; Hill and Ransley 1983).

Surgically, ureterosigmoidostomy is a much less demanding undertaking than many forms of urinary diversion. Such patients do, however, have to undergo a lifelong follow-up in the form of regular colonoscopies, since the incidence of malignant change within the sigmoid colon is high (varying from 6% to 29%). This malignancy often occurs on the bowel wall opposite the ureteric anastomosis and may occur 10–20 years after urinary diversion. The mechanism is thought to be due to the presence of nitrosamino compounds in contact with the sigmoid mucosa for prolonged periods.

## Ileocaecal sigmoidostomy

Animal experiments have suggested that the development of bowel malignancy after ureterosigmoidostomy resulted from the presence of faecal carcinogens in contact with juxtaposed transitional and colonic epithelium. In an attempt to overcome this, an ileocaecal conduit can be constructed with the ureters anastomosed to the ileum, while the caecal margin is anastomosed to the anti-mesenteric border of the sigmoid colon (Rink and Retick 1987). However, the incidence of reflux is common, since the ileocaecal valve is often incompetent. At present insufficient data are available to determine whether the upper tracts are adequately protected by this technique. In addition, long-term follow-up in large numbers of patients is required to determine whether the long-term colonic cancer risk is decreased.

## Rectal bladder urinary diversions

A variety of ingenious surgical techniques have been described in an attempt to utilise the rectum as a reserve for urine, while separating it from the faecal stream. Although a number of variations exist, the basic principle involves anastomosis of the ureter to the rectum while the proximal sigmoid colon is disconnected and either brought to the skin as a colostomy (Mauclaire 1895) or brought down to the perineum (Heitz-Boyer 1912). Bowel and urinary control is achieved by utilising the anal sphincter. However, this procedure presents a formidable surgical challenge and the incidence of complications is high. Possibly the most devastating is the development of urinary and faecal incontinence.

## CONTINENT CUTANEOUS DIVERSIONS

In the majority of patients where a continent bladder replacement is required, continent cutaneous reservoirs have been employed. Although a number of different techniques are available, several general principles apply to all the techniques. For example, the reservoir is emptied by ISC and, thus, the patients must have sufficient hand–eye co-ordination to accomplish this task.

The site for the catheterisable stoma varies. The two favourite sites are at the umbilicus or the lower quadrant, through the rectus sheath and below the 'bikini line'. In between catheterisation the patient wears a small dressing or Elastoplast over the stoma site. The most demanding feature of any catheterisable stoma is the construction of the continence mechanism. A number of techniques have been used to achieve this. Tunnelling of the appendix is probably the simplest and involves the appendix being tunnelled into the caecum, creating a valve mechanism, which maintains continence

while the stoma is emptied by ISC (Duckett and Snyder 1986). However, a number of problems may arise. In some patients the appendix may have been removed at previous appendicectomy, or may be too short to reach the anterior abdominal wall after sufficient length allowed for tunnelling. In addition, only small diameter catheters of 12–14 Fr can be used rather than the more usual 20–22 Fr. This may lead to problems with mucus retention and cutaneous stenosis.

Another major type of continence mechanism is the use of a tapered segment of terminal ileum, including the ileocaecal valve, which is plicated to achieve continence. However, the ileal segment becomes elongated over time and the loss of the ileocaecal segment may lead to diarrhoea.

A further surgical principle used in constructing the continence mechanism is the formation of an intussuscepted nipple valve. The creation of such nipple valves is, however, technically demanding and a number of different techniques are available. One technique used is the Kock pouch (Ghoneim *et al.* 1987). Approximately 70 cm of distal ileum is mobilised and resected with its blood supply. Bowel continuity is restored. The middle portion of the ileum is folded in the shape of a 'U', with each limb of the 'U' measuring 20–25 cm. The medial borders of the 'U' are sutured to one another on the serosal surface with running Vicryl sutures prior to opening this central portion with electrocautery along its anti-mesenteric border. At this point, an intussusception of the afferent and efferent limbs is required. About 3 cm from either end of the mesenteric attachment is freed by electrocautery over a 6–8 cm distance. Intussusception is performed to create at least a 5 cm intussuscipiens. This is stapled in two quadrants with a TA55 (Auto Suture Co.) urological stapler which has the inner four staples missing to avoid deposition of staples at the distal aspect of the nipple valve which, otherwise, could act as a nidus for stone formation (Skinner, Boyd and Lieskowsky 1984). A further staple line is used to attach the intussuscipiens to the side wall of the reservoir and pinholes from the stabilising pin are then oversewn with absorbable sutures. The ureters are anastomosed to the nipple valve with absorbable sutures over ureteric stents. The anterior wall of the pouch is then closed with running sutures of Vicryl. The efferent limb is then sutured to the skin to create a continent cutaneous catheterisable stoma.

Absorbable mesh collars are advocated by some investigators to anchor the base of the nipple valve to the anterior abdominal wall. The authors' own preference is to use a mesh, but rather than attachment to the nipple valve, the mesh is attached to the mesentery of the pouch and this is subsequently used to anchor the efferent limb. Ureteric stents are routinely used and, as for the orthotopic Kock pouch, a contrast study is performed on the fourteenth postoperative day and the stents removed if the study confirms that there is no leakage of contrast.

The patient then commences ISC (Figure 3), initially every two hours, and gradually increases this period as pouch capacity increases.

A number of other continence mechanisms and pouches are sometimes created. These include the Benchekroun valve, the Mainz pouch and a variety of pouches which utilise the right colon with intussusception of the terminal ileum. However, the principles of all these techniques are similar, with the creation of a large capacity, low pressure, continent pouch with an anti-reflux mechanism.

Common to all pouches is the low initial capacity. Initial pouch capacity is 200–300 ml, but this increases to 750 ml over a period of

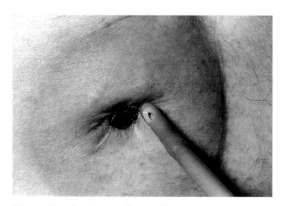

**Figure 3**  *Continent catheterisable cutaneous stoma*

time. The most common complication is failure of the continence valve mechanism. In Kock's original series this failure rate exceeded 80%, but in most current series averages 15% or less.

## ORTHOTOPIC BLADDER REPLACEMENT

A number of surgical techniques have been developed to provide orthotopic voiding diversions. However, in the treatment of patients with intractable incontinence such a technique has a limited role, since many patients with abnormal bladder function which required bladder replacement (e.g. patients with neuropathic bladders) will also have co-existing bladder neck and urethral disorders.

These techniques share a number of characteristics. They all involve providing a non-refluxing pouch of low pressure and high capacity which allows voiding, preferably by a Valsalva manoeuvre or, failing this, by clean ISC.

The hemi-Kock pouch is one of the orthotopic pouches commonly employed which illustrates the above principles. The technique is similar to that described for creating a continent cutaneous Kock pouch except that a slightly shorter length of distal ileum (55 cm) is required. In addition, an intussusception is only required for the proximal limb, since the efferent limb is anastomosed to the bladder neck. The anastomosis to the bladder neck is completed with interrupted Vicryl sutures and a large-bore catheter is placed immediately prior to completion of the anastomosis. The ureteric catheters are tied to the urethral catheter to facilitate their subsequent removal.

Postoperatively, twice daily wash-outs of the pouch are performed. The patient is commenced on $H_2$ antagonists to reduce mucus production. Once oral fluids are commenced, patients are encouraged to drink cranberry juice to further reduce mucus production. A cystogram is performed on the fourteenth postoperative day and the catheter and ureteric stents are removed if there is no pouch leakage.

The majority of patients achieve complete continence during the day, but nocturnal enuresis may occur with all orthotopic bladder reconstructions. The reason for enuresis is that nervous control between the new bladder and sphincter does not exist. Thus, external sphincteric recruitment can only occur under voluntary control. Timed voiding, however, helps the majority of patients, as does the increase in pouch capacity over time.

Such orthotopic bladder reconstructions were originally devised for male patients with reliance on the external urethral sphincter to maintain continence. However, they can be used in women by preserving the bladder neck to serve as the continence mechanism. A number of different pouches (including the Camey II operation) have been described, but they all share the basic principles of the hemi-Kock pouch.

## SUMMARY

An extensive array of surgical procedures exist to treat patients suffering from intractable incontinence. Many of these procedures are technically demanding. However, meticulously planned surgery appropriate for the individual patients carried out in specialised units has a high degree of success. The rewards for both the surgeon involved and the previously incontinent patient are extremely gratifying. Before such patients are condemned to a lifelong existence with their incontinence, when standard surgical treatments have failed, such specialised advice and assistance should always be sought.

# References

Appell, R. A. (1990) Injectables for urethral incompetence. *World J Urol* 8, 208–11

Berry, J. L. (1961) A new procedure for correction of urinary incontinence: preliminary report. *J Urol* 85, 771

Bramble, F. J. (1982) The treatment of adult enuresis and urge incontinence by enterocystoplasty. *Br J Urol* 54, 693

Bricker, E. M. (1950) Bladder substitution after pelvic evisceration. *Surg Clin North Am* 30, 1511–21

Chute, R. and Sallade, R. L. (1961) Bilateral side to side cutaneous ureterostomy in the midline for urinary diversion. *J Urol* 85, 280–3

Duckett, J. W. and Snyder, H. M. (1986) Use of the Mitrofanoff principle in urinary reconstruction. *Urol Clin North Am* 13, 271–4

Elder, D. D., Moisey, C. U. and Rees, R. W. M. (1979) A long-term follow up of the colonic conduit operation in children. *Br J Urol* 51, 462–5

Fishman, I. J., Shabsigh, R. and Scott, F. B. (1989) Experience with the artificial urinary sphincter model AS 800 in 148 patients. *J Urol* 141, 307

Ghoneim, M. A., Kock, N. G., Kycke, G. and Shebab, El-Din A. B. (1987) An applicance-free, sphincter controlled bladder substitute: the urethral Kock pouch. *J Urol* 138, 1150–4

Golimbu, M. and Morales, P. (1975) Jejunal conduits: technique and complications. *J Urol* 113, 787–95

Gundian, J. C., Barrett, D. M. and Parulkar, B. G. (1989) Mayo Clinic experience with the use of AMS 800 artificial urinary sphincter for urinary incontinence following radical prostatectomy. *J Urol* 142, 1459

Herzog, A. R. and Fultz, N. H. (1990) Prevalence and incidence of urinary incontinence in community dwelling populations. *J Am Geriatr Soc* 38, 273–81

Hill, J. T. and Ransley, P. G. (1983) The colonic conduit: a better method of urinary diversion? *Br J Urol* 55, 629–31

Hinman, F. Jr (1989) 'Bladder augmentation', in: F. Hinman Jr (Ed.). *Atlas of Urologic Surgery*, p.534. Philadelphia: W. B. Saunders

Hu, T. W. (1990) Impact of urinary incontinence on health care costs. *J Am Geriatr Soc* **38**, 292–5

Husmann, D. A., McLorie, G. A. and Churchill, B. M. (1989) Non-refluxing colonic conduits: a long-term life table analysis. *J Urol* **142**, 1201–3

Resnick, N. M. (1988) 'Voiding dysfunction in the elderly' in: S. V. Yalla, E. J. McGuire, A. El-badawi and J. G. Blaivas (Eds.). *Neurology and Urodynamics: Principles and Practice*, pp. 303–30. New York: Macmillan

Rink, R. C. and Retick, A. B. (1987) 'Uretero-ilealcaecalsigmoidostomy and avoidance of carcinoma of the colon' in: L. R. King, A. R. Stone and G. D. Webster (Eds.). *Bladder Reconstruction and Continent Urinary Diversion*, pp. 172–8. Chicago: Year Book Medical Publishers

Scott, F. B., Bradley, W. E. and Timm, G. W. (1973) Treatment of urinary incontinence by implantable prosthetic sphincter. *Urology* **1**, 252

Seiffert, L. (1935) Die 'Darm-siphonblase'. *Arch F Klin Chir* **183**, 569–74

Shapiro, S. R., Lebowitz, R. and Colodny, A. H. (1975) Fate of 90 children with ileal conduit urinary diversions a decade later: analysis of complications, pyelography, renal function and bacteriology. *J Urol* **114**, 289–95

Skinner, D. G., Boyd, S. and Lieskovsky, G. (1984) Clinical experience with the Kock continent ileal reservoir for urinary diversion. *J Urol* **132**, 1101–7

Smith, T. (1879) An account of an unsuccessful attempt to treat extroversion of the bladder by a new operation. *St Bartholomew Hosp Rep* **15**, 29–35

Tizzoni, G. and Foggi, A. (1888) Die wiederherstellung der harnblase. *Zentbl Chir* **15**, 921

# 15

# Subtotal vaginal hysterectomy

*Anthony Davies and Adam L. Magos*

Hysterectomy can be classified as a total or sub-total (or supracervical) hysterectomy and can be performed abdominally, vaginally or laparoscopically. The title of this chapter refers to a technique of performing subtotal hysterectomy described by Magos and his colleagues in 1995 (Magos *et al.* 1995a). Before detailing this new operation, it will be necessary to discuss two controversies surrounding current hysterectomy practice: namely, which route should be employed and what should be removed during the operation.

## HISTORICAL BACKGROUND

The first subtotal hysterectomy was performed using an abdominal approach by Heath in 1843 at the Manchester School of Medicine in England (Thom, Dunne and Livornesse 1967). Compared with total hysterectomy, the procedure was relatively simple, with a significantly reduced operating time and injuries to ureters and bladder. Blood loss and infection were also minimised, which was especially important in the era when there was a lack of adequate blood products for transfusion and before antibiotics. Supracervical amputation of the uterus remained the standard technique of hysterectomy for benign pelvic lesions until the 1960s. Gradually, total hysterectomy became the preferred procedure, with subtotal hysterectomy being reserved for cases where technical difficulties meant that conservation of the cervix became a safer option (e.g. where there was an elongated cervix, severe endometriosis with dense pelvic adhesions or a Caesarean hysterectomy was required).

In recent years there has been renewed interest in conserving the cervix at hysterectomy as a result of two reasons:

(1) The results of research which have reported advantages of the subtotal operation compared with total; and

(2) Its adoption by laparoscopic surgeons because of the increased safety and ease of the operation.

## ADVANTAGES AND DISADVANTAGES

A series of studies by Kilkku in the 1980s suggested that conservation of the cervix at the time of hysterectomy may be associated with several functional advantages in terms of reduced posthysterectomy urinary, bowel, sexual and psychological dysfunction. For instance, he reported that total hysterectomy was associated with a reduction in orgasmic frequency not seen with the supravaginal procedure, although the effects of libido, coital frequency and dyspareunia were similar between the two operations (Kilkku 1983; Kilkku *et al.* 1983). He also reported that adverse psychological symptoms, including nervousness, irritability and depression, were less frequent after the more conservative procedure (Kilkku *et al.* 1987). Finally, he found that urinary symptoms, such as the sensation of residual urine following micturition and incontinence, were also less common following subtotal hysterectomy (Kilkku 1985).

The main criticism of these results is that the data were not collected within the setting of a randomised study for the two types of hysterectomies, and the patient groups may therefore not have been similar in baseline characteristics. Although there may be theoretical reasons for such differences in outcome, perhaps linked to local nervous injury (Mundy 1982; Parys et al. 1990; Prior et al. 1992a; Varma 1992) or changes in the elasticity and compliance of surrounding tissues secondary to dissection and excision of the cervix during total hysterectomy (Vervest et al. 1989a; Ilio et al. 1993), studies utilising objective measures of urinary and bowel function have come to conflicting conclusions with respect to the effects of total hysterectomy. Most attention has been focused on the urodynamic evaluation of urethrovesical function, with some investigators reporting adverse effects following hysterectomy (Parys et al. 1989; Parys, Wolfenden and Parson 1990), while others have not (Coughlan, Smith and Moriarty 1989; Vervest et al. 1989b; Langer et al. 1989). Yet others have shown a poor correlation between subjective symptoms and urodynamic findings (Hansen et al. 1989). Similarly, conflicting data are available concerning bowel motility (Roe, Bartola and Mortensen 1988; Taylor, Smith and Fulton 1989; Prior et al. 1992b).

As for the psychosexual sequelae of hysterectomy, preoperative factors are probably much more important than the type of hysterectomy carried out (Oates and Gath 1989). Whereas early and poorly controlled studies tended to conclude that a considerable proportion of women undergoing total hysterectomy experienced a deterioration in sexual functioning (Munday and Cox 1967; Dennerstein, Wood and Burrows 1977), more accurate prospective studies have shown that the psychosexual outcome is either unchanged or, indeed, improved in the majority of women (Martin, Roberts and Clayton 1980; Gath, Cooper and Day 1981; Gath et al. 1981).

Another theoretical advantage of subtotal hysterectomy is the preservation of the pelvic floor supports, with the cardinal and uterosacral ligaments remaining intact. This should eliminate the risk of vault prolapse that can occur following total hysterectomy, and other complications, such as Fallopian tube prolapse (Muntz, Falkenberry and Fuller 1988), small bowel prolapse (Astill 1982) and vaginal cuff cysts (Davis et al. 1986) become a physical impossibility.

Interestingly, doubts about the relative advantages and disadvantages of subtotal hysterectomy are dramatically illustrated in the institution in which Kilkku works: 53% of abdominal hysterectomies were subtotal in the period 1981–1986, whereas in 1991 the rate of subtotal hysterectomies was no more than 13% (Virtanen, Mäkinen and Kiilholma 1995). This change was based on the observations that more pelvic relaxation occurred after subtotal than total hysterectomy (Virtanen and Mäkinen 1993). Furthermore, total hysterectomy was found not to provoke urinary or sexual symptoms but, on the contrary, to have beneficial effects (Virtanen et al. 1993).

It would seem in the light of these results that any possible difference between total and subtotal hysterectomy is likely to be extremely small and probably clinically insignificant. Ultimately, only carefully controlled, prospective studies can provide the definitive answers to these issues.

There are, however, some advantages to subtotal hysterectomy which do not require further proof. The reduced need for dissection in the region of the uterine isthmus and uterine vessels means that ureteric damage and the development of vault haematomas are less likely with the supracervical procedure (Kuhn and de Crespigny 1985). Conversely, retention of a cervical stump can lead to complications such as inflammatory disease, endometriosis, cervical prolapse (Adamian, Kulakov and Dzhabrailova 1991) and the development of an obstructive mucocoele (Malviya et al. 1988). In one series, 11 out of 12 women required cervicectomy after subtotal hysterectomy (Van Coeverden de Groot and Zabow 1983).

Finally, there is still the fear of cervical malignancy, although cytological screening and colposcopy should mean that high-risk cases are not offered cervical conservation at the time of hysterectomy. Kilkku (1987) demonstrated that the incidence of carcinoma in a cervix that has shown repeated benign Papanicolaou smears is extremely low, and it is even lower if the endocervical epithelium has been surgically removed and the remnant endometrial epithelium and exocervix has been electro-cauterised at the time of the supravaginal hysterectomy. He found that out of 2712 subtotal hysterectomies performed in this manner for benign condition, only three patients (0.11%) developed carcinoma of the cervical stump (usual incidence, 0.4–1.9%). Although this incidence is very small, the risk still exists, and is eliminated only by total hysterectomy.

## LAPAROSCOPIC TECHNIQUES

Laparoscopic total hysterectomy was first performed in 1988 (Reich, DeCaprio and McGlynn 1989) and has become an established alternative to abdominal hysterectomy. In common with the vaginal route of surgery, there are major advantages to the patient by avoiding a laparotomy, including reduced surgical risk and postoperative pain, shorter recovery time and cost. Subtotal laparascopic hysterectomy was subsequently introduced to make the procedure easier by reducing the dissection required in the region of the uterine arteries and ureter. In addition to the advantages already described, performing a subtotal hysterectomy avoided opening the vagina and therefore made the procedure completely laparoscopic.

One of the first descriptions of a laparoscopic subtotal hysterectomy was described by Semm (1991) and called the classical intrafascial SEMM hysterectomy (CISH) technique for which he uses a serrated-edge macromorcellator. The first stage of this procedure is to straighten the axis of the uterus by inserting a straight, metal, perforation probe into the uterine cavity. The uterine fundus is then deliberately perforated under laparoscopic control. In the original CISH technique the ovarian pedicles are secured with a suture and divided with laparoscopic scissors. Next, the anterior leaf of the peritoneum is opened and the bladder reflected so that a series of three Roeder loops can be passed over the fundus of the uterus and tightened once a cylinder of tissue has been removed from the centre of the cervix and the uterus with a calibrated uterine resection tool (CURT) macromorcellator. The uterine body is then amputated above the level of the Roeder loops from the retained cervix. Haemostasis is secured with an electrical coagulation probe applied to the cervical stump. The round ligaments are tied into the vault of the vagina and the vault is reperitonealised. The uterus is morcellated with the macromorcellator and removed via a 15- or 20-mm suprapubic cannula. Ewen and Sutton (1994) used a similar technique, but used staples for the upper pedicles. Others have described subtotal laparoscopic hysterectomy using conventional instruments without the need for coring the uterus (Donnez and Nisolle 1993; Lyons 1993).

In the few comparative studies that have been reported, it has been found that the operating time is less with subtotal than total laparoscopic hysterectomy, the hospital stay is shorter, the time before a return to work is less (Lyons 1993) and there is reduced operative blood loss (Hasson et al. 1993).

## VAGINAL ROUTE

The available evidence shows that since the widespread introduction of prophylactic antibiotics, vaginal hysterectomy is associated with less febrile morbidity, less bleeding requiring transfusion, shorter hospitalisation and faster convalescence compared with abdominal hysterectomy (Dicker et al. 1982). Despite these obvious advantages, all large-scale surveys of hysterectomy practice have shown that 70–80% of hysterectomies are performed by the abdominal approach (Dicker et al. 1982; Easterday, Grimes and Riggs 1983; Pokras 1989; Vessey et al. 1992; Wilcox et al. 1994). The exception to this is the management of uterovaginal prolapse for which the vaginal route is normally used, but this indication only accounts for approximately 10% of patients.

The unpopularity of vaginal approach stems from a combination of factors which should really no longer apply. Concern about postoperative vault sepsis has been addressed by the use of prophylactic antibiotics (Allen, Rampone and Wheeler 1972; Ohm and Galask 1975; Glover and Van Nagell 1976). Factors widely held to be contraindications to vaginal hysterectomy, such as nulliparity (Sheth 1993), absence of uterine prolapse (Sheth 1991), enlarged uterus (Kovac 1986; Grody 1989; Stovall, Washington and Ling 1994; Magos *et al.* 1996), previous pelvic surgery which includes Caesarean section (Coulam and Pratt 1973; Hoffman and Jaeger 1990) and a need to perform oophorectomy (Capen *et al.* 1983; Sheth and Malpani 1991; Magos *et al.* 1995; Davies, O'Connor and Magos 1996) have all been shown to be inappropriate in most cases. Related to this, inadequate training and experience in vaginal surgery have played a major role in determining the bias towards abdominal hysterectomy (Kovac 1995).

As stated earlier, laparoscopic hysterectomy has distinct advantages over abdominal hysterectomy, but this is not the case when compared with vaginal hysterectomy. The operating time for laparoscopic hysterectomy is considerably longer and the use of disposable laparoscopic instruments makes it a more expensive procedure without any benefits in terms of postoperative pain or recovery (Summitt *et al.* 1992); Richardson, Bournas and Magos 1995). Even surgeons who are keen proponents of laparoscopic hysterectomy agree that the vaginal approach is the optimum route of hysterectomy (Jones 1993; Querleu *et al.* 1993).

Having studied the various laparoscopic procedures, including the modified Doderlein–Kronig hysterectomy described by Saye *et al.* (1993), it became apparent to us that subtotal hysterectomy could be performed vaginally without any need for additional laparoscopic surgery.

## VAGINAL SUBTOTAL HYSTERECTOMY

Vaginal subtotal hysterectomy is carried out using a modification of the technique originally described by Doderlein and Kronig in 1906. The bladder is first catheterised and left on free drainage. After cervical infiltration with 10 ml of 0.5% lignocaine containing 1:200,000 adrenaline, a semicircular incision is made in the anterior vaginal fornix (Figure 1) and the uterovesical fold of peritoneum opened (Figure

2). A lateral vaginal wall retractor is inserted anteriorly to protect and elevate the bladder, while the uterine fundus is directed towards the colpotomy using an acutely curved uterine sound within the uterine cavity (Figure 3). Tissue forceps (e.g. Littlewoods) are then

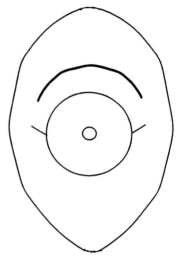

**Figure 1** *Anterior colpotomy is made in the anterior vaginal fornix above the cervix. (Reproduced from Magos, A. L., Bournas, N., Richardson, R. E., Sinha, R. and O'Connor. H. O. (1995a) Subtotal vaginal hysterectomy. Minimally Invasive Ther 4, 91–7, with permission of the editor and Blackwell Science Ltd)*

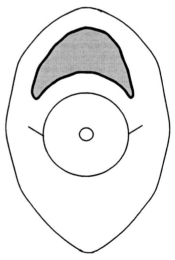

**Figure 2** *Uterovesical fold is opened to gain entry into the peritoneal cavity. (Reproduced from Magos et al. 1995a [full reference details in the legend to Figure 1] with permission of the editor and Blackwell Science Ltd)*

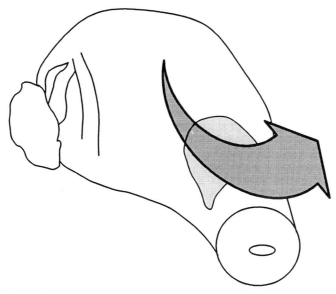

**Figure 3** *Uterus is pulled through the anterior colpotomy into the vagina. (Reproduced from Magos et al. 1995a [full reference details in the legend to Figure 1] with permission of the editor and Blackwell Science Ltd)*

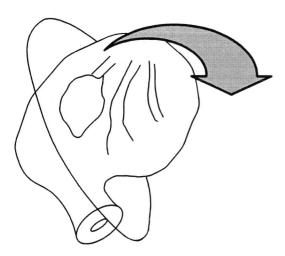

**Figure 4** *Uterine fundus is pulled further towards the vaginal introitus to gain access to the vascular pedicles. (Reproduced from Magos et al. 1995a [full reference details in the legend to Figure 1] with permission of the editor and Blackwell Science Ltd)*

applied progressively up the anterior uterine wall until the body of the uterus could be drawn through the vaginal incision towards the introitus (Figure 4). Alternatively, a '1' prolene suture on a large, wide-bored, curved needle is inserted deep into the anterior wall of the uterus and traction applied, bringing more of the uterus into view. The needle is then reinserted higher up the uterus and further traction applied so more of the uterus is pulled through the colpotomy incision. This is continued until the uterus is delivered.

After examining the cul-de-sac and ensuring there are no adhesions to the uterus or adnexa, the ovarian and uterine pedicles are clamped, divided and ligated (Figure 5). The uterine body is cut off the cervix using a cone-shaped incision to leave a concavity in the stump. Any obvious bleeding points are cauterised and the cut anterior and posterior edges of the cervix approximated with sutures (Figure 6). The cervical stump is then returned to the peritoneal cavity (Figure 7). If a salpingo-oophorectomy is required it can be performed at this stage by pulling the Fallopian tubes and ovaries medially with soft tissue clamps so that vascular clamps can be applied laterally on to the infundibulopelvic ligaments. Finally, the vaginal incision is closed, ensuring that peritoneum is included in the suture line for good haemostasis (Figure 8).

Since the authors' initial report, they have performed nine subtotal hysterectomies. They do not actively recruit patients for this operation, but it is offered to patients who

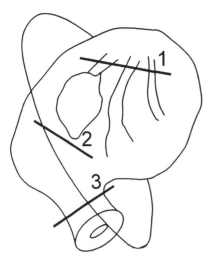

**Figure 5** *Ovarian (1) and uterine artery (2) pedicles are clamped, ligated and divided, followed by amputation of the uterine body from the cervix at the level of the uterine isthmus (3). (Reproduced from Magos et al. 1995a [full reference details in the legend to Figure 1] with permission of the editor and Blackwell Science Ltd)*

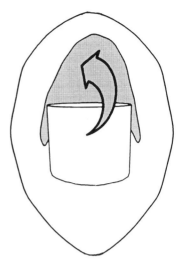

**Figure 7** *Cervical stump is returned to peritoneal cavity. (Reproduced from Magos et al. 1995a [full reference details in the legend to Figure 1] with permission of the editor and Blackwell Science Ltd)*

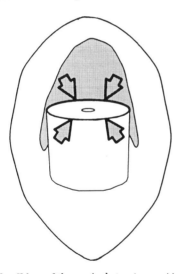

**Figure 6** *Edges of the cervical stump are approximated. (Reproduced from Magos et al. 1995a [full reference details in the legend to Figure 1] with permission of the editor and Blackwell Science Ltd)*

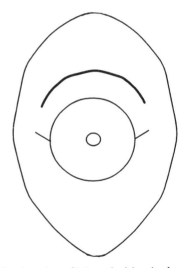

**Figure 8** *Anterior colpotomy incision is closed. (Reproduced from Magos et al. 1995a [full reference details in the legend to Figure 1] with permission of the editor and Blackwell Science Ltd)*

request conservation of their cervix. The prerequisites for performing the operation are:

(1) A clinically and cytologically healthy cervix;

(2) A patient who is reliable, highly motivated and well informed of the need for subsequent cytological follow-ups;

(3) The absence of uterine or associated genital prolapse;

(4) A uterus enlarged no greater than 12 weeks' gestational size;

(5) Uterine mobility;

(6) Adequate vaginal access; and

(7) Conditions in which the removal of the cervix is not essential to the surgical treatment of the patient's primary pelvic problem.

The mean age of the authors' patients was 46.5 years. One was nulliparous, two had previous Caesarean births (one had two) and another had previous pelvic surgery. The indications for the hysterectomy were dysfunctional uterine bleeding (six patients), fibroids (two patients) and haematometra (one patient). The average uterine size was equivalent to seven weeks' gestation (range four to 12 weeks). Three patients had concomitant vaginal oophorectomy performed. The mean operative time was 76.3 minutes (range 35–150 minutes) and the mean estimated blood loss was 302 ml (50–1000 ml). The patient with the longest operating time and largest operative blood loss was grossly obese and had undergone two Caesarean deliveries, which made opening the uterovesical fold difficult. The only post-operative complication in this series was of urinary retention, for which the patient required catheterisation for 24 hours. The average post-operative stay was 3.1 days (range two to four days).

## CONCLUSIONS

The vaginal approach is a suitable alternative route to subtotal hysterectomy in selected patients, even in nullipara and after previous pelvic surgery. While there is no comparative data with respect to abdominal and laparoscopic techniques, vaginal subtotal hysterectomy is a relatively simple procedure and it is likely that it would have the same advantages as conventional (total) vaginal hysterectomy. Nonetheless, further work still needs to be done to determine whether hysterectomies should be total or subtotal.

# References

Adamian, L. V., Kulakov, V. I. and Dzhabrailova, S. S. (1991) Characteristics of surgical treatment of pathological conditions of the cervical stump. *Akusherstvo i Gynekologiyas* 60–2

Allen, J. L., Rampone, J. F., Wheeles, C. R. (1972) Use of prophylactic antibiotics for vaginal hysterectomies. *Obstet Gynecol* **39**, 218–24

Astill, A. N. (1982) Small bowel prolapse through the vaginal vault. *Aust NZ J Obstet Gynaecol* **22**, 59–60

Capen, C. V., Irwin, H., Magrina, J. and Masterson, B. J. (1983) Vaginal removal of the ovaries in association with vaginal hysterectomy. *J Reprod Med* **28**, 589–91

Coughlan, B. M., Smith, J. M. and Moriarty, C. T. (1989). Does simple hysterectomy affect lower urinary tract function — a urodynamic investigation. *Irish J Med Sci* **158**, 215–16

Coulam, C. and Pratt, J. H. (1973) Vaginal hysterectomy: is previous pelvic operation a contraindication? *Am J Obstet Gynecol* **116**, 252–60

Davies, A., O'Connor, H. and Magos, A. (1996) Oophorectomy at vaginal hysterectomy. *Br J Obstet Gynaecol* (in press)

Davis, M. C., Fishman, E. K., Cameron, J. L., Magid, D. and Siegelman, S. S. (1986) Computed tomography of vaginal cuff cyst: a late complication of hysterectomy. *J Comput Assist Tomogr* **10**, 354–6

Dennerstein, L., Wood, C. and Burrows, G. D. (1977) Sexual response following hysterectomy and oophorectomy. *Obstet Gynecol* **49**, 92–6

Dicker, R. C., Greenspan, J. R., Strauss, L. T. *et al.* (1982) Complications of abdominal and vaginal hysterectomy among women of reproductive age in the United States. *Am J Obstet Gynecol* **144**, 841–8

Doderlein, A. and Kronig, S. (1906) *Die Technik der Vaginalen Bauchholen-operationen.* Leipzig: Verlag von S Hirzel

Donnez, J. and Nisolle, M. (1993) Laparoscopic supracervical (subtotal) hysterectomy. *J Gynecol Surg* **2**, 91–4

Easterday, C. L., Grimes, D. A. and Riggs, J. A. (1983) Hysterectomy in the United States. *Obstet Gynecol* **62**, 203–12

Ewen, S. P. and Sutton, C. J. G. (1994) Initial experience with supracervical laparoscopic hysterectomy and removal of the cervical transformation zone. *Br J Obstet Gynaecol* **101**, 225–8

Gath, D., Cooper, P. and Day, A. (1981) Hysterectomy and psychiatric disorder: levels of psychiatric morbidity before and after hysterectomy. *Br J Psychiatry* **140**, 335–52

Gath, D., Cooper, P., Bond, P. and Edmonds, G. (1981) Hysterectomy and psychiatric disorder: demographic, psychiatric and physical factors in relation to psychiatric outcome. *Br J Psychiatr* **140**, 385–8

Glover, M. W. and Van Nagell, J. R. (1976) The effect of prophylactic ampicillin on pelvic infection following vaginal hysterectomy. *Am J Obstet Gynecol* **126**, 395–8

Grody, T. H. M. (1989) Vaginal hysterectomy: the large uterus. *J Gynecol Surg* **5**, 301–12

Hansen, B. M., Bonnesen, T., Hvidberg, J. E., Eliasen, B. and Nielsen, K. (1989) Changes in symptoms and colpocysturethrography in 35 patients before and after total abdominal hysterectomy: a prospective study. *Urologia* **40**, 224–6

Hasson, H. M., Rotman, C., Rana, N. and Asakura H. (1993) Experience with laparoscopic hysterectomy. *J Am Assoc Gynecol Laparosc* **1**, 1–11

Hoffman, M. S. and Jaeger, M. (1990) A new method for gaining entry into the scarred anterior cul-de-sac during transvaginal hysterectomy. *Am J Obstet Gynecol* **162**, 1269–70

Ilio, S., Yoshioka, S., Yokoyama, M., Iwata, H. and Takeuchi, M. (1993) Urodynamic evaluation for bladder dysfunction after radical hysterectomy. *Nippon Hinyokika Gakkai Zasshi* **84**, 535–40

Jones, R. A. (1993) Laparoscopic hysterectomy — a technique. *Aust NZ J Obstet Gynaecol* **33**, 290–5

Kilkku, P. (1983) Supravaginal uterine amputation *vs.* hysterectomy. Effects of coital frequency and dyspareunia. *Acta Obstet Gynecol Scand* **62**, 141–5

Kilkku, P. (1985) Supravaginal uterine amputation versus hysterectomy with reference to subjective bladder symptoms and incontinence. *Acta Obstet Gynecol Scand* **64**, 375–9

Kilkku, P. (1987) 'Total versus subtotal abdominal hysterectomy' in: C. R. Garcia, J. J. Mikuta and N. G. Rasenblum (Eds.). *Current Therapy in Surgical Gynecology*, p. 58. Toronto, Canada: B. C. Decker Inc

Kilkku, P., Gronroos, M., Hirvonen, T. and Rauramo, L. (1983) Supravaginal uterine amputation *vs.* hysterectomy. Effects on libido and orgasm. *Acta Obstet Gynecol Scand* **62**, 147–52

Kilkku, P., Lehtinen, V., Hirvonen, T. and Gronroos, M. (1987) Abdominal hysterectomy versus supravaginal uterine amputation: pyschic factors. *Ann Chir Gynaecol* **202**, 62–7

Kovac, R. S. (1986) Intramyometrial coring as an adjunct to vaginal hysterectomy. *Obstet Gynceol* **67**, 131–6

Kovac, R. S. (1995) Guidelines to determine the route of hysterectomy. *Obstet Gynecol* **85**, 18–23

Kuhn, R. J. and de Crespigny, L. C. (1985) Vault haematoma after vaginal hysterectomy: an invariable sequel? *Aust NZ J Obstet Gynaecol* **25**, 59–62

Langer, R., Neuman, M., Ron-el, R. *et al.* (1989) The effect of total abdominal hysterectomy on bladder function in asymptomatic women. *Obstet Gynecol* **74**, 205–7

Lyons, T. L. (1993) Laparoscopic supracervical hysterectomy using the contact Nd YAG laser. *Gynaecol Laparosc* **2**, 79–81

Magos, A. L., Bournas, N., Sinha, R., Lo, L. and Richardson, R. E. (1995) Transvaginal endoscopic oophorectomy. *Am J Obstet Gynecol* **172**, 123–4

Magos, A. L., Bournas, N., Richardson, R. E., Sinha, R. and O'Connor, H. O. (1995a) Subtotal vaginal hysterectomy. *Minimally Invasive Ther* **4**, 91–7

Magos, A. L., Bournas, N., Sinha, R., Richardson, R. E. and O'Connor, H. (1996) Vaginal hysterectomy for the enlarged fibroid uterus. *Br J Obstet Gynaecol* **103**, 246–51

Malviya, V. K., Budev, H., Drabecki, T. and Stephenson, C. D. (1988) Obstructive mucocoele of the cervix after subtotal hysterectomy. A case report. *J Reprod Med* **33**, 480–1

Martin, R. R., Roberts, W. V. and Clayton, P. J. (1980) Psychiatric status after hysterectomy — a one-year prospective follow-up. *J Am Med Assoc* **244**, 350–3

Munday, R. N. and Cox, L. W. (1967) Hysterectomy for benign lesion. *Med J Aust* **17**, 814–17

Mundy, A. R. (1982) An anatomical explanation for bladder dysfunction following rectal and uterine surgery. *Br J Urol* **54**, 501–4

Muntz, H. G., Falkenberry, S. and Fuller, A. F. Jr (1988) Fallopian tube prolapse after hysterectomy. A report of two cases. *J Reprod Med* **33**, 467–9

Oates, M. and Gath, D. (1989) Psychological aspects of gynaecological surgery. *Bailliere's Clin Obstet Gynaecol* **3**, 729–49

Ohm, M. J. and Galask, R. P. (1975) The effect of antibiotic prophylaxis on patients undergoing vaginal operations. 1. The effect on morbidity. *Am J Obstet Gynecol* **123**, 590–6

Parys, B. T., Haylaen, B. T., Hutton, J. L. and Parsons, K. F. (1989) Urodynamic evaluation of lower urinary tract function in relation to total hysterectomy. *Aust NZ J Obstet Gynaecol* **30**, 161–5

Parys, B. T., Woolfenden, K. A. and Parsons, K. F. (1990) Bladder dysfunction after simple hysterectomy: urodynamic and neurological evaluation. *Eur J Urol* **17**, 129–33

Pokras, R. (1989) Hysterectomy, past, present, and future. *Stat Bull Metrop Insur Co* **70**, 12–21

Prior, A., Stanley, K. M., Smith, A. R. and Read, N. W. (1992a) Effect of hysterectomy on anorectal and urethrovesical physiology. *Gut* **33**, 262–7

Prior, A., Stanley, K. M., Smith, A. R. and Read, N. W. (1992b) Relation between hysterectomy and the irritable bowel: a prospective study. *Gut* **33**, 814–17

Querleu, D., Cosson, M., Parmentier, D. and Debodinance, P. (1993) The impact of laparoscopic surgery on vaginal hysterectomy. *Gynaecol Endosc* **2**, 89–91

Reich, H., DeCaprio, J. and McGlynn, F. (1989) Laparoscopic hysterectomy. *J Gynecol Surg* **5**, 213–16

Richardson, R. E., Bournas, N. and Magos, A. L. (1995) Is laparoscopic hysterectomy a waste of time? *Lancet* **345**, 36–41

Roe, A. M., Bartolo, D. C. and Mortensen, N. J. (1988) Slow transit constipation. Comparison between patients with or without previous hysterectomy. *Dig Dis Sci* **33**, 1159–63

Saye, W. B., Espy, G. B., Bishop, M. R. *et al.* (1993) Laparoscopic Doderlein hysterectomy: a rational alternative to traditional abdominal hysterectomy. *Surg Laparosc Endosc* **3**, 88–94

Semm, K. (1991) Hysterectomy via laparotomy or pelviscopy: a new CASH method without colpotomy. *Geburtshilfe Frauenheilkd* **51**, 996–1003

Sheth, S. S. (1993) 'Vaginal hysterectomy' in: J. Studd (Ed.). *Progress in Obstetrics and Gynaecology*, Vol. 10, pp. 317–40. Edinburgh: Churchill Livingtone

Sheth, S. S. (1991) The place of oophorectomy at vaginal hysterectomy. *Br J Obstet Gynaecol* **98**, 662–6

Sheth, S. S. and Malpani, A. (1991) Vaginal hysterectomy for the management of menstruation in mentally retarded women. *Int J Gynaecol Obstet* **35**, 319–21

Stovall, R. L., Washington, S. A. and Ling, F. W. (1994) Gonadotrophin-releasing hormone agonist use before hysterectomy. *Am J Obstet Gynecol* **170**, 1744–51

Summitt, R. L., Stovall, T. G., Lipscomb, G. H. and Ling, F. W. (1992) Randomized comparison of laparoscopy-assisted vaginal hysterectomy with standard vaginal hysterectomy in an outpatient setting. *Obstet Gynecol* **80**, 895–901

Taylor, T., Smith, A. N. and Fulton, M. (1989) Effect of hysterectomy on bowel function. *BMJ* **229**, 300–1

Thom, C. H., Dunne, T. J. and Livornesse, G. (1967) Vaginal cervicectomy. *Obstet Gynecol* **30**, 473–80

Van Coeverden de Groot, H. A. and Zabow, P. (1983) The cervical stump. *S Afr Med J* **64**, 745–6

Varma, J. S. (1992) Autonomic influences on colorectal motility and pelvic surgery. *World J Surg* **16**, 811–19

Vervest, H. A., Van Venrooji, G. E., Barents, J. W., Haspels, A. A. and Debruyne, F. M. (1989a) Non-radical hysterectomy and the function of the lower urinary tract. I: Urodynamic quantification of changes in storage function. *Acta Obstet Gynecol Scand* **68**, 221–9

Vervest, H. A., Van Venrooji, G. E., Barents, J. W., Haspels, A. A. and Debruyne, F. M. (1989b) Non-radical hysterectomy and the function of the lower urinary tract. II: Urodynamic quantification of changes in evacuation function. *Acta Obstet Gynecol Scand* **68**, 231–5

Vessey, M. P., Villard-Mackintosh, L., McPherson, K., Coulter, A. and Yeates, D. (1992) The epidemiology of hysterectomy: findings in a large cohort study. *Br J Obstet Gynaecol* **99**, 402–7

Virtanen, H. S. and Mäkinen, J. I. (1993) Retrospective analysis of 711 patients operated on for pelvic relaxation in 1983–1989. *Int J Gynaecol Obstet* **42**, 109–15

Virtanen, H. S., Mäkinen, J. I. and Kiilholma, P. J. A. (1995) Conserving the cervix at hysterectomy. *Br J Obstet Gynaecol* **102**, 587

Virtanen, H. S., Mäkinen, J., Tenho, T., Kiilholma, P. and Hirvonen, T. (1993) Effects of abdominal hysterectomy on urinary and sexual symptoms. *Br J Urol* **72**, 868–72

Wilcox, L. S., Koonin, L. M., Pokras, R. *et al.* (1994) Hysterectomy in the United States, 1988–1990. *Obstet Gynecol* **83**, 549–55

# 16

# Laparoscopic colposuspension

*Edward J. Shaxted*

Burch colposuspension (Burch 1968) has been the standard treatment for urinary stress incontinence in women for many years now. The procedure has been shown time and again to be superior to anterior repair and other vaginal operations in terms of long-term cure of stress incontinence (Stanton 1986). The procedure is usually performed through a Pfannensteil incision under a general anaesthetic. Usually between two and four sutures are placed either side of the bladder neck and base and used to elevate the bladder base towards the ileopectineal ligament. Many surgeons use a non-absorbable suture of either braided polyester (Ethibond) or monofilament nylon or prolene. Others use an absorbable suture such as polygycolic acid (Vicryl) or PDS (polydioxanone). Bow-stringing of the sutures is common and not thought to be important (Stanton 1986). Voiding difficulties are common after this type of surgery and many surgeons routinely use a suprapubic catheter postoperatively. A postoperative hospital stay of five to seven days is common, with four to eight weeks off work.

Laparoscopic bladder neck suspension was first described by Vancuille and Schuessler (1991). They attempted to emulate the Kranz procedure rather than the Burch colposuspension. It is now possible to perform the Burch operation laparoscopically with many of the benefits of minimal access surgery. In particular, there is minimal tissue trauma, little postoperative pain and an early discharge from hospital.

However, laparoscopic colposuspension is not easy and should only be attempted by gynaecologists who are experienced in advanced laparoscopic techniques. The Royal College of Obstetricians and Gynaecologists places laparoscopic colposuspension as a level four procedure.

There is the problem of access to the retropubic space and the inherent difficulty of suturing laparoscopically, as well as the problem of placing sutures in the limited retropubic space. A lack of three-dimensional vision adds to the difficulties. Indeed, some would say that laparoscopic suturing is perhaps one area where the development of a three-dimensional cameras might be of significant help.

Laparoscopic suturing needs to be practised on simulators before the surgeon attempts it on patients. Surgeons are reminded that colposuspension should only be attempted after appropriate training and supervised experience.

Whether or not the laparoscopic approach provides as good a long-term cure as does the traditional open procedure is still to be determined, but the short-term results are promising.

Although laparoscopic colposuspension can be performed under regional anaesthesia it is usual to use a general anaesthetic. The airway may need the protection of a laryngeal mask, but there is no need for controlled ventilation.

## THE APPROACH TO THE CAVE OF RETZIUS

The patient should be placed on the operating table in a flat Lloyd-Davies position. The bladder should be emptied and a Foley catheter inserted. A combined laparotomy and lithotomy draping is used so as to allow access to the vagina during the operation. As with all laparoscopic operations, the equipment must be checked and tested before starting because the absence or malfunction of even the simplest item can make the operation impossible. Blue dye in the bladder, commonly used during an open operation, may be omitted during a laparoscopic procedure — the bladder edge is usually easy to visualise. However, in case of doubt, it is probably best to use dye to ensure that sutures are not inadvertently passed through the bladder. Curiously, the cave of Retzius seems to bleed very little during a laparoscopic colposuspension and haemostatic techniques or lavage are rarely needed.

There are a number of different methods described for approaching and dissecting the cave of Retzius laparoscopically. Each has advantages and disadvantages.

### Transperitoneal

The transperitoneal approach to laparoscopic colposuspension has been well described by Lui (1993). Using this technique a pneumoperitoneum is created and laparoscopy performed in the usual fashion. The reflection of bladder on to the anterior abdominal wall is identified and the peritoneum divided at this position. This part of the operation may be facilitated if there is a small amount of fluid in the bladder. A combination of blunt and sharp dissection into the retroperitoneal tissue between bladder and symphysis pubis enables the cave of Retzius to be entered from the peritoneal cavity (Figure 1).

This approach has the advantage of allowing inspection of the intra-abdominal viscera and is useful if colposuspension is to be combined with another endoscopic procedure (e.g. hysterectomy). However, finding the right plane between bladder and abdominal wall can be quite difficult and it is easy to make a hole in the bladder during the dissection. Bleeding from veins in the region of the bladder base may be more of a problem with the transperitoneal approach. If a suprapubic catheter is used postoperatively, urine can leak out of the cystotomy hole into the peritoneal cavity and, occasionally, out of the abdominal port sites.

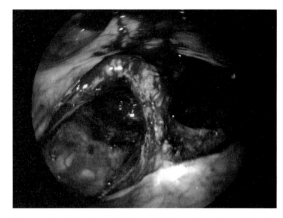

**Figure 1** *The transperitoneal approach to the retropubic space*

### Direct insufflation of the cave of Retzius and direct laparoscopic approach

Using this technique, a Veress needle is passed through the lower abdominal wall behind the symphysis pubis and carbon dioxide insuflated directly into the cave of Retzius. A Foley catheter needs to be placed in the bladder prior to this insufflation to ensure that gas is not being instilled into the bladder. After partial dissection of the cave of Retzius with carbon dioxide, a trocar can be passed either directly into this space through the abdominal wall, or, alternatively, a cutting device (e.g. Visiport made by Auto Suture, Ascot, Berkshire) can be used to cut a channel from the umbilicus through the subcutaneous fat and via the sheath immediately suprapubically.

This procedure works quite well and is particularly useful for patients who have had previous abdominal surgery and who may, therefore, have some scar tissue on the anterior abdominal wall. However, on entering the cave of Retzius which has been insufflated with carbon dioxide, the anatomy is far from clear and the initial dissection can be daunting with no landmarks being immediately available. The initial appearance is that of the inside of a sponge (Figure 2).

### Balloon dilatation of the cave of Retzius

Balloon dissection of the extraperitoneal space has been used for several extraperitoneal laparoscopic procedures. These include reno-scopy and renal biopsy, lymph node biopsy, nephrectomy ligation of varicocoele and hernia repair (Guar 1994).

Using this technique the rectus sheath is identified and incised as an open procedure through a small vertical subumbilical incision. Care must be taken, especially in patients who have had a previous laparoscopy, not to open the peritoneal cavity at this point. A disposable transparent balloon tipped canula (Origin Medsystems Inc., Menlo Park, CA) is passed under direct vision through the sheath at the level of the umbilicus and passed between the rectus muscles without puncturing the peri-toneum to lie on top of the symphysis pubis. Lubrication of the balloon with sterile petroleum jelly (e.g. KY) assists the smooth passage of the balloon tipped canula. Care must be taken not to puncture the balloon.

The balloon is dilated using air and a hand pump, deflated and then passed behind the symphysis pubis and distended yet further. Because the balloon is transparent, a laparo-scope can be left in the balloon to ensure that the dissection is taking place in the right area. The back of the symphysis pubis and the dome of the bladder can usually be identified easily. This technique works extremely well in display-ing the structures in the cave of Retzius and the balloon creates a far more complete dissection than does carbon dioxide alone. There is surprisingly little bleeding when the dissection is performed in this way and bladder trauma is rare.

Unfortunately, this technique does not work well with patients who have had previous lower abdominal surgery. The peritoneum may be adherent to the back of the rectus muscles at the site of previous scars and the dissection is often incomplete or the perineum transgressed inadvertently. If the peritoneal cavity is inadver-tently opened in the course of this procedure, it should be closed to avoid gas leaking into the peritoneal cavity; if this proves to be impossible, a Veress needle may be left in the peritoneal cavity to vent off leaking carbon dioxide. Alter-natively, the procedure can be converted into a transperitoneal approach. A gasless technique

using a device to elevate the abdominal wall is available, but has few advantages over the traditional method other than avoiding the risk of surgical emphysema.

## THE OPERATION

After entering the cave of Retzius, the first step is to orientate yourself. Usually the back of the symphysis pubis and the upper pubic rami are clearly visible. The next step is to identify and to clean the ileopectineal ligament of the fatty areolar tissue (Figure 3). Haemostatic measures are rarely needed, but bipolar diathermy will usually coagulate any small vessel bleeding. Care

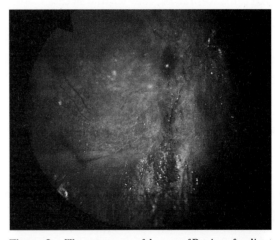

**Figure 2** *The appearance of the cave of Retzius after direct insufflation with carbon dioxide; there are no guiding landmarks visible*

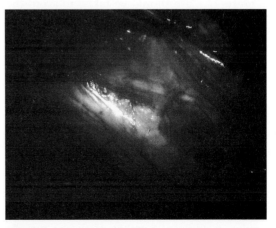

**Figure 3** *The ileopectineal ligament above the superior pubic ramus*

must be taken to avoid the inferior superficial epigastric vessels. The bladder edge and urethrovesicle angle must be identified and reflected medially. The vaginal fascia is easily identified by its white appearance. This dissection is facilitated by the presence of a Foley catheter in the bladder and can usually be accomplished quite easily with blunt dissection using either a small pledgelet or simply with metallic instruments alone.

As with all endoscopic operations, positioning of the lower secondary ports is vital. These ports can usually be positioned at the ends of where an imaginary Pfannensteil incision would be located. Care must be taken not to extend it too far laterally so that access to the ileopectineal ligament is difficult. If an entirely extraperitoneal approach is favoured, then the ports must not be positioned too high, or the peritoneal cavity will be punctured (blindly and dangerously). The size of ports used will be determined by the instruments and suturing method used. The author uses a 5-mm port on the left and an 11-mm port on the right. A J-shaped needle can just be passed down the larger port. If suturing is performed using a short, straight needle, then two 5-mm ports will suffice.

The author attempts to recreate an open Burch colposuspension endoscopically. Sutures of either prolene or Ethibond on a J-shaped needle are used, elevating and approximating the vaginal fascia to the ileopectineal ligaments (Figure 4). Care should be taken to avoid the periosteum, as this is associated with the development of postoperative periostitis (Lui 1993). Other surgeons use a small straight needle with Ethibond sutures, but both techniques attempt to emulate the open procedure.

Tying the knot can be done in a variety of ways. Perhaps the easiest is to tie it extracorporeally. A Roder knot can be tied, run down into position and tightened. Prior to attempting this it is essential to practise on a simulator. Different suture materials need slight variations of technique with this suture; in particular, a different number of throws may be needed with different materials. An alternative

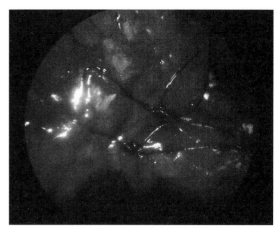

**Figure 4** *Good elevation of the bladder base with just two nylon sutures*

is to run down successive throws of half hitches. For the experts, intracorporeal knot tying will cause no difficulties. However, with this technique an assistant will be required to elevate the vagina during the knot tying.

For those who cannot suture laparoscopically, a number of other techniques have been described using staplers to staple mesh between the ileopectineal ligament and the vaginal fascia. How this compares in terms of long-term or short-term cure with suturing is unknown, but short-term results seem comparable (Ou, Presthus and Beadle 1993).

Infiltration of the port sites with 0.5% Marcain, and the use of non-steroidal anti-inflammatory drug routinely at the end of the operation reduces the need for narcotic analgesics and aids early mobilisation.

## PATIENT SELECTION

As with other operations for urinary incontinence, it is important to select patients with genuine stress incontinence. It is therefore important to perform appropriate bladder pressure and flow studies before the operation. Patients are selected who fulfil the following criteria:

(1) They should have genuine stress incontinence without any evidence of bladder instability.

(2) They should have reasonable urinary flow rates to avoid the risk of permanent retention postoperatively.

(3) In my view, patients who have had a previous failed operation for stress incontinence should currently be offered an open operation. The long-term results of the laparoscopic approach are still unknown.

(4) Patients should understand that this operation is still relatively new and untried.

(5) Patients who have had previous pelvic surgery, which might inhibit access to the cave of Retzius, should be warned of the possible need to convert the operation to an open one.

Although it is customary to avoid surgery in patients with bladder instability, recent work suggests that patients with incontinence of mixed cause (stress incontinence and detrusor overactivity) may also benefit considerably from Burch colposuspension (Colombo *et al.* 1996). This is because these patients may represent a significant percentage of women with incontinence, and the laparoscopic approach may also benefit them.

Patients in the author's unit are routinely given prophylactic subcutaneous heparin with the premed and antibiotics intraoperatively. Consent includes written permission to transfer to an open operation if this becomes necessary.

In my view, patients should currently be warned that the laparoscopic approach to this procedure is not proven from a long-term point of view. As a result it is of vital importance that surgeons performing the operation laparoscopically should make arrangements for the long-term follow-up of their patients.

## POSTOPERATIVE MANAGEMENT

There is little point in performing the colposuspension laparoscopically unless the patient recovers and is discharged home more rapidly than following the open procedure. We have found that early discharge has been facilitated by a rigid adherence to the postoperative protocol in Table 1. Using this protocol of high fluid load immediately intra- and postoperatively, fol-

**Table 1** *Management protocol after laparoscopic colposuspension*

| |
|---|
| Give 2 litres of fluid intravenously on the operating table |
| Remove the drip before the patient returns to the ward and encourage mobilisation immediately |
| Remove the drain on the evening of the operation |
| Remove the catheter the morning after the operation |
| Assuming the patient has voided, and does not clinically have urinary retention, allow home the day after the operation |
| Patient returns to the ward or clinic on day 4 or 5 for suture removal check on an ultrasound scan of the bladder while it is being emptied |

lowed by a rapid removal of all drains, drips and catheters, encourages early patient mobilisation and has enabled us to discharge all patients home either one or two days after surgery. Other authors have performed the operation on a day case basis (Ou, Presthus and Beadle 1993), but we have not yet been this adventurous.

The author sees the patient on about day 5 for removal of skin sutures and to check both clinically and ultrasonically that the bladder is empty.

## PROBLEMS AND COMPLICATIONS

In addition to the usual complications of laparoscopic surgery, it is important to mention those problems peculiar to laparoscopic colposuspension. Surgical emphysema occurs frequently, especially in the vulval area, but is rarely a major problem. Mention has already been made of bladder injury, the most likely of which is tearing a hole in the fundus of the bladder early in the dissection process. Usually this can be repaired laparoscopically, but the patient's recovery will be delayed by the necessity of prolonged catheterisation. Voiding difficulties seem much less common than after an open operation, possibly reflecting the lesser degree of tissue trauma and postoperative pain.

## LONG-TERM RESULTS

So far there are no long-term (i.e. five years or more) results of laparoscopic colposuspension and no direct comparative trials available for open colposuspension.

A 1979 review of open colposuspension performed on 180 patients produced a cure rate of 87% at one year and 86% at two years (Stanton and Cardozo 1979). Needle suspension operations (Shortliffe and Stamey 1986; Gaur 1994) have been represented as less invasive operations. However, lower long-term cure rates of 53% at four years in patients under 65 years of age and 76% in those over 65 years (Hilton and Mayne 1991) have contributed to a decline in the popularity of these procedures. If the laparoscopic approach to colposuspension proves to have long-term results that are as good as the open procedure, then there will be genuine advantage in using this approach.

Early operations in the author's unit were performed transperitoneally. Results were not good. Of the seven patients operated on in this way, two suffered from bladder trauma with holes in the bladder. These were repaired laparoscopically. Three patients have returned with recurrent symptoms. It seems likely that many of these problems were due to the learning curve as much as to any intrinsic failure of the operation method.

**Table 2** *The characteristics of patients who underwent laparoscopic colposuspension by the extraperitoneal approach*

| | |
|---|---|
| Total number of patients | 53 |
| Mean age (years) | 43 |
| Age range (years) | 27–65 |
| Mean weight (kg) | 75 |
| Weight range (kg) | 53–119 |
| Previous hysterectomy | 15 |
| Previous bladder neck surgery | 4 (all for prolapse) |

However, early experience of the extraperitoneal approach to the operation is encouraging. Fifty-seven patients have been operated on in this way. Patient characteristics are shown in Table 2.

Two patients had to convert to open operation; in both cases previous surgery had resulted in excessive scarring, rendering the extraperitoneal access to the cave of Retzius impossible. Of the 43 patients in the author's unit who have had an entirely extraperitoneal approach and on whom there is at least three-month follow-up, all have had their stress incontinence cured, two have returned with partial urinary retention and required recatheterisation and two have had symptoms of urgency and frequency which have settled with medical treatment. Long-term follow-up continues.

# References

Burch, J. C. (1968) Cooper's ligament urethrovesical suspension for stress incontinence. *Am J Obstet Gynecol* **100**, 764–74

Colombo, M., Zanetta, G., Vitobello, D. and Milani, R. (1996) The Burch colposuspension for women with and without detrusor overactivity. *Br J Obstet Gynaecol* **103**, 225–60

Guar, D. D. (1994) Retroperitoneoscopy: the balloon technique. *Ann R Coll Surg Engl* **76**, 259–63

Hilton, P. and Mayne, G. J. (1991) The Stamey endoscopic bladder neck suspension: a clinical and urodynamic investigation, including actuarial follow up over four years. *Br J Obstet Gynaecol* **98**, 1141–9

Lui, C. Y. (1993) Laparoscopic retropubic colposuspension (Burch procedure). *J Reprod Med* **38**, 526–30

Ou, C., Presthus, J. and Beadle, E. (1993) Laparoscopic bladder neck suspension using heria mesh and surgical staples. *J Laparosc Surg* **6**, 563–6

Shortliffe, L. M. and Stamey, T. A. (1986) 'Urinary incontinence in the female' in: P. C.

Walsh, R. F. Gittes, A. D. Perlmutter and T. A. Stamey (Eds.). *Cambell's Urology,* p. 2699. Philadelphia: W. B. Saunders

Stanton, S. L. (1986) 'Colposuspension' in: S. L. Stanton (Ed.). *Surgery of Female Incontinence,* 2nd edn, pp. 95–103. New York: Springer-Verlag

Stanton, S. L. and Cardozo, L. R. (1979) Results of colposuspension operation for incontinence and prolapse. *Br J Obstet Gynaecol* **86** 693–7

Vancuille, T. G. and Schuessler, W. (1991) Laparoscopic bladder neck suspension. *J Laparoendosc Surg* **3**, 169–73

# 17

# The current place of laparoscopic hysterectomy

*Anthony R. B. Smith*

In 1993/1994 in England and Wales 73,517 hysterectomies were performed in the National Health Service for the treatment of menorrhagia. On follow-up most women are satisfied with hysterectomy as a definitive form of treatment for their menstrual problems (Sculpher *et al.* 1996). In the Mersey region, despite a sixfold increase in the use of endometrial resection/ablation since 1989, the number of hysterectomies performed has remained unchanged (Department of Health 1995). In the Mersey region the introduction of endometrial resection/ablation led the life chance of a woman receiving surgical treatment for dysfunctional uterine bleeding to increase from 6.5% to 11%, with no reduction in the number of hysterectomies performed (Bridgman 1996).

The first laparoscopic hysterectomy was reported in the English literature in 1989 by Reich (Reich, DeCaprio and McGlynn 1989). The development of laparoscopic hysterectomy has been encouraged for three main reasons: the large improvements made in laparoscopic surgical equipment, the benefit seen from performing minor laparoscopic procedures (e.g. removal of ectopic pregnancy) and the potential to convert an abdominal to a vaginal hysterectomy with accompanying reduction in time for convalescence. The current Royal College of Obstetricians and Gynaecologists audit of hysterectomy in England, Wales and Northern Ireland indicates that 5% of hysterectomies in both the private and the National Health Service sectors are performed with laparoscopic assistance and 21% vaginally without laparo-

scopic assistance (personal communication, unvalidated data, October 1994–April 1995).

The key question which should be addressed is: what proportion of hysterectomies *should* be performed vaginally, abdominally or with laparoscopic assistance? Whether future years will witness an increase in the use of laparoscopic assistance will depend on the answer to this question. There is a risk that laparoscopic hysterectomy will be performed because it is possible to do it that way, when a vaginal hysterectomy would have been simpler and of equal benefit. It is probable that there are cases in which laparoscopic assistance will either make a vaginal hysterectomy safer or enable a uterus to be removed vaginally when otherwise an abdominal hysterectomy would be required.

## TYPES OF LAPAROSCOPIC HYSTERECTOMY

The laparoscope may be used solely to confirm that there is no pathology, precluding straightforward vaginal hysterectomy or as part of the surgical procedure. The following classification was recommended by Garry and Reich (1994) and it goes a long way in reducing the confusion which surrounds the terminology:

(1) *Vaginal hysterectomy assisted by laparoscopy*: a standard vaginal hysterectomy following diagnostic laparoscopy.

(2) *Laparoscopic-assisted vaginal hysterectomy (LAVH)*: the ovarian pedicle is secured laparoscopically, but the remaining pedicles

including the uterine artery pedicles are secured vaginally.

(3) *Laparoscopic hysterectomy (LH)*: the ovarian and uterine artery pedicles are secured laparoscopically.

(4) *Total laparoscopic hysterectomy (TLH)*: all three pedicles are secured laparoscopically and the uterus is removed through the vagina or morcellated and removed laparoscopically.

(5) *Laparoscopic supracervical hysterectomy (LSH)*: the top two pedicles are secured laparoscopically and the uterus morcellated and removed laparoscopically or through the pouch of Douglas.

(6) *Classical intrafascial serrated-edge macromorcellation (SEMM) hysterectomy (classic intrafascial SEMM hysterectomy [CISH]/classic abdominal SEMM hysterectomy)*: laparoscopic securing of top two pedicles with central conisation of the cervix. The uterus removed laparoscopically following morcellation.

(7) *Radical laparoscopic hysterectomy (RLH)*: total laparoscopic removal of uterus, adnexae and lymph nodes.

A scoring system for determining the optimum surgical approach to hysterectomy has been devised but has not been widely adopted (Garry and Reich 1994).

## METHODS OF SECURING PEDICLES

Laparoscopic securing of the major pedicles may be achieved in four different ways: monopolar diathermy, bipolar diathermy, sutures and staples. These will now be discussed in turn.

### Monopolar diathermy

Monopolar diathermy may be used for coagulation and cutting major pedicles, but the heating effect is such that there is significant risk to adjacent structures. Electrical accidents with monopolar diathermy were first reported during tubal occlusion at sterilisation and have continued with the growth of laparoscopic

surgery. In addition to heat injury to adjacent structures, injuries to more distant structures from the field of view from capacitance coupling is a potential hazard.

### Bipolar diathermy

This technique has been used most frequently because of its availability. Cheap, reusable equipment (Kleppinger forceps) can be used to secure both ovarian and uterine vessel pedicles. Generally, the pedicles undergo diathermy until the area is fully desiccated, before being cut with scissors. It is believed that heat spread from bipolar diathermy is less than monopolar diathermy and there are fewer risks of other electrical problems such as capacitance coupling.

### Sutures

Laparoscopic suturing, whether intra- or extracorporeal, requires additional skills. Suturing has the advantage of avoiding electrical safety issues and is cheap. However, additional time is involved.

### Staples

Staples may be delivered as single metal clips applied to skeletalised vessels or from a multiple staple device with linear cutter incorporated. Absorbable clips are also available in single-clip applicators. The main advantage of the multiple-clip applicator with linear cutter is the speed of securing the pedicle, but the disadvantages are the cost and the width of the delivery device, which is particularly important in the uterine artery pedicle.

## INDICATIONS FOR LAPAROSCOPIC HYSTERECTOMY

It is generally accepted that recovery from vaginal hysterectomy is quicker than abdominal hysterectomy. Protagonists of laparoscopic hysterectomy advocate that laparoscopic hysterectomy is a method of converting an abdominal hysterectomy into a vaginal hysterectomy. Since most hysterectomies are performed abdominally, this deserves closer scrutiny — including the indications for abdominal rather than vaginal hysterectomy. There is no evidence that a laparoscopic hysterectomy will be of greater benefit to the patient than a vaginal hysterectomy (Summitt *et al.* 1992). Possible indications for laparoscopic hysterectomy include:

(1) Hysterectomy for benign disease;

(2) Removal of the ovaries;

(3) As part of another laparoscopic procedure;

(4) Hysterectomy for carcinoma;

(5) Fewer surgical complications;

(6) Reduced postoperative pain;

(7) Reduced length of stay in hospital; and

(8) Earlier return to work.

## Hysterectomy for benign disease

There is no doubt that laparoscopic assistance will enable some uteri to be removed vaginally that would otherwise have required abdominal removal. Since there is evidence that the morbidity following abdominal hysterectomy is greater than following vaginal hysterectomy (Dicker *et al.* 1982), the use of the laparoscope should be part of the gynaecologist's armamentarium if he or she is involved in pelvic surgery. What is not clear, however, is what proportion of hysterectomies should be removed by each of the three methods available. Currently, the great majority are removed abdominally and, since it has been shown that it is possible to remove a greater proportion vaginally with or without laparoscopic assistance, our efforts should be directed at establishing what reasonable rates of standard vaginal hysterectomy are achievable. Kovac (1995) prospectively assigned 617 women to vaginal, abdominal or laparoscopically assisted hysterectomy on the basis of uterine size, presumptive risk factors and uterine or adnexal immobility or inaccessibility. Sixty-three of the 617 cases underwent laparoscopy prior to hysterectomy due to risk factors and in 12 of these laparoscopic surgery was employed to enable vaginal removal of the uterus. In only six cases of 617 was abdominal hysterectomy required. Therefore, in his series Kovac employed laparoscopic surgery to remove the uterus in only 2% of cases. Surgical complications in the two groups, which contained greatly different numbers of women, occurred in a similar percentage of cases and the time to return to normal activity was equal in the two vaginal groups and doubled in the abdominal group. Querleu *et al.* (1993a) also considered the impact of laparoscopic surgery on vaginal hysterectomy. In a 12-month period they performed a prospective study on 149 women who were scheduled for hysterectomy. Cases with genital prolapse were excluded. Vaginal hysterectomy was completed without laparoscopic assistance in 77% of cases. Laparoscope-assisted vaginal hysterectomy (LAVH) was performed in 17% of cases and abdominal hysterectomy in only 6%. The main difference between the Querleu and the Kovac series was the exclusion of prolapse in the former, which probably explains the increased need for laparoscopic assistance reported by Querleu.

The most important factors in determining the route of removal of the uterus at hysterectomy are: the angle of the subpubic arch, the size of the uterus, uterine descent and previous pelvic infection or endometriosis. These are now discussed in turn.

### The angle of the subpubic arch

A wide arch makes access to the uterus easier and is probably the most important factor in determining the ease with which a uterus can be removed.

### The size of the uterus

Most gynaecologists regard the larger uterus as an indication to elect for abdominal removal. The studies of Kovac (1995) and Querleu *et al.* (1993) demonstrate that with frequent use of facilitating procedures such as coring, hemisection and morcellation, the larger uterus may be removed safely by the vaginal route. Magos *et al* (1996) in a series of 14 consecutive cases demonstrated that a uterus enlarged to a size equivalent to 20 weeks' gestation can be removed safely by the vaginal route without laparoscopic assistance. There are no data analysing whether laparoscopic assistance makes the vaginal removal of the large uterus any safer for the patient.

### Uterine descent

Descent of the cervix and uterus within the vagina is probably the factor which most influences the gynaecologist in deciding whether vaginal hysterectomy is possible. Generally, descent is greater if the woman is parous. Descent may be improved by securing the ovarian and uterine pedicles laparoscopically, but it is often the uterosacral ligament pedicle which limits uterine mobility. A possible remedy is to partially divide the uterosacral ligaments laparoscopically before proceeding to vaginal removal.

### Previous pelvic infection or endometriosis

Women who have a history of previous pelvic inflammatory disease or endometriosis may have adhesions between the uterus and appendages and bowel and omentum. In addition, mobility of the uterus may be impaired. Some gynaecologists use the laparoscope to ensure that safe vaginal hysterectomy would not be impeded by adhesions, while others use laparoscopic assistance to divide adhesions and one or more pedicles. When there is limited descent of the uterus in the pelvis, division of the uterosacral ligaments alone may enable the surgeon to proceed to vaginal hysterectomy. This may be of particular use when endometriosis has produced scarring and fixity of the ligaments.

## Removal of the ovaries

Adnexal removal is frequently performed with hysterectomy. In the Thames region oophorectomy, usually bilateral, was performed in 50% of cases (Jones and Lapsley 1994). Laparoscopic division of the ovarian pedicle prior to vaginal hysterectomy has probably been the most widely applied use of the laparoscope at hysterectomy. Oophorectomy is often performed because of the risk of developing ovarian cancer, but

increasingly vocal conservation arguments are being heard and this may influence the rate in future. The problems subsequent to poor compliance with hormone replacement therapy should be considered before ovaries are removed in premenopausal women.

Removal of the ovaries may be difficult at vaginal hysterectomy, although there are series published which demonstrate that it is feasible (Wright 1974; Smale et al. 1978; Capen et al. 1983) and techniques using the laparoscope vaginally with endoloops have been described.

## As part of another laparoscopic procedure

If hysterectomy is being performed with laparoscopic colposuspension, the hysterectomy may be aided laparoscopically. In addition, the laparoscopic visualisation enables careful approximation of the uterosacral ligaments which helps to prevent enterocoele, a recognised problem after colposuspension.

## Hysterectomy for carcinoma

Laparoscopic pelvic lymphadenectomy has been described prior to hysterectomy for both carcinoma of the cervix and carcinoma of the endometrium. Laparoscopic lymphadenectomy has been shown to be feasible and safe in the staging of carcinoma of the cervix (Querleu, Leblanc and Castelain 1991). Kadar (1994) reported a series of eight cases in which laparoscopic vaginal radical hysterectomy was performed for women with stage IA2–IIA carcinoma cervix. While at an early stage, and for a proper evaluation, Kadar used well-evaluated techniques with regard to removal of nodes and uterine issues, he essentially used the laparoscope to facilitate performing a vaginal radical hysterectomy described by Schauta.

The value of the laparoscope for carcinoma of the endometrium is similarly under evaluation. Although pelvic and aortic lymphadenectomy have been shown to be technically possible, there is not uniform agreement among oncologists about the value of staging by lymphadenectomy. There is evidence that staging on histological grading of myometrial invasion may be inadequate (Kindemann 1991). Use of the laparoscope enables full examination of the peritoneal cavity and cytological examination in addition to lymphadenectomy and hysterectomy with removal of appendages. Long-term follow-up is required to determine whether the use of laparoscopic assistance is of benefit to the patient.

## Fewer surgical complications

The Royal College of Obstetricians and Gynaecologists Audit Unit is currently conducting a study into hysterectomy in England and Wales in both the National Health Service and the private sector. (It is called VALUE, which stands for vaginal, abdominal and laparoscopic uterine excision.) The impetus for the study came from the publicity arising from complications of laparoscopic hysterectomy and the subsequent realisation that the complication rate of abdominal hysterectomy is not known. Many of the complications of laparoscopic hysterectomy are common to all types of hysterectomy, but some are new. Garry and Phillips (1995) considered the surgical complications associated with laparoscopic hysterectomy and produced a metaanalysis of 3189 cases from 29 studies; they then compared the series with the complication rate reported by Dicker *et al.* (1982). This report noted that bowel injury occurred in 0.5% of laparoscopic hysterectomies compared with 0.6% vaginal and 0.3% abdominal hysterectomies. Urinary tract injury occurred in 1.6% of

laparoscopic hysterectomies, compared with 1.6% vaginal hysterectomy and 0.5% abdominal hysterectomies (Table 1).

Garry and Phillips concede that the series for the meta-analysis is comprised of cases from acknowledged experts in laparoscopic surgery and probably represents an underestimate of the complication rate. In addition, later complications such as incisional hernia, which are rare in open surgery, have been reported in 21 per 100,000 cases in laparoscopic surgery and are associated with significant morbidity, are not included in the analysis (Montz, Holschneider and Munro 1994). The complications from laparoscopic surgery often do not present immediately and Querleu (1993b) noted in a retrospective review of over 18,000 cases of laparoscopic surgery that the need for laparotomy was not recognised until after the initial operation in 60% of cases.

The use of ureteric stents (including illuminated stents) has been described to reduce the risk of ureteric injury (Phipps 1993a). This has been a particular concern with the use of linear cutting stapling devices which secure a wider pedicle than a conventional clamp. Ureteric stents carry their own risks, however, and postoperative pyelocalyceal obstruction has been reported (Phipps 1993a).

## Reduced postoperative pain

Phipps (1993a) reported that women recovering from laparoscopic hysterectomy required

**Table 1** *Comparison of complication rates of laparoscopic* (n = 3189), *vaginal* (n = 568) *and abdominal* (n = 1283) *hysterectomy. (Reproduced from Garry and Phillips 1995\* with permission of Academic Press Inc.)*

| Complication | Laparoscopic (%) | Vaginal (%) | Abdominal (%) |
|---|---|---|---|
| Febrile morbidity | 4.3 | 15.3 | 32.3 |
| Transfusion | 1.2 | 8.3 | 15.4 |
| Bowel trauma | 0.5 | 0.6 | 0.3 |
| Urinary tract trauma | 1.4 | 1.6 | 0.5 |
| Bladder | 1.1 | 1.6 | 0.3 |
| Ureter | 0.3 | 0 | 0.2 |
| Pulmonary embolus | 0.2 | 0 | 0.2 |
| Overall | 15.6 | 24.5 | 42.8 |

\*Garry, R. and Phillips, G. (1995) How safe is the laparoscopic approach to hysterectomy [editorial]? *Gynecol Endosc* **4**, 77–9 one dose of opiate analgesia for every four requested by patients recovering from abdominal hysterectomy. This presumably is a reflection of pain produced by the abdominal incision. Summitt *et al.* (1992) reported that the analgesia requirement following laparoscopic hysterectomy was greater than that requested following vaginal hysterectomy. The reasons for this are less clear, but may represent pain from the abdominal port wounds.

### Reduced length of stay in hospital

The length of postoperative hospitalisation depends on many factors, including the philosophy of health care delivery. In North America length of stay is generally much shorter because of financial penalties of a longer stay. In a recent study on postoperative hospitalisation following abdominal hysterectomy the author noted a dramatic increase in early discharge following the introduction of a simple policy of informing the patient that they would remain in hospital for only three or four days after surgery (Mac-Kenzie 1996). In reality there is little medical justification for keeping a patient in hospital for more than 48 hours after uncomplicated vaginal hysterectomy and 72 hours following uncomplicated abdominal hysterectomy. Reports of early discharge following laparoscopic hysterectomy should be interpreted in this context. Studies in which laparoscopic hysterectomy have been compared to vaginal hysterectomy have demonstrated similar lengths of hospital stay (Summitt *et al.* 1992).

### Earlier return to work

In his study comparing recovery from laparoscopic and abdominal hysterectomy, Phipps (1993b) noted that a recovery time of two weeks was required before returning to work following laparoscopic hysterectomy, compared with a six-week period following abdominal hysterectomy. Other studies report comparable times before return to work between laparoscopic and vaginal hysterectomy, with a more prolonged recovery for the abdominal route.

### SURGICAL TRAINING

Laparoscopic surgery requires training in techniques, of which many are unfamiliar to the conventional surgeon. Lack of familiarity with these techniques has undoubtedly contributed to some of the surgical accidents which have been widely reported in the press. The establishment of minimal access surgical training centres has helped provide the opportunity to learn the techniques involved, although the difficulties of being tutored *in vivo* have not yet been resolved. The Calman reforms could be seen as an opportunity to reorganise our surgical training programmes to ensure a more structured and uniform training is achieved. The wide variation in the use of the vaginal route to remove the uterus might be seen as evidence of clinical freedom, but may also be seen to expose deficiencies in surgical training in the specialty. The readiness with which laparoscopic hysterectomy has been adopted without first considering the vaginal route is also of concern.

The importance given to each of the above factors will vary with each surgeon. In the 1993/1994 National Health Service survey (Sculpher *et al.* 1996), 19% of hysterectomies were performed vaginally and this mirrors North American and Australian experience. In an audit of hysterectomy in the North-West Region in 1992 (which included 24 gynaecology units and contains unpublished data) the use of the vaginal route varied from 1% to 48% of cases, indicating a wide variety of expertise and practice. Current evidence suggests that the training and surgical skills of the gynaecologist are the most important determinant of the route of uterine removal. With improvement in training in vaginal surgery many more women could undergo conventional vaginal hysterectomy. Laparoscopic assistance could be reserved for more difficult cases, with significantly less than 50% of women requiring abdominal hysterectomy.

# References

Bridgman, S. A. (1996) Trends in endometrial ablation and hysterectomy for dysfunctional uterine bleeding in Mersey Region. *Gynaecol Endosc* **5**, 5–8

Capen, C. V., Irwin, H., Margina, J. and Materson, B. J. (1983) Vaginal removal of ovaries in association with vaginal hysterectomy. *J Reprod Med* **28**, 589–91

Department of Health (1995) *Hospital Episode Statistics*, Vol. 1, *Finished Consultant Episodes by Diagnosis, Operation and Specialty*. London: HMSO

Dicker, R. G., Greenspan, J. R., Strauss, L. T. *et al.* (1982) Complications of abdominal and vaginal hysterectomy among women of reproductive age in the United States. *Am J Obstet Gynecol* **144**, 841–8

Garry, R. and Phillips, G. (1995) How safe is the laparoscopic approach to hysterectomy [editorial]? *Gynecol Endosc* **4**, 77–9

Garry, R. and Reich, H. (1994) Laparoscopic hysterectomy — definitions and indications. *Gynecol Endosc* **3**, 1–3

Jones, I. and Lapsley, H. (1994) Quality assurance applied to laparoscopically assisted hysterectomy: a pilot study. *J Qual Clin Practice* **14**, 121–9

Kadar, N. (1994) Laparoscopic vaginal radical hysterectomy: an operative technique and its evolution. *Gynecol Endosc* **3**, 109–122

Kadar, N. (1995) Transient ureteric obstruction following ureteral catheterisation for laparoscopic hysterectomy. *Gynecol Endosc* **4**, 289–91

Kindemann, G. (1991) Differenziertes operative Therapie des Endometriumkarzinoms. *Verh Dtsch Ges Pathol* **75**, 378–80

Kovac, R. (1995) Guidelines to determine the route of hysterectomy. *Obstet Gynecol* **85** (1), 18–22

MacKenzie, I. Z. (1996) Reducing hospital stay after abdominal hysterectomy. *Br J Obstet Gynaecol* **103**, 175–8

Magos, A., Bournas, N., Sinha, R., Richardson, R. E. and O'Connor, H. (1996) Vaginal hysterectomy for the large uterus. *Br J Obstet Gynaecol* **103**, 246–51

Montz, F. J., Holschneider, S. H. and Munro, M. G. (1994) Incisional hernia following laparoscopy: a survey of the American Association of Gynecological Laparoscopists. *Obstet Gynecol* **84** (5), 881–4

Phipps, J. H. (1993a) *Laparoscopic Hysterectomy and Oophorectomy*, p. 43. Edinburgh: Churchill Livingstone

Phipps, J. H. (1993b) Laparoscopic hysterectomy and oophorectomy, p. 65. Edinburgh: Churchill Livingstone

Querleu, D., Cosson, M., Parmentier, D. and Debodinance, P. (1993a) The impact of laparoscopic surgery on vaginal hysterectomy. *Gynecol Endosc* **2**, 89–91

Querleu, D., Chevallier, L., Chapron, C. and Bruhat, M. (1993b) Complications of gynaecological laparoscopic surgery. A French multicentre collaborative study. *Gynecol Endosc* **2**, 3–6

Querleu, D., Leblanc, E. and Castelain, B. (1991) Laparoscopic lymphadenectomy in the staging of early carcinoma cervix. *Am J Obstet Gynecol* **164**, 579–81

Reich, H., DeCaprio, J. and McGlynn, F. (1989) Laparoscopic hysterectomy. *J Gynaecol Surg* **5**, 213–16

Sculpher, M. J., Dwyer, N., Byford, S. and Stirratt, G. M. (1996) Randomised trial comparing hysterectomy and transcervical endometrial resection: effect on health related quality of life and costs two years after surgery. *Br J Obstet Gynaecol* **103** 142–9

Smale, L. E., Smale, M. L., Wilkening, R. L., Mundy, C. F. and Ewing, T. L. (1978) Salpingo-oophorectomy at the time of vaginal hysterectomy. *Am J Obstet Gynecol* **131**, 122–6

Summitt, R. L. Jr, Stovall, T. G., Lipscomb, G. H. and Ling, F. W. (1992) Randomised comparison of laparoscopic assisted vaginal hysterectomy with standard vaginal hysterectomy in an outpatient setting. *Obstet Gynecol* **80**, 895–901

Wright, R. C. (1974) Vaginal oophorectomy. *Am J Obstet Gynecol* **120**, 759–63

# 18

# Surgical recovery of sperm for intracytoplasmic sperm injection

*Mark Vandervorst, Herman Tournaye and Paul Devroey*

Major progress has been made in infertility treatment in the last decade, especially in the field of assisted reproductive technology (ART). The introduction of intracytoplasmic sperm injection (ICSI) has completely changed the approach to severe male-factor infertility (Palermo *et al.* 1992).

Until recently, azoospermic couples were recommended to consider donor-sperm insemination. Since the introduction of the possibility of fertilising oocytes with sperm obtained from different parts of the male genital tract, the use of donor sperm has been reduced to a position of second choice.

At first, surgically retrieved sperm from the vas deferens (Pryor *et al.* 1984) was used for *in vitro* fertilisation (IVF). Standard IVF procedures were then performed with epididymal sperm (Temple-Smith *et al.* 1985) and testicular sperm (Hirsh *et al.* 1993), while Schoysman *et al.* (1993a) reported the first fertilisation after subzonal insemination (SUZI) using testicular sperm. Pregnancy rates have been increasing since the introduction of ICSI using epididymal sperm (Silber *et al.* 1994; Tournaye *et al.* 1994; Devroey *et al.* 1996) and testicular spermatozoa (Craft, Bennett and Nicholson 1993; Silber *et al.* 1995; Tournaye *et al.* 1996a).

This paper focuses on ART with both surgical and non-surgical sperm retrieval.

## AZOOSPERMIA

Azoospermia refers to a clinical condition which is characterised by the absence of spermatozoa in an ejaculate after masturbation (World Health Organisation 1992). Real azoospermia should be differentiated from virtual azoospermia, in which a few spermatozoa can be found in the semen after centrifugation. Retrograde ejaculation should first be ruled out. Conditions leading to azoospermia can be divided into two categories: either normal spermatogenesis with an obstructed genital outflow is involved, or an intrinsic testicular failure, leading to a decreased sperm production.

*Obstructive* or *excretory azoospermia*, characterised by a normal testicular size (< 15 ml) and follicle stimulating hormone (FSH) level is present in 46.7–60% of all azoospermic males. Congenital bilateral absence of the vasa deferentia (CBAVD) accounts for 9.3–11.9% of genital tract obstructions, while post-infectious blockage accounts for 7.8–14% (Jequier 1985; Micic 1987; Matsumiya *et al.* 1994). Young's syndrome (sinopulmonary disease with obstructive azoospermia) is not common (Hughes, Skolnick and Belker 1987). The Sperm Microaspiration Retrieval Technique Study Group (1994) has found a failed vasectomy reversal to be responsible in 17% of the cases.

In cases of *non-obstructive* or *secretory azoospermia*, males often have small (< 15 ml) and soft testes and/or elevated FSH levels. Germ cell hypoplasia (hypospermatogenesis), maturational arrest, germ cell aplasia (Sertoli cell-only syndrome) and sclerosing tubular degeneration (Klinefelter's syndrome) are the most common testicular histological diagnoses which occur with azoospermia (Levin 1979).

## TREATMENT MODALITIES

### Obstructive azoospermia

Sperm duct obstruction after infection or vasectomy can be treated by microsurgical reconstruction. However, complete patency, allowing sperm transport from the testicle through the rete testis, epididymis and vas deferens cannot always be re-established. In cases of CBAVD or extended damage to the sperm ducts, the only means towards a pregnancy is IVF, with spermatozoa recovered proximally to the obstruction.

### Sperm retrieval

Surgical sperm retrieval can be performed on several parts of the male genital tract: namely, the vas deferens, the epididymal caput, the corpus or cauda, the vasa efferentia and the testicle (Pryor *et al.* 1984; Jequier *et al.* 1990; Silber *et al.* 1990; Bladou *et al.* 1991; Craft, Bennett and Nicholson 1993; Silber *et al.* 1994).

Pryor *et al.* reported in 1984 on the first pregnancy after conventional IVF with surgically retrieved spermatozoa from the vas deferens of a man with inguinal vas obstruction. He had 0.15 ml of fluid, containing 17.7 million spermatozoa with 70% motility, aspirated. Six oocytes were incubated with the sperm, giving rise to four four-cell embryos, which were all transferred into the patient's wife. A twin pregnancy was diagnosed by ultrasound, ending at nine weeks' gestation in a missed abortion. Temple-Smith *et al.* (1985) achieved the first pregnancy by regular IVF with sperm aspirated from the distal part of epididymal corpus after failed vasectomy reversal in 1985, while Silber *et al.* (1988) reported the first pregnancies with sperm aspirated from the most proximal region

of the epididymal caput in two men with CBAVD.

The efficacy of conventional IVF after microscopic epididymal sperm aspiration (MESA) has been the subject of several papers. Table 1 lists the fertilisation and pregnancy rates of regular IVF after MESA.

### Special micromanipulation techniques

After the disappointing fertilisation and pregnancy rates from conventional IVF, oocyte insemination with micromanipulation was introduced. At first epididymal sperm was used in conjunction with SUZI and partial zona dissection. Schlegel *et al.* (1994) reported on the importance of micromanipulation in 11 couples who underwent both standard oocyte insemination and micromanipulation during IVF-embryo transfer (ET) using cohort eggs. Fertilisation was achieved only after SUZI procedure or partial zona dissection.

The introduction of ICSI to treat severe oligo-astheno-teratospermia resulted in high fertilisation and pregnancy rates (Palermo *et al.* 1992; Van Steirteghem *et al.* 1993a; 1993b). It was, therefore, only a short time before oocytes were inseminated after micromanipulation with spermatozoa obtained by MESA. Tournaye *et al.* (1994) reported the first pregnancies after a MESA/ICSI procedure. Twelve couples with husbands suffering from CBAVD underwent 14 MESA procedures. One hundred and twenty-seven metaphase-II oocytes were injected with epididymal sperm resulting in 71 zygotes with normal fertilisation (i.e. two-pronuclear oocytes). Between 3.3 and 2.5% of the zygotes contained one and three pronuclei, respectively. In 10 transfers, 26 embryos were replaced, giving rise to five pregnancies. A pregnancy rate

**Table 1** *Outcome of microscopic epididymal sperm aspiration/*in vitro *fertilisation cycles in cases of obstructive azoospermia*

| Study | Cycles (n) | Fertilisation rate (%) | Transfer rate (%) | Pregnancy rate/transfer (%) | Pregnancy rate/cycle (%) | Ongoing pregnancy/cycle (%) |
|---|---|---|---|---|---|---|
| Silber *et al.* (1990) | 32 | 26 | 66 | 48 | 31 | 22 |
| Bladou *et al.* (1991) | 14 | 32 | 36 | 40 | 14 | 0 |
| Hirsch *et al.* (1994) | 46 | 11 | 50 | 9 | 4 | 2 |
| Silber *et al.* (1994) | 67 | 7 | — | — | 9 | 4.5 |

**Table 2** *Outcome of intracytoplasmic sperm injection/microscopic epididymal sperm aspiration cycles in cases of obstructive azoospermia*

| Study | Cycles (n) | Fertilisation rate (%) | Transfer rate (%) | Pregnancy rate/transfer (%) | Pregnancy rate/cycle (%) | Ongoing pregnancy/cycle (%) |
|---|---|---|---|---|---|---|
| Tournaye *et al.* (1994) | 14 | 58 | 71 | 50 | 36 | 14 |
| Silber *et al.* (1994) | 17 | 41 | 88 | 53 | 47 | 30 |
| Silber *et al.* (1995) | 16 | 45 | 100 | 75 | 75 | 50 |
| Devroey (1996) | 127 | 52 | 91 | 42 | 39 | — |

of 35.7% per started MESA/ICSI cycle and 50% per transfer was achieved. Embryo wastage was high. Two pregnancies were ongoing at the time of publication, while one was biochemical and two ended in miscarriages. After frozen–thawed ET, another confirmed pregnancy and a biochemical pregnancy were obtained, resulting in a general ongoing pregnancy rate of 21.4% and early pregnancy wastage of 57% per started cycle. Silber *et al.* (1994) compared MESA cycles with conventional IVF and ICSI retrospectively. Pregnancy rates per cycle were 4.5% and 47%, respectively.

Table 2 shows the efficacy of ICSI in conjunction with surgically retrieved epididymal sperm in cases of obstructive azoospermia.

## Cryopreservation

One sperm cell is enough to inject one egg. Supernumerary spermatozoa can be cryopreserved and thawed for a subsequent treatment cycle. Devroey *et al.* (1995a) demonstrated that, despite the fact that freezing and thawing of fresh spermatozoa involves loss of quality, enough thawed epididymal spermatozoa retain their fertilisation capacity after injection into the oocytes. The already impaired motility of the fresh samples with absence of progressive motility (World Health Organisation type A) decreased dramatically after the freezing–thawing procedure, leading to almost complete immotility in all samples. No differences were observed in the two-pronuclear fertilisation rates or cleavage rates between the fresh and frozen sperm samples in seven patients. Embryo quality was comparable in the two groups. Three ongoing pregnancies (two singleton and one twin) were obtained with frozen–thawed samples, while in these same patients previous

**Table 3** *Comparison between the use of fresh and frozen–thawed epididymal spermatozoa in intracytoplasmic sperm injection cycles. (Reproduced from Devroey et al. 1995a with permission of Oxford University Press)*

| Epididymal spermatozoa | Fresh | Frozen–thawed |
|---|---|---|
| Concentration (mean $\times 10^6$) | 12.3 | 1.9 |
| Total motility (%) | 19.1 | 0 |
| Percoll technique: | | |
| concentration ($\times 10^6$) | 7.4 | 0.46 |
| total motility | 38.7 | 0 |
| Fertilisation rate (%) | 57 | 45 |
| Cleaved embryos | 79 | 82 |
| Embryo quality: | | |
| excellent | 5 (19%) | 1 (5%) |
| good | 18 (69%) | 14 (63%) |
| fair | 3 (12%) | 7 (32%) |

*Devroey, P., Silber, S., Nagy, Z. *et al.* (1995a) Ongoing pregnancies and birth after intracytoplasmic sperm injection with frozen–thawed epididymal spermatozoa. *Hum Reprod* **10**, 903–6

attempts with fresh epididymal spermatozoa had failed to lead to pregnancy (Table 3).

Oates *et al.* (1996) propose dissociating the time of surgical sperm retrieval and the ICSI procedure by cryopreserving all epididymal spermatozoa. In this way pointless female stimulation cycles can be avoided. They report a two-pronuclear fertilisation rate of 37%, with an ongoing pregnancy rate of 40% per couple (or 29% per cycle) with frozen–thawed spermatozoa.

## Use of testicular sperm

While either the epididymis is absent or completely damaged or the MESA procedure fails to recover enough spermatozoa to inject all the oocytes, spermatozoa must be found at a more proximal level (the testicle itself). After incision in the scrotal skin, tunica vaginalis and tunica albuginea, a small piece of extruding testicular tissue can be excised from which spermatozoa are extracted (Devroey *et al.* 1995b).

At first there was much concern about the fertilising capacity of this sperm, because testicular spermatozoa have not undergone the functional maturing process which takes place during epididymal transit (Turner 1995). The first fertilisation with testicular sperm obtained by *testicular sperm extraction* (TESE) in conjunction with standard IVF was reported in 1993 by Hirsh *et al.*, while Schoysman *et al.* (1993a) and Craft, Bennett and Nicholson (1993) reported fertilisation after SUZI and ICSI procedures. In the same year Schoysman *et al.* (1993b) reported the first pregnancy after inseminating the oocytes with SUZI and ICSI using testicular spermatozoa. Although several case reports deal with TESE in association with ICSI (Devroey *et al.* 1994; Abuzeid *et al.* 1995), the literature is scarce as regards data on large series. The results of combined TESE/ICSI cycles in cases of obstructive azoospermia are listed in Table 4.

### Non-obstructive azoospermia

Primary testicular failure results in an extremely bad fertility prognosis. Levin (1979) pointed out that azoospermic males with a histological diagnosis of germ-cell aplasia (Sertoli cell-only syndrome) or maturation arrest can still retain sporadic points of spermatogenesis. This opened the possibility of exploring the testicles in several open biopsies, in the hope of retrieving an active spot. Testicular spermatozoa obtained by the TESE procedure are used for ICSI. Results from the literature are summarised in Table 5.

## DISCUSSION

### Surgically-retrieved sperm

Untreated azoospermia leads unconditionally to definite male sterility. It is clear that if spermatozoa are lacking in a semen sample, there is either an obstruction on the excretory duct (post-infection, failed vasectomy re-anastomosis, congenital absence of the vas deferens), or an intrinsic defective spermatogenesis. The progress of assisted reproduction technologies led to the possibility of using surgically retrieved epididymal or testicular sperm cells to micro-inseminate oocytes obtained in artificial super-ovulation cycles. Before this evolution, such couples' desire for a child could only be fulfilled by artificial insemination using a donor's sperm. Today, the husband's own sperm is used in conjunction with ICSI treatment, avoiding the psychological and relational stress.

At first there was much concern about the fertilising capacity of testicular and epididymal sperm. Animal experiments support the view that spermatozoa should initially undergo maturation and require the motility-improving

**Table 4** *Results of combined testicular sperm extraction/intracytoplasmic sperm injection cycles in cases of obstructive azoospermia*

| Study | Cycles (n) | Fertilisation rate (%) | Transfer rate (%) | Pregnancy rate/transfer (%) | Pregnancy rate/cycle (%) | Ongoing pregnancy/cycle (%) |
|---|---|---|---|---|---|---|
| Silber *et al.* (1995) | 12 | 46 | 75 | 67 | 50 | 43 |
| Tournaye *et al.* (1996a) | 70 | 63 | 89 | 59 | 53 | 39 |
| Kahraman *et al.* (1996) | 16 | 65 | 100 | 62 | 62 | 44 |

**Table 5** *Outcome of combined testicular sperm extraction/intracytoplasmic sperm injection cycles in cases of non-obstructive azoospermia*

| Study | Cycles (n) | Fertilisation rate (%) | Transfer rate (%) | Pregnancy rate/transfer (%) | Pregnancy rate/cycle (%) | Ongoing pregnancy/cycle (%) |
|---|---|---|---|---|---|---|
| Tournaye *et al.* (1996a) | 54 | 45 | 76 | 54 | 41 | 33 |
| Kahraman *et al.* (1996) | 16 | 34 | 75 | 42 | 31 | 25 |

effects of epididymal transit (Turner, Gleavy and Harris 1990). However, in 1988 Silber described two pregnancies after efferentio-vasostomy because of failed vasectomy reversal in two couples (Silber 1988). As the paternity of the two husbands was never tested, the credibility of the two cases is in doubt. Weiske (1994), on the other hand, achieved a pregnancy after microsurgical anastomosis between the vas deferens and the rete testis. The paternity was confirmed by DNA fingerprinting. These two reports, therefore, contradict the previous animal observations in which epididymal transit was thought to be essential to induce the fertilising capacity of spermatozoa.

It is possible to bypass most cases of epididymal or vasal obstruction, although the outcome is unpredictable. Pregnancy rates after bilateral vasovasostomy and vasoepididymostomy are around 53% and 15%, respectively (Belker, Thomas and Fuchs 1991). In cases of CBAVD, or when damage to the epididymis or vas deferens is too extensive, microsurgical restoration is not possible and the surgical retrieval of spermatozoa for IVF treatment is the only option. Microscopic epididymal sperm aspiration, as well as TESE, may be used. However, MESA with regular IVF yields low and unpredictable fertilisation and pregnancy rates. No ongoing pregnancy rate per started MESA/IVF cycle higher than 22% has ever been reported (Table 1). Only one-third of the classically inseminated oocytes reach the two-pronuclear zygote state. The success rate of standard IVF remains highly dependent on the number and motility of retrieved epididymal spermatozoa (Hirsh et al. 1994).

The pattern of sperm motility in a chronically obstructed epididymis is the inverse of the normal state, in which motility is strictly dependent on the epididymal distance that has been completed. Silber et al. (1990) observed that in an obstructed system the proximal caput and vasa efferentia contain the largest number of motile spermatozoa. This is probably the result of intraluminal sperm absorption by macrophages, which occurs primarily in the distal segment of the obstructed epididymis (Schlegel et al. 1994). The adverse effect of dying and dead

sperm occurs predominantly in the distal part of the obstructed epididymis. Consequently, sperm from men with a longer epididymis yields higher fertilisation rates (Sperm Microaspiration Retrieval Techniques Study Group 1994). Microscopic epididymal sperm aspiration should, therefore, be carried out at the most proximal part of the epididymis. When only immotile spermatozoa are exposed, the surgeon should try to move on to a more proximal part of the epididymis or even the vasa efferentia.

The differences between the pregnancy and ongoing pregnancy rates of standard IVF procedures with epididymal sperm (Table 1) show that pregnancy wastage is significant. Hirsh et al. (1994) hypothesised that a 'male factor' is required for normal embryo implantation, possibly conferred on spermatozoa by passage through the epididymis.

As morphology, count and progressive motility are not crucial to ICSI results (Nagy et al. 1995), it is clear that better results are expected with combined MESA/ICSI cycles. Even senescent distal epididymal spermatozoa have fertilising capacity (Tournaye et al. 1994), although even for ICSI it is preferable to use sperm cells with at least minor motility to assess sperm vitality, when vitality staining is not routinely performed. Tournaye et al. (1994) found that almost all immotile spermatozoa recovered in small concentrations after centrifugation were dead, as shown by eosine vitality testing. No pregnancies occurred with totally immotile sperm after centrifugation.

Fertilisation rates, transfer rates, pregnancy rates and ongoing pregnancy rates per started cycle are almost twice as high after MESA/ICSI cycles than after MESA/IVF cycles (Tables 1 and 2). As it is impossible to determine in advance which MESA cases are likely to result in good fertilisation rates with regular IVF, it is therefore mandatory to combine MESA procedure only with ICSI (Silber et al. 1994).

There is no need to biopsy the testicles in obstructive azoospermia in order to evaluate spermatogenesis prior to the MESA procedure. Silber, Patrizio and Asch (1990) found no correlation between the quantity or quality of spermatozoa retrieved during MESA and actual sperm production. In obstructive azoospermia, it is secondary pressure-induced inspissation and obstruction in the rete testis collecting system, rather than reduced spermatogenesis, which induce poor epididymal sperm retrieval.

Intracytoplasmic sperm injection requires only a few sperm cells, offering the possibility of cryopreserving supernumerary spermatozoa retrieved during a fresh MESA cycle. After thawing, these spermatozoa can be used for subsequent cycles. Equivalent fertilisation rates with fresh and cryopreserved spermatozoa have been reported (Table 3) (Devroey et al. 1995a; Oates et al. 1996). In this way a single scrotal incision provides an opportunity to perform multiple ICSI cycles.

Absence of the epididymis or failure to retrieve epididymal sperm creates a particular problem. The only way to retrieve sperm from this location is to go to the testicle itself. Testicular sperm extraction/ICSI cycles in obstructive azoospermia yield fertilisation and ongoing pregnancy rates comparable to those for MESA/ICSI cycles (Tables 2 and 4). It is not now possible to determine the most appropriate technique, because there is a lack of prospective randomised trials comparing these two treatments. Certainly, TESE appears to be an easier and quicker method than MESA which requires less surgical expertise and does not always need general anaesthesia. The number and motility of testicular spermatozoa have to be assessed to see whether it is worth cryopreserving them for a following treatment cycle. Except for some case reports no large series are known. Romero et al. (1996) came to a fertilization rate of 57% and 63% in two couples after ICSI with frozen–thawed testicular spermatozoa. No clinical pregnancies were achieved.

When spermatogenesis itself is deficient, the concentration of sperm cells in the epididymis is far too low for MESA. Besides, MESA always presents the risk of an iatrogenic obstruction in non-obstructive cases. As in non-obstructive azoospermia active spots of spermatogenesis can be present (Levin 1979), TESE should be carried out in conjunction with ICSI. No pregnancies have been reported in cases after TESE procedure with regular IVF. Fertilisation

rates, transfer rates and ongoing pregnancy rates per sperm retrieval are situated around 40%, 75% and 30%, respectively (Table 5) (Devroey et al. 1995b; 1996). These figures mean that the outcome after TESE/ICSI cycles for non-obstructive and obstructive azoospermia are comparable. In a recent paper, Tournaye et al. (1996a) have pointed out the correlation between the histological testicular changes and the outcome after ICSI using testicular spermatozoa in non-obstructive azoospermic males. Spermatozoa were retrieved in 84% and 76% of patients with either incomplete germ-cell aplasia or maturation arrest. Compared to men with normal testicular histology (55%), a significantly lower fertilisation rate was observed in couples in which the husband suffered from germ-cell aplasia (36%) and maturation arrest (27%). These differences were not reflected in embryonic quality. The implantation rate and pregnancy rate were lowest in couples among whom the men showed maturation arrest. These differences, however, were not significant statistically.

Until recently, testicular biopsy as a diagnostic tool was considered useless in males suffering from hypergonadotrophic hypogonadism, since this clinical condition reflects an untreatable testicular pathology (Schoysman 1980; Comhaire 1992). Recent work, however, has demonstrated that clinical diagnosis of non-obstructive azoospermia based on the classical triad (azoospermia, small testicles and high FSH levels) does not always correlate with the histological diagnosis. Hauser et al. (1995) found a histological normal spermatogenesis in seven out of 31 patients with a clinical condition suggestive of primary testicular failure. This finding was confirmed in a paper by Tournaye et al. (1995). These observations underline the importance of testicular biopsy in differentiating obstructive from non-obstructive azoospermia.

If an intrinsic testicular pathology is proven on biopsy, will this have predictive value for the success of the TESE procedure? In cases of germ-cell hypoplasia or normal spermatogenesis, a preliminary testicular biopsy will be strongly predictive of a positive TESE procedure. On the contrary, when the biopsy shows complete or incomplete maturation arrest or germ cell aplasia, then spermatozoa can be present or absent in the set preparation (Tournaye *et al.* 1996a). A hypothetical explanation of this discrepancy lies in the fact that only a few active spots of spermatogenesis are distributed throughout the testicle. Only one preliminary biopsy is usually taken, while TESE procedure is normally continued until a few possible motile spermatozoa are recovered. The main question, however, remains — how far should we go? Despite a low sensitivity, histological examination of a random testicular biopsy remains a better parameter than semen analysis, measurement of testicular volume or FSH levels (Tournaye *et al.* 1996b).

## Non-surgical sperm retrieval

The invasive nature of MESA limits the number of procedures that a patient can undergo. Besides, the success rate of MESA is highly dependent on the microsurgical skill of the surgeon. Postoperative haematoma formation, infection and secondary fibrotic reaction can complicate further surgery. A non-invasive method of retrieving sperm from obstructive azoospermic males was developed to reduce peri- and postoperative morbidity and to increase patients' ability to undergo several subsequent procedures with minimal discomfort. At the Tenth Annual Meeting of the European Society of Human Reproduction and Embryology in 1994, Tsirigotis *et al.* (1994) presented a percutaneous epididymal aspiration technique, named PESA. In seven out of nine patients epididymal spermatozoa were recovered percutaneously by fine-needle aspiration and syringe suction. Monospermic fertilisation was achieved in 19% of injected oocytes, leading to six ETs, with an ongoing pregnancy rate of 33% per couple or 22% per started cycle. Compared to results with MESA/ICSI cycles this fertilisation rate and ongoing pregnancy rate per started cycle are less favourable. However, unlike MESA, PESA can be performed several times under local anaesthesia without inconvenience to the patient.

The technique is simple, not needing an operating microscope, and can be easily acquired. Only minimal equipment is needed (Tsirigotis and Craft 1995). A 21-gauge butterfly needle connected to a syringe is introduced into the epididymal caput or corpus, after fixation between the fingers, so that the epididymis is felt as a distended structure free of the testicle. Minimal negative syringe pressure aspirates the epididymal fluid, which is washed out through the needle and tubing. Contamination with blood cells happens only sporadically if the tubing is clamped to keep up the negative pressure while the needle is retracted from the testicle and skin.

Schrivastav *et al.* (1994) combined PESA with gamete intrafallopian transfer (GIFT) where spermatozoa showed active forward progression. Where motility was severely impaired, ICSI with intrauterine ET was performed. In all seven patients suffering from obstructive azoospermia and undergoing the PESA procedure, epididymal spermatozoa were recovered. Concentrations ranged between 0.8 and $100 \times 10^6$/ml. Active progressive motility was present in three cases, so that GIFT could be carried out. Two patients became pregnant after the PESA/GIFT procedure, resulting in one live birth of twins and one miscarriage. In four patients undergoing PESA/ICSI, only one biochemical pregnancy was observed. Craft, Tsirigotis and Schrivastav (1995) reported an overall pregnancy rate of 20.8% when combining PESA with GIFT and ICSI in couples where the male partner had an obstruction of the excretory duct.

Epididymal percutaneous puncture is clearly a blind manoeuvre. The operator cannot know if an epididymal blood vessel has been punctured. Furthermore, the epididymis is not microsurgically sutured and remains open. To resolve this issue and yet avoid substantial microsurgical and anaesthetic complications, Bassil *et al.* (1995) proposed a compromise between MESA and PESA. The minimal surgical approach under locoregional anaesthesia uses only a minimal scrotal incision, while epididymal spermatozoa can be aspirated under microscope magnification. The epididymis is then closed microsurgically. This method failed to recover spermatozoa in only one-quarter of the couples. No complications occurred in 16 patients.

If PESA fails to recover spermatozoa, the epididymal tubules will probably not contain any spermatozoa at all. If classical MESA procedure is performed in these cases, it will mostly end unsuccessfully. An attempt to recover spermatozoa from the testicle should then be performed. Although no objective facts are known with regard to this problem, it is the strong belief of Craft, Tsirigotis and Schrivastav (1995) and Tsirigotis and Craft (1995) that in the negative PESA procedures the next step is to look for testicular rather than epididymal spermatozoa.

Results of fine-needle aspiration (FNA) of the testicles were convincing in obtaining testicular tissue for cytological (Foresta, Varotto and Scandellari 1992) and histological analysis (Mallidis and Baker 1994). However, Gottschalk-Sabag *et al.* (1995) reported that several punctures are needed for a conclusive cytological diagnosis. This can be carried out as an out-patient procedure under locoregional anaesthesia. Foresta, Varotto and Scandellari (1992) demonstrated the various steps of spermatogenesis (from spermatogonia to spermatozoa) on testicular cytological smears obtained with FNA. Postoperative complications are rare: especially there is no testicular volume increase or elevated concentration of antisperm antibodies. Currently, these observations together with the experience of TESE/ICSI have prompted some investigators to search for spermatozoa in cases of obstructive azoospermia on wet preparations of tissue obtained by means of testicular FNA.

Bourne *et al.* (1995) reported the first two pregnancies after testicular FNA/ICSI treatment in two couples where the male suffered from genital tract obstruction. Punction was done with a 20-gauge Mencini needle, previously tested by Mallidis and Baker (1994). On the other hand, Sherins and co-workers (1996, personal communication) have detected sper-matozoa in the testicular fluid obtained by means of FNA in 63% of patients with suspected non-obstructive azoospermia. They achieved similar fertilisation and ongoing pregnancy rates for TESE/ICSI and FNA/ICSI cycles within patients with obstructive and non-obstructive azoospermia. Future research on a larger scale should concentrate on comparing FNA with open testicular biopsy and MESA in obstructive TESE in non-obstructive azoospermia. If non-surgical sperm retrieval with ICSI entails results identical to those from the surgical approach, the former offers a gentler and non-aggressive alternative for obtaining sperm. Multiple consecutive treatment cycles can be carried out because of their non-invasive character and the use of locoregional anaesthesia, reducing the need to cryopreserve sperm samples.

## CONCLUSIONS

The following conclusions can be drawn:

(1) Surgical sperm retrieval in conjunction with ART has almost completely superseded donor insemination as a way to treat azoospermic males.

(2) Conventional IVF with both epididymal and testicular spermatozoa yields low fertilisation and pregnancy rates. It is mandatory to perform only ICSI with these sperm samples.

(3) Both the MESA and TESE procedures can be done in cases of obstructive azoospermia, although the best treatment option in these cases has to be assessed in large controlled trials.

(4) The very bad fertility prognosis for non-obstructive azoospermia is improving since the introduction of the TESE/ICSI procedure. In these cases, testicular histology turns out to be the best prognostic parameter.

# References

Abuzeid, M. I., Chan, Y. M., Sasy, M. A., Basata, S. and Beer, M. (1995) Fertilisation and pregnancy achieved by intracytoplasmic injection of sperm retrieved from testicular biopsies. *Fertil Ster* **64**, 644–6

Bassil, S., Gordts, S., Otero, E. *et al.* (1995) 'Sperm epididymal aspiration. The value of a minimal surgical approach' in: *The Abstract Book for International Symposium on Human Reproduction and Male Subfertility,* October 18–21, 1995, Genk, Belgium

Belker, A. M., Thomas, A. J. and Fuchs, E. F. (1991) Results of 1469 microsurgical vasectomy-reversals by the Vasovasostomy Study Group. *J Urol* **145**, 505

Bladou, F., Grillo, J. M., Rossi, D. *et al.* (1991) Epididymal sperm aspiration in conjunction with *in vitro* fertilisation and embryo transfer in cases of obstructive azoospermia. *Hum Reprod* **6**, 1284–7

Bourne, H., Watkins, W., Spiers, A. and Baker, G. (1995) Pregnancies after intracytoplasmic injection of sperm collected by fine needle biopsy of the testis. *Fertil Steril* **64**, 433–6

Comhaire, F. H. (1992) 'An approach to the management of male infertility' in: D. M. de Kretser (Ed.). *Baillière's Clinical Endocrinology and Metabolism,* Vol. 6, pp. 435–50. London: Baillière Tindall

Craft, I., Bennett, V. and Nicholson, N. (1993) Fertilising ability of testicular spermatozoa. *Lancet* **342**, 864

Craft, I., Tsirigotis, M. and Schrivastav, P. (1995) Value of percutaneous epididymal sperm aspiration? *Fertil Steril* **63**, 208–9

Devroey, P. (1996) 'De aanpak van de azoösperme man en op welke 'evidence' is deze gebaseerd' in: *Proceedings Infertiliteit, Gynaecologie en Obstetrie anno 1996,* pp. 65–8. Rotterdam: Organon

Devroey, P., Liu, J., Nagy, Z. *et al.* (1994) Normal fertilization of human oocytes after testicular sperm extraction and intracytoplasmic sperm injection. *Fertil Steril* **62**, 639–41

Devroey, P., Liu, J., Nagy, Z. *et al.* (1995b) Pregnancies after testicular sperm extraction and intracytoplasmic sperm injection in non-obstructive azoospermia. *Hum Reprod* **10**, 1457–60

Devroey, P., Nagy, Z., Tournaye, H. *et al.* (1996) Outcome of intracytoplasmic sperm injection with testicular spermatozoa in obstructive and non-obstructive azoospermia. *Hum Reprod* (in press)

Devroey, P., Silber, S., Nagy, Z. *et al.* (1995a) Ongoing pregnancies and birth after intracytoplasmic sperm injection with frozen–thawed epididymal spermatozoa. *Hum Reprod* **10**, 903–6

Foresta, C., Varotto, A. and Scandellari, C. (1992) Assessment of testicular cytology by fine needle aspiration as a diagnostic parameter in the evaluation of the azoospermic subject. *Fertil Steril* **57**, 858–65

Gottschalk-Sabag, S., Weiss, D. B., Folb-Zacharow, N. and Zukerman, Z. (1995) Is one testicular specimen sufficient for quantitative evaluation of spermatogenesis? *Fertil Steril* **64**, 399–402

Hauser, R., Temple-Smith, P. D., Southwick, G. J. and de Kretser, D. (1995) Fertility in cases of hypergonadotropic azoospermia. *Fertil Steril* **63**, 631–6

Hirsh, A., Montgomery, J., Mohan, P. *et al.* (1993) Fertilisation by testicular sperm with standard IVF techniques. *Lancet* **342**, 1237–8

Hirsh, A. V., Mills, C., Bekir, J. *et al.* (1994) Factors influencing the outcome of *in vitro* fertilization with epididymal spermatozoa in irreversible obstructive azoospermia. *Hum Reprod* **9**, 1710–16

Hughes, T. M., Skolnick, J. L. and Belker, A. M. (1987) Young's syndrome: an often unrecognised correctable cause of obstructive azoospermia. *J Urol* **137**, 1238–40

Jequier, A. M. (1985) Obstructive azoospermia: a study of 102 patients. *Clin Reprod Fertil* **3**, 21–36

Jequier, A. M., Cummins, J. M., Gearon, C. *et al.* (1990) A pregnancy achieved using sperm from the epididymal caput in idiopathic obstructive azoospermia. *Fertil Steril* **53**, 1104–5

Kahraman, S., Özgür, S., Alatas, C. *et al.* (1996) High implantation and pregnancy rates with testicular sperm extraction and intracytoplasmic sperm injection in obstructive and non-obstructive azoospermia. *Hum Reprod* **11**, 673–6

Levin, H. S. (1979) Testicular biopsy in the study of male infertility. Its current usefulness, histologic techniques, and prospects for the future. *Hum Pathol* **10**, 569–84

Mallidis, C. and Baker, G. (1994) Fine needle tissue aspiration biopsy of the testis. *Fertil Steril* **6**, 367–75

Matsumiya, K., Namiki, M., Takahara, S. *et al.* (1994) Clinical study of azoospermia. *Int J Androl* **17**, 140–2

Micic, S. (1987) Incidence of aetiological factors in testicular obstructive azoospermia. *Int J Androl* **10**, 681–4

Nagy, Z. P., Liu, J., Joris, H. *et al.* (1995) The result of intracytoplasmic sperm injection is not related to any of the three basic sperm parameters. *Hum Reprod* **10**, 1123–9

Oates, R. D., Lobel, S. M., Harris, D. H. *et al.* (1996) Efficacy of intracytoplasmic sperm injection using intentionally cryopreserved epididymal spermatozoa. *Hum Reprod* **11**, 133–8

Palermo, G., Joris, H., Devroey, P. and Van Steirteghem, C. C. (1992) Pregnancies after intracytoplasmic sperm injection of single spermatozoon into an oocyte. *Lancet* **340**, 17–18

Pryor, J., Parsons, J., Goswamy, R. *et al.* (1984) *In-vitro* fertilisation for men with obstructive azoospermia. *Lancet* **ii**, 762

Romero, J., Remohi, J., Minguez, Y. *et al.* (1996) Fertilization after intracytoplasmic sperm injection with cryopreserved testicular spermatozoa. *Fertil Steril* **65**, 877–9

Schlegel, P. N., Berkeley, A. S., Goldstein, M. *et al.* (1994) Epididymal micropuncture with *in vitro* fertilization and oocyte micromanipulation for the treatment of unreconstructable obstructive azoospermia. *Fertil Steril* **61**, 895–901

Schoysman, R. (1980) The interest of testicular biopsy in the study of male infertility. *Acta Eur Fertil* **11**, 1–32

Schoysman, R., Vanderzwalmen, P., Nijs, M., Segal-Bertin, G. and van de Casseye, M. (1993a) Successful fertilization by testicular spermatozoa in an *in-vitro* fertilization programme. *Hum Reprod* **8**, 1339–40

Schoysman, R., Vanderzwalmen, P., Nijs, M. *et al.* (1993b) Pregnancy after fertilisation with human testicular spermatozoa. *Lancet* **342**, 1237

Shrivastav, P., Nadkarni, P., Wensvoort, S. and Craft, I. (1994) Percutaneous epididymal sperm aspiration for obstructive azoospermia. *Hum Reprod* **9**, 2058–61

Silber, S. J. (1988) Pregnancy caused by sperm from vasa efferentia. *Fertil Steril* **49**, 373–5

Silber, S. J., Balmaceda, J., Borrero, C., Ord, T. and Asch, T. (1988) Pregnancy with sperm aspiration from the proximal head of the epididymis: a new treatment for congenital absence of the vas deferens. *Fertil Steril* **50**, 525–8

Silber, S. J., Nagy, Z. P., Liu, J. *et al.* (1994) Conventional *in-vitro* fertilisation versus intracytoplasmic sperm injection for patients requiring microsurgical sperm aspiration. *Hum Reprod* **9**, 1705–9

Silber, S. J., Ord, T., Balmageda, J., Patrizio, P. and Asch, R. H. (1990) Congenital absence of the vas deferens. The fertilizing capacity of human epididymal sperm. *N Engl J Med* **323**, 1788–92

Silber, S. J., Patrizio, P. and Asch, R. H. (1990) Quantitative evaluation of spermatogenesis by testicular histology in men with congenital absence of the vas deferens undergoing epididymal sperm aspiration. *Hum Reprod* **5**, 89–93

Silber, S. J., Van Steirteghem, A. C., Liu, J. *et al.* (1995) High fertilization and pregnancy rate after intracytoplasmic sperm injection with spermatozoa obtained from testicle biopsy. *Hum Reprod* **10**, 148–52

Sperm Microaspiration Retrieval Techniques Study Group (1994) Results in the United States with sperm microaspiration retrieval techniques and assisted reproductive technologies. *J Urol* **151**, 1255–9

Temple-Smith, P. D., Southwick, G. J., Yates, C. A., Trounson, A. D., de Kretser, D. M. (1985) Human pregnancy by *in vitro* fertilization (IVF) using sperm aspirated from the epididymis. *J In Vitro Fertil Embryo Transfer* **2**, 119–22

Tournaye, H., Camus, M., Goossens, A. *et al.* (1995) Recent concepts in the management of infertility because of non-obstructive azoospermia. *Hum Reprod* **10** (Suppl. 1), 115–19

Tournaye, H., Devroey, P., Liu, J. *et al.* (1994) Microsurgical epididymal sperm aspiration and intracytoplasmic sperm injection: a new effective approach to infertility as a result of congenital bilateral absence of the vas deferens. *Fertil Steril* **61**, 1045–51

Tournaye, H., Goossens, A., Ubaldi, F., Silber, S., Van Steirtegham, A. and Devroey, P. (1996b) 'Are there any predictive factors for successful testicular sperm recovery in azoospermic patients?' in: *European Society of Human Reproduction and Embryology (ESHRE)*, Maastricht 30 June–3 July, 1996

Tournaye, H., Liu, J., Nagy, P. Z. *et al.* (1996a) Correlation between testicular histology and

outcome after intracytoplasmic sperm injection using testicular spermatozoa. *Hum Reprod* **11**, 127–32

Tsirigotis, M., Bennett, V., Hodewind, G., Pelekanos, M. and Craft, I. (1994) Percutaneous epididymal sperm aspiration simplified sperm recovery of obstructive azoospermia. *Hum Reprod* **9** (Suppl. 4), 169–70

Tsirigotis, M. and Craft, I. (1995) Sperm retrieval methods and ICSI for obstructive azoospermia. *Hum Reprod* **10**, 758–60

Turner, T. T. (1995) On the epididymis and its role in the development of the fertile ejaculate. *J Androl* **16**, 292–8

Turner, T. T., Gleavy, J. L. and Harris, J. M. (1990) Fluid movement in the lumen of the rat epididymis: effect of vasectomy and subsequent vasovasostomy. *J Androl* **11**, 422–8

Van Steirteghem, A. C., Nagy, Z. and Joris, H. *et al.* (1993a) High fertilization and implantation rates after intracytoplasmic sperm injection. *Hum Reprod* **8**, 1061–6

Van Steirteghem, A. C., Liu, J., Joris, H. *et al.* (1993b) Higher success rate of intracytoplasmic sperm injection than by subzonal insemination. Report of the second series of 300 consecutive treatment cycles. *Hum Reprod* **8**, 1055–60

Weiske, W. H. (1994) Pregnancy caused by sperm from vasa efferentia. *Fertil Steril* **62**, 642–3

World Health Organisation (1992) *Laboratory Manual for the Examination of Human Semen and Semen–Cervical Mucus Interaction*, 3rd edn. Cambridge: Cambridge University Press

# 19

# Chronic pelvic pain and endometriosis

*Olusegun A. Odukoya and Ian D. Cooke*

There is no universally accepted definition for chronic pelvic pain (CPP). Generally, it refers to pain which is present, either intermittently or constantly, for at least six months and which is severe enough to interfere with the quality of life of the woman. The perception of pain varies considerably between one individual and another and is not related to the magnitude or duration of the pain-producing stimulus. Although a number of possible organic factors has been considered, no physical abnormality can be documented in many women who report CPP. Furthermore, factors such as social and family background, cultural differences, anxiety and stress levels which influence an individual's personality affect individual perception of pain.

In Britain, pelvic pain is the most common complaint among women seeking gynaecological consultation (Morris and O'Neil 1958). In a survey undertaken by the Royal College of Obstetricians and Gynaecologists in Britain involving almost 21,000 laparoscopies, the primary indication was CPP in 11,000 patients (52%) (Chamberlain and Brown 1978). In the United States, a prevalence of 35% was reported (Reiter 1990a). An Australian study of 717 women with endometriosis for whom the chief complaint was recorded, revealed dysmenorrhoea as the chief complaint, followed by dyspareunia and pelvic pain (O'Connor 1987; Table 1). While endometriosis may be asymptomatic, the most common presenting symptom is pelvic pain, classically starting in the third decade. The pain may be in the form of dysmenorrhoea or dyspareunia. To enhance understanding of endometriosis-associated CPP, a brief description of the nerve supply of the pelvis and the possible mechanisms of pain are given, followed by a review of the various treatment modalities.

## PELVIC AND LOWER ABDOMINAL NERVE SUPPLY

The autonomic nerves (sympathetic and parasympathetic) supply the abdominopelvic organs. Damage to any of these nerves can simulate pelvic pain. Pain impulses from the uterus, medial part of the Fallopian tube, broad ligament and upper vagina are conducted via visceral afferents to the Frankenhauser's paracervical plexus from where it is transmitted to the inferior, middle and superior hypogastric plexus to enter the thoracolumbar sympathetic chain. The afferents then enter the spinal cord via the posterior nerve route to the level of T10–L1 (Ripkin 1990). The afferent pathway from the ovary, lateral part of the Fallopian tube and peritoneum enters the main sympathetic

**Table 1** *Symptom distribution in endometriosis. (Adapted from O'Connor 1987\*, reproduced with permission of Churchill Livingstone)*

| Symptom | Number (n = 717) | Percentage |
|---|---|---|
| Dysmenorrhoea | 227 | 32 |
| Dyspareunia | 188 | 26 |
| Pelvic pain | 114 | 16 |
| Infertility | 64 | 9 |
| Asymptomatic | 155 | 22 |

\*O'Connor, D. T. (1987) 'Clinical features in diagnosis' in: A. Jordon and A. Singer (Eds.). *Endometriosis*, pp. 68–78. Edinburgh: Churchill Livingstone nerve chain at the fourth lumbar sympathetic ganglion and ascends with the sympathetic to enter the spinal cord at the ninth and tenth thoracic segment. The pelvic parasympathetic fibres travel in the pudendal nerves and enter the spinal cord via the nervi erigentes (S2–S4). Pain originating from pelvic organs may be experienced in the skin areas supplied by the somatic afferent fibres of the same spinal segment. This phenomenon is known as 'referred' pain.

## PAIN PHYSIOLOGY

The pelvis is supplied by somatic and visceral nerves. Pain perception is dependent on the stimulation of nerve endings (nociceptors) with the transmission of impulses via the spinal cord to the brain. There are two types of nociceptors: The $A\delta$ and the C types. The afferent axons of $A\delta$ receptors which are often associated with somatic nerves are small, myelinated with rapid impulse conduction. The pain generated by such receptors tends to be of acute onset, well localised and circumscribed. The afferent axons of the C receptors which are distributed in deep (visceral) tissues are unmyelinated with slow transmission of impulses. Pain signals are poorly localised, causing a vague dull pain or ache, diffuse and sometimes described as 'deep' or 'numb'. They are typical of that experienced in endometriosis. The impulses from the nociceptor fibres synapse in the grey matter of the dorsal horn of the spinal cord at the same or adjacent segment of the spinal cord. The impulses are relayed via ascending fibres in the contralateral spinothalamic tract to the reticular formation and thalamic nuclei in the brain. The information may then be transmitted to the postcentral gyrus of the cerebral cortex.

Pain signals may be modified either pharmacologically or surgically at all levels before and within the spinal cord and the brain. Pharmacological agents such as prostaglandin synthetase inhibitors decrease the amount of prostaglandins. Opiate receptor stimulation may inhibit spinal neurones at the dorsal root ganglion or stimulate the midbrain, which in turn causes an inhibition of the descending pathway. The variation in pain perception is probably due to the degree of inhibitory modification rather than differences in nociceptor activity.

## MODELS OF PAIN PERCEPTION

The management of CPP is often diverse due to our poor understanding of its pathogenesis and maintenance. Management is based on the various proposed theories of pain perception.

### Medical model (Cartesian theory)

Pain perception is a direct result of tissue trauma and its perception is directly related to the severity of the trauma. This model supposes that eradication of the source of the tissue injury ameliorates the pain, hence the intensity of the investigation to find and treat the cause. When such a cause is not identified, a spurious or psychogenic cause is attached. This model is overtly simplistic as multiple psychological factors have been demonstrated in many patients, leading to the development of gate control theory.

### Gate control theory

The theory integrates the peripheral stimuli to cerebral cortex variables such as mood and anxiety in the pain perception. In this model, pain and depression are argued to occur simultaneously through an interlocking mechanism. Certainly, the gate control theory is a better predictor of short- and long-term outcomes in CPP populations than the Cartesian model. The latter model fails to incorporate the myriad social variables which may affect the perception of pain (Steege, Staut and Somkuti 1992).

### Biopsychosocial model

This is a combination of chronic nociceptive stimuli and multiple psychological and social determinants. It supposes that, although nociceptive stimuli (e.g. dysmenorrhoea) are prevalent in the population, they will not lead to harmful outcomes in the absence of specific psychological conditions. Thus, the eradication of nociceptive stimuli without alteration of the predisposing psychological state in a chronic pain patient would lead to a temporary improvement in the symptoms followed by recurrent disabling symptoms, sometimes involving an alternate site such as chronic fatigue and headache. The latter is called symptom shift. The biopsychosocial model provides for the multidisciplinary team approach to the management of CPP.

## CAUSES OF CPP

An understanding of the aetiology of CPP is important because of the dehabilitating effect it has on women. The main causes are as shown in Table 2. In about 30–75% of patients no aetiology could be found (Beard 1986; Reiter 1990b). It interferes with the daily life of those affected ranging from absence from work to serious marital disharmony. Furthermore, these patients have a high prevalence of emotional disturbance ranging between lassitude, depression, chronic anxiety, loss of interest in social activities, hypochondriasis, sleep disturbances, multiple drug use and abuse (Wood, Wiesner and Reityer 1990). Duncan and Taylor (1952) noted that 29 (80%) of 36 patients with unexplained pelvic pain had an unfavourable family environment in childhood, which they suggested led to emotional disturbance in later life. In the United Kingdom, the estimated cost of diagnosis and treatment of CPP in 1991 to the National Health Service (NHS) was £158.4 million per annum (Beard, Gangar and Pearce 1994).

## CLASSIFICATION OF PAIN

This could be embryological, physiological or clinical (Kumazao 1986). These will now be discussed in turn.

### Embryological

Pain arising from tissues of ectoderm origin (e.g. skin and mucous membrane) is sharp, with well-defined localisation. Those of mesoderm

**Table 2**  *Causes of chronic pelvic pain*

*Gynaecological:*
  pelvis
    endometriosis
    pelvic congestion syndrome
    pelvic adhesions
    chronic pelvic infammatory disease
  ovary
    benign cysts (endometrioma)
    polycystic ovarian disease
    ovarian remnant syndrome
    'ovarian enlargement'
  uterus
    dysmenorrhoea (congestive and spasmodic)
    intrauterine contraceptive device
    uterovaginal prolapse
  cervix
    stenosis
  others
    vulvodynia
    malignancies of the genital tract

*Non-gynaecological:*
  neuromusculoskeletal
    myofascial and trigger point pain
    illioinguinal nerve entrapment
    ventral hernia
    rectus tendon strain
    pain-associated postural change
    pelvic floor tension myalgia
    prolapsed intervertebral disc
    lumbosacral osteoarthritis
  gastrointestinal tract
    irritable bowel syndrome
    inflammatory bowel disease
    diverticulitis
  urinary tract
    calculus
    chronic retention
    interstitial cystitis
    malignancy

*Psychogenic*

*Idiopathic*

origin (e.g. muscles, ligaments, bone and joint) have poor localisation, are often deep and are not as sharp. Tissues which originate from the endoderm give rise to pain which is dull, aching and ill defined.

### Physiological

Pain could be classified as neuropathic, nociceptive or idiopathic (Arner and Meyerson 1988;

Hamman 1993). Neuropathic pain is caused by destruction of function in peripheral nerves, pain receptors (nociceptors) or the central pain pathway. This destruction is caused by mechanical trauma, ischaemia, degeneration or inflammation of the peripheral or central pain pathway. Nociceptive pain is caused by stimulation of peripheral nociceptors. The pain is often in response to mechanical distortion, thermal damage or in response to the release of chemical substances such as serotonin, 5-hydroxytryptamine, bradykinin, prostaglandins and substance P (Iggo 1983). Idiopathic pelvic pain is a condition in which a thorough evaluation has failed to disclose a plausible aetiology.

## Clinical

Based on the duration of symptoms, pain could be either acute or chronic. Chronic pelvic pain in women is defined as non-cyclic pelvic pain of greater than six months' duration which is not relieved by non-narcotic analgesics (Reiter 1990a). It can occur with or without pelvic pathology. It is a non-specific term which clinicians associate with laparoscopically evident pelvic pathology (e.g. endometriosis), occult somatic pathology (e.g. irritable bowel syndrome) or non-somatic (psychogenic) disorders.

## PAIN MECHANISMS IN ENDOMETRIOSIS

This often depends on whether the visceral or the somatic pathway is involved. The involvement may be direct or indirect. Direct involvement may be by the deposition of endometriosis deposits or the seqealae of the deposit such as degenerative scarring with fibrotic reaction. The indirect pathway is suggested to be via chemical substances produced by eutopic or ectopic endometrium. Suggested mechanisms are:

(1) The retrograde passage of menstrual blood containing prostaglandin through the Fallopian tubes into the peritoneum may sensitise the nociceptors in the peritoneum causing pain. However, almost all women in the reproductive age group experience retrograde menstruation, most of whom have no pain (Halme *et al.* 1984). This suggests that menstrual effluent alone may not be responsible for the pelvic pain.

(2) The provocation of inflammatory changes following endometrial implantation into the peritoneum with the release of chemical mediators (e.g. serotonin, histamine, bradykins and cytokines) which stimulate the sympathetic nociceptors, leading to pain (Denzlinger *et al.* 1985; Cunha *et al.* 1991).

(3) Deep infiltrating endometriosis provokes tissue damage (Cornillie *et al.* 1990). Direct involvement of the autonomic nerves by endometriotic deposits may be a possible mechanism. This may explain why small deposits of endometriosis in the uterosacral ligament produce pain in some women.

(4) Organ distension as in an endometriotic cyst may cause capsular stretch and nociceptor stimulation resulting in pain. Furthermore, chronic leakage or rupture of such a cyst may predispose to chemical peritonitis and chronic pain.

(5) Tissue tethering resulting from scarring and subsequent retraction may lead to pelvic pain of prolonged standing.

(6) Fixity of the uterus from adhesion formation resulting in retroversion, or displacement and fixity of the ovaries in the pouch of Douglas, may result in coital ache. Endometriotic nodule deposition in the uterosacral ligament and rectovaginal pouch causing scarring may be associated with dyspareunia.

(7) Endometriotic deposit in the bowel may cause distension from fibrosis and retraction. This may result in pain at defecation (dyschezia) and explain the difficulty in distinguishing irritable bowel syndrome from endometriosis. Fixity of the bowel to a nodule in the rectovaginal pouch may further explain the deep dyspareunia experienced by patients.

## PAIN SYMPTOMS ASSOCIATED WITH ENDOMETRIOSIS

The prevalence of endometriosis in patients who had a laparoscopic investigation for CPP ranged from 3% to 45% with an average of around 15% (Tables 3 and 4). The extent to which endometriosis is associated with CPP is controversial. Patients who have extensive disease may have no symptoms, whereas patients with minimal disease may complain of disabling symptoms. In a study of 100 women who had diagnostic laparoscopy for pelvic pain, 32% had endometriosis, while this diagnosis was made in 15% of 50 women who had no pain during laparoscopic tubal ligation (Kresch *et al.* 1984). Cunanan, Courey and Lippes (1983) studied 1194 women with pelvic pain, of whom 43 (4.6%) were found to have endometriosis. If endometriosis is indeed a cause of CPP, the severity of pain symptoms should be proportional to the *location*, severity *(stage)* and *extent* of the disease.

**Table 3** *Prevalence of previous surgery in endometriosis associated pelvic pain at the Jessop Hospital for Women in Sheffield, United Kingdom*

| Previous surgery | Number | Percentage (%) |
|---|---|---|
| Laparotomy* | 35 | 31 |
| Laparoscopy† | 31 | 28 |
| Laparoscopy† and laparotomy* | 10 | 9 |
| None | 36 | 32 |
| Total | 112 | 100 |

*The indications for laparotomy include hysterectomy, previous adhesiolysis for endometriosis, oophorectomy, ovarian cystectomy and excision of rectosigmoid endometriosis. † Laparoscopy was mainly for diagnostic purposes in the referral hospital

## Location

In a prospective study of 160 women in which the location of endometriosis was related to the symptom of pelvic pain to test the hypothesis that if endometriosis were a cause of pain then it should cause pain at the site(s) of implantation, no correlation was obtained between location of endometriosis and pelvic pain (Fedele *et al.* 1990). In another study of 89 patients with pelvic pain of whom 59 had endometriosis, 45 (76%) patients had some correlation between implant localisation and focal tenderness on pelvic examination (Ripps and Martin 1991). It is noted in this study that 26 (59%) of the 45 patients had areas of endometriosis that were not tender on pelvic examination, suggesting that the presence of the lesion is not always associated with symptoms. A non-gynaecological location of ectopic endometrium may present with apparent symptoms such as cyclical pain and bleeding (surgical or umbilical scar) and cyclical haemoptysis (lung deposits) or haematuria (bladder deposit). However, the severity of the symptoms bears no relation to that of the lesion (Shaw 1993).

## Severity

An attempt to explain the variability of pain with endometriosis is based on the production of prostaglandins (PG). The peritoneal fluid of patients with endometriosis contains significant amounts of prostaglandin $E_2$ ($PGE_2$) and $PGF_{2\alpha}$ (Badawy, Marshall and Cuenca 1985; Schmidt 1985; Deleon *et al* 1986). Jansen and Russell (1986) classified endometriosis into non-pigmented and pigmented lesions based on laparoscopic evaluation of the peritoneum.

**Table 4** *Prevalence of endometriosis in patients with chronic pelvic pain*

| Authors | Chronic pelvic pain (n) | Endometriosis n | % |
|---|---|---|---|
| Lundberg, Wall and Mathers (1973) | 95 | 13 | 14 |
| Cunanan, Courey and Lippes (1983) | 1194 | 43 | 3.6 |
| Kresch *et al.* (1984) | 100 | 32 | 32 |
| Goldstein (1989) | 282 | 126 | 45 |
| Moen and Muss (1991) | 107 | 24 | 22 |

Non-pigmented lesions are white, opacified, glandular, or red flame-like in appearance. These lesions have been shown by light microscopy and by both scanning and electron microscopy to be composed of highly differentiated endometrial glands with well vascularised ectopic stroma, suggesting that these minimal lesions are active and may directly stimulate nociceptive nerve endings eliciting pain (Stripling et al. 1988; Cornillie et al. 1990). Furthermore, Vernon et al. (1986) showed that these lesions had a greater capacity for synthesising PGF than the pigmented ones, which have the classical puckered scar fibrosis or powder-burn effect. The biochemical activity of ectopic endometriotic implants may correlate with the severity of the symptoms, although there are no current data to support this view. It is possible that these chemical compounds cause vasospasm, with consequent release of pain producing substances such as serotonin or bradykinin. This is further supported by the knowledge that prostaglandin inhibitors are sometimes effective in treating endometriosis pain.

## Extent

The American Fertility Society (AFS) classification score of endometriosis of 1985 was specifically developed for the evaluation of fertility on weighted scales based on the severity of ovarian and tubal involvement. However, a poor correlation exists between the extent of endometriosis and the severity of disease symptoms. The extent of the disease can be estimated either by the depth of infiltration, the number of implants or the anatomical and functional damage to tissue structures (usually in the form of adhesion formation). Koninckx and Martin (1992) showed that deep endometriosis, defined as endometriosis that infiltrated more than 5 mm, is associated with pelvic pain. In another study of 59 patients with endometriosis, an average infiltration depth greater than 5 mm was associated with focal areas of pelvic tenderness (Ripps and Martin 1991). These studies, although suggestive, require further prospective work to evaluate the relation between depth

of infiltration and the symptom of pelvic pain as proposed by the more recent AFS endometriosis pain score (American Fertility Society 1993). The relationship between the number of implants and pain symptoms was investigated by Perper et al. in 1995. In this prospective study of 70 patients who had a laparoscopy for pain or infertility, 39 (56%) had menstrual pain. There was a significant association between the intensity of pain and the number of ectopic implants (pigmented and non-pigmented).

There is inadequate evidence to support abdominopelvic adhesions as a cause of CPP. In a retrospective study of 100 patients who underwent laparoscopic investigation for CPP and 88 for infertility, there was no difference between these groups regarding the presence (26% versus 39%) or severity of adhesions (Raplan 1986). On the other hand, Chan and Wood (1985), demonstrated a partial or total improvement in the pain symptom in 65% of patients following laparotomy for adhesiolysis, while a 67% improvement rate was shown with laparoscopic adhesiolysis (Daniel 1989). This is further compounded by anecdotal clinical experience in which a single tense band of adhesion producing CPP is relieved by surgical removal. In a review of 112 patients with CPP who were diagnosed to have endometriosis at the Jessop Hospital for Women in Sheffield, United Kingdom, between 1985 and 1994, 45 (59%) of the 76 patients with previous pelvic surgery had had a laparotomy (Table 4). Among the latter group, 33 (89%) patients had lower central abdominal pain with adhesions involving the adnexa, bowel and uterus in different combinations (unpublished data). These data suggest that laparotomy is associated with adhesion formation in patients with endometriosis and concur with the suggestion that if adhesiolysis is to be undertaken where possible, the laparoscopic route seems to be associated with a lower degree of adhesion formation and reformation (Donnez et al. 1992). The value of adhesiolysis is further called into question by the demonstration of the placebo effect of laparoscopy in the relief of pelvic pain (Baker and Symonds 1992). The authors suggested that attributing a psychogenic cause to CPP should only be contemplated after diagnostic laparoscopy.

## MANAGEMENT OF ENDOMETRIOSIS ASSOCIATED CPP

The management of CPP depends on the identification of problem areas which are targets for intervention, the development of a treatment plan and the establishment of baseline information to allow progress in evaluation and treatment effectiveness. The value of an adequate, detailed and meticulous history taken by a sympathetic listener cannot be overemphasised in these patients, many of whom have passed through more than one practitioner. Ideally information should be obtained from both patient and partner or family. Particular attention is paid to composure, fluency of narration, derailment of thought and emotions (including the 'body language') which may give valuable clues to psychological state. Her attitudes towards the discussion of her past, including parental and sexual relationships, may give vital clues to hidden causes of pelvic pain. The characteristics of the pain including site, duration, mode on onset, radiation and relationship to coitus and menstrual cycle should be explored. Memoirs of childhood experience and bereavement, including past psychiatric disturbances, should be explored with caution and diplomacy. Attention should be paid to abnormalities of the urinary and gastrointestinal tracts. In our experience, symptoms of irritable bowel syndrome (IBS) commonly occur with endometriosis-associated CPP, often due to paracolic adhesions which improve when the adhesions are dealt with.

There may be no abdominal sign on palpation. Sometimes a 'trigger point' is elicited. The sigmoid colon and caecum may be palpably enlarged and tender suggesting IBS. Cystic swelling with or without tenderness of the fossae may suggest an ovarian endometrioma. Bimanual vaginal examination may show positive cervical excitation tenderness, with or without adnexal masses. The uterosacrals may be tender from endometriotic nodule deposits. The rectovaginal septum may contain endo-metriotic nodules, which are better assessed by simultaneous vagina and rectal examinations.

Laparoscopy complemented by directed biopsy is the hallmark of diagnosis of endometriosis. Ultrasonographic imaging technique is unique in that it is non-invasive and readily available in most centres. It may be important in the diagnosis of endometrioma, although its sensitivity is poor. Magnetic resonance imaging (MRI) has been suggested to improve diagnostic sensitivity (71–90%) in endometriosis (Zawin et al. 1989; Togashi et al. 1991). A modification of conventional MRI with fat saturation of tissues in 51 patients with endometriosis increased the sensitivity to 97% (Takahashi et al. 1994). However, this procedure is expensive, not readily available and of little value in detecting small lesions. Proctoscopy, sigmoidoscopy and/or barium studies may be useful investigations if there is bowel or rectovaginal septum involvement.

## TREATMENT

Most patients believe that CPP due to endometriosis is an indication of progressive damage to pelvic structures. It is the duty of the attending physicians to educate the patient that this is not necessarily the case. Physical and emotional factors play a role in endometriosis associated CPP (Low, Edelman and Sutton 1994). The treatment approach should be multidisciplinary involving the gynaecologist, health psychologist, counsellor and an anaesthetist. The treatment should be concurrent. Having diagnosed endometriosis in a patient with CPP the options include medical, surgical or combination therapy.

### Medical therapy

Conservative management in the form of medical therapy is indicated when there is a need to preserve reproductive potential or when the patient wishes to retain her reproductive organs for personal, social or psychological reasons. Furthermore, the proponents of medical therapy explain that all lesions, whether microscopic or macroscopic, are exposed to the pharmacological agent as long as there is a reasonable blood supply. The principle behind hormonal medical therapy is to mimic the hypo-oestrogenic serum profile that is associated with the menopause or pregnancy which is hostile to the growth and development of ectopic endometrium. It is believed that the superficial implants respond better than the deep ones to hormone therapy (Shaw 1991). Symptom relief is similar with most medical therapies, and in almost half of the patients a return to pretreatment level occurs after six months (Dlugi, Miller and Knittle 1990). The hormonal treatments which have been demonstrated to be effective in the relief of pain in endometriosis are low-dose oral contraceptive pills, progestogens, androgenic steroids and gonadotrophin hormone releasing hormone analogues (GnRHa).

### Low-dose combined oral contraceptive pill

The combined pills exert their effect by suppressing ovarian function. In a randomised trial of 50 patients with either danazol or Enavid (75 µg of menstranol and 5 mg of norethisterone), 89% and 35%, respectively, experienced partial or complete relief of their symptoms (Noble and Letchworth 1980). However, 87% of the Enavid group had severe side effects of weight gain, nausea, vomiting, breathlessness and thromboembolic effects. These side effects made its use unpopular. A recent randomised study involving 57 patients on low-dose cyclic oral contraception (0.02 mg of ethinyloestradiol and 0.15 mg of desogestrel per day) and goserelin by monthly injection showed similar relief in pain symptoms in the two groups (Vercellini et al. 1993). Further prospective work needs to be done in this area in view of the low cost, relative safety and availability of oral contraception.

### Progestogens

Progestogens are effective in causing decidualisation and atrophy of ectopic endometrium. Derivatives of 19-nortestoterone (norethisterone, norgestrel and megestrol) or of prog-esterone (medroxyprogesterone acetate [MPA], dydrogesterone) have been shown to be effective in the relief of pelvic pain. Schlaff and co-workers (1990) treated 29 patients with megestrol (40 mg per day) and reported 86% relief in pelvic pain after six months' therapy. In a prospective, placebo-controlled trial comparing danazol with MPA (100 mg per day), comparable relief of pelvic pain which was significantly better than the placebo was reported (Telima et al. 1987). Common side effects of progestogen therapy include breakthrough bleeding, fluid retention, nausea and breast tenderness. Progestogens also cause a rise in the serum concentration of low-density lipoprotein with a tendency toward atherogenicity. Although the progestogens are relatively cheap and readily available, the long-term effects of this group of drugs on the cardiovascular system need further evaluation.

### Danazol

Danazol is an isoxazol derivative of 17 α-ethinyl testosterone. It is mildly androgenic with anabolic properties. Its effectiveness in relieving pelvic pain varies from 60–100% (Henzl et al. 1988; Kennedy et al. 1990). It is used in doses of 200–800 mg per day. Common side effects include weight gain, acne, oily skin, fluid retention, muscle cramps and mood changes. Other less common effects are depression, hot flushes, hirsutism, skin rash and deepening of voice. These side effects are dose related. Furthermore, danazol therapy is known to cause an increase in low-density lipoprotein and a decrease in high-density lipoprotein cholesterol, an indicator of future risk of developing heart disease (Fahraeus et al. 1984; Bergquist 1990). The atherogenic effect is not dose dependent and is reversible after cessation of therapy (Lemay et al. 1991). Periodic evaluation of serum lipid is advisable in patients who are on long-term danazol therapy.

### Gonadotrophin releasing hormone analogues

The use of GnRHa results in reversible 'medical oophorectomy'. This is because the continued administration of GnRHa leads to desensitisation and down-regulation of the pituitary GnRH receptors, followed by reduction of the serum gonadotrophin concentrations, which results in low serum oestrogen levels and, consequently, the inhibition of ovarian steroidogenesis. Several randomised studies have shown decreased pain in 70–90% of patients after six months of therapy (Rolland and Van der Heijden 1990; Nafarelin European Endometriosis Trial (NEET) Group 1992). In a prospective, randomised, double-blind study of 179 patients given three or six months' nafarelin for endometriosis-associated pelvic pain, no difference was detected between the two drugs while on therapy and 92% of patients experienced clinical improvement. The pain score at the end of 12 months' follow-up remained significantly below the baseline in both groups of patients (Hornstein et al. 1995). There is evidence that three months of either danazol or leuprolide acetate is efficacious in the relief of endometriosis-associated pain (Wright et al. 1995). The side effects of GnRHa are those related to hypo-oestrogenic states often in the form of hot flushes, reduction in libido, vaginal dryness, headaches, emotional instability and depression. Given the cost and side effects of GnRHa, an effective, short-duration treatment would be of considerable clinical and economic importance. Furthermore, greater than six months' use is associated with bone loss. An attempt to maintain a therapeutic improvement in symptoms but minimise bone loss has led to the suggestion of add-back therapy in patients with endometriosis who may require more than six months of treatment (Barberi 1992). A recent study showed a good correlation between pain relief and serum oestradiol level of less than 40 pg/ml compared to those with concentrations greater than 40 pg/ml (Hornstein et al. 1995). Whether this level is sufficient to prevent bone loss and serve as an 'oestrogen therapeutic window' requires further investigation.

## Surgery

Surgical therapy for endometriosis related CPP could be conservative or radical. The aims of conservative surgery include: reduction in the volume of ectopic endometrial tissue, restoration of normal pelvic anatomy, removal of ovarian endometrioma and interruption of afferent sensory pain pathways. These can be achieved by surgery to peritoneal and ovarian endometriosis, excision of deep-infiltrating endometriosis (including resection of the rectovaginal septum), and treatment of ureteral and gastrointestinal deposits. These procedures could be performed by laparoscopy or laparotomy (Bateman, Kolp and Mills 1994). Peritoneal endometriosis which is associated with pelvic pain is treated with coagulation, laser vaporisation or excision. In a double-blind, prospective study of 21 patients with endometriosis who had laser uterine nerve ablation (LUNA), nine of 11 (82%) reported relief of pain after three months' therapy while improvement was sustained in 45% at the end of one year. None of the 10 women in the control group had relief of symptoms (Lichten and Bombard 1987). Malinak (1985) suggested that LUNA may be particularly useful in situations where a nodule is present at the base of the uterosacral ligament, which may require excision, when there is inadequate exposure of the presacral nerves to allow presacral neurectomy and when pain recurs after presacral neurectomy. Furthermore, in a review of 13 reports of 633 cases of LUNA, 73.5% were reported to have pain relief after treatment. The authors suggested that presacral neurectomy may have an adjunctive role, albeit small, in the treatment of a centrally located pelvic pain which is associated with endometriosis, adhesive disease or chronic pelvic inflammatory disease (Lee et al. 1986).

The superficial ovarian endometriotic cyst as well as the deep endometrioma can be treated via the laparoscope. In the case of a deep endometrioma that is greater than 3 cm, drainage of the cyst (laparoscopic cystotomy and biopsy) followed by three months of GnRHa has been shown to be effective (Donnez et al. 1994). Endometriosis of the rectovaginal septum can be removed by laparoscopy if discrete and well localised (Nezhat, Nezhat and Pennington 1992; Nezhat et al. 1995). In the authors' opinion, most require laparotomy with or without temporary colostomy. It is the authors' practice to administer preoperative GnRHa for three months to reduce vascularity and volume of the tumour. Total abdominal hysterectomy and bilateral removal of the ovaries with hormone replacement therapy may be contemplated in those patients who have completed their family, although this does not guarantee a cure. In a study of 99 patients who had hysterectomy for CPP, 22 patients had no remission after a mean follow-up of 22 months (Stovall, Ling and Crawford 1990).

Other non-conventional methods of pain relief include radiofrequency currents, electrical nerve stimulation and acupuncture. Interruption of the pathways in the central nervous system (anterolateral cordotomy) appears an attractive way of relieving pain, but the results are disappointing as the pain returns either due to nerve regeneration or by development through alternative pathways.

### Psychological

There is evidence, albeit inconclusive, that psychological abnormalities such as depression, neuroticism, substance and drug abuse, poor marital relationship and childhood and adult sexual abuse exist in women with CPP when compared with the controls (Walker *et al.* 1988; Steege, Stout and Somkuti 1991). The treatment regimens often include cognitive–

behavioural pain therapy. These methods include relaxation techniques such as hypnotherapy, pain behaviour modification, physical exercise, marital and family counselling (Milburn, Reiter and Rhomberg 1993). The goals of management are to control pain, reduce disability, promote wellbeing and treat specific psychological abnormalities such as depression. A randomised study of 106 patients comparing multidisciplinary treatment with a Cartesian therapy approach showed a better control of CPP in the former when compared with the latter (Peter *et al.* 1991). Such an approach which breaks the endometriosis– fibrosis–pain vicious cycle may minimise the use of hysterectomy for the treatment of CPP.

### CONCLUSION

Endometriosis is associated with various forms of abdominopelvic pain. While endometriosis may play a role in the pathophysiology of CPP its severity does not correlate with the degree of pain. However, the depth of invasion and the number of ectopic implants correlate with pain severity. Various forms of therapy are advocated with equal efficacy. The multidisciplinary approach, although costly to set up and run, is associated with better relief of symptoms with low recurrence rate. A randomised controlled trial is needed to assess the various methods of treatment with long-term follow-up to assess the return of symptoms.

# References

American Fertility Society (1993) Management of endometriosis in the presence of pelvic pain. *Fertil Steril* **60**, 952–5

Arner, S. and Meyerson, B. A. (1988) Lack of analgesic effect of opioids on neuropathic and idiopathic forms of pain. *Pain* **33**, 11–23

Badawy, S. Z. A., Marshall, L. and Cuenca, V. (1985) Peritoneal fluid prostaglandin in various stages of the menstrual cycle: role in infertile patients with endometriosis. *Int J Fertil* **30**, 48–53

Baker, P. N. and Symonds, E. M. (1992) The resolution of chronic pain after normal laparoscopy finding. *Am J Obstet Gynecol* **166**, 835–37

Barberi, R. (1992) Hormone treatment of endometriosis: the estrogen theshold hypothesis. *Am J Obstet Gynecol* **166**, 740–5

Bateman, B., Kolp, L. and Mills, S. (1994) Endoscopic versus laparotomy management of endometriomas. *Fertil Steril* **62**, 690–5

Beard, R. W. (1986) Pelvic pain in women. *BMJ* **293**, 1160–2

Beard, R. W., Gangar, K. and Pearce, S. (1994) 'Chronic gynaecological pain' in: P. D. Wall and R. Melzack (Eds.). *Textbook of Pain*, pp. 597–614. Edinburgh: Churchill Livingstone

Bergquist, C. (1990) Effects of nafarelin versus danazol on lipid and calcium metabolism. *Am J Obstet Gynecol* **162**, 589–891

Chamberlain, G. and Brown, J. C. (1978) Gynaecological laparoscopy: report of the working party of the confidential enquiry into gynaecologic laparoscopy. London: Royal College of Obstetricians and Gynaecologists

Chan, C. L. K. and Wood, C. (1985) Pelvic adhesiolysis — the assessment of symptom relief by 100 patients. *Aust NZ J Obstet Gynaecol* **25**, 295–9

Cornillie, F. J., Oosterlynck, D., Lauweryns, J. M. and Koninckx, P. R. (1990). Deeply infiltrating pelvic endometriosis: histology and clinical significance. *Fertil Steril* **53**, 978–83

Cunanan, R., Courey, N. and Lippes, J. (1983) Laparoscopy findings in patients with pelvic pain. *Am J Obstet Gynecol* **146**, 589–91

Cunha, F. Q., Lorenzetti, B. B., Poole, S. and Ferreira, S. H. (1991) Interleukin-8 as a mediator of sympathetic pain. *Br J Pharmacol* **104**, 765–7

Daniel, J. F. (1989) Laparoscopy enterolysis for chronic abdominal pain. *J Gynecol Surgery* **5**, 61–5

Deleon, F. D., Vijayakumar, R., Brown, M. *et al.* (1986) Peritoneal fluid volume in patients with and without endometriosis. *Obstet Gynecol* **68**, 189–94

Denzlinger, C., Rapp, S., Hagmann, W. and Keppler, D. (1985) Leukotrienes as mediators in tissue trauma. *Science* **230**, 330–2

Dlugi, A. M., Miller, J. D. and Knittle, J. (1990) Lupron acetate depot in the treatment of endometriosis: a randomised, placebo-controlled double blind study. *Fertil Steril* **54**, 419–27

Donnez, J. Nisolle, F., Casanas-Roux, F. and Clerckx, F. (1992) 'Endometriosis: rationale for surgery' in: I. Brosens and J. Donnez (Eds.). *The Current Status of Endometriosis Research and Management*, pp. 385–96. New York: Parthenon

Donnez, J., Anaf, V., Nisolle, M., Clerckx-Braun, F. and Casanas-Roux, F. (1994) Ovarian endometrial cysts: the role of gonadotrophin-releasing hormone agonist and/or drainage. *Fertil Steril* **62**, 63–6

Duncan, H. Q. and Taylor, H. C. (1952) A psychosomatic study of pelvic congestion. *Am J. Obstet Gynecol* **64**, 1–12

Fahraeus, L., Larsson-Cohn, U., Ljungbert, S. and Wallentine, L. (1984) Profound alteration of the lipoprotein metabolism during danazol treatment in premenopausal women. *Fertil Steril* **42**, 52–7

Fedele, L., Parazzini, F., Bianchi, S., Arcaini, L. and Candiani, G. (1990) Stage and localisation of pelvic endometriosis and pain. *Fertil Steril* **53**, 155–8

Goldstein, D. P. (1989) Acute and chronic pelvic pain. *Adol Gynecol* **36**, 573–9

Halme, J., Hammond, M. G., Hulka, J. F., Raj, S. J. and Talbert, L. M. (1984) Retrograde menstruation in healthy women and in patients with endometriosis. *Obstet Gynecol* **64**, 151–4

Hamman, H. (1993) Neuropathic pain: a condition which is not always well appreciated. *Br J Anaesth* **71**, 799–81

Henzl, M. Corson, S., Moghisi, K. *et al.* (1988) Adminstration of nasal as compared with oral danazol for the treatment of endometriosis. A multicentre double blind comparative clinical trial. *N Engl J Med* **318**, 485–9

Hornstein, D., Yuzpe, A., Burry, K. *et al.* (1995) Prospective randomised double-blind trial of three versus six months of nafarelin therapy for endometriosis associated pelvic pain. *Fertil Steril* **63**, 955–62

Iggo, A. (1983) 'Mechanisms of nociception in persistent pain' in: S. Lipton and J. Miles (Eds.). *Persistent Pain: Modern Methods of Treatment,* Vol. 3, pp. 1—16. London: Academic Press

Jansen, R. S. and Russell, P. (1986) Non-pigmented endometriosis: clinical, laparoscopic and pathological definition. *Am J Obstet Gynecol* **155**, 1154–9

Kennedy, S., Williams, I., Brodribb, J., Barlow, D. and Shaw, R. (1990) A comparison of nafarelin acetate and danazol in the treatment of endometriosis. *Fertil Steril* **53**, 998–1002

Koninckx, P. and Martin, D. (1992) Deep endometriosis: a consequence of infiltration or retraction of possibly adenomyosis externa? *Fertil Steril* **58**, 924–8

Kresch, A. J., Seifer, D. B., Sach, L. B. and Barvese, I. L. (1984) Laparoscopy in 100 women with chronic pelvic pain. *Obstet Gynecol* **64**, 672–4

Kumazao, T. (1986) 'Sensory innervation of reproductive organs' in: F. Cervero and J. F. B. Morison (Eds.). *Visceral Sensation,* pp. 115–18. New York: Elsevier Science

Lee, R. B., Stone, K., Magelssen, D., Belts, R. and Benson, W. (1986) Presacral neurectomy for chronic pelvic pain. *Obstet Gynecol* **68**, 517–21

Lemay, A., Brideau, N. A., Forest, J. C., Dodin, S. and Maheux, R. (1991) Cholesterol fraction and apoprotein during endometriosis treatment by a gonadotrophin releasing hormone (GnRH) agonist implant or danazol. *Clin Endocrinol* **35**, 305–10

Lichten, E. M. and Bombard, J. (1987) Surgical treatment of dysmenorrhoea with laparoscopic uterine nerve ablation. *J Reprod Med* **32**, 37–42

Low, W. Y., Edelman, R. J. and Sutton, C. J. (1994) Patients with chronic pelvic pain and/or infertility: psychological differences pre- and post-treatment. *J Psychosom Obstet Gynecol* **15**, 45–52

Lundberg, W. I., Wall, J. E. and Mathers, J. (1973) Laparoscopy in evaluation of pelvic pain. *Obstet Gynecol* **42**, 872–5

Malinak, L. R. (1985) Pelvic pain — when is surgery indicated? *Contemp Obstet Gynaecol* **26**, 43–6

Milburn, A., Reiter, R. and Rhomberg, A. (1993) Multidisciplinary approach to chronic pelvic pain. *Obstet Gynecol Clin North Am* **20**, 643–59

Moen, H. M. and Muss, K. M. (1991) Endometriosis in pregnant and non-pregnant women at tubal sterilisation. *Hum Reprod* **6**, 699–702

Morris, N. and O'Neil, D. (1958) Out-patient gynaecology. *BMJ* **ii**, 1038–40

Nezhat, C., Nezhat, F., Nezhat, C. H. and Seidman, D. (1995) Severe endometriosis and operative laparoscopy. *Curr Opin Obstet Gynecol* **7**, 299–306

Nezhat, C., Nezhat, F. and Pennington, E. (1992) Laparoscopic treatment of lower colorectal and infiltrative rectovaginal septum endometriosis by the technique of videolaseroscopy. *Br J Obstet Gynaecol* **99**, 664–7

Nafarelin European Endometriosis Trial (NEET) Group (1992) Nafarelin for endometriosis: large scale, danazol-control trial of efficacy and safety with one-year follow up. *Fertil Steril* **57**, 524–432

Noble, A. D. and Letchworth, A. T. (1980) Treatment of endometriosis: a study of medical management. *Br J Obstet Gynaecol* **87**, 726–8

O'Connor, D. T. (1987) 'Clinical features in diagnosis' in: A. Jordan and A. Singer (Eds.). *Endometriosis,* pp. 68–78. Edinburgh: Churchill Livingstone

Perper, M. M., Nezhat, F., Goldstein, H., Nezhat, C. H. and Nezhat, C. (1995) Dysmenorrhoea is related to the number of implants in endometriosis patients. *Fertil Steril* **63**, 500–3

Peter, A. W., Van Dorst, E., Jellis, B. *et al.* (1991) A randomised clinical trial to compare two different approaches in women with chronic pelvic pain. *Obstet Gynecol* **77**, 740–4

Raplan, A. J. (1986) Adhesions and pelvic pain: a retrospective study. *Obstet Gynecol* **68**, 13–18

Reiter, R. (1990a) Chronic pelvic pain. *Clin Obstet Gynecol* **33**, 117–18

Reiter, R. C. (1990b) Occult somatic pathology in women with chronic pelvic pain. *Clin Obstet Gynecol* **33**, 154–60

Ripkin, A. J. (1990) Neuroanatomy, neurophysiology and neuropharmacology of pelvic pain. *Clin Obstet Gynecol* **33**, 119–29

Ripps, B. A. and Martin, D. C. (1991) Focal pelvic tenderness, pelvic pain and dysmenorrhea in endometriosis. *J Reprod Med* **36**, 470–5

Rolland, R. and Van der Heijden, P. (1990) Nafarelin versus danazol in the treatment of endometriosis. *Am J Obstet Gynecol* **162**, 586–8

Schlaff, W. D., Dugoff, L., Damewood, M. and Rock, J. (1990) Megestrol acetate for the treatment of endometriosis. *Obstet Gynecol* **75**, 646–8

Schmidt, C. (1985) Endometriosis: a reappraisal of pathogenesis and treatment. *Fertil Steril* **44**, 157–73

Shaw, R. W. (1991) 'Treatment of endometriosis' in: J. Studd (Ed.). *Progress in Obstetrics and Gynaecology*, Vol. 9, pp. 273–87. London: Churchill Livingstone

Shaw, R. W. (Ed.) (1993) *An Atlas of Endometriosis*, pp. 17–18. Carnforth, Lancashire: Parthenon Publishing Group

Steege, J. F., Stout, A. L. and Somkuti, S. G. (1991) Chronic pelvic pain in women: toward an integrative model. *J Psychosom Obstet Gynaecol* **12**, 3–30

Steege, J. F., Stout, A. L. and Somkuti, S. G. (1992) Chronic pelvic pain in women: towards an integrative model. *Obstet Gynecol Survey* **48**, 95–110

Stout, A. L., Steege, J. F., Dodson, W. C. and Hughes, C. L. (1991) Relationship of laparoscopic finding to self-report of pelvic pain. *Am J Obstet Gynecol* **164**, 73–9

Stovall, T. G., Ling, F. and Crawford, D. (1990) Hysterectomy for chronic pelvic pain of presumed uterine etiology. *Obstet Gynecol* **75**, 676–9

Stripling, M. C., Martin, D. C., Chatman, D. L., Vanderzwaag, R. and Poston, W. M. (1988) Subtle appearance of pelvic endometriosis. *Fertil Steril* **49**, 427–31

Takahashi, K., Okada, S., Ozaki, T., Kitao, M. and Sugimura, K. (1994) Diagnosis of pelvic endometriosis by magnetic resonance imaging using 'fat saturation' technique. *Fertil Steril* **62**, 973–7

Telima, S., Puolakka, J., Ronnuberg, L. and Kaupilla, A. (1987) Placebo-controlled comparison of danazol and high dose medoxyprogesterone acetate in the treatment of endometriosis. *Fertil Steril* **60**, 75–9

Togashi, K., Nishimura, K., Kimura, I. *et al.* (1991) Endometrial cysts: diagnosis with MR imaging. *Radiology* **180**, 73–8

Vercellini, P., Tresoidi, L., Colombo, A. *et al.* (1993) A gonadotropin-releasing hormone agonist versus a low dose oral contraceptive for pelvic pain associated with endometriosis. *Fertil Steril* **60**, 75–9

Vernon, M. W., Beard, J. S., Graves, K. and Wilson, E. A. (1986) Classification of endometriosis implants by morphological appearance and capacity to synthesize prostaglandin F. *Fertil Steril* **46**, 801–5

Walker, E., Katon, W., Harrop-Griffiths, J. *et al.* (1988) Relationship of chronic pelvic pain to psychiatry diagnosis and childhood sexual abuse. *Am J Psychiatry* **145**, 75–80

Wood, P. D., Wiesner, M. G. and Reityer, C. R. (1990) Psychogenic chronic pelvic pain: diagnosis and management. *Clin Obstet Gynecol* **33**, 179–95

Wright, S., Valdes, C., Dunn, R. and Franklin, R. (1995) Short term lupron or danazol therapy for pelvic endometriosis. *Fertil Steril* **63**, 504–7

Zawin, M., McCarthy, S. M., Scoutt, L. and Comite, F. (1989) Endometriosis: appearance and detection at MR imaging. *Radiology* **171**, 693–6

# 20

# Treatment options in women with unexplained chronic pelvic pain

*Kevin M. Smith and Philip W. Reginald*

Pelvic pain is one of the most common problems encountered in clinical practice, with about one-third of patients attending the gynaecology clinic reporting pelvic pain as their major symptom (Morris & O'Neil 1958; Henker 1979). Despite the prevalence of pelvic pain in younger women, its aetiology is poorly understood and specific diagnosis to enable targeted treatment is often elusive. A number of women have an identifiable gynaecological cause for the pain, such as endometriosis or pelvic inflammatory disease. In a few, the pain can be attributed to non-gynaecological causes such as inflammatory bowel disease, irritable bowel syndrome, ureteric calculus or diverticulitis. A review of the literature, however, reveals that up to 67% of diagnostic laparoscopies for pelvic pain reveal no pathological findings (see Table 1) and so management becomes a challenge. The role of this chapter is to outline and discuss some of the current ideas on treatment of this distressing condition.

## ROLE OF LAPAROSCOPIC MANAGEMENT

The diagnostic role of laparoscopy has long been accepted and the laparoscope has become one of the most useful tools in the gynaecologist's practice. A two-year review of the laparoscopies performed at the University of Iowa Hospital (Reiter 1990) showed that 34% of these procedures were to investigate chronic pelvic pain. In addition, a survey by the Royal College of Obstetricians and Gynaecologists into gynaecological laparoscopy (Chamberlain and Brown 1978) showed that over 50% of diagnostic laparoscopies in the United Kingdom were done to investigate pelvic pain. As mentioned previously, up to two-thirds of laparoscopies for pelvic pain show no obvious pelvic disease. However, it is important to be careful when diagnosing a normal pelvis as both Redwine *et al.* (1978) and Stripling, Martin and Poston (1988) have shown that histologically proven endometriosis can appear as black, white, red, brown, yellow or clear lesions. It is eminently easy, therefore, to miss a potential cause for pelvic pain at laparoscopy. Similarly, it is easy to ascribe pelvic pain to supposed pelvic pathology which may not be the cause, as it is well known that at least 30% of women with endometriosis do not complain of pelvic pain. Kresh *et al.*

**Table 1** *A literature review of the number of patients who underwent diagnostic laparoscopy for pelvic pain but for whom no pathological condition was found*

| Authors | No. patients in series | No. with a normal pelvis at laparoscopy (%) |
|---|---|---|
| Liston, Bradford and Kerr (1972) | 134 | 67 |
| Lundberg, Wall and Mathers (1973) | 95 | 39 |
| Cunanan, Courey and Lippes (1983) | 1194 | 30 |
| Stacey and Munday (1984) | 81 | 59 |

(1984) described a series of 100 laparoscopies performed on women with pelvic pain and compared the findings with 50 controls (represented by asymptomatic women attending for laparoscopic sterilisation) and found that nearly 30% of the control group had abnormal findings at laparoscopy. However, it is the woman with pelvic pain and no pelvic pathology that presents such a dilemma in terms of diagnosis and treatment.

A report by Baker and Symonds (1992) suggests that laparoscopy itself may have a therapeutic role in the management of patients with pelvic pain but no discernible pelvic pathology. Sixty women with pelvic pain underwent laparoscopy at which no pelvic pathology was evident. The patients were all reassured postoperatively that there was no serious pelvic disease, and they were followed up six weeks and six months after the procedure and questioned on the nature of their symptoms. Six weeks after surgery, 62% reported an absence or improvement of their pelvic pain. Six months postoperatively, 58% reported that they were pain-free and a further 39% reported that their pain had diminished. This study can be criticised because the authors made minimal efforts to quantify the pain before and after the procedure by any of the recognised pain assessment methods. In addition, there was no control group (i.e. a cohort of patients with similar pain who did not undergo laparoscopy). Despite these faults, this study highlights a role for laparoscopy in the management of patients with unexplained pelvic pain. Stacey and Munday (1984) showed that pelvic inflammatory disease is overdiagnosed clinically and this condition, along with endometriosis, carries with it fears about infertility and it is possible that the reassurance of a negative laparoscopy enables women to cope better with their symptoms. If nothing else, it highlights the placebo effect of laparoscopy in this condition and it is important to bear this in mind when drawing conclusions from the many, often retrospective, observational studies which claim that a particular procedure had been successful in alleviating symptoms.

## PRESACRAL NEURECTOMY

Pelvic organs have both a sympathetic and parasympathetic nerve supply. Pain impulses from the uterus, medial part of the Fallopian tubes and upper part of the vagina travel through visceral afferents to Frankenhauser's paracervical plexus of nerves. From this plexus, the impulses travel to the inferior, middle and superior hypogastric plexus and enter the lumbar and lower thoracic sympathetic chain, entering the spinal cord through the posterior nerve roots at the level of T10–L1.

The idea of presacral nerve resection to eliminate painful visceral afferent stimuli in women with severe dysmenorrhoea was independently described by Ruggi and Jaboulay in 1899 (quoted in Vercellini et al. 1991) and it came into vogue during the first half of this century. The advent of non-steroidal anti-inflammatory drugs heralded a fall in the number of pelvic denervations, but during the 1980s interest in the technique was rekindled as non-steroidals failed to be the panacea that was originally hoped.

Black (1964) reviewed 9937 cases that appeared in the literature worldwide and reported that 75–80% of patients experienced significant relief of dysmenorrhoea after the operation. However, most studies into the efficacy of pre-sacral neurectomy in relieving pelvic pain are retrospective and non-randomised. The denervation was usually performed as an adjunct to conservative surgery for endometriosis and all the studies have been criticised (Vercellini et al. 1991) for the authors' lack of specification of the stage of the disease. Ripps and Martin (1992), however, have since shown that reported symptoms in patients with endometriosis show poor correlation with the extent of the disease at surgery. The results in terms of pain relief in this series are variable: some are encouraging (Tjaden et al. 1990) and others less so (Puolakka, Kauppila and Ronnberg 1980). These results are summarised in Table 2.

Garcia and David (1977) reported a retrospective analysis of 71 patients who underwent conservative surgery for endometriosis, 35 of

**Table 2**  *A literature review of the reported relief from chronic pelvic pain following presacral neurectomy. (Adapted from Vercellini* et al. *1991\*, with permission of Mosby-Year Book Inc.). CSEL, conservative surgery for endometriosis at laparotomy; PSN, presacral neurectomy*

| Author(s) | Treatment | No. with dysmenorrhoea | Report relief of dysmenorrhoea (n) | Type of study |
|---|---|---|---|---|
| Garcia and David (1977) | CSEL + PSN | 35 | 97 | Retrospective, |
| | CSEL | | 72 | non-randomised |
| Puolakka, Kauppila and | CSEL + PSN | 51 | 90 | Retrospective, |
| Ronnberg (1980) | CSEL | 45 | 80 | non-randomised |
| Polan and DeCherney (1980) | CSEL + PSN | 20 | 70 | Retrospective, |
| | CSEL | 19 | 26 | non-randomised |
| Tjaden *et al.* (1990) | CSEL + PSN | 17 | 88 | Prospective, partially |
| | CSEL | 9 | 0 | randomised |

*Vercellini, P., Fedde, L., Bianchi, S. and Candiani, G. B. (1991) Pelvic denervation for chronic pain associated with endometriosis: fact or fancy. Am J Obstet Gynecol **165**, 745–9

whom also underwent presacral neurectomy. Ninety-seven per cent of the presacral neurectomy group reported relief of their pain compared with 72% of the control group. Puolakka, Kauppila and Ronnberg (1980), however, in a similar retrospective series reported a less impressive difference of only 10% between the presacral neurectomy and the control group.

In a study by Polan and DeCherney (1980), again retrospective and non-randomised, the combination of presacral neurectomy with conservative surgery increased the total postoperative pain relief from 26% in the control group to an impressive 75%. Interpretation of these results, however, is confounded by both the design of the study and the inclusion of patients with a range of pelvic disorders, including pelvic inflammatory disease and endometriosis.

On the grounds that the afferent nerve pathway from the ovary travels along the ovarian artery rather than to the superior hypogastric plexus, Tjaden *et al.* (1990) divided dysmenorrhoea 'midline' and 'lateral' pain. They observed that midline pain was abolished in four patients randomised to neurectomy versus none of the four controls who underwent only resection of endometrial lesions. They combined these data with the findings in a group of 18, non-randomised women and showed that

the symptoms of 88% of those with midline pain were relieved by presacral neurectomy compared with no improvement at all in the control group. These impressive data led the monitoring committee for this trial to discontinue the study on the grounds that it was:

> '*unethical to deprive patients with midline dysmenorrhoea of the benefit of pain relief that could be afforded with presacral neurectomy.*'

These impressive results may form the basis of an argument in favour of using presacral neurectomy to treat patients with midline pelvic pain. However, the number of randomised patients in the trial was small and the findings are at odds with those of Stovall, Ling and Crawford (1990). These authors followed up 99 women who underwent hysterectomy for midline pelvic pain of presumed uterine aetiology. Histology confirmed uterine pathology in only 34% of these patients, and almost 25% continued to suffer pelvic pain after the operation. This study gives an indication that the reported site of the pain is an unreliable indicator of the anatomical cause.

In an analysis of these various series, Vercellini *et al.* (1991) concluded that, owing to weak study design, variable follow-up, lack of an objective evaluation of pain symptoms and limited sample sizes, definitive comments on efficacy of presacral neurectomy in relieving pelvic pain could not be made. Furthermore, the procedure is not without its risks. Heavy bleeding has been reported (Lee *et al.* 1986) from accidental laceration of the middle sacral vein and other complications resulting from the inevitable transection of efferent nerve fibres to the bladder and bowel, including transient retention of urine, small bowel obstruction and constipation (Frier 1965; Ingersoll and Meigs 1948; Buttram and Reiter 1985). While the results of series by Tjaden (1990) are encouraging, the need for prospective, blinded, randomised studies in this field is necessary before the procedure can be widely revived.

Encouraging results have been reported by de-Leon-Casasola, Kend and Lema (1993), who describe a technique of administering a percutaneous neurolytic superior hypogastric plexus block using 10% phenol. The subjects were 26 patients with extensive gynaecological, colorectal or genitourinary cancer who suffered uncontrolled, incapacitating pelvic pain. All had received a successful diagnostic block using 0.25% bupivicaine. All patients reported a visual analogue pain score (VAS) of 10 out of 10 before the nerve block. Sixty-nine per cent of patients reported satisfactory pain relief (VAS < 4 out of 10). Fifty-seven per cent reported relief after one block and a further 12% after a second block. The remaining patients had moderate pain control (VAS 4–7 out of 10). This level of response was maintained throughout the follow-up period of six months. This study introduces two interesting ideas:

(1) Giving a test block using a short-lived anaesthetic agent to see if the more definitive procedure is likely to be successful; and

(2) The possibility of producing a satisfactory nerve block using a percutaneous technique rather than at laparotomy.

In 1992 Nezhat and Nezhat described a method of laparoscopic presacral neurectomy. Eighty-five women with central pelvic pain due to endometriosis underwent laparoscopic ablation of the endometriotic lesions followed by laparoscopic presacral neurectomy. Ninety-four per cent reported an improvement of their symptoms. There were no operative complications in this series; however, as there was also no control arm to study, the results, while encouraging, cannot be used to draw definitive conclusions.

The need for controlled, randomised, prospective trials in this field is obvious. The description of a less invasive method of presacral nerve block in patients with cancer-related pain by de-Leon-Casasola, Kend and Lema (1993) may provide an interesting path forward in the exploration of techniques to relieve non-cancer pain.

## LAPAROSCOPIC UTEROSACRAL NERVE ABLATION

Laparoscopic uterosacral nerve ablation (LUNA) is a procedure related to presacral neurectomy which involves the resection or ablation of the uterosacral ligaments in patients with dysmenorrhoea or pelvic pain. Sympathetic axons, including the Aδ and C pain fibres, to and from the uterus are resected, together with some of the parasympathetic axons and their pain fibres (Doyle 1955).

Lee *et al.* (1986) observed that amputation of the uterosacral ligaments in patients who also underwent presacral neurectomy, perhaps unsurprisingly, did not improve the outcome in terms of relief. The question really is whether resection of the uterosacral ligaments alone, which would be a simpler and possibly safer procedure than presacral neurectomy, will produce relief of pelvic pain.

The technique was first described by Doyle (1955) who transected the uterosacral ligaments transvaginally in patients with dysmenorrhoea and reported symptomatic improvement in 70% of cases. Since this original study, a number of observational studies have been reported in the literature, utilising a variety of methods to ablate the uterosacral ligaments (see Table 3). All these are observational studies with follow-up periods ranging from six months (Daniell 1989) to up to six years (Sutton

**Table 3**   *A literature review of the reported relief from chronic pelvic pain following laparoscopic uterosacral nerve ablation*

| Author | Method | No. with symptoms | Reports of symptom relief (%) | Type of Study |
|---|---|---|---|---|
| Feste (1985) | CO$_2$ laser | 32 | 72 | Observational |
| Daniell (1989) | KTP laser | 80 | 75 | Observational |
| Sutton and Hill (1990) | CO$_2$ laser | 100 | 86 | Observational |
| | | | 80 | Observational |
| Perez (1990) | Nd: YAG laser | 25 | | |

CO$_2$, carbon dioxide; KTP, potassium/titanium/platinum; Nd: YAG, neodynium: yttrium/argon/garnet

and Hill 1990). All report a success rate of around 70–80% in terms of pain but, unfortunately, all were uncontrolled and, bearing in mind the potential placebo effect of laparoscopy in patients with pelvic pain described by Baker and Symonds (1992), it is difficult to draw conclusions from these studies. As pointed out by Sutton and Hill (1990):

> '*Sceptics can quite reasonably argue that there is a massive placebo effect with this kind of symptom, especially if it is treated with the sort of high tech wizardry that is implicit in laser beam procedures.*'

Lichten and Bombard (1987) have probably conducted the only randomised, prospective, double-blind study to evaluate the efficacy of LUNA. The study is particularly interesting in that co-existent psychiatric illness was evaluated and those with abnormal psychological profiles were excluded from the study. Only patients with macroscopically normal pelvis at laparoscopy were admitted to the study, so eliminating the influences of different pathology and stages of disease which confused most of the studies on presacral neurectomy. Twenty-one such patients with pelvic pain were randomised to either the group undergoing LUNA (performed by means of bipolar cautery and scissors transection) or the control group who only underwent laparoscopy. Neither the patient nor the physician conducting the follow-up interviews was aware of the group to which the patient had been allocated. Three months after the procedure, none of the patients in the control group reported relief from dysmenorrhoea, whereas 81% of the LUNA group reported almost complete pain relief. One year after the operation, the satisfaction rate with the procedure had decreased to 45%. Although the number of patients was small, this remains the seminal paper investigating the efficacy of LUNA in relieving pelvic pain. Interestingly, Lichten and Bombard did not show the placebo effect of laparoscopy alone that was described by Baker and Symonds (1992), as none of the control group reported any improvement of symptoms at all. It would seem, also, that the follow-up period after such procedures needs to be quite long in order to reflect the true outcome of the operation. Perhaps most significantly, however, this study shows that LUNA may have some therapeutic effect in around half the patients who undergo the procedure. It is perhaps unsurprising that the success rate was only around the 50% mark, in view of the possible ovarian involvement in the pathogenesis of pelvic pain in a proportion of women with macroscopically normal pelvis (to be discussed later in this chapter). Furthermore, the success of LUNA in rendering patients completely pain-free depends on the erroneous assumption that uterine innervation is confirmed to the uterosacral ligaments. Reginald and Stones (1992) have clearly shown that the uterus also derives innervation via the cardinal ligaments and there is no difference in distribution of nerve fibres in the uterosacral compared with the lateral paracervical ligaments.

Although Lichten and Bombard have shown that a certain degree of long-term benefit can be derived from LUNA, the number of patients in their series was quite small and would probably not be sufficient to adequately display the potential complication rate of this procedure. This complication rate is potentially high in view of the proximity of the ureters, rectosigmoid and uterine vessels. Two deaths have occurred in North America as a result of bleeding from the uterosacral ligaments (Daniell 1989) and cases of procidentia have also been reported following LUNA (Good, Copas and Doody 1992) In view of this, larger prospective studies should be undertaken to confirm the benefits of the procedure over and above its complications before it is widely embraced by gynaecologists.

## TREATMENT OF PELVIC VENOUS CONGESTION

Gooch (1831) described 'a morbid state of blood vessels indicated by their fullness' in women with pelvic pain. He was probably the first to introduce the concept of vascular congestion as a cause for pelvic pain. Taylor (1949a) and Duncan and Taylor (1952) gave a detailed account of pelvic pain with vascular congestion and hyperaemia. This venous congestion can sometimes be seen at laparoscopy, but it must be remembered that dilated veins often disappear because of the combined effects of raising the intra-abdominal pressure with gas and the head-down tilt used by most gynaecologists for this procedure. The pelvis of patients with this condition often, therefore, appear normal at laparoscopy. Beard *et al.* (1984) confirmed that venous congestion exists as an entity in such patients when they performed venograms on 45 such women and found significantly higher venogram scores in these patients compared with two control groups: one made up of women with no pelvic pain and the second comprising women with pelvic pain thought to be due to other pelvic pathology found at laparoscopy.

Reginald *et al.* (1987) produced further evidence to implicate congested pelvic veins in the pathogenesis of pelvic pain. They successfully used the selective venoconstrictor dihydroergotamine (DHE) to reduce both venous congestion and pelvic pain in six women complaining of pelvic pain. Pain was significantly diminished for up to four days after the intravenous administration of DHE. Unfor-

tunately, the manufacturers have withdrawn the oral preparation of this drug and further studies of drugs with similar venoconstrictor activity in the treatment of pelvic pain are needed before their general use can be advocated.

The exact cause of venous congestion remains uncertain, but indirect evidence suggests that it may be caused by ovarian hormones, possibly oestrogen. Pelvic pain and congestion are only observed in the reproductive years (Taylor 1949b; Renaer *et al.* 1980); these women tend to have dysfunctional bleeding (Beard, Reginald and Wadsworth 1988) and, in 56% of cases, polycystic changes in the ovary (Adams *et al.* 1990). They also tend to have an enlarged uterus and thicker endometrium, implying either excess oestrogen or increased target organ response to oestrogen. With this in mind, Reginald (1989) performed a pilot study in which ovarian function was suppressed, resulting in the reduction of oestrogen in 22 women with pelvic pain due to venous congestion. This was achieved using 30 mg of medroxyprogesterone acetate (MPA) daily for six months. There was a reduction of pelvic congestion demonstrated by venography in 17 (77%) of these women. The improvement in pelvic pain in these 17 women was significantly higher than in the five women who showed no reduction in pelvic congestion. Three of the five women who showed no reduction in pelvic congestion were not rendered amenorrhoeic by the MPA, indicating that ovarian activity was probably not suppressed. A significant association between ovarian suppression and reduction in pelvic congestion was noted. Ovarian hormones, therefore, appear to be implicated in pelvic pain and suppression of ovulation and reduction of oestrogens improved symptoms.

In the light of this pilot study, a double-blind, randomised, control trial of treatment with MPA and/or psychotherapy was performed (Farquhar *et al.* 1989). It showed a statistically significant benefit in terms of a reduction of pain after four months of treatment with MPA alone (Figure 1). Six months after stopping treatment, the beneficial effects of treatment with MPA were still present, but were no longer greater than the effects of placebo.

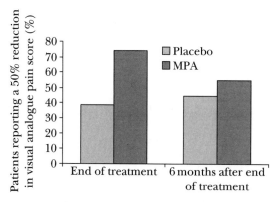

**Figure 1** *Some results from a double-blind, randomised control study which evaluated the treatment of chronic pelvic pain with medroxyprogesterone acetate (MPA) and/or psychotherapy. The long-term efficacy of MPA over placebo is shown. (Adapted from Farquhar C. M., Rogers, V., Franks, S. et al. (1989) A randomised controlled trial of medroxyprogesterone acetate and psychotherapy for the treatment of pelvic congestion. Br J Obstet Gynaecol **96**, 1153–62)*

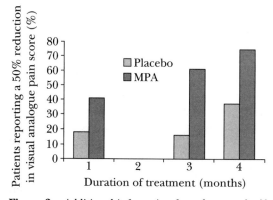

**Figure 2** *Additional information from the same double-bind, randomised control study which evaluated the treatment of chronic pelvic pain with medroxyprogesterone acetate (MPA) and/or psychotherapy discussed in Figure 1. The effect of the treatment duration on the efficacy of MPA over placebo is shown. (Adapted from Farquhar et al. 1989 [full reference details in the legend to Figure 1])*

Figure 2, also taken from the results of Farquhar *et al.* (1989) shows two interesting points:

(1) The efficacy of MPA increases over the treatment period, indicating that treatment should not be abandoned if found to be ineffective in the first two months; and

(2) It highlights the extraordinary effect of placebo in such cases, indicating the need for therapeutic trials to be carefully controlled before conclusions can be reliably drawn.

Hobbs (1990) and Lechter and Alvarez (1986) have independently treated small groups of patients with pelvic venous congestion by ovarian vein ligation with good results. In addition, Edwards *et al.* (1993) published a case report in which pelvic pain in a woman with venous congestion was successfully treated by embolisation of the ovarian vein using small steel coils inserted into the femoral vein via a catheter. Sichlau, Yao and Vogelzang (1994) published a small series of three patients who were successfully treated using a similar technique. These observations support the theory that venous congestion is a likely aetiological factor in pelvic pain experienced by these women and that transcatheter ovarian vein embolotherapy may be a surgical approach to the treatment of this condition.

## HYSTERECTOMY, WITH OR WITHOUT OOPHORECTOMY

Stovall, Ling and Crawford (1990) evaluated the long-term outcome of 99 women who underwent hysterectomy for pelvic pain of at least six months' duration. All had symptoms and physical examination findings suggestive of disease confined to the uterus. Subsequent histological examination revealed uterine pathology in only 34% of these patients, and long-term follow-up showed that almost 25% of these patients continued to suffer pelvic pain despite the operation. None of these patients underwent diagnostic laparoscopy prior to hysterectomy and this may have meant that extrauterine pathology may have been missed. The point, however, is that although a 75% chance of a cure for a patient who has endured pelvic pain of assumed uterine pathology may seem appealing, about one-quarter of patients will not be cured by hysterectomy alone.

This observation is probably a reflection of the fact that either non-gynaecological pathology, particularly irritable bowel syndrome, can be a cause for the pain in a proportion of patients (Longstreth, Preskill and Youkeles 1990), or that the ovaries are implicated in the pathogenesis. Reginald (1989) showed that ovarian suppression improved pelvic pain and this was supported by the results of a prospective, double-bind, randomised, controlled trial of ovarian suppression in patients with pelvic pain by Farquhar *et al.* (1989).

Beard *et al.* (1991) performed a prospective study to determine whether bilateral oophorectomy combined with hysterectomy is an effective treatment for chronic pelvic pain. Thirty-six women underwent the operation and the median pain score on visual analogue scale fell from a preoperative value of 10 to 0 at one year postoperatively. Although this study did not have a control arm for comparison (e.g. a group who underwent hysterectomy without oophorectomy), it would appear that, if radical surgery for pelvic pain caused by pelvic congestion is contemplated, a bilateral oophorectomy as well as hysterectomy should be considered. This would be particularly relevant to women whose pelvic pain recurred, having improved during treatment with ovarian suppression. However, it has great implications, as the average age of a patient presenting with pelvic pain is 32 years (Beard, Reginald and Wadsworth 1988) and obviously fertility and the effect of long-term hormone replacement must be taken into consideration.

## ILIOHYPOGASTRIC/ILIOINGUINAL NERVE ENTRAPMENT

So far we have considered visceral pain, but somatic pain originating in the anterior abdominal wall, in particular that caused by ilioinguinal or iliohypogastric nerve entrapment, may also present as pelvic pain. Typically, the pain follows a Pfannenstiel or an appendicectomy incision and is intermittent, sharp and induced by physical activity. The pain is usually felt at the incision site, radiating into the labia and upper aspect of the thigh. It is suggested that nerve entrapment occurs as a result of nerve damage

by the incision or suture, leading to information of a neuroma or entrapment of the nerve by scar tissue. Local anaesthetic can be injected into the soft tissue 2 cm medial and below the anterior superior iliac spine and, if this temporarily resolves the pain, Hahn (1989) has described more permanent results by transecting the nerve.

## PSYCHOLOGICAL/ MULTIDISCIPLINARY APPROACH TO THE TREATMENT OF CHRONIC PELVIC PAIN

The common finding of normal pelvic organs in women with chronic pelvic pain has led to the exploration of the possibility of psychological causes that may somehow contribute to the genesis or perception in pain. Both Walker and Stenchever (1993) and Walling *et al.* (1994) showed a specific association between sexual victimisation and chronic pelvic pain, while Fry *et al.* (1993) reported that patients with chronic pelvic pain have a higher incidence of paternal overprotection, lower maternal care, more depression and anxiety than normal. The levels are similar to those found in other out-patient populations presenting with migraine and irritable bowel syndrome. The question is whether or not the implication of psychosocial factors in chronic pelvic pain can be utilised in the management of the condition.

Pearce, Knight and Beard (1992) randomly allocated 32 patients with pelvic pain to three treatment groups and a no-treatment control group. The women in the control groups had either relaxation training, behavioural counselling or non-directive psychotherapy. All three treatment groups showed a significant increase in the number of pain-free days between the initial assessment and the three-month follow-up. The control group also showed an improvement, but this was not significant. This study showed that psychological intervention may provide some benefit to chronic pelvic pain patients, although the mechanisms are unclear.

Another study by Pearce (1986) compared stress analysis with pain analysis using a minimal intervention control group. Women allocated to the stress analysis group were assessed in interviews when potential areas of stress (financial, marital or housing) were identified. The therapist identified the patients' reaction to the stressors and discussed alternative responses. The use of relaxation strategies in stressful situations was encouraged. The women in the pain analysis group were encouraged to monitor antecedent and consequent events associated with the pain. Therapy was aimed at identifying patterns associated with pain episodes and alternative strategies for avoiding or reducing pain episodes were discussed. Patients in the control group were given the same explanations as the treatment group about the frequency of their disorder and the absence of a medical or surgical treatment approach. Results showed that women in both treatment groups responded significantly better than the control group at the six-month follow-up. This study suggests that psychosocial approaches designed to cope with stress and pain prove beneficial to women with chronic pelvic pain, but long-term follow-up would be necessary to determine the lasting effect of such an adaptation.

Evidence for the benefits of integrating psychotherapy with a more standard treatment regimen is provided by Farquhar *et al.* (1989), who randomised 102 women with chronic pelvic pain into four treatment groups: placebo, placebo with psychotherapy, MPA and MPA with psychotherapy. The psychotherapy was similar to that used by Pearce (1986) and consisted of six sessions of about 45 minutes at two-week intervals. Six months after the end of the treatment period there was no overall significant benefit of MPA or psychotherapy alone over placebo, but there was a statistically significant improvement in the patients who received MPA with psychotherapy (see Figure 3).

Peters *et al.* (1991) showed that there may be a role for disciplines other than the gynaecologist and psychotherapist in the management of chronic pelvic pain. One hundred and six patients with chronic pelvic pain were randomised into either a group which underwent evaluation and treatment from a team including a gynaecologist, psychologist, physiotherapist and nutritionist, or a group which underwent

the more standard approach of diagnosis and treatment under the gynaecologist alone. The study showed that the integrated approach to management was more successful than the standard approach. It did not, however, reveal whether the involvement of physiotherapists and nutritionists conferred any more benefit than the combined gynaecologist/psychotherapist approach advocated by Farquhar *et al.* (1989).

It would seem that the diagnosis and management of chronic pelvic pain may be facilitated by an approach which integrates specific medical interventions with cognitive–behavioural pain strategies (Milburn, Reiter and Rhomberg 1993; Rosenthal 1993). Such collaboration is difficult to organise from a general gynaecology clinic, which is where most of these patients will present, and so may nesessitate the introduction of clinics specifically for patients with pelvic pain. Walker, Sullivan and Stenchever (1993), while recognising a lack of formal evidence for their efficacy, advocate the use of antidepressants in the treatment of chronic pelvic pain as part of this multidisciplinary treatment package. They feel that the relative safety of these medicines and the high prevalence of depression in this population (Hodgkiss, Sufraz and Watson

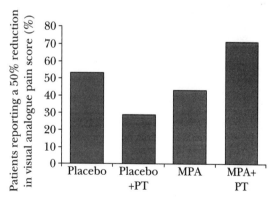

**Figure 3** *Further results from the double-bind, randomised control study which evaluated the treatment of chronic pelvic pain with medroxyprogesterone acetate (MPA) and/or psychotherapy (PT) also discussed in Figures 1 and 2. The efficacy of the various treatment options at six-month follow up. (Adapted from Farquhar* et al. *1989 [Full reference details are shown in the legend to Figure 1])*

1994) make their routine empirical use a justifiable strategy.

## CONCLUSION

Unexplained chronic pelvic pain is a challenging management problem. While both medical and surgical approaches are available, a multidisciplinary approach involving psychotherapy in conjunction with these medical and surgical therapies would seem to offer the maximum benefit to patients.

# References

Adams, J., Reginal, P. W., Franks, S., Wadsworth, J. and Beard, R. W. (1990) Uterine size and endometrial thickness and the significance of cystic ovaries in women with pelvic pain due to congestion. *Br J Obstet Gynaecol* **97**, 583–7

Baker, P. N. and Symonds, E. M. (1992) The resolution of chronic pelvic pain after normal laparoscopic findings. *Am J Obstet Gynecol* **166**, 835–6

Beard, R. W., Highman, J. H., Pearce, S. and Reginald, P. W. (1984) Diagnosis of pelvic varicosities in women with chronic pelvic pain. *Lancet* **ii**, 946–9

Beard, R. W., Reginald, P. W. and Wadsworth, J. (1988) Clinical features of women with lower abdominal pain and dilated pelvic veins. *Br J Obstet Gynaecol* **95**, 153–61

Beard, R. W., Kennedy, R. G., Gangar, K. F. *et al.* (1991) Bilateral oophorectomy and hysterectomy in the treatment of intractible pelvic pain associated with pelvic congestion. *Br J Obstet Gynaecol* **98**, 988–92

Black, W. T. (1964) Use of presacral neurectomy on the treatment of dysmenorrhoea. *Am J Obstet Gynecol* **89**, 16

Buttram, V. C. J. and Reiter, R. C. (1985) 'Endometriosis' in: V. C. J. Buttram and R. C. Reiter (Eds.). *Surgical Treatment of the Infertile Female*, pp. 89–147. Baltimore: Williams and Wilkins

Chamberlain, G. and Brown, J. C. (Eds.) (1978) *Gynaecological Laparoscopy. Reports of the Working Party of the Confidential Enquiry into Gynaecological Laparoscopy.* London: RCOG

Cunanan, R. G., Courey, N. G. and Lippes, J. (1983) Laparoscopic findings in patients with pelvic pain. *Am J Obstet Gynecol* **146**, 589

Daniell, J. F. (1989) 'Fibreoptic laser laparoscopy' in: C. J. G. Sutton (Ed.). *Clinical Obstetrics and Gynaecology*, 3rd edn, pp. 545–62. London: Baillière Tindall

de-Leon-Casasola, O. A., Kend, E. and Lema, M. J. (1993) Neurolytic superior hypogastric plexus block for chronic pelvic pain associated with cancer. *Pain* **54**, 145–51

Doyle, J. B. (1955) Paracervical uterine denervation by transection of the cervical plexus for the relief of dysmenorrhoea. *Am J Obstet Gynecol* **70**, 1–16

Duncan, C. H. and Taylor, H. C. (1952) A psychosomatic study of pelvic congestion. *Am J Obstet Gynecol* **64**, 1–12

Edwards, R. D., Robertson, I. R., MacLean, A. B. and Hemingway, A. P. (1993) Case report: pelvic pain syndrome — successful treatment of a case of ovarian vein embolisation. *Clin Radiol* **47**, 429–31

Farquhar, C. M., Rogers, V., Franks, S. *et al.* (1989) A randomised controlled trial of medroxyprogesterone acetate and psychotherapy for the treatment of pelvic congestion. *Br J Obstet Gynaecol* **96**, 1153–62

Feste, J. R. (1985) Laser laparoscopy. A new modality. *J Reprod Med* **30**, 413–17

Frier, A. (1965) Pelvic neurectomy in gynaecology. *Obstet Gynecol* **25**, 48

Fry, R. P., Crisp, A. H., Beard, R. W. and McGuigan, S. (1993) Psychosocial aspects of chronic pelvic pain, with special reference to sexual abuse. A study of 164 women. *Postgrad Med J* **69**, 566–74

Garcia, C. R. and David, S. S. (1977) Pelvic endometriosis: infertility and pelvic pain. *Am J Obstet Gynecol* **129**, 740–7

Gooch, R. (1831) *On Some of the Most Important Diseases Peculiar to Women.* London: republished by Sydenham Society (1859)

Good, M. C., Copas, P. R. and Doody, M. C. (1992) Uterine prolapse after laparoscopic uterosacral transection: a case report. *J Reprod Med Obstet Gynaecol* **37**, 995–8

Hahn, L. (1989) Clinical findings and results of operative treatment in ilioinguinal nerve entrapment. *Br J Obstet Gynaecol* **96**, 1080–3

Henker, F. O. (1979) Diagnosis and treatment of nonorganic pelvic pain. *South Med J* **72**, 1132–4

Hobbs, J. T. (1990) The pelvic congestion syndrome. *Br J Hosp Med* **43**, 200–6

Hodgkiss, A. D., Sufraz, R. and Watson, J. P. (1994) Psychiatric morbidity and illness behaviour in women with chronic pelvic pain. *J Psychosom Res* **38**, 3–9

Ingersoll, F. M. and Meigs, J. V. (1948) Presacral neurectomy for dysmenorrhoea. *N Engl J Med* **238**, 357

Kresh, A. J., Seifer, D. B., Sachs, L. B. and Barrese, I. (1984) Laparoscopy in 100 women with chronic pelvic pain. *Obstet Gynecol* **64**, 672

Lechter, A. and Alvarez, A. (1986) 'Pelvic varices and gonadal veins' In: D. Negus and G. Jantet (Eds.). *Phlebology*, pp. 225–8. London: John Libbey

Lee, R. B., Stone, K., Magelssen, D., Belts, R. P. and Benson, W. L. (1986) Presacral neurectomy for chronic pelvic pain. *Obstet Gynecol* **69**, 517–21

Lichten, E. M. and Bombard, J. (1987) Surgical treatment of primary dysmenorrhoea with laparoscopic uterine nerve ablation. *J Reprod Med* **32**, 37–41

Liston, W. A., Bradford, J. and Kerr, M. G. (1972) Laparoscopy in a general gynecologic unit. *Am J Obstet Gynecol* **113**, 672

Longstreth, G. F., Preskill, D. B. and Youkeles, L. (1990) Irritable bowel syndrome in women having diagnostic laparoscopy or hysterectomy; relation to gynecologic features and outcome. *Dig Dis Sci* **35**, 1285–90

Lundberg, W. I., Wall, J. E. and Mathers, J. E. (1973) Laparoscopy in the evaluation of pelvic pain. *Obstet Gynecol* **42**, 872

Milburn, A., Reiter, R. C. and Rhomberg, A. T. (1993) Multidisciplinary approach to pelvic pain. *Obstet Gynecol Clin North Am* **20**, 643–61

Morris, N. and O'Neil, D. (1958) Outpatient gynaecology. *BMJ* **ii**, 1038–9

Nezhat, C. and Nezhat, F. (1992) A simplified method of laparoscopic prescral neurectomy for the treatment of central pelvic pain due to endometriosis. *Br J Obstet Gynaecol* **99**, 659–3

Pearce, S. (1986) A psychological investigation of chronic pelvic pain in women. *PhD Thesis*, University of London

Pearce, S., Knight, C. and Beard, R. W. (1982) Pelvic pain — a common gynaecological problem. *J Psychosom Obstet Gynaecol* **1**, 12–17

Perez, J. J. (1990) Laparoscopic prescral neurectomy. *J Reprod Med* **35**, 625–30

Peters, A. A. W., vanDorst, E., Jellis, B. *et al.* (1991) A randomized clinical trial to compare two different approaches in women with chronic pelvic pain. *Obstet Gynecol* **77**, 740–4

Polan, M. I. and DeCherney, A. (1980) Presacral neurectomy for pelvic pain in infertility. *Fertil Steril* **34**, 557–60

Puolakka, J., Kauppila, A. and Ronnberg, L. (1980) Results in the operative treatment of pelvic endometriosis. *Acta Obstet Gynecol Scand* **59**, 429–31

Redwine, D. B. (1987) Age related evolution in colour appearance of endometriosis. *Fertil Steril* **48**, 62

Reginald, P. W. (1989) Investigation of pelvic pathology. *MD Thesis*, University of London.

Reginald, P. W., Beard, R. W., Kooner, J. S. *et al.* (1987) Intravenous dihydroergotamine to relieve pelvic congestion with pain in young women. *Lancet* **ii**, 351–3

Reginald P. W. and Stones, W. (1992) 'Division of uterosacral ligaments — is there a scientific basis?' in: *26th British Congress of Obstetrics and Gynaecology Abstracts*' **Part 1**, 97 (abstract)

Reiter, R. C. (1990) A profile of women with pelvic pain. *Clin Obstet Gynecol* **33**, 130–6

Renaer, M., Nijs, P., Van Asshe, A. and Vertommen, H. (1980) Chronic pelvic pain without obvious pathology in women. Personal observations and a review of the problem. *Eur J Obstet Gynaecol Reprod Biol* **10**, 415–63

Ripps, B. A. and Martin, D. C. (1992) Correlation and focal pelvic tenderness with implant dimension and stage of endometriosis. *J Reprod Med* **37**, 620–4

Rosenthal, R. H. (1993) Psychology of chronic pelvic pain. *Obstet Gynecol Clin North Am* **20**, 627–42

Sichlau, M. J., Yao, J. S. and Vogelzang, R. L. (1994) Transcatheter embolotherapy for the treatment of pelvic congestion syndrome. *Obstet Gynecol* **83**, 892–96

Stacey, C. M. and Munday, P. E. (1994) Abdominal pain in women attending a genitourinary medicine clinic: who has PID? *Int J STD AIDS* **5**, 338–42

Stovall, T. G., Ling, F. W. and Crawford, D. A. (1990) Hysterectomy for chronic pelvic pain of presumed uterine etiology. *Obstet Gynecol* **75**, 676–9

Stripling, M. C., Martin, D. C. and Poston, W. M. (1988) Does endometriosis have a typical appearance? *J Reprod Med* **879**

Sutton, C. and Hill, D. (1990) Laser laparoscopy in the treatment of endometriosis. A five year study. *Br J Obstet Gynaecol* **97**, 181–5

Taylor, H. C. (1949a) Vascular congestion and hyperemia. I. Psychologic basis and history of the concept. *Am J Obstet Gynecol* **57**, 211–30

Taylor, H. C. (1949b) Vascular congestion and hyperemia. III. Etiology and therapy. *Am J Obstet Gynecol* **57**, 654–68

Tjaden, B., Schlaff, W. S., Kinball, A. and Rock, J. A. (1990) The efficacy of presacral neurectomy for the relief of midline dysmenorrhoea. *Obstet Gynecol* **76**, 89–91

Vercellini, P., Fedele, L., Bianchi, S. and Candiani, G. B. (1991) Pelvic denervation for chronic pain associated with endometriosis: fact or fancy. *Am J Obstet Gynecol* **165**, 745–51

Walker, E. A. and Stenchever, M. A. (1993) Sexual victimisation and chronic pelvic pain. *Obstet Gynecol Clin North Am* **20**, 795–807

Walker, E. A., Sullivan, M. D. and Stenchever, M. A. (1993) Use of antidepressants in the management of women with chronic pelvic pain. *Obstet Gynecol Clin North Am* **20**, 743–51

Walling, M. K., Reiter, R. C., O'Hara, M. W., Milburn, A. K., Lilly, G. and Vincent, S. D (1994) Abuse history and chronic pain in women: I. Prevalences of sexual abuse and physical abuse. *Obstet Gynecol* **84**, 193–99

# 21

# Endometriosis, pelvic pain and psychological functioning

*Kathleen G. Waller*

Many patients with endometriosis present to the gynaecologist complaining of pain symptoms such as dysmenorrhoea, pelvic pain and dyspareunia. However, other individuals with the same amount of disease do not complain of any pain symptoms and endometriosis is discovered as a result of laparoscopy for other reasons. These women are said to have asymptomatic disease. Women with pelvic pain have, in general, been shown to be more likely than controls to suffer from mild disorders of psychological functioning. It has also been suggested that psychological factors may play a part in the aetiology of the endometriosis. The relationship between endometriosis, pelvic pain symptoms and psychological factors is complex and has not been studied to any great extent.

The clinical symptoms of endometriosis were first described in detail by King in 1924. One hundred and twenty-two women were studied, all of whom had histological confirmation of their disease. In 17 cases, the disease was of the uterus, and thus would today be classified as adenomyosis. The most common complaint was abdominal pain, which was present in 63% of those who had symptoms. It was generally described as 'shooting', 'gripping' or 'aching' pain of the lower abdomen. Usually it was worse during menstruation. Dysmenorrhoea itself was described as being very severe in half the cases, although 25% had either no dysmenorrhoea or only mild pain during menses. A most characteristic feature of the dysmenorrhoea was that it was of sudden onset in women who had previously been free of pain.

Among this group of patients, there was an actual record of dyspareunia in only 8% of cases, but King commented that '*it would probably have been much more frequently recorded if it had been desirable to make routine enquiries concerning it*'. Sixteen per cent of patients were asymptomatic and the disease was found at operation undertaken for other conditions.

Endometriosis is therefore characterised by pelvic pain symptoms, but these symptoms occur more frequently than the disease in the general population.

## PELVIC PAIN IN THE GENERAL POPULATION

### Dysmenorrhoea

Coppen and Kessel (1963) reported a 45% incidence of dysmenorrhoea in 500 unselected women. Other authors have reported on the prevalence of dysmenorrhoea in specific populations only, such as industrial workers (Bergsjo, Jensson and Vellar 1975). The prevalence of dysmenorrhoea was most effectively studied in a random sample of women who were 19 years old living in Goteberg, Sweden (Andersch and Milson 1982). The same women were asked to complete a further questionnaire when they were 24 years of age (Sundell, Milson and Andersch 1990). The prevalence of dysmenorrhoea was 72% at 19 years and 67% at 24 years. The prevalence and severity of dysmenorrhoea were reduced in women who were nulliparous at

19 years and parous at 24 years, but unchanged in women who remained nulliparous. The proportion of women who had severe dysmenorrhoea, which limited their daily activities, fell from 15% in the women aged 19 years to 10% in the women aged 24 years. The prevalence and severity of dysmenorrhoea were significantly reduced in women using the oral contraceptive pill.

### Dyspareunia

Detailed descriptions of dyspareunia first occurred in the Egyptian Raesseum papyri scrolls, and the word is derived from the Greek meaning 'difficulty mating' or 'badly mated'. The prevalence of dyspareunia has been reported in gynaecology clinic populations as between 1.5% (Frank 1948) and 40% (Semmens and Semmens 1974). Dyspareunia was studied in a group of 428 women in their early thirties who had all been college students (Glatt, Zinner and McCormack 1990). Dyspareunia was defined as pain or discomfort in the labia, vaginal or pelvic area during or after intercourse. At the time of the study 33.5% of women had dyspareunia, and a further 27.5% had had dyspareunia at some time in their lives, which had either spontaneously resolved or had got better with treatment. Of those women who had dyspareunia, 23.8% had it frequently or virtually all the time. Of those with dyspareunia at the time of the study, 33.7% reported who it was having an important adverse effect on their relationships. Although the definition of dyspareunia was broad in this study, and one-third of women had superficial dyspareunia only, it still appeared to be a very common and important symptom in the general population.

### Pelvic pain

Chronic pelvic pain can be defined as non-cyclical pain of at least six months' duration. The prevalence of chronic pelvic pain in a randomly selected group of women is not well described.

## PELVIC PAIN IN THE ENDOMETRIOSIS POPULATION

### Uncontrolled studies

Many authors have commented on the prevalence of symptoms of endometriosis in their own series of patients. O'Connor in 1987 listed the symptoms of endometriosis in order of occurrence and found that, although dysmenorrhoea was the most common symptom followed by dyspareunia, the third most frequent presentation was a complete lack of symptoms, and this was found in 155 of 717 patients (22%). Buttram in 1979 described, retrospectively, the symptomatology in 206 infertile women with endometriosis. Sixty-two per cent of these women had dysmenorrhoea and 27.2% described their dysmenorrhoea as severe. For women with mild, moderate and severe disease the prevalence rates for severe dysmenorrhoea were 21.6%, 26.5% and 35.3%, respectively. For deep dyspareunia, the prevalence rates were 22.7%, 28.0% and 33.8% for mild, moderate and severe disease.

Cramer et al. (1986) analysed the menstrual characteristics of women with and without endometriosis in a large, case–controlled study. They documented a greater probability of the disease in women with menstrual pain. The relative risk (RR) for women with mild, moderate and severe dysmenorrhoea in relation to those without dysmenorrhoea was 1.7, 3.4, and 6.7, respectively. Although a large number of controls were used in this study, the absence of endometriosis in controls was only presumed.

Prospective studies have been performed to investigate pelvic pain symptoms in women with endometriosis. Fedele et al. (1990) administered 160 women with a questionnaire prior to laparoscopic diagnosis. A total of 78% reported dysmenorrhoea, 39% had pelvic pain and 32% had deep dyspareunia. The presence and severity of the symptoms had no relationship to the stage of disease. The pain profile of patients with ovarian lesions was similar to that of patients with peritoneal disease, and a more detailed analysis according to the peritoneal location of disease did not reveal important differences in pain symptomatology.

## Controlled studies

Prevalence rates for particular symptoms in populations of endometriosis patients, whether evaluated prospectively or retrospectively, are useful, but as pelvic pain symptoms are common in the general population, properly controlled studies are essential. The following studies have utilised laparoscoped control groups. Lim, Fisk and Templeton in 1989 found no difference in the prevalence of dysmenorrhoea, pelvic pain and dyspareunia in 19 patients with minimal or mild endometriosis and 18 normal controls. Mahmood *et al.* (1991) performed the largest study on menstrual symptoms in women with endometriosis. One thousand two hundred women were given questionnaires prior to laparoscopy or hysterectomy, of whom 201 (17%) were found to have endometriosis. Deep dyspareunia and pelvic pain unrelated to menses were found with greater frequency in women with endometriosis, and women with pelvic adhesions, than in controls. Dysmenorrhoea was found with greater frequency in women with endometriosis, than in controls and women with pelvic adhesions. There was no relationship between symptomatology and the stage of endometriosis in this study. Symptoms were not analysed according to severity, and were only recorded as present or absent.

Fedele *et al.* (1992) reported on pain symptoms associated with endometriosis in 124 infertile women with the disease and 67 infertile women with normal pelvic findings. They found that the severity of some symptoms increased according to disease stage, as classified by the American Fertility Society (1985). The severity of dysmenorrhoea was greater in women with moderate (stage III) or severe (stage IV) disease, compared with minimal (stage I) or mild (stage II) endometriosis or no disease. However, the frequency of dysmenorrhoea was similar in patients and controls. Pelvic pain was found more frequently in women with stage III and IV endometriosis, whereas dyspareunia was more frequent in patients than in controls, regardless of the stage of disease, but was not analysed in terms of severity. An association of two or more pain symptoms was more common in women with endometriosis than those with a normal pelvis (RR = 3.1). Secondary dysmenorrhoea is considered to be one of the hallmarks of endometriosis. This study found a greater frequency of secondary dysmenorrhoea compared with primary dysmenorrhoea in patients with disease stages III and IV compared with controls. Fedele and co-workers therefore found both greater frequency and severity of pelvic pain symptoms in women with stage III and IV disease in their controlled 1992 study, in contrast to the results of their uncontrolled study of 1990, when the severity of the pelvic pain symptoms was not related to disease stage.

## Pathogenesis for endometriosis pain

Some authors have suggested that retrograde menstruation is the cause of dysmenorrhoea. However, Liu and Hitchcock (1986) sterilised 75 women during menstruation. Seventy-six per cent of women had retrograde menstruation at laparoscopy, and this was not associated with the occurrence of dysmenorrhoea or observed endometriosis.

Large amounts of prostaglandin (Vernon *et al.* 1986) and other mediators of inflammation are thought to be produced by peritoneal endometriotic lesions, causing irritation to the peritoneal surface. Other proposed mechanisms by which endometriosis may produce pain symptoms, such as scarring, retraction of the peritoneal surface and endometriomas leaking irritant material, are discussed by Burns and Schenken (1989).

It has also been proposed that the depth of the endometriotic implant is an important factor in the causation of symptoms. Cornillie *et al.* in 1990 found that very deep (> 10 mm) endometriotic implants correlated strongly with pelvic pain symptoms. Disease was more active in these deep lesions compared with more superficial disease. The excisional biopsies of deep endometriosis were said to contain nerve fibres and inflammatory cells in and around the implants, which may explain the association of these implants with pelvic pain.

## Asymptomatic endometriosis

One of the greatest enigmas of endometriosis is the fact that some patients with severe disease have no symptoms at all, while others with minimal disease suffer incapacitating pelvic pain. It is thought that for some individuals with more severe disease, the endometriosis itself has disrupted the afferent nerves of the pelvis and so the pain symptoms are minimal or absent. Furthermore, some women may not complain of crippling dysmenorrhoea, for example, as they consider such symptoms to be normal. There may also be psychological differences between women with asymptomatic and symptomatic endometriosis. However, before considering whether aspects of psychological functioning may be important in some women with endometriosis, it must be remembered that there are many studies which have shown abnormal psychological parameters in women with pelvic pain and a normal pelvis at laparoscopy.

## PSYCHOLOGY OF WOMEN WITH PELVIC PAIN ALONE

Several investigators have found psychological differences between women with an 'organic' cause for pelvic pain and women with pain and no apparent pelvic pathology. Beard *et al.* in 1977 reported on 35 women with pelvic pain, of whom 17 had abnormalities at laparoscopy (including three with endometriosis) and 18 had a normal pelvis. The women with no cause demonstrable for pelvic pain tended to be more neurotic, and were shown to have negative attitudes towards themselves and their partners. Women with a negative laparoscopy did not rate their relationship with their husband or partner as highly.

Women with chronic pain and a normal pelvis have also been found to be significantly depressed when compared with a group with positive laparoscopy findings (Magni *et al.* 1984). Rapkin and co-workers (1990) compared patients with chronic pelvic pain with women who had chronic pain in other locations and normal controls. Within the pelvic pain group,

65% of patients had identifiable pelvic pathology in the form of endometriosis or pelvic adhesions. Thirty-nine per cent of women in the pelvic pain group had been physically, although not sexually, abused in childhood. This percentage was significantly greater than that observed in other chronic pain patients (18.4%) or controls (9.4%). Reiter *et al.* (1991) compared two groups of laparoscopically normal women; 47 had a probable somatic cause for pain, of which the most common diagnosis was myofascial pain, and 52 women had no identifiable somatic cause for pain. The latter group of women had an earlier age at first intercourse, a higher lifetime number of partners, and a higher prevalence of sexual abuse before the age of 20 years.

## PSYCHOLOGY OF WOMEN WITH ENDOMETRIOSIS

Few studies exist which look at the psychological functioning of women with endometriosis, which perhaps is surprising in that endometriosis is a common relapsing condition which can trouble sufferers throughout their reproductive lives. The relationship, if any, between endometriosis and psychological factors is, therefore, not well understood. Two previous studies have looked at the association between affective disorder and endometriosis. Lewis *et al.* (1987) studied 16 women who were treated for endometriosis, and found that 12 met the diagnostic criteria for bipolar or major depressive disorders, which usually had started prior to the diagnosis of the disease. However, that study was uncontrolled and Walker *et al.* (1989) compared 14 women with endometriosis with 55 women without the disease and found no difference in the prevalence of affective disorder.

### Psychological abnormalities from chronic pain

It is not known whether abnormal psychological or psychiatric functioning makes it more likely that a woman will develop endometriosis or, indeed, more likely that the disease is discovered and pain be attributed to its presence. Psychological abnormalities may, however, occur as a consequence of endometriosis which can be a chronic painful condition. Renaer and co-workers in 1979 used only patients with endometriosis in their pelvic pathology group in a study comparing women with pelvic pain and pelvic pathology, women with pelvic pain and no pelvic pathology and normal controls. The authors were surprised to find that the psychological profile of women with endometriosis did not differ significantly from the profile of women with no organic cause for pain. Both the endometriosis group and the group with a normal pelvis and pelvic pain differed significantly from controls in that there were inflated scores for hypochondriasis, hysteria, psychasthenia and social inversion, as well as lower scores on ego strength using the Minnesota Multiphasic Personality Inventory (MMPI) (Hathaway and McKinley 1951). The authors concluded that, as endometriosis is unlikely to occur in neurotic people, pain itself is likely to lead to neuroticism.

## Psychological abnormalities and vulnerability to endometriosis

In contrast, Low, Edelman and Sutton (1994) proposed that psychological abnormalities may make women more vulnerable to developing endometriosis. They studied 40 women with pelvic pain and endometriosis and compared them with 41 women with pelvic pain due to other gynaecological causes. Both pain groups were found to have neuroticism and psychiatric morbidity scores elevated in relation to normative data as measured using the General Health Questionnaire (GHQ) (Goldberg and Williams 1988). However, endometriosis patients were found to be significantly more introverted and have higher scores for measures of psychoticism than women with pelvic pain from other causes as measured by the Eysenck Personality Inventory (Eysenck and Eysenck 1975), although all scores were within the normal range. Endometriosis patients were also found to have significantly higher transient state anxiety and dispositional trait anxiety as measured by the Stait–Trait Anxiety Inventory

(Speilberger 1983), when compared to women with pelvic pain from other causes or normative data. The authors argued that there would be no grounds for expecting differences between groups as a consequence of pain, and that psychological abnormalities (such as anxiety) serve as vulnerability factors for endometriosis.

## Further research

Waller and Shaw (1995) aimed to examine further the relationship between endometriosis, pelvic pain symptoms and psychological functioning by directly comparing women whose endometriosis was symptomatic with women with asymptomatic disease. All women in this study had only minimal or mild endometriosis according to the American Fertility Society classification of 1985. It was reasoned that if only the women with symptomatic endometriosis were found to have abnormalities of psychological functioning, then these results would concur with those of Renaer and co-workers (1979) — that is, chronic pelvic pain can lead to abnormal psychological functioning. However, if both groups of women with endometriosis were found to have similar abnormalities on psychometric testing, this could mean that abnormalities in psychological functioning (such as increased anxiety) act as vulnerability factors for the development of endometriosis, as proposed by Low, Edelmann and Sutton in 1994.

Women admitted for laparoscopy for pelvic pain symptoms, infertility or sterilisation were administered with psychometric tests as well as an endometriosis symptom questionnaire. This enabled multidimensional pelvic pain scores to be calculated. Patients were then divided into four groups according to the findings at operation. The controls (group 1, $n = 38$) consisted of patients admitted for sterilisation and found to have a normal pelvis. Group 2 ($n = 31$) consisted of patients who only complained of infertility but were found to have minimal or mild endometriosis. Group 3 ($n = 18$) were patients found to have minimal or mild endometriosis and complained of one or more pelvic pain symptoms. Group 4 ($n = 30$)

were patients with pelvic pain symptoms but no obvious pathology at laparoscopy.

When multidimensional pain scores were analysed, it was found that infertile women with endometriosis (group 2) had significantly more dysmenorrhoea and pelvic pain than the normal controls (group 1). However, women with symptomatic endometriosis (group 3) had significantly higher scores for dyspareunia and pelvic pain than their infertile counterparts with the same amount of disease. Symptomatic women with a normal pelvis (group 4) reported the highest pain scores for all parameters.

## Depression

Waller and Shaw (1995) found that women in both pain groups (groups 3 and 4) had significantly higher total Beck Depression Inventory (BDI) (Beck and Steer 1987) scores than women in both control groups (groups 1 and 2). Two subscales are contained within the BDI. The first 13 items create a cognitive–affective subscale for estimating depression in persons whose vegetative and somatic symptoms might overestimate the severity of their depression. The final eight items create a subscale to measure somatic–performance complaints. Women in both pain groups had significantly higher scores for the somatic–performance items of the BDI when compared with both control groups, but there was no difference when compared with women with asymtomatic mild endometriosis (group 2) for the cognitive–affective items. These results are similar to those of Raener et al. (1979) who used the MMPI to evaluate depression. Low, Edelmann and Sutton (1994) also found that women with endometriosis and women with pelvic pain from other causes had similar scores on the BDI.

## Anxiety

Waller and Shaw (1995) found no significant differences between groups for the Speilberger Stait–Trait Anxiety Inventory (Speilberger 1983). The results for all scales were normal for all groups. These results are in contrast to the study of Renaer and co-workers (1979), in which

both pain groups had higher anxiety scores on the clinical scale of the MMPI than the pain-free control group. Low, Edelmann and Sutton (1994), however, found that women with endometriosis had an elevated Stait–Trait Anxiety Inventory score when compared with women with pelvic pain from other causes and normative data.

## Sexual functioning

The female scale of the Golombok Rust Inventory of Sexual Satisfaction (GRISS) (Rust and Golombok 1986) was used as a measure of sexual functioning by Waller and Shaw. Total GRISS scores were similar for all groups. However, when subscales of the GRISS were analysed separately, some significant differences were observed between groups. Women in both pain groups scored significantly higher than both control groups for infrequency of sexual intercourse. Women with pelvic pain and no pathology (group 4) scored higher for nonsensuality than women in both control groups, and group 4 women scored higher on the scale for vaginismus than women being sterilised. These differences were not accounted for by the greater frequency of dyspareunia in both pelvic pain groups. There were no differences found between groups for age at coitarche (age at first interourse) and lifetime number of sexual partners. No other studies have specifically investigated sexual functioning in women with endometriosis.

Therefore, it appears that the psychological profile of women with endometriosis is similar to the profile of women with no organic cause for pain (Renaer et al. 1979; Waller and Shaw 1995). Women in chronic pain, whatever its cause, appear to have substantial distress which may lead to abnormalities of psychological functioning. There is some evidence, however, that psychological abnormalities may act as vulnerability factors for the development of endometriosis (Low, Edelmann and Scott 1994), and further research is needed. Women with so-called asymptomatic disease, however, have been shown to have significantly more dysmenorrhoea and pelvic pain than normal controls and it is possible that differences in psychological characteristics act to alter perception and reporting of pain.

## MANAGEMENT OF SYMPTOMATIC ENDOMETRIOSIS

Women with pelvic pain symptoms and moderate and severe endometriosis can usually be effectively treated using conservative surgical modalities or hysterectomy. Medical treatment can also be useful, although recurrence rates can be high once ovarian activity returns (Waller and Shaw 1993). However, it often seems that women with more mild disease can present a difficult management problem.

### Surgical treatment

Sutton *et al.* in 1994 reported on the effectiveness of laser laparoscopy for the treatment of symptomatic endometriosis in a prospective, double-blind, randomised, controlled trial involving 63 patients. The results for women with minimal disease were poorest, with only 38% reporting improvement compared with 69% for those with mild disease and 100% for those with moderate disease. The authors speculated on whether endometriosis was the cause for pain in all their patients with minimal disease.

### Medical treatment

Psychological abnormalities may be compounded by the fact that medical treatment for endometriosis can itself cause mood changes in some women. Depression is a well-known side effect when gonadotrophin releasing hormone analogues (GnRHa) and danazol are used to treat endometriosis, although the proportion of patients reported with this side effect varies considerably with different clinical trials (Shaw 1992). Depression can also occur as a side effect of progestogen treatment for endometriosis (Telimaa *et al.* 1987). Patients can also become distressed as a result of other side effects of medications (e.g. weight gain), which commonly occur in women taking danazol (Telimaa *et al.* 1987).

Antidepressants such as amitriptyline have been shown to be superior to a placebo in double-blind studies in non-gynaecological patients complaining of chronic pain (McQuay, Carroll and Glynn 1992). Perhaps these medications would be useful in the management of some women with more mild disease who do not respond well to conventional therapy alone, particularly if they also exhibit symptoms of depression.

## CONCLUSION

It is important to be aware that mild psychological abnormalities, particularly depression, may coexist with pain symptoms in women with endometriosis. A psychologist working with the gynaecologist may be helpful in the management of some cases, and a supportive attitude on the part of the gynaecologist is especially important.

# References

American Fertility Society (1985) Revised American Fertility Society classification of endometriosis. *Fertil Steril* **43**, 351–2

Andersch, B. and Milson, I. (1982) A epidemiologic study of young women with dysmenorrhoea. *Am J Obstet Gynecol* **144**(6), 655–60

Beard, R. W., Belsey, E. M., Lieberman, B. A. and Wilkinson, J. C. M. (1977) Pelvic pain in women. *Am J Obstet Gynecol* **128**, 566–70

Beck, A. T. and Steer, R. A. (1987) *Beck Depression Inventory Manual.* The Psychological Corporation/San Antonio: Harcourt Brace Jovanovich Inc.

Bergsjo, P., Jensson, H. and Vellar, O. D. (1975) Dysmenorrhoea in industrial workers. *Acta Obstet Gynecol Scand* **54**, 255–9

Burns, W. N. and Schenken, R. S. (1989) 'Pathophysiology' in: R. S. Schenken (Ed.). *Endometriosis. Contemporary Concepts in Clinical Management*, pp. 83–118. Philadelphia: J. B. Lippincott Co.

Buttram, V. C. (1979) Conservative surgery for endometriosis in the infertile female: a study of 206 patients with implications for both medical and surgical therapy. *Fertil Steril* **31**(2), 117–23

Coppen, A. and Kessel, N. (1963) Menstruation and personality. *Br J Psychiatry* **109**, 711

Cornillie, F. J., Oosterlynck, D., Lauweryns, J. M. and Koninckx, P. R. (1990) Deeply infiltrating pelvic endometriosis: histology and clinical significance. *Fertil Steril* **53**, 978–83

Cramer, D. W., Wilson, E., Stillman, R. J., Berger, M. J. and Belisle, S. (1986) The relation of endometriosis to menstrual characteristics, smoking and exercise. *J Am Med Assoc* **255**, 1904–8

Eysenck, H. J. and Eysenck, S. B. G. (1975) *Manual of the Eysenck Personality Questionnaire.* London: Hodder and Stoughton

Fedele, L., Parazzini, F., Bianchi, S., Arcaini, L. and Candiani, G. B. (1990) Stage and localization of pelvic endometriosis and pain. *Fertil Steril* **53**, 155–8

Fedele, L., Bianchi, S., Bocciolone, L., Di Nola, G. and Parazzini, F. (1992) Pain symptoms associated with endometriosis. *Obstet Gynecol* **79**, 767–9

Frank, R. T. (1948) Dyspareunia: a problem for the general practitioner. *J Am Med Assoc* **136**, 361

Glatt, A. E., Zinner, S. H. and McCormack, W. M. (1990) The prevalence of dyspareunia. *Obstet Gynecol* **75**, 433–6

Goldberg, D. P. and Williams, P. (1988) *A User's Guide to the General Health Questionnaire.* Windsor: NFER-Nelson

Hathaway, S. R. and McKinley, J. C. (1951) *Minnesota Multiphasic Personality Inventory:* *Manual.* New York: The Psychological Corporation

King, W. W. (1924) The clinical symptoms of pelvic adenomyomata. *BMJ* **ii**, 573–5

Lewis, D. O., Comite, F., Mallouh, C. and Zadunaisky, L. (1987) Bipolar mood disorder and endometriosis: preliminary findings. *Am J Psychiatry* **144**, 1588–91

Lim, B. H., Fisk, N. M. and Templeton, A. A. (1989) Early endometriosis: does it cause symptoms? *J Obstet Gynaecol* **9**, 332–3

Liu, D. T. and Hitchcock, A. (1986) Endometriosis: its association with retrograde menstruation. *Br J Obstet Gynaecol* **93**, 859–62

Low, W. Y., Edelmann, R. J. and Sutton, C. (1994) A psychological profile of endometriosis patients in comparison to patients with pelvic pain of other origins. *J Psychosom Res* **37**, 111–16

Magni, G., Salmi, A., De Leo, D. and Ceola, A. (1984) Chronic pelvic pain and depression. *Psychopathology* **17**, 132–6

Mahmood, T. A., Templeton, A. A., Thomson, L. and Fraser, C. (1991) Menstrual symptoms in women with pelvic endometriosis. *Br J Obstet Gynaecol* **98**, 558–63

McQuay, H. J., Carroll, D. and Glynn, C. J. (1992) Low dose amitriptyline in the treatment of chronic pain. *Anaesthesia* **48**, 281–5

O'Connor, D. T. (1987) 'Clinical features in diagnosis' in: Jordan, A. and Singer, A. (Eds.). *Endometriosis*, pp. 68–78. Edinburgh: Churchill Livingstone

Rapkin, A. J., Kames, L. D., Drake, L. L., Stampler, F. M. and Naliboff, B. D. (1990) History of physical and sexual abuse in women with chronic pelvic pain. *Obstet Gynecol* **76**, 92–6

Reiter, R. C., Shakerin, L. R., Gambone, J. C. and Milburn, A. K. (1991) Correlation between sexual abuse and nonsomatic chronic pelvic pain. *Am J Obstet Gynecol* **165**, 104–9

Renaer, M., Vertommen, H., Nijs, P., Wagemans, L. and Van Hemelrijck, T. (1979)

Psychological aspects of chronic pelvic pain in women. *Am J Obstet Gynecol* **134**, 75–80

Rust, J. and Golombok, S. (1986) *The Golombok Rust Inventory of Sexual Satisfaction.* Windsor: NFER-Nelson

Semmens, J. P. and Semmens, J. F. (1974) Dyspareunia. Brief guide to office counselling. *Med Aspects Hum Sexual* **8**, 85

Shaw, R. W. (1992) Treatment of endometriosis. *Lancet* **340**, 1267–71

Speilberger, C. D. (1983) *Manual for the Stait–Trait Anxiety Inventory.* Palo Alto, CA: Consulting Psychologists Press Inc.

Sundell, G., Milson, I. and Andersch, B. (1990) Factors influencing the prevalence and severity of dysmenorrhoea. *Br J Obstet Gynaecol* **97**, 588–94

Sutton, C. J. G., Ewen, S. P., Whitelaw, N. and Haines, P. (1994) Prospective, randomized, double-blind, controlled trial of laser laparoscopy in the treatment of pelvic pain associated with minimal, mild and moderate endometriosis. *Fertil Steril* **62**(4), 696–700

Telimaa, S., Puolakka, J., Ronberg, L. and Kauppila, A. (1987) Placebo-controlled comparison of danazol and high dose medroxyprogesterone acetate in the treatment of endometriosis. *Gynecol Endocrinol* **1**, 393–71

Vernon, M. W., Beard, J. S., Graves, K. and Wilson, E. A. (1986) Classification of endometriotic implants by morphologic appearance and capacity to synthesize prostaglandin F. *Fertil Steril* **46**, 801–6

Walker, E., Katon, W., Jones, L. M. and Russo, J. (1989) Relationship between endometriosis and affective disorder. *Am J Psychiatry* **146**, 380–1

Waller, K. G. and Shaw, R. W. (1993) Gonadotropin-releasing hormone analogues for the treatment of endometriosis: long-term follow-up. *Fertil Steril* **59**, 511–15

Waller, K. G. and Shaw, R. W. (1995) Endometriosis, pelvic pain and psychological functioning. *Fertil Steril* **63**, 796–800

# 22

# Taking a sexual history

*Lynne Webster*

Sexual problems of all kinds are common in clinic attenders and in the general population (Bancroft 1989). Community surveys of sexual problems are difficult to design and implement, but Osborn, Hawton and Gath (1988) in a large representative sample of middle-aged women in Oxford found that one-third of them suffered from significant sexual dysfunction. When patients attending some hospital out-patient clinics or general practitioner surgeries are surveyed, even higher rates emerge (Table 1). Much of this suffering can be relieved by appropriate reassurance and information about aspects of sexual anatomy and physiology. Failing this, specific advice or more intensive treatment is likely to help. Besides pharmacological and surgical interventions where indicated, there are psychological therapies of proven effectiveness available for couples and individuals with sexual problems (Hawton 1995). Contrary to some popular beliefs about psychotherapy, most of the treatment programmes based on cognitive, behavioural or systemic therapy for individuals and couples

with psychosexual problems are short term, showing beneficial changes within 12 sessions (Crowe and Ridley 1990). Many patients with sexual worries do not need specialist therapy and are simply relieved to be able to talk about their concerns with a sympathetic and knowledgeable doctor or nurse. In either case, there is no longer any excuse for avoiding discussion of sex with patients on the grounds that nothing can be done about their symptoms, as we now have a range of helpful treatment approaches to offer.

## AIMS

The aim of taking a sexual history is to get an accurate picture of what has been happening to cause the patient concern, in order to produce a formulation of the problem which will lead to the most appropriate and helpful treatment plan. This may seem obvious when stated, but it is surprising how often even the simple requirements of accuracy, overall formulation and eventual treatment plan are not achieved by otherwise experienced interviewers. A common mistake when trying to assess a sexual problem is to confuse the levels of information that are being gathered during the history taking. The four levels are:

(1) What has actually been happening?

(2) What does the patient feel about it?

(3) What is the underlying 'meaning' of the symptom?

(4) What does the interviewer think and feel about it?

**Table 1** *Sexual problems in clinic attenders. (Data from Bancroft 1989\*, with permission of Churchill Livingstone)*

| Type of patient | % | Sexual problem Type |
|---|---|---|
| Psychiatric first-attenders | 26 | Sexual/marital problems |
| Gynaecology out-patients | 28 | Sexual problems |
| Medical out-patients | 34 | Erectile problems |
| General practice attenders | 20 | Sexual problems |

\*Bancroft, J. (1989) *Human Sexuality and its Problems.* Edinburgh: Churchill Livingstone

The first level concentrates on a factual account of the symptoms, their duration, severity and consistency. This is a history just as any clinician would gather from any patient, whether they present with chest pain or pain on penetration. This may be more difficult than it seems, because the choice of language used by both the doctor and patient to describe sexual feelings and functions can lead to misunderstandings. For example, it is quite common for patients to use the word 'discharge' to describe ejaculation, whereas to a genitourinary physician this would mean something quite different. The second and third levels take account of the patient's reactions to and beliefs about the symptom. This may entail a closer look at cultural, family and relationship factors with a psychosexual developmental history going back as far as childhood. The final level adds the reactions, intuitions and judgements of the interviewer, acknowledging that the encounter with the patient is a two-way process. It is so easy to be drawn into the fascinating areas of levels two, three and four that the basic information on level one is overlooked. Conversely, a history which concentrates solely on the mechanics of the patient's sexual symptoms and neglects the more subtle areas of feeling and meaning will often lead to a very partial formulation and a simplistic treatment plan which fails.

## Overlooking basic information

An example of the first mistake would be Mrs J., aged 47 years. At the menopause clinic where she has been referred because her general practitioner has not been able to find a hormone replacement regimen that suits her, she is visibly distressed then starts crying. By gentle and sympathetic interviewing, the doctor elicits that she is very worried about her marriage. Her husband no longer seems interested in her sexually. Concerns about ageing emerge and she reveals that both her two older sisters' husbands left for younger women. Although Mrs J. is no longer distressed now that she has talked about this, the doctor is reluctant to enquire more directly about the frequency and quality of the couple's sexual contact. The fact that the problem started after Mr J. began experiencing retrograde ejaculation following a transurethral prostatectomy is missed, along with Mrs J.'s belief that he cannot find her sexually attractive any more because he does not produce an ejaculation of semen. In this case the doctor elicited the patient's feelings and the underlying meaning of the symptom to the patient, but neglected to gather basic information which would have led to a quite different formulation and treatment plan.

## Neglecting psychological considerations

An example of the second category of mistake is Mrs K., a woman of 25 years who has not yet consummated her five-year marriage. She is referred to a psychosexual specialist who proceeds to take a detailed history. A full account is recorded concerning the patient's inability to use tampons, reluctance to insert her own finger into her vagina and panic symptoms whenever her husband approaches her genitalia. Although the background history reveals no evidence of previous psychological or physical trauma, and on examination a vaginismic spasm is evident. Ignoring a nagging feeling that the history does not seem sufficient to explain the intensity of the patient's symptoms, the specialist confidently diagnoses primary vaginismus and just as confidently embarks on a behavioural programme of treatment using relaxation techniques and vaginal dilators. The specialist has ignored clear evidence in the interview that the patient expresses anger when talking about her husband's meek obedience to her domineering mother-in-law, and her desperate wish to leave the in-laws' house and get a home of their own. It only emerges much later after the planned treatment has failed how much the patient hates her interfering mother-in-law, and that allowing her husband entry into her vagina would be like losing her own identity and surrendering to the older woman's powerful need for grandchildren. In this case, the doctor's anxiety to get a detailed and accurate history screened out the important levels of feeling and meaning.

## PROFESSIONAL FEARS

Since the mid-1970s the department of psychiatry in Manchester has offered postgraduate training and qualifications in psychosexual counselling. Courses are attended by professionals from a wide range of disciplines, including general practice, obstetrics and gynaecology, psychiatry, genitourinary medicine, urology, diabetology, clinical psychology, social work and occupational therapy. It is a recurring source of surprise to the tutors that mature and knowledgeable trainees are often so anxious that they have palpitations and a tremor when faced with doing their first assessments with patients in the psychosexual training clinic. A number of possible reasons that have been identified from discussions with trainees: namely embarrassment, lack of time, fear of opening the floodgates, getting out of one's depth, being stigmatised, difficulty handling intimacy and problems coping with couples. Each of these factors will now be discussed in turn.

### Embarrassment

Trainees fear that they will be embarrassed by having to discuss explicit and intimate aspects of the patient's sexual experience. Indeed, they feel this would not only be uncomfortable for the trainee, but it will be noticed by the patient, who will then lose confidence in the interviewer. Trainees also fear that their enquiries will embarrass their patient, so that assessment cannot proceed. In fact, relatively simple interview techniques for dealing with embarrassment can be learned which overcome the problem in most cases.

### Lack of time

This is a legitimate concern that it might not be possible to take a full sexual history in the time allocated. Doctors used to working within the constraints of general practice or the hospital out-patient clinic feel under great pressure to complete their assessment and produce a treatment plan within a maximum of 15 minutes. This contrasts with trainees from counselling backgrounds such as Relate, where therapists are taught that a full psychosexual assessment takes four one-hour sessions. Clearly, the assessment needs to be modified to take account of circumstances, but there is no doubt that taking an excellent basic history is possible in a short time, judging by the referral letters received from busy clinics (Figure 1).

### Fear of opening the floodgates

Sex is a topic associated with strong emotions. Passionate love, painful loss, humiliation, guilt, shame and unbearable jealousy are just some of the feelings that may be attached to the patient's story of their symptoms. Doctors fear that discussion of sexual matters will risk bringing all these messy and uncontrollable feelings into the surgery or clinic. The doctor is then left with a situation in which they have elicited all these feelings, but feel powerless

---

Dear Dr Webster,

I would be grateful if you could send an appointment to this 25-year-old lady. She has one child aged four and has been married five years. For the past two years she has not been able to have intercourse with her husband and she has sought help because she feels that this is not normal and that it is not fair on him. She is not concerned for herself, however, and she says she would be quite content never to have sex again for the rest of her life.

She says she had a very strict upbringing from elderly parents who were prohibitive about sex, and I think this has left her a bit inhibited about sexual matters. She has always felt that sex and genitals were dirty. She has never been able to use tampons and is reluctant to have physical examinations.

I would be grateful for any help you can give her.

Yours sincerely,

**Figure 1** *This letter, modified to protect confidentiality, was sent by a busy general practitioner. It contains all the levels of information in two short paragraphs*

to help. This is largely overcome by acquiring more knowledge of sexual medicine and the treatments that are available for sexual problems. In addition, most patients are only too aware of the constraints of time and resources that make it inappropriate to delve deeply into these areas unless the therapeutic setting supports this, as it does in counselling or psychotherapy.

## Getting out of one's depth

This fear follows on from the previous one, with the trainee imagining that it will be impossible to deal with the distressing emotions experienced on both sides when painful issues such as childhood sexual abuse emerge. This concern is well-founded, and anyone working with patients who present with sexual problems should have access to a clinical supervisor or peer group where cases can be discussed, along with how best to handle the feelings that arise. This is somewhat against the culture that still prevails in some areas of medicine, where we have been notoriously bad at supporting junior staff and each other. However, we are gradually coming to realise that there is no advantage for the doctor or the patient in shouldering huge emotional and clinical burdens alone.

## Fear of being stigmatised

If we gain extra skills in some area of our chosen field of medicine, such as expertise in the management of diabetic patients or knowledge of the latest hormonal treatments, we will undoubtedly earn the respect of our colleagues and the gratitude of our patients. This is not entirely true, however, of skills in psychosexual medicine. Trainees on the postgraduate courses report mixed attitudes from colleagues, sometimes including mockery or outright hostility. This reflects society's deep discomfort with sexuality which also emerges in the medical profession. For many years, the psychosexual clinic in Central Manchester was housed in the clock tower of the old maternity hospital, as far away from the rest of the hospital's clinical activities as was geographically possible.

## Difficulty in handling intimacy

It is true that talking with patients about their sexual problems requires a greater degree of openness and trust in the consultation than discussing more neutral symptoms, such as abdominal pain or dizziness. Some patients (and clinicians) find it difficult to return to a more business-like interaction after the patient has confided about sexual problems, and routine complaints are subsequently taken to another colleague. At the extreme end of the scale, the intimacy and trust can overstep the boundaries of professional conduct, leading to sexual exploitation of the patient. Fahy and Fisher (1992) remarked that gynaecologists and psychiatrists might be more at risk of this type of involvement as their work necessitates 'the most extreme invasion of the patient's physical or emotional privacy'. Reassuringly, there is some evidence that extra training in psychosexual therapy makes this less likely, presumably because these issues are tackled more explicitly in training (Schover 1989).

## Problems coping with couples

Many sexual problems that lead patients to seek help occur in the context of a sexual relationship with another person. Sometimes it is vital to see both partners, separately and together, before a full picture of the difficulties can be obtained. Professionals who are accustomed to working with individuals may be anxious about interviewing couples, with some justification. It takes additional skills to manage the increased number of possible interactions in the consulting room. The interviewer may feel distinctly uncomfortable as each partner tries to recruit sympathy for their partial view of the problem by criticising the behaviour of the other. The interviewer may grow increasingly alarmed as the consultation degenerates into a slanging match and full-scale row. Couple therapists are trained in the observation and therapeutic management of such interactions, and for anyone working in the field of sexual medicine it is worth acquiring some of these extra skills.

## APPROACHES

When faced with their first formal psychosexual assessment in the training clinic, most trainees want to arm themselves with a comprehensive check list of symptoms to ask about and areas of enquiry to cover. Reluctantly, the course tutors provide a printed history sheet which is almost purely for the purpose of reducing the trainees' initial anxiety. On the surface, it addresses their fears that they will miss out something of importance in the interview, but in reality it acts as a shield and talisman that they can clutch to protect themselves in the encounter. With a little more experience, these props can be discarded as they lead at best to stilted, if comprehensive, interviews. At worst they encourage questioning that is nonsensical to the point of being insulting. A devoted man and wife in their sixties who cannot manage intercourse because of the husband's vascular disease will not appreciate being asked if either of them has ever had an extramarital homosexual affair just because the interviewer needs to tick a box on an over-inclusive history schedule. As with most other clinical accomplishments, sexual history taking requires application of common sense allied to background knowledge and good inter-personal skills. Anyone who wants a thorough basic framework from which to develop these skills will find excellent examples by Hawton (1989), in Table 2 and by Bancroft (1989).

Some traditions of psychosexual medicine that have grown out of a more psychoanalytic theoretical framework have a tendency to fall into the opposite trap of using a very unstructured interview technique (Mathers *et al.* 1994). In these cases it is only by good fortune that they gather any relevant information at all. Patients emerging from such a consultation may well feel that they have been listened to respectfully and that the nature of their problem has been understood by a wise and sympathetic doctor, but they are unlikely to be any nearer to getting a treatment plan that will help them solve their problem. It is all very well to help a man with a diabetic neuropathy gain insight into why his loss of erections is a blow to his masculinity, but it is of more practical use to give him a leaflet about vacuum pumps to induce erections. As a general rule, we have found that people with medical training need practice in asking more open questions and avoiding a premature rush to diagnosis and treatment. Those from

**Table 2** *Areas to cover during the assessment interviews with each partner. (Reproduced from Hawton 1989\* with permission of Oxford University Press)*

The sexual problem — its precise nature and development, desired changes in the sexual relationship (i.e. goals)
Family background and early childhood — including relationships with parents, parental relationship, family attitudes to sexuality
Sexual development and experiences — including attitudes to puberty, onset of sexual interest, previous sexual experiences and problems, masturbation, traumatic sexual experiences (e.g. sexual abuse) and homosexuality
Sexual information — source, extent, whether the person thinks he or she lacks information, and the therapist's assessment of level of sexual knowledge
Relationship with partner — including its development, previous sexual adjustment, general relationship, children and contraception, infidelity, commitment to the relationship, feelings and attraction towards the partner
School, occupation, interests, religious beliefs
Medical history — including any current medication
Psychiatric history
Use of alcohol and drugs
Appearance and mood (mental state)
Physical examination (if appropriate)

\*Hawton, K. (1989) 'Sexual dysfunction' in: K. Hawton, P. M. Salkovskis, J. Clark and D. M. Kirk (Eds.). *Cognitive Behaviour Therapy for Psychiatric Problems.* Oxford: Oxford University Press counselling backgrounds often need more training in focusing their enquiries to gather specific information and acquiring a more problem-solving approach. Training groups and clinical teams where a mix of disciplines and skills can contribute may speed up this process of learning.

## PITFALLS (WITH EXAMPLES)

Having disposed of the idea of check lists, it may still be useful to draw attention to some areas of the history that can be important, but are often overlooked.

## Drugs

It is well known that commonly prescribed drugs affect all aspects of sexual function in men, but recent research shows that they can also profoundly affect women (Riley and Riley 1986). In particular, β-blockers and benzodiazepines can reduce arousal and most of the routinely-used antidepressants can suppress libido (Harrison *et al.* 1985). It is not uncommon for patients to present with distress about sexual dysfunction that has affected their relationship when there is a clear link to the use of medication. A comprehensive drug history is therefore essential in all cases of sexual dysfunction. Particularly in younger patients, we need to be aware of the extent of use of recreational drugs and anabolic steroids for body-building, as these have definite, but as yet largely unresearched, effects on sexual function.

## Alcohol

It is well worth enquiring about alcohol intake in both sexes. Sometimes sexual and relationship problems are the presenting symptoms of underlying alcohol abuse and dependence. If this is the case and it is not detected, the chances of any therapeutic intervention being successful are virtually zero while the patient is still drinking heavily. Patients are used to doctors being concerned about health promotion and are not offended by questions about such aspects of their lifestyle.

## Work

Too much or too little of this can have a devastating effect on sexuality, particularly on libido. The middle-aged man made redundant and convinced he might never work again may not yet meet the criteria for clinical depression, but his loss of self-esteem and the role of provider upsets the balance of his relationship and sexual interest is lost. Likewise, the young woman who has given up the companionship and status of the workplace for isolation with a new baby may be similarly affected. The following conversation took place in the clinic:

Doctor: '*Tell me what your work entails, Mr G.*'
Patient: '*Well, I'm self-employed as a salesman since the company went bust, so there's no alternative. Every day this week I've driven a minimum of 500 miles round trip to see clients. I need to work late at home most nights to get the paperwork done and the last three weekends I have been in Brussels trying to secure a contract.*'

This man wondered why his libido had declined. It is clear from the annual surveys of British households that women do not fare any better, often struggling to combine full-time work with domestic and childcare responsibilities. A careful look at their weekly schedule makes loss of libido seem like a perfectly normal response to their circumstances rather than a pathological entity.

## Ethnic background

There is relatively little published work available on transcultural aspects of sexual and relationship therapy. Most therapists working in multicultural settings have learned about this area from their mistakes in clinical practice. D'Ardenne (1988) points out that patients from non-western cultures may have very different expectations and assumptions when consulting a doctor about sexual problems. They may not share our view that past history, going back as far as childhood, is of importance in explaining a sexual dysfunction experienced later in life. There may be an exaggerated respect for 'experts' and a powerful belief in physical remedies, leading them to seek the advice of herbalists and other traditional healers. It is less likely for women from these cultures to be the presenting partner when there is a sexual dysfunction, except where there is a question of infertility (Bhugra and Cordle 1988). Taking the sexual history needs to be modified, sometimes considerably, to make the process useful and meaningful when dealing with patients from different cultures.

## Age

When assessing sexual problems in older patients (and patients in their seventies and eighties are increasingly asking for help with sexual dysfunction), we need to bear in mind their different pattern of sexual practices. For instance, it has emerged from the British Survey of Sexual Attitudes and Lifestyles (Johnson *et al.* 1994) that people under 40 are twice as likely to have partaken of oral sex in the past year than older age groups. A similar trend is evident in the much smaller number of people who have tried anal intercourse. Power-Smith (1991) makes a thoughtful case, entreating us to consider the different experiences and concerns of patients in old age as regards their sexual relationships. Our stereotype of older people as being asexual acts as a barrier against them receiving appropriate help with sexual and relationship problems.

## CONCLUSIONS

Taking a sexual history should not present any difficulty for an otherwise competent clinician, but we have to acknowledge that this can be a delicate area for both doctor and patient. The medical profession functions within wider social and cultural parameters, and our society is very mixed in its attitudes to sex. We seem to be able to combine fascination, prurience, hypocrisy, condemnation, exploitation and delight in this least objective area of human experience. We cannot help but take our attitudes into the clinical setting, and only reflection on long experience or specific training are likely to modify this to make us more efficient and effective when discussing sexual symptoms with patients. This can be addressed by training in interview technique and regular update in the field of sexual medicine, particularly the rapidly-expanding options for treatment that are becoming available. We also need to be aware of the difficulties that trainees at both undergraduate and postgraduate levels experience when dealing with patients' sexual and relationship problems. Sometimes the culture of the departments and organisations we work within discourages trainees from expressing their fears and embarrassments, and if this is the case it is hard for us to teach them useful and creative ways to overcome these barriers so they can become more effective in taking sexual histories.

# References

Bancroft, J. (1989) *Human Sexuality and its Problems.* Edinburgh: Churchill Livingstone

Bhugra, D. and Cordle, C. (1988) A case control study of sexual dysfunction in Asian and non-Asian couples, 1981–1985. *Sex Marital Ther* **3**, 71–6

Crowe, M. and Ridley, J. (1990) *Therapy with Couples.* Oxford: Blackwell Scientific Publications

D'Ardenne, P. (1988) 'Sexual dysfunction in a transcultural setting' in: M. Cole and W. Dryden (Eds.). *Sex Therapy in Britain.* Milton Keynes: Open University Press

Fahy, T. and Fisher, N. (1992) Sexual contact between doctors and patients. *BMJ* **304**, 1519–20

Harrison, W. M., Stewart, J., Ehrhardt, A. A. *et al.* (1985) A controlled study of the effects of antidepressants on sexual function. *Psychopharmacol Bull* **21**, 85–8

Hawton, K. (1989) 'Sexual dysfunction' in: K. Hawton, P. M. Salkovskis, J. Kirk and D. M. Clark (Eds.). *Cognitive Behaviour Therapy for Psychiatric Problems*. Oxford: Oxford University Press

Hawton, K. (1995) Treatment of sexual dysfunctions by sex therapy and other approaches. *Br J Psychiatry* **167**, 307–14

Johnson, A. M., Wadsworth, J., Wellings, K. *et al.* (1994) *Sexual Attitudes and Lifestyles*. Oxford: Blackwell Scientific Publications

Mathers, N., Bramley, M., Draper, K. *et al.* (1994) Assessment of training in psychosexual medicine. *BMJ* **308**, 969–72

Osborn, M., Hawton, K. and Gath, D. (1988) Sexual dysfunction among middle-age women in the community. *BMJ* **296**, 959–62

Power-Smith, P. (1991) Problems in older people's longer term sexual relationships. *Sex Marital Ther* **6**, 287–96

Riley, A. J. and Riley, E. J (1986) The effect of single dose diazepam on female sexual response induced by masturbation. *Sex Marital Ther* **1**, 49–53

Schover, L. R. (1989) 'Sexual exploitation by sex therapists' in: G. O. Gabbard (Ed.). *Sexual Exploitation in Professional Relationships*. Washington: American Psychiatric Press

# 23

# Female sexual problems

*Fran Reader*

Female sexuality is multifaceted, involving biological, physiological, cultural and ethical dimensions. A normal physiological response to sexual arousal takes place when the physical and psychological components are healthy and when the experience conforms to the woman's cultural beliefs and ethical values. Within this environment a woman can choose and enjoy a wide range of sexual behaviours with herself (masturbation) or a person of the same or opposite sex. When another person is involved they bring into the sexual relationship their own physical, psychological, cultural and ethical sexual dimensions. Sexual likes and dislikes need to be communicated so that the outcome is mutually pleasurable. Sex can be procreational, recreational or a means of expressing affection and confirming bonding. When there is a sexual problem this cannot happen and the failure can be devastating for the individual and the relationship.

## WHAT SEXUAL PROBLEMS?

The *International Classification of Disorders–10* (World Health Organisation 1994) classifies sexual problems not caused by organic disease according to the phases of the sexual response cycle of drive, desire, arousal, orgasm and problems with penetration (Table 1). The sexual problems secondary to organic disease are classified by the particular pathological condition.

The prevalence of female sexual problems in the population is unknown. A variety of studies, whether scientifically based on general (Kinsey *et al.* 1953; Garde and Lunde 1980) or clinic populations (Levine and Youst 1976; Golombok, Rust and Pickford 1984), or non-scientifically based from, for example, sampling through magazines (Saunders 1985) or questionnaires (Hite 1976; Quilliam 1994), have attempted to quantify the frequency of sexual problems. In Saunders' study (1985) on 4000 women responding to a questionnaire in *Woman* magazine, 59% reported a sexual problem sometime during their life and 23% were troubled by a sexual problem at the time of response. Referrals to clinics specialising in treatment of sexual problems (Bancroft and Coles 1976; Hawton 1985; Draper, Bramley and Snead 1994) show that problems of sexual desire or pleasure are the most frequent female problem to present, followed by orgasmic problems and problems with penetration due to either vaginismus or dyspareunia.

Two recent studies on sexual behaviour have extended knowledge of female sexual behaviour in the United States (Janus and Janus 1993) and Great Britain (Wellings *et al.* 1994). Women are experiencing first intercourse at a younger age. Vaginal intercourse is the most common activity, but non-penetrative sex (including fellatio and cunnilingus) contributes to

**Table 1**  *The International Classification of Disorders for non-organic female sexual problems*

| | |
|---|---|
| F52.0 | Lack or loss of sexual desire |
| F52.1 | Sexual aversion and lack of sexual enjoyment |
| F52.2 | Failure of genital response |
| F52.3 | Orgasmic dysfunction |
| F52.5 | Non-orgasmic vaginismus |
| F52.6 | Non-organic dyspareunia |
| F52.7 | Excessive sexual drive |

the sexual experiences of most women, while anal sex is a minority activity. Younger women tend to have more partners than the older cohort, but serial monogamy remains the main pattern. Homosexual activity is reported by a minority of women, with 4.5% reporting a sexual attraction to a woman, 3.5% sexual contact and 1.5% genital contact with a woman (Wellings *et al.* 1994). Hite (1976) and Quilliam (1994) in their questionnaires confirm the importance of masturbation for women. In Quilliam's study over 90% of women reported difficulty with orgasm through penetration alone; most preferred to combine penetration with direct clitoral stimulation. Women also reported they tend to take longer to reach the peak of arousal than men and are not orgasmic as frequently as men. Between 5% and 10% of women never become orgasmic. Both sexes reported that sexual activity, arousal response and intensity of orgasm decline with age.

The current classification of sexual problems and attitudes to sexual behaviour have been defined within our own cultural framework which is based on a medicalised, heterosexual and penetration-focused concept of female sexuality. Ussher and Baker (1993) in their book *Psychological Perspectives on Sexual Problems* provide a refreshing challenge to this model, recognising the importance for women of non-genital sensuality as well as genital sexuality.

## HOW DO THESE WOMEN PRESENT?

Some women are comfortable with their sexuality and openly discuss their problems, while others present indirectly, either in their own right or via their partner. Alternatively, some women present because it is their partner who has the problem. The sexual problem may be acknowledged inwardly, but embarrassment prohibits a direct request for help. Indeed, sex may be such a shameful topic that the problem is unconsciously denied and presents as a psychosomatic disorder. Body language when discussing sexual health issues or expressions of embarrassment, shame, revulsion or fear when an examination of the genital parts of the body is proposed or performed can give an important insight into whether a sexual problem is present (Tunnadine 1992). It is, therefore, not uncommon for sexual problems to emerge directly or indirectly during an obstetric, gynaecological, contraceptive or sexual health consultation. Due to their reproductive role, women have greater exposure to the medical profession and this may be the reason for the higher prevalence of reported sexual problems in women (Read 1995).

## SEXUAL PROBLEMS AND THEIR MANAGEMENT

### Physiological factors

*After childbirth*

Many women experience reduced interest in sex in the first six months after childbirth (Kumar, Brant and Mordecai-Robson 1981) and many couples do not return to previous sexual activity until one year later, if at all. Exhaustion and sleep deprivation play a part, as can the raised prolactin and low oestrogen levels in women who are breast-feeding. Following a vaginal delivery physical changes to the labia minora and introitus may affect the woman's ability to grip the penis and achieve the same sensations during penetration, because it reduces the indirect stimulation to the clitoral head from the tugging effect on the clitoral hood produced by the thrusting penis. This mechanical change may adversely affect the woman's ability to achieve orgasm with penetration. Another factor after childbirth can be the temporary incontinence of urine, flatus or even faeces. Embarrassment may lead to sexual avoidance. Possible management strategies could involve:

(1) Reading self-help information about sex after childbirth (Rix 1995);

(2) Using the female superior position and the simultaneous manual stimulation of the clitoris may overcome a difficulty with achieving coital orgasm; and

(3) Improving pelvic floor muscle tone with Kegal exercises or, more effectively, with Femina cones.

## The menopause

The loss of oestrogen and testosterone have been linked psychologically with loss of sexual interest (Montgomery and Studd 1991; Sherwin 1994). Physical factors, such as night sweats and atrophic changes to the urogenital tissues, can lead to sexual avoidance because of exhaustion or fear of pain. Women may present problems with arousal or orgasm because with increasing age it takes longer to become aroused and orgasm becomes less intense. Some women have described touch impairment with the menopause that leads to sexual avoidance (Riley 1989). Stress incontinence can also present at this time and lead to sexual avoidance (Cardoza and Kelleher 1994). The women concerned can be helped by:

(1) Reading self-help information about the menopause and changes to the female sexual response (Stoppard 1994);

(2) Taking hormone replacement therapy for night sweats, atrophic urogenital changes and touch impairment;

(3) Using testosterone implants to increase interest;

(4) Using Femina cones to overcome stress incontinence; and

(5) Undergoing surgery for persistent stress incontinence.

## Organic/iatrogenic factors

Organic disease can lead to sexual problems because of physical factors. For example:

(1) The disease process affects the sexual response (e.g. multiple sclerosis);

(2) Surgery affects the sexual response (e.g. vulvectomy);

(3) The disease process affects mobility for sexual activity (e.g. cerebrovascular accident, cerebral palsy and spinal cord injury);

(4) Pain limits sexual activity (e.g. organic dyspareunia, arthritis and back problems); and

(5) Lethargy affects sexual interest (e.g. anaemia and renal failure).

Or psychological factors, such as:

(1) Poor body image and low self-esteem (e.g. after a mastectomy, or due to ostomies or psorasis); and

(2) Fear that sex could make the illness worse (e.g. myocardial infarction, asthma and epilepsy);

or due to drug side effects (Riley, Peet and Wilson 1993). Organic and iatrogenic factors and their relationship to sexual problems are fully reviewed by Bancroft (1989) and Sapire (1990); the latter was revised and adapted for the United Kingdom by Belfield and Guillebaud. Tables 2 and 3 outline the sexual problems that can be associated with specific gynaecological disorders or follow surgical procedures. Management of such problems can include:

(1) Treatment of the specific pathological condition.

(2) Individual/couple counselling and support.

(3) Providing information about the disease and/or treatment effect on the sexual response.

(4) Giving practical advice about, for example, adapting sexual activity to the limitations of the disease process. A good organisation for this is the Association to Aid the Sexual and Personal Relationships of People with a Disability (SPOD), 286 Camden Road, London N7 0BJ (telephone 0171-607-8851/2).

(5) Undertaking couple therapy to open up communication about the sexual relationship which may otherwise be avoided for fear of hurting or being hurt.

## Psychosocial factors

### Lack of, or incorrect information about, sex

Knowledge about sexual anatomy, physiology and behaviour is often lacking or incorrect.

**Table 2**  *The sexual problems associated with different gynaecological disorders*

| Gynaecological disorder | Sexual problem |
| --- | --- |
| Dysfunctional uterine bleeding | Reduced frequency/loss of interest (anaemia) |
| Endometriosis/pelvic inflammatory disease | Deep dyspareunia |
| Adenomyosis/endometriosis | Deep dyspareunia/orgasmic pain |
| Fibroid polyp | Orgasmic pain |
| Chronic pelvic congestion | Deep dyspareunia and lingering pain after sex |
| Sub/infertility | Loss of interest or sexual avoidance if feeling under 'performance pressure' or unconscious conflict about relationship/parenting |
| Candida/herpes/vulval dermatological conditions | Superficial dyspareunia |

**Table 3**  *The sexual problems associated with different surgical procedures*

| Surgical procedure | Sexual problems |
| --- | --- |
| Episiotomy | Superficial dyspareunia |
| Hysterectomy | Reduced sensations of pelvic fullness with arousal. Reduced orgasmic intensity. Less ability to reach multiple orgasm |
| Anterior repair | Reduced sensations over anterior vaginal wall. Can be significant and reduce arousal if 'G' spot was a pleasurable source of sexual arousal |
| Posterior repair | Creation of vaginal 'bridge' may cause dyspareunia |
| Wertheim's hysterectomy | Length of vagina reduced (elasticity and capacity compromised if treated with radiotherapy). Loss of interest because of diagnosis |
| Vulvectomy | Difficulty in reaching orgasm. Superficial dyspareunia due to introital scarring. Loss of interest. Poor body image |

Access to information may have been limited due to family or cultural sexual guilt and repression of information. Alternatively, information may have been received via dirty jokes or media sensationalism. Either can lead to sexual problems, both in the act itself or in unrealistic expectations. It should be managed by:

(1) Providing information verbally, with or without the help of pictures;

(2) *In vivo* education with the use of a hand-held mirror during an examination of the woman's external genitalia; and

(3) Self-help books (Dickson 1985; Fenwick and Walkery 1994).

*Sexual myths and taboos*

Beliefs and attitudes are formed within family, social and cultural and religious frameworks. Each have their own myths and taboos about sexual behaviour. Where myths and taboos feed performance pressure or lead to feelings of fear, guilt or shame, then sexual problems are common. Some common sexual myths are:

(1) It is performance that counts;

(2) The man takes charge;

(3) A woman who initiates sex is loose;

(4) Good sex is spontaneous;

(5) All physical contact leads to sex;

(6) Sex equals intercourse; and

(7) 'If he really loved me he'd know what I like'.

These myths should be challenged with sensitivity to cultural issues and open, non-judgemental, unembarrassed discussion should take place about sexual matters.

## Communication problem

Many sexual difficulties present because of poor communication, either generally or specifically. A common communication problem centres around failure to be assertive and let a partner know what actions are not enjoyed. The fear is that the other person will hear criticism and be hurt. We cannot read each other's minds and so, unless we can communicate our dislikes, the other person can hardly be blamed for getting it wrong. General communication problems within a relationship can also be expressed as a sexual problem, as shown in Figure 1.

It is important to make the couple aware that:

(1) Good communication requires clear verbal messages, congruent body language and active listening skills;

(2) Communication problems are best approached as part of couple work; and

(3) Communication and assertion skills can also help in individual work to bring about a shift out of a vicious circle.

## Differing expectations and appetites

One partner may want sex every night and the other once a month. One may enjoy oral sex and the other dislike it. Such differences in expectations and sexual preferences can lead to difficulties unless a mutually acceptable compromise can be reached. Unrealistic expectations can lead to sexual problems when the sexual act is goal orientated and, therefore, leads performance pressure. Examples include expecting no change in sexual interest when ill, tired or bereaved; expecting always to achieve orgasm during intercourse; expecting to reach orgasm together; expecting to return to the same interest in sex after childbirth; and expecting performance to remain unchanged with age. Management would involve:

(1) Giving information.

(2) Challenging unrealistic expectations.

(3) Improving communication skills. Where there are differing expectations and appetites the couple can be helped to negotiate a compromise (Crowe and Ridley 1990).

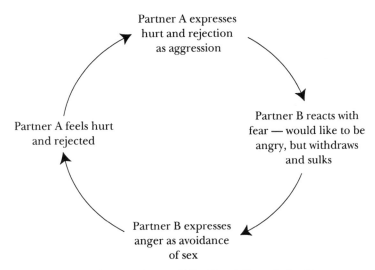

**Figure 1** *An example of how general communication difficulties within a relationship are expressed as a sexual problem*

(4) Initiating a sensate focus. This is a behavioural/cognitive strategy that helps remove performance pressure by banning penetrative sex and allows couples to share and communicate their non-genital sensual needs and to take responsibility for their own pleasure (Kaplan 1974).

## Precipitating events

Sexual problems are often precipitated by a specific event such as redundancy, bereavement, becoming a parent or learning that the partner has been unfaithful. Women respond differently to such events. For some the problem will resolve spontaneously, but for others the difficulty will persist once the cycle of failure and fear of failure has become established. Examples of precipitating and predisposing factors are shown in Table 4.

Individual or couple psychodynamic therapeutic approaches may help to bring about insight into predisposing or precipitating factors. Insight into the past does not always lead to change in the here and now. More directive behavioural/cognitive strategies may be required.

## SPECIFIC LIFE CYCLE ISSUES

### Puberty

The physiological changes that occur to the body around puberty can be disturbing for some young women who are in conflict about their adult sexual identify, gender identity or sexual orientation. This group may present with menstrual problems, sexually transmitted diseases, contraceptive problems or unplanned pregnancy. They may avoid sex, or may be sexually hyperactive, seeking reassurance in themselves in sexual relationships only to confirm their undesirability by pushing their partners away with their overdependency. This conflict may also present as eating disorders, drug problems or other forms of self-abuse. Individual therapy may help the young woman to resolve these conflicts. Within this group may also present

**Table 4** *Examples of factors that could precipitate, or predispose, a woman to sexual problems*

*Precipitating factors:*
adolescence
parenthood
menopause
illness
random failure
life stresses/bereavement
performance pressure
loss of trust in relationship
traumatic sexual experience

*Predisposing factors:*
physical, emotional or sexual abuse in childhood
restrictive upbringing
poor self-esteem
lack of information
poor body image
communication problems
uncertain sexual identity
psychiatric illness

young women who have been victims of child sexual abuse. Draper, Bramley and Snead (1994) reported 38% of women under 20 presenting with sexual problems within a National Health Service setting over a one-year period. Frequently help requires long-term psychiatry or psychotherapy.

### Parenthood

The transition to motherhood involves enormous changes to a woman's sense of self, her lifestyle, roles and probably career opportunities. Conflict over the parenting role may arise with her partner who may be feeling marginalised or jealous. The woman may be afraid of future pregnancies, particularly if she experienced a traumatic pregnancy or childbirth. Her body is likely to have changed and she may experience doubts about her sexual attractiveness. These factors coupled with the physiological and organic factors already discussed can precipitate sexual problems, particularly loss of interest or sexual avoidance. In this situation the following management strategies may prove effective:

(1) Brief counselling, helping her to realise that emotional upheaval is normal;

(2) Couple work to negotiate new roles and communicate changing sexual needs and preferences, thus reducing relationship tensions which are often part of the problem;

(3) Simple contraceptive advice to take away the fear of future pregnancy and give the woman time to come to terms with her birth experience; and

(4) Longer term individual therapy may be required (Brockington and Kumar 1982).

## The menopause

McKinlay and McKinlay in 1989 undertook a prospective longitudinal study of 2300 women and found that more than 70% reported relief or neutral feelings related to the menopause. The main factor to affect their feelings negatively was the persistence of hot flushes. Although the declining hormone levels may be responsible for depression and loss of sexual interest around the menopause, McKinlay and McKinlay's study suggests that the depression is associated with life events and consequent stress rather than the menopause. It is not uncommon for women at this time of life to be coping with several major life events. The resulting stress could affect their ability to relate sexually to their partner. Many of these life events involve loss or role change such as children leaving home, death of parents, moving to a new neighbourhood, retirement or redundancy. Furthermore, the ending of fertility may re-awaken grief of past infertility and for most women it is a time to confront their own future mortality (Griffin 1995). In this situation it is best to:

(1) Take a holistic approach to the management of sexual problems around the menopause; this is important so that the need for hormone replacement therapy is balanced by the opportunity for women to explore the meaning of their individual life crises and look at strategies for coping with them (Griffin 1995).

(2) Initiate couple work. Men may also be experiencing similar losses and sexual problems may arise related to difficulty in maintaining or achieving an erection.

(3) Suggest sexual therapy for individuals or couples as, at this time in life, it often focuses on broadening the definition of sex to include non-penetrative sensual options. Many couples respond positively to the idea of increasing quality rather than quantity of sexual activity.

## SPECIFIC SEXUAL PROBLEMS

### Lack or loss of desire

The problem may have always existed or may develop after a period of normal sexual interest. It is possible for low desire to exist in isolation, but commonly it is secondary to some other sexual problem so that repeated unsatisfactory experiences lead to a loss of desire. Deep-seated personal problems or relationship difficulties often present in this way. Chronic physical illness frequently leads to low desire because of fatigue, loss of self-esteem, altered body image or as a side effect of medication (Kaplan 1979). In this situation:

(1) Exclude physical factors if they exist, recognise their significance to the maintenance of the sexual problem.

(2) Initiate individual or couple therapy.

(3) Suggest self-pleasuring or sensate focus exercises to improve understanding and communication of sexual needs.

(4) Drug options are: (a) bromocriptine for hypoprolactinaemia; (b) testosterone implants for postmenopausal women (especially if the menopause occurs prematurely through a natural or iatrogenic loss of ovarian function); and (c) antidepressants if clinically depressed.

## Sexual aversion and lack of sexual enjoyment

Sexual avoidance, aversions and phobias often stem from some traumatic sexual experience such as childhood sexual abuse, rape or other abusive sexual experience in adult life. They may also stem from receiving strongly negative messages about sex so that sex is feared as it leads to feelings of guilt or shame. Sexual aversion may present as low desire because frequency of sexual activity is low. There is a difference between sexual interest being present but the activity avoided, rather than no interest and therefore no activity. Sexual aversion and phobias can be total, in which case all sexual activity is avoided or situational when specific sexual activities trigger the aversion or phobic response. For example, the woman may be phobic about the male penis, semen, penetration, breast stimulation or oral sex. The sense of impending loss of control with mounting arousal can trigger a panic response. For a woman who needs to remain in control the experience of sexual pleasure can trigger panic when childhood conditioning has enforced the idea that sexual pleasure is wrong. Such women may benefit from:

(1) Individual therapy to help to discover the predisposing or precipitating factors.

(2) Where a traumatic past sexual experience is responsible then abuse resolution work is required before dealing with the sexual problem (Jehu 1988).

(3) A process of gradual desensitisation to sexual activities that lead to the aversive response.

(4) Drugs such as: (a) serotonin re-uptake inhibitors can reduce the physical phobic response; and (b) β-blockers one hour prior to exposure (Kaplan 1987).

## Failure of genital response

The physiological arousal response in the female is invisible, unlike the male erection. It is common for both men and women to be unaware of the physical changes that accompany female arousal. Most know and understand that vaginal lubrication indicates arousal, but have no knowledge of the pelvic congestion and ballooning of the inner two-thirds of the vagina that occurs with high arousal.

It is uncommon for women to present with arousal problems in isolation. It is usually linked to low desire, sexual avoidance or orgasmic dysfunction (Segrave and Segrave 1991). Arousal problems often present as painful sex. Lack of lubrication makes penetration sore and lack of vaginal ballooning can lead to the woman experiencing deep discomfort with penile thrusting. The problem is rarely one of inability to become aroused, but rather that her partner is ahead of her in his arousal and penetrated her too soon, and the woman is unable to communicate the problem. This can be managed by:

(1) Self-discovery, self-pleasuring exercises.

(2) Sensate focus.

(3) Use of fantasy (Friday 1991).

(4) Reading self-help books (Yaffe and Fenwick 1992).

(5) Individual therapy (Hiller 1996).

(6) Drugs such as: (a) hormone replacement therapy if oestrogen deficiency is a factor in failure of lubrication; and (b) other lubricants (e.g. Replens or Senselle).

## Orgasmic dysfunction

This problem is related to either inadequate stimulation or to difficulty in letting go and losing control. It is often situational so that orgasm may occur with masturbation, but not with a partner, and can be resolved by:

(1) Exploring the use of fantasy, erotic material and sexual aids (e.g. vibrators);

(2) Reading self-help books (Heiman and LoPiccolo 1988); and

(3) Using nipple stimulation during sexual arousal to enhance orgasmic response due to oxytocin release (Riley 1988).

## Vaginismus

In this condition the woman has an involuntary spasm of the pubococcygeus muscle. Muscle tightens in anticipation of pain and, if penetration is forced through the tight muscle, then pain is certainly experienced reinforcing the problem. The vaginal spasm may also be accompanied by spasm of the adductor muscles of the thigh. The reasons for vaginismus are various, such as traumatic past experiences, or growing up with negative or over-romanticised messages about sex leading to fear of intimacy or loss of control. Another common link is seen with women of small stature who believe that their vagina is too small (Adler 1989). Women with vaginismus can be helped if they:

(1) Read information about genital anatomy and the female sexual response.

(2) Use individual therapy to explore predisposing factors (Hiller 1996).

(3) Undertake couple therapy where couples collude to maintain the problem.

(4) Gradually desensitise using: (a) such items as cotton buds, one finger, tampon covers of increasing size, two fingers, etc., with plenty of lubrication; (b) specifically designed vaginal trainers in different sizes (Stanley 1981); or (c) visualisation techniques;

(5) Gradually move to penile penetration with the woman maintaining control (she is likely to feel most relaxed in the female superior or side-to-side position).

(6) Use drugs, such as serotonin re-uptake inhibitors which may be useful to help overcome the strong physical phobic response if this is blocking progress.

## Dyspareunia

In women there are many physical causes for superficial and deep dyspareunia, but about 70% will have no obvious disease process. Emotional pain related to penetrative sex can also be expressed as genuine physical pain (Black 1988; Mira 1988). This may be due to past traumatic experiences such as sexual abuse or difficult childbirth, or may be an expression of problems within a relationship and part of an attempt to avoid intimacy with a partner. It is important to note that for these women:

(1) The management is similar to vaginismus.

(2) Adaptation of sexual positions will minimise pain.

(3) The drug options are: (a) adequate lubrication is essential and use of artificial lubricant is beneficial; (b) topical steroids may help if dermatological problems exist; (c) topical oestrogens may improve atrophic changes; or (d) local anaesthetic gel can be applied locally to a specific sore spot with the aid of a cotton bud or specifically placing a strip of gel along a tampon or finger which can then rest for five minutes against the spot to be anaesthetised. This local directed approach is preferable to applying the gel generally which then removes all sensation and can adversely affect penile sensation for the male partner.

## EXCESSIVE SEXUAL DESIRE

This sexual problem is also referred to as sexual addiction (Carnes 1992). This type of sexual behaviour is self-destructive and compulsive and, like other addictions, can lead to loss of family, money, job and even life. Most sexual addicts come from dysfunctional families and were abused as children, sexually, physically or emotionally. Many exhibit other addictions such as alcohol, drugs or gambling. Sexual addicts are powerless to control their compulsion to be sexual, despite the negative consequences. They will require:

(1) Long-term individual therapy.

(2) Group therapy. Most groups function along similar lines to Alcoholics Anonymous (AA) with a 12-step recovery programme (e.g. Sex Addicts Anonymous, telephone 0171-402-7278).

(3) Self-help information (Norwood 1985).

# References

Adler, E. (1989) Vaginismus — its presentation and treatment. *Br J Sex Med* **16**(11), 420–4

Bancroft, J. (1989) *Human Sexuality and its Problems*. Edinburgh: Churchill Livingstone

Bancroft, J. and Coles, M. (1976) Three years experience in a sexual problems clinic. *BMJ* i, 1575–7

Black, J. (1988) Sexual dysfunction and dyspareunia in the otherwise normal pelvis. *Sex Marital Ther* **3**(2), 213–22

Brockington, F. and Kumar, R. (1982) *Motherhood and Mental Illness*. London: Academic Press

Cardozo, L. and Kelleher, C. (1994) 'Estrogen deficiency and urinary incontinence' in: G. Berg and M. Hammar (Eds.). *The Management of the Menopause*, pp. 187–99. New York: Parthenon

Carnes, P. (1992) *Don't call it love. Recovery from Sexual Addiction*. London: Piatkus

Crowe, M. and Ridley, J. (1990) *Therapy with Couples*. London: Blackwell

Dickson, A. (1985) *The Mirror Within*. London: Quartet

Draper, K., Bramley, M. and Snead, S. (1994) Child sexual abuse in a retrospective survey of psychosexual referrals. *Br J Fam Plann* **20**, 17–20

Fenwick, E. and Walker, R. (1994) *How Sex Works*. London: Dorling Kindersley

Friday, N. (1991) *Women on Top*. London: Quartet

Garde, K. and Lunde, J. (1980) Female sexual behaviour: a study in a random sample of 40 year old women. *Maturitas* **2**, 225–40

Golombok, S., Rust, J. and Pickford C. (1984) Sexual problems encountered in general practice. *Br J Sex Med* **11**, 210–12

Griffin, M. (1995) The sexual health of women after the menopause. *Sex Marital Ther* **10**(3), 277–92

Hawton, K. (1985) *Sex Therapy: A Practical Guide*. Oxford: Oxford University Press

Heiman, J. and LoPiccolo, J. (1988) *Becoming Orgasmic: A Sexual Growth Program for Women*. London: Piatkus

Hiller, J. (1996) Female sexual arousal and its impairment: the psychodynamics of non-organic coital pain. *Sex Marital Ther* **11**(1), 55–76

Hite, S. (1976) *The Hite Report*. New York: Dell

Janus, S. and Janus, C. L. (1993) *The Janus Report on Sexual Behavior*. New York: Wiley

Jehu, D. (1988) *Beyond Sexual Abuse*. Chichester: Wiley

Kaplan, H. S. (1979) *Disorders of Sexual Desire*. New York: Brunner/Mazel

Kaplan, H. S. (1974) *The New Sex Therapy: Active Treatment of Sexual Dysfunction*. New York: Brunner/Mazel

Kaplan, H. S. (1987) *Sexual Aversion, Sexual Phobias and Panic Disorders*. New York: Brunner/Mazel

Kinsey, A. C., Pomeroy, W. B., Martin, C. E. and Gebhard, P. H. (1953) Sexual behaviour in the human female. Philadelphia: W. B. Saunders

Kumar, R., Brant, H. A. and Mordecai-Robson (1981) Childbearing and maternal sexuality: a prospective survey of 119 primiparae. *J. Psychosom Res* **25**(5), 373–83

Levine, S. B. and Youst, M. A. (1976) Frequency of sexual dysfunction in a general gynaecological clinic: an epidemiological approach. *Arch Sex Behaviour* **5**, 229–38

Montgomery, J. C. and Studd, J. W. W. (1991) Psychological and sexual aspects of the menopause. *Br J Hosp Med* **45**, 300–2

McKinlay, S. M. and McKinlay, J. B. (1989) 'The impact of menopause and social factors on health' in: C. B. Hammond, F. P. Haseltine and J. Schiff (Eds.). *Menopause: Evaluation, Treatment and Health Concerns*, pp. 137–61. New York: Alan R. Liss

Mira, J. J. (1988) A therapeutic package for dyspareunia: a three case example. *Sex Marital Ther* **3**(2), 77–82

Norwood, R. (1985) *Women Who Love Too Much*. London: Arrow

Quilliam, S. (1994) *Women on Sex*. London: Smith Gryphon

Read, J. (1995) Female sexual dysfunction. *Int Rev Psychol*, **7**, 175–82

Riley, A. (1988) Oxytocin and coitus. *Sex Marital Ther* **3**(1), 29–36

Riley, A. (1989) Post menopausal touch impairment presenting as sexual avoidance: a case report. *Sex Marital Ther* **4**(2), 189–93

Riley, A., Peet, M. and Wilson, C. (1993) *Sexual Pharmacology*. Oxford: Oxford University Press

Rix, J. (1995) *Is there Sex after Childbirth?* London: Thorsons

Sapire, E. K. (1990) *Contraception and Sexuality in Health and Disease* [UK edition/revision and adapted by T. Bellfield and J. Guillebaud]. Maidenhead: McGraw-Hill

Saunders, D. (1985) *The Woman's Book of Love and Sex*. London: Joseph

Segrave, R. T. and Segrave, K. B. (1991) Diagnosis of female arousal disorder. *Sex Marital Ther* **6**(1), 9–14

Sherwin, B. B. (1994) 'Hormonal influences on sexuality in the menopause' in: G. Berg and M. Hammar (Eds.). *The Modern Management of the Menopause*, pp. 589–98. Carnforth, Lancashire: Parthenon Publishing

Stanley, E. (1981) Sex problems in practice: vaginismus. *BMJ* **282**, 1435–7

Stoppard, M. (1994) *Menopause*. London: Dorling Kindersley

Tunnadine, P. (1992) *Insight into Troubled Sexuality*. London: Chapman and Hall

Ussher, J. and Baker, E. (1993) *Psychological Perspectives on Sexual Problems*. London: Routledge

Wellings, K. Field, J. Johnson, A. and Wadsworth, J. (1994) *Sexual Behaviour in Britain*. London: Penguin

World Health Organisation (1994) *International Classification of Disorders – 10*. Geneva: World Health Organisation

Yaffe, M. and Fenwick, E. (1992) *Sexual Happiness for Women*. London: Dorling Kindersley

# 24

# Libido

*Alessandra Graziottin*

---

Sexual appetite, desire and drive, sexual impulse and interest: many psychosexual and behavioural terms are used to describe basic human mental states — and their biological counterparts — involved in sexuality (Levin 1994).

'Libido', a more comprehensive term, is a Latin word that means 'desire'. It was first used by Sigmund Freud (1877) to indicate the energy correspondent to the psychic side of the sex drive. In 1938 Carl Jung defined libido in a wider sense, as the psychic energy present in all that is '*appetitus*', a kind of 'desire towards', not necessarily sexual (McGuire and Hull 1977). Since then, the realm of libido has grown to include a deeper understanding of its *biological* roots (Levine 1984; Bloom and Kupfer 1995), both endocrine and neurochemical, of the *motivational* and *relational* components (Kaplan 1979; Talmadge and Talmadge 1986; Beck Gayle, Bozman and Qualtrough 1991; Graziottin and Defilippi 1995; Macphee, Johnson and Van der Veer 1995), and of its vulnerability to personal factors and external agents.

Human beings undertake sexual activity for two primary reasons: to procreate (reproductive sex) and to give themselves pleasure (recreational sex) (Levin 1994). A study in Sweden carried out in the 1970s showed that only about 2% of sexual activity was performed with the conscious purpose of procreation (Linner 1972). A third reason that widely runs through our sexual behaviour and includes a host of motives (Neubeck 1974) is 'instrumental sex'. This is a means to obtain advantages and express motivations different from pleasure and/or procreation. It happens when coitus is used to confirm a person's identity, to achieve sexual competence, to rebel against authority, to control and dominate, to degrade and hurt, to overcome loneliness or boredom, to show that sexual access was possible, to obtain favours such as a better position or role in life, to satisfy masochistic needs or even for livelihood. It is therefore evident that, in our species, libido has several roots, with a complex interplay among biological, motivational and relational factors, all of which have both an inhibiting or enhancing role.

Libido, or sexual desire, is considered different from sexual arousal. Sexual desire is an attitude toward an object, while sexual arousal is a state with specific feelings, usually attached to the genitals. There can be sexual arousal without sexual desire, and sexual desire without arousal. A working definition was produced by Levin (1994). It states that:

> '*Sexual desire is normally an activated, unsatisfied mental state of variable intensity, created by external — via the sensory modalities — or internal stimuli — fantasy, memory, cognition — that induces a feeling of a need or want to partake of sexual activity (usually with the object of desire) to satisfy the need.*'

Human sexual arousal can be characterised by three components: a central arousal, a non-genital peripheral arousal and a genital arousal (Levin 1994). Sexual desire and sexual arousal should, therefore, be kept separate for sake of clarity and practical usefulness.

From the clinical point of view, gynaecologists are more interested in the biological and endocrinological side of libido, while psychologists and sexologists focus on motivational and relational dynamics. This chapter will discuss the first issue, with a few notes for the psychosexual side.

## BIOLOGICAL ROOTS OF LIBIDO

### Hormones

Hormones are the necessary, but not sufficient, factors to maintain a satisfying human libido. In women, oestrogens prime the central nervous system, acting as neurotrophic and psychotrophic factors (Birge 1994; Pfaus and Everitt 1995) during the female life. They also prime the sensory organs, including skin with its sebaceous and sweat glands, that are the key receptors for external sexual stimuli. Sensory organs transmit the basic information that, mixed with emotional and affective messages, contributes to the structuring of core sex identity and self-image, so relevant for the personal perception of being an 'object of desire' and for the direction (homo or heterosexual) of the libido itself (Money and Ehrhardt 1972).

The interplay between oestrogens and the dopaminergic system is the key process in determining the *appetitive* side of sexual behaviour (Bloom and Kupfer 1995), which can be further thrilled by the peak of androgens at ovulation. Oestrogens contribute to neuro- and psychoplasticity that can be considered as the neuroscientific translation of the 'psychic energy' involved in libido.

Prolactin has an inhibiting effect on libido and on the sexual cascade of neurovegetative and vascular responses, via the same dopaminergic system (Pfaus and Everitt 1995). Progestins act as sedatives, through a complex mechanism that is both central and, probably, peripheral. Androgens have a definite thrilling role, in women (Sands and Studd 1995) as well as in men (Bloom and Kupfer 1995). Hypothyroidism may inhibit libido, while hyperthyroidism seems to increase most the biopsychological rhythms, without a specific positive effect on sexual desire.

Hormones, in their complex interplay, seem to control the *intensity* of libido and sexual behaviour, rather than its direction (Levine 1984).

### Sensory organs

Sensory organs are well known windows for the environmental sexual stimuli. Less attention is paid to the effect of hormones on the function and morphology of sensory organs, both as sexual targets and sexual determinants of libido. A growing body of evidence shows that sexual hormones have a specific effect on smell, taste, touch, hearing and vision. These will now be discussed in turn.

### Smell

Chemoreception is the ability to receive chemical messages from the environment. In complex multicellular organisms, specialised structures are devoted to receive chemical stimuli and to transmit them as nervous impulses to the central nervous system. The sense of smell (olfaction) is the most refined sense based on chemoreception. The receptor organ, the olfactory epithelium, is made of specialised neurons localised in an exceptionally peripheral position. The olfactory epithelium is a perfect example of hormone-dependent neuroplasticity. It is made of three cell types:

(1) The olfactory neurones, whose axons form the 'fila olfactoria';

(2) The supporting cells; and

(3) The basal cells (Balboni *et al.* 1991).

Castration elicits detrimental structural alterations of the olfactory epithelium that can improve after administration of sexual hormones (Balboni *et al.* 1991; Arimondi, Vannelli and Balboni 1993). Moreover, in female Rhesus monkeys, the olfactory epithelium presents some changes during the preovulatory phase of the ovarian cycle that could explain the increased olfactory sensitivity occurring at the time of ovulation. In animals, and in humans, the olfactory epithelium shows different appearance and different behaviour of the olfactory, supporting and basal cells in pre- and postpuberty (Balboni *et al.* 1991). A close relationship between olfaction and gonadal activity has been clinically confirmed in Kalman's syndrome (Kalman, Schoenfeld and Barrera 1994), which is characterised by anosmia, eunochoidism and hypogonadotrophic hypogonadism due to a functional deficiency of the gonadotrophic hypothalamic centres. The luteinising hormone releasing hormone (LHRH) cells take rise in the olfactory placode and migrate via the nervus terminalis, preoptic septal area, to the hypothalamus. The hypogonadism in Kalman's syndrome could, therefore, be due to a defective migration of the LHRH cells to the hypothalamus. These data can explain the close relationship between olfaction, the endocrine system and sexual activity.

The involutional morphological changes of the olfactory epithelium in hypo-oestrogenic states (long lasting functional amenorrhoea and menopause) could also contribute to the biologically determined reduction of libido so often reported in these conditions.

These changes could also reduce the responsivity to pheromones, chemical messages emitted by animals, and be able to influence behaviour and physiology of other animals of the same species (Balboni *et al.* 1991; Arimondi, Vannelli and Balboni 1993; Pfaus and Everitt 1995). The invisible cloud of pheromones that envelops humans as a second dress is a potent factor in subliminal attraction that enhances libido and activates sexual arousal. In women, reduction in the production of chemically attractive substances that contribute to the 'scent of woman', typical of the fertile age, could be responsible both for the reduced self-perception as an object of sex desire and for the reduced attractiveness for the partner. Therefore, even in a microsmatic animal, such as a human being, hormone-dependent olfactory modifications may be important biological and functional contributors to the variation of libido in different phases of a woman's life. Moreover, the functional model of cyclical neuroplasticity in the olfactory epithelium may add further information to the role of oestrogens as central neurotrophic factors.

## Taste

Gustative receptors can also perceive pheromones (Balboni *et al.* 1991). Taste is another key biological and emotional factor in the thrill of sex drive, especially in women. Increase of salivary secretion during sexual desire and arousal, and the pleasure in the taste of skin and of kisses, are strong predictive factors for the quality of sex. Functional mouth dryness, more frequent in hypo-oestrogenic states, could be another understudied and underevaluated factor in the biological modulation of libido.

## Touch

A highly sexually communicative skin depends on a happy mixture of good genes, optimal endocrine impregnation, good pheromone production and reception, plus excellent brain activity in the processing of peripheral information from the sensory organ enhanced with internal sexual and emotional stimuli: love, beyond libido, is the strongest attachment factor in the couple bonding through skin touch (Bowlby 1988; Shaver and Hazan 1995). Oxytocin seems to be a key neurochemical factor enhanced in response to a desired skin touch and a potent brain mediator of attachment needs and dynamics (Pfaus and Everitt 1995; Rinaman, Sherman and Stricker 1995). Touch, taste and smell contribute to the 'cenesthetic channel', which is considered the most important sensory contributor of libido in women. The sensory and emotional side of libido is deeply rooted in the quality of cenesthetic and loving bonding between mother and child from early infancy (Bowlby 1988).

## Hearing

This is a variable, usually strong attractive sense for women, mostly for the emotional vibration of the voice (the so called 'feeling tone'), beyond the emotional, loving or sexual content of the message. Hormonal variations of hearing function are far from clear.

## Vision

This is the most potent sexual sense in men, less in women. Oestrogenic responsiveness of ophthalmic structures is now well recognised for the anterior part of the eye (conjunctiva and lacrimal glands). According to Metka *et al.* (1991), 35% of postmenopausal women complain of ophthalmic disturbances secondary to the lack of oestrogens. Most of them improve with hormone replacement therapy. However, whether the variations of eyes' wellbeing contribute to modulation of libido is far from being defined. It is possible that all these subtle changes in sensory organ function and morphology could contribute to the deterioration of libido with age and to the accelerated reduction in many women in early postmenopausal years (Appleby, Montgomery and Studd 1991; Dennerstein *et al.* 1994; Graziottin 1995; Myers 1995; Graziottin 1996).

## Brain

The brain is the very first sex organ, as it is the biological and emotional realm of libido. It is the brain that associates sensory stimuli and emotions (just think how important smell and touch *memories* are for love, affection, emotions and nostalgia). Furthermore, it anticipates the pleasures of love, colours our erotic and emotional life with fantasies, dreams, erotic fantasms and sexual daydreams, and maintains the internal coherence of our Ego, which is the basis of sex identity, self-image and self-esteem (Money and Ehrhadt 1972; Bowlby 1988; Levin 1992; Pfaus and Everitt 1995).

Sex hormones are potent neurotrophic factors (Birge 1994). Gynaecologists should, therefore, pay more attention to the functional (and morphological) modifications of the brain and psychosexual behaviour during long-lasting hypo-oestrogenic states which are seen, for example, in girls with persistent functional amenorrhoea (Schmidt 1995; Treasure 1995)

and in postmenopausal women (Channon and Ballinger 1986; Frock and Money 1992; Busch, Zanderman and Costa 1994; Pearlstein 1995). They should provide optimal hormone replacement therapy (Palinkas and Barrett-Connor 1992; Birge 1994; Sands and Studd 1995) to minimise these subtle damages that may contribute to a deterioration of the libido, the 'vital energy' in the Jungian sense, that is the most exciting fuel for the joy of living and the quality of life (Graziottin 1995; 1996).

## Quality of physical and mental health

Other biological factors which doctors should inquire about when there is a variation in libido are physical diseases and treatment, psychiatric affective disorders, pelvic floor problems, lifestyle and substances taken (or smoked). These will now be discussed in turn (Graziottin and Defilippi 1995).

## Physical diseases and treatment

A detailed clinical history could reveal anaemia, hyperprolactinaemia or hypothyroidism. Moreover, the reactive depression that frequently follows physical diseases may also explain a transitory, parallel fall in libido.

## Psychiatric affective disorders

These may contribute to variations of libido in both directions.

For example, an increase is seen in manic states (leading to promiscuous behaviour), a reduction during depression, and variation in cyclothymic states (Gabbard 1995). *Diagnostic and Statistical Manual of Mental Disorders* (American Psychiatric Association 1995) further differentiates the modifications of libido *per se* from those associated to axis I disorders. Binge-eating disorders (BID) are a peculiar, increasing problem (mostly among adolescents) that deserves the gynaecologist's attention (Treasure 1995). One-third of bulimic patients have an history of sexual harassment (Schmidt 1995); indeed, sometimes they show periods of promiscuous behaviour, a kind of 'sexual bulimia', with low libido. Similarly to the bulimic attack that happens without appetite, sexual bulimia is a compulsive behaviour, more or less consciously devoted to lessen anxiety and anguish (Graziottin and Defilippi 1995). Anorexic women generally have a low libido, with a delay in all the normative events that characterise sexual life.

## Pelvic floor problems

This is, unfortunately, an underdiagnosed as a cause of secondary loss of libido. Hypertonus of the pubococcygeus muscle, from whatever cause, may provoke dyspareunia to the degree of frank vaginism. If intercourse is obtained, a painful postcoital cystitis that appears 24–72 hours after coitus may further complicate the situation (Graziottin 1996). Pain itself can cause a defensive spasm of the muscle that worsens the dyspareunia, reduces libido and vaginal lubrication, and blocks the orgasm, in a vicious circle that often ends in a total avoidance of sexual intimacy. The situation is equally poor with hypotonus which frequently follows delivery of macrosomic newborns or vaginal operative deliveries: vaginal hypaesthesia to the point of coital anorgasmia is a frequent complaint (more usually reported to a gynaecologist with sexological training) that anticipates a later stress incontinence (Graziottin 1996). Appropriate psychiatric rehabilitation of the pelvic floor could be easily taught by the gynaecologist him- or herself, with the aim of modulating an optimal muscular function tone. Recovery of the normal tone will help the woman to rediscover coital pleasure. If pain, or hypaesthesia, is the only cause of reduced libido, normalisation of sex drive will follow without the need for further psychotherapies.

## Lifestyle

Sleep patterns and rhythms are extremely important in recovery from the daily fatigue. Chronic inadequacy of sleep quality may cause tiredness, mood depression, chronic stress and fading of libido. Workaholic, diet-aholic or sport-aholic women and men (Graziottin 1992) may invest all their energy in these activities,

leading to a biological and psychological chronic stress, until they are deprived of any sensual and sexual resource (Graziottin and Defilippi 1995).

### Substance taken

Alcohol, drugs, medicines (Martindale 1993), aphrodisiacs and smoking (Bloom and Kupfer 1995) may further modulate the complex interplay of factors that contribute to human libido.

## MOTIVATIONAL ROOTS OF LIBIDO

Contributing to this aspect of sexual desire are sexual identity (gender and role identity) (Money and Ehrhardt 1972), quality of non-sexual relationships (attachment need and its relation to the ability to trust, to share intimacy, to love) (Bowlby 1988; Shaver and Hazan 1993), non-sexual motivation to sexual behaviour (Neubeck 1974) and the quality and intensity of transfer from past significant relationships (Graziottin and Defilippi 1994). All these aspects contribute to the sexual relationship that is a vital part of the 'personality of marriage' (Talmadge and Talmadge 1986).

## RELATIONAL ROOTS OF LIBIDO

Fears, vulnerability, passive–aggressive styles, commitment dynamics, intimacy problems, love sickness are major issues in emotional involvement and trust for good sexual adjustment (Kaplan 1979; Talmadge and Talmadge 1986; Graziottin and Defilippi 1995; MacPhee, Johnson and Van der Veer 1995).

An apparently banal, often underevaluated relational factor is the *real* desirability of the partner: lack of attention to good hygiene, to self-care and cure, to the subtle courting atmosphere that should be cultivated even in a long-lasting relationship, may precipitate the rapid 'perceptive wear and tear' of the partner as an object of sex desire, leading to indifference or frank aversion.

The partner's sexual problems (e.g. low libido, premature ejaculation or erectile deficits) may also contribute to the deterioration of female libido: in these cases it is appropriate to talk about the 'sexual dyad', with the more or less unconscious interplay between the 'symptom inducer' and the 'symptom carrier' (Kaplan 1979). In cases of inhibited sexual desire, the practical advice is to ask if the partner has a sexual symptom, if he/she sabotages the sexual atmosphere, if the intensity of quarrelling or frank conflicts are so strong that they paralyse the libido (Kaplan 1979; Graziottin and Defilippi 1995).

## COGNITIVE ROOTS OF LIBIDO

They are mostly involved in the cognitive evaluation of the wish and risk to behave sexually. It can have a paralysing effect when the perception of risks is exaggerated because of irrational fears, anxiety, anguish and/or inhibitions, or an enhancing effect when the risk is perceived as an aphrodisiac leading to 'acting out' (Levin 1994; Beck Gayle, Bozman and Qualtrough 1991; Graziottin and Defilippi 1995).

## MENOPAUSAL CHANGES IN LIBIDO

Lack of oestrogen deprives the brain and all the female body of the natural lymph that contributes to the perception of the *female sex identity*, of a satisfying *sexual function* and to the sensuality and seductivity that improve the quality of *sexual relationships*, causing a progressive loss of libido and a crisis of the self-perception as an object of desire (Birge 1994; Sands and Studd 1995; Graziottin 1996).

Moreover, as previously mentioned, the lack of oestrogens deprives sweat and sebaceous glands of the stimulus to produce the peculiar chemical secretion (pheromones) responsible for the 'scent of woman', so critical in sexual attraction (Balboni *et al.* 1991; Arimondi, Vannelli and Balboni 1993). Oestrogens are the permitting factors for the action of the vasointestinal peptide (VIP), the key neurotransmitter for the endothelial and vasal changes that lead to vaginal lubrication (Levin 1992). That is why the absence of oestrogens causes vaginal dryness and pain (dyspareunia) that can further inhibit libido through a negative feedback mechanism.

Obviously, enhancing and inhibiting factors (medicines, drugs, alcohol [Bloom and Kupfer 1995], plus other health problems) can modify the biological impact of menopause on libido.

*Motivational–affective* and *relational* factors, implications and quality of *couple relationship*, and the partner's attitude and problems, may further modulate the intensity and *direction* of libido (Levine 1984).

The doctor's increasing attention to sexual problems of perimenopausal women will dramatically improve female quality of life during this delicate transition (Myers 1995).

## CLINICAL INTERVIEW

The clinician interested in a proper evaluation of libido should, therefore, look for potential biological factors responsible for the motivational and affective dynamics and for a cognitive evaluation. A simple diagnostic set of questions to differentiate at least the most important problems is as follows (Beck Gayle, Bozman and Qualtrough 1991; Graziottin and Defilippi 1995):

(1) What is the frequency of erotic dreams, sexual day dreams and voluntary sex fantasies? If they are present and satisfying, the biological and emotional central side of libido can be considered good.

(2) How is sexual arousal? If it is easy, with a normal lubrication and orgasm, it excludes central and peripheral endocrine problems, as well as neurological and vascular ones.

(3) Is there any autoerotic activity? Satisfying masturbation usually indicates good libido, good relationship with one's body and lack of inhibition. Only when compulsive and/or too frequent may it suggest a narcissistic disorder, difficulty in establishing relationships, difficulty in intimacy;

(4) Does the patient prefer sexual contacts to be non-coitus-orientated? This may suggest the presence of a phobia towards coitus, dyspareunia or vaginism (when the phobia is combined with a marked

hypertonus of the pubococcygeus), post-coital cystitis, vestibolitis and vulvodynia, other painful vulvar conditions and muscular problems (myofascial trigger points) that all could cause a secondary fall of libido. Vaginal hypoaesthesia should also be considered.

(5) What is the frequency of intercourse? This rough indicator should be analysed using a further set of questions. Who begins the intercourse? How do you perceive your partner? What is your prevalent role in the intercourse? Which are your motivations to the intercourse? Do you have sex fantasies during coitus? How is the quality of your arousal? How is your orgasm? How do you feel after intercourse? Obviously with this intimate clinical dialogue it is better if the gynaecologist has personal sexological

training to analyse and treat sexual disorders. Such a role is frequently performed better by a woman.

## CONCLUSION

Problems in libido are increasingly reported during the gynaecological consultation, especially if the clinician is willing to listen and to look at the patient as a person who is suffering emotionally. A basic sexological training should become part of routine gynaecological training, to enable physicians to diagnose properly the biological conditions they could adequately treat and to encourage the patient to consult a psychosexologist if the problem reported during the consultation seems to be more rooted in intrapsychic, motivational or relationship bases.

# References

American Psychiatric Association (1995) *Diagnostic and Statistic Manual of Mental Disorders.* Washington, DC: American Psychiatric Association

Appleby, L., Montgomery, J. and Studd, J. (1991) 'Oestrogens and affective disorders' in: J. Studd (Ed.). *Progresses in Obstetrics and Gynaecology*, Vol.9, pp. 289–302. Edinburgh: Churchill Livingstone

Arimondi, C., Vannelli, G. B. and Balboni, G. C. (1993) Importance of olfaction in sexual life: morpho-functional and psychological studies in man. *Biomed Res (India)* **4**, 43–52

Balboni, G. C., Gheri, G., Ghery Bryk, S., Barni, T., Arimondi, C. and Vannelli, G. B. (1991) 'New trends in olfaction' in: Firenze (Ed.). *Proceedings of the 45th Congress of the Italian Society of Anatomy*, pp. 14–16. Firence: Mozzon

Beck Gayle, J., Bozman, A. W. and Qualtrough, T. (1991) The experience of sexual desire: psychological correlates in a college sample. *J Sex Res* **28**(3), 443–56

Birge, S. J. (1994) 'The role of estrogen deficiency in the aging of the central nervous system' in: R. A. Lobo (Ed.). *Treatment of Postmenopausal Women: Basic and Clinical Aspects*, pp. 153–77. New York: Raven Press

Bloom, F. E. and Kupfer, D. (1995) *Psychopharmacology*. New York: Raven Press

Bowlby, J. (1988) *A Secure Base*. London: Routledge

Busch, C. M., Zonderman, A. B. and Costa, P. T. Jr (1994) Menopausal transition and psychological distress in a nationally representative sample: is menopause associated with psychological distress? *J Aging Health* **6**(2), 209–28

Channon, L. D. and Ballinger, S. E. (1986) Some aspects of sexuality and vaginal symptoms during menopause and their relation to anxiety and depression. *Br J Med Psychol* **59**(2), 173–80

Dennerstein, L., Smith, A. M., Morse, C. A. and Burger, H. G. (1994) Sexuality and the menopause. *J. Psychol Obstet Gynecol* **15**(1), 59–66

Freud, S. (1877) 'On sexuality' in: A. Richards (Ed.). *Three Essays on the Theory of Sexuality and Other Works*, The Pelican Freud Library, Vol. 7. London: Penguin Books

Frock, J. and Money, J. (1992) Sexuality and menopause. *Psychother Psychosom* **57**, 29–33

Gabbard, G. O. (1995) *Psychodynamic Psychiatry in Clinical Practice*. Washington, DC: American Psychiatric Association

Graziottin, A. (1992) Life span perspective in psychogenic impotence. *Int J Impot Res* **4**, 165–73

Graziottin, A. and Defilippi, A. (1995) 'Disfunzioni del desiderio sessuale' in: P. Marandola (Ed.). *Andrologia e Sessuologia Clinica*, pp. 229–37. Pavia: La Goliardica

Graziottin, A. (1995) 'Menopausa e sessualità' in: P. Marandola (Ed.). *Andrologia e Sessuologia Clinica*, pp. 255–60. Pavia: La Goliardica

Graziottin, A. (1996) 'Terapie ormonali sostitutive e terapie sessuologiche in post menopausa' in: A. R. Genazzani and L. Zichella (Eds.). *Atti del Primo Convegno Nazionale di Consenso e Formazione in Scienze Ginecologiche e Ostetriche*, Madonna di Campiglio, 18–24 Marzo, 1996

Kalman, F., Schoenfeld, W. A. and Barrera, S. E. (1994) The genetic aspects of primary eunuchoidism. *Am J Ment Defic* **48**, 203–36

Kaplan, H. S. (1979) *Disorders of Sexual Desire*. New York: Simon and Schuster

Levin, R. J. (1992) The mechanisms of human female sexual arousal. *Ann Rev Sex Res* **3**, 1–48

Levin, R. J. (1994) 'Human male sexuality: appetite and arousal, desire and drive' in: C. Legg and D. Boott (Eds.). *Human Appetite: Neural and Behavioural Bases*, pp. 127–64. Oxford: Oxford University Press

Levine, S. B. (1984) An essay on the nature of sexual desire. *J Sex Marital Ther* **10**(2), 83–96

Linner, B. (1972) *Sex and Society in Sweden*. New York: Harper and Row

Macphee, D. C., Johnson, S. M. and Van der

Veer, M. M. (1995) Low sexual desire in women: the effect of marital therapy. *J Sex Marital Ther* **21**(3), 159–82

Martindale, W. (1993) *The Extra Pharmacopeia*. London: The Pharmaceutical Press

McGuire, W. and Hull, R. F. C. (Eds.) (1977). *C. G. Jung Speaking*. Princeton University Press

Metka, M., Enzelsberger, H., Knogler, W., Schurz, B. and Aichmair, H. (1991) Opthalmic complaint as a climacteric symptom. *Maturitas* **14**(1), 3–8

Money, J. and Ehrhardt, A. (1972) *Man and Woman, Boy and Girl*. Baltimore: The John Hopkins University Press

Myers, L. S. (1995) Methodological review and meta-analysis of sexuality and menopause research. *Neurosci Biobehav Rev* **19**(2), 331–41

Neubeck, G. (1974) 'The myriad of motives for sex' in: L. Gross (Ed.). *Sexual Behaviour — Current Issues*, pp. 89–97. Flushing: Spectrum

Palinkas, L. A. and Barrett-Connor, E. (1992) Estrogen use and depressive symptoms in postmenopausal women. *Obstet Gynecol* **80**(1), 30–6

Pearlstein, T. B. (1995) Hormones and depression: what are the facts about premenstrual syndrome, menopause and hormone replacement therapy? *Am J Obstet Gynecol* **173**(2), 646–53

Pfaus, J. G. and Everitt, B. J. (1995) 'The psychopharmacology of sexual behaviour' in: F. E. Bloom and D. Kupfer (Eds.). *Psychopharmacology*, Chapter 65, pp. 743–58. New York: Raven Press

Rinaman, L., Sherman, T. G. and Stricker, E. M. (1995) 'Vasopressin and oxytocin in the central nervous system' in: F. E. Bloom and D. Kupfer (Eds.). *Psychopharmacology*, Chapter 47, pp. 531–42. New York: Raven Press

Sands, R. and Studd, J. (1995) Exogenous androgens in postmenopausal women. *Am J Med* **98**(1A), 76–9

Schmidt, H. (1995) Anorexia nervosa and psychosexual development. *Psychol Med* **25**, 112–24

Shaver, P. R. and Hazan, C. (1995) 'Adult romantic attachment process: theory and evidence' in: D. Perlman and W. Jones (Eds.). *Advances in Personal Relationship Outcomes*, Vol. IV, pp. 29–70. London: J. Kingsey

Talmadge, L. D. and Talmadge, W. C. (1986) Relational sexuality: an understanding of low sexual desire. *J Sex Marital Ther* **12**, 1–8

Treasure, J. L. (1995) 'Eating disorders' in: J. Studd (Ed.). *Yearbook of the Royal College of Obstetricians and Gynaecologists.* London: RCOG Press

# 25

# Premenstrual syndrome

*Abha Govind, Changulanda M. Joshi and P. M. Shaughn O'Brien*

Premenstrual syndrome (PMS) is the cyclical recurrence, in the luteal phase of the menstrual cycle, of any combination of distressing physical, psychological and/or behavioural change of sufficient severity to result in deterioration of interpersonal relationships and/or interference with normal activities (Reid and Yen 1981). It is a complex psychoneuroendocrine disorder of unknown aetiology. Recent understanding of its pathophysiology has increased and it is now possible to offer some treatment options that have been scientifically assessed.

It is only in 2–10% of women in their reproductive years that PMS poses a significant health problem (Logue and Moos 1986; Woods, Most and Dery 1982), although almost 90% of women experience some mild physical and psychological alteration in the premenstrual phase some time during their lives. Consequently, it becomes essential to discern true PMS from milder and more common *physiological symptoms*. Women with PMS must also be distinguished from those with psychiatric disorders whose symptoms are non-cyclical and unrelated to ovarian endocrine cycle. Failing to do this may lead to unsuitable and ineffectual treatment.

## CLASSIFICATION

Women may fall into the following possible groups (O'Brien 1987), with just 5% being entirely free from symptoms (see also Figure 1):

(1) Asymptomatic;

(2) Physiological premenstrual changes;

(3) Primary premenstrual syndrome;

(4) Secondary premenstrual syndrome; and

(5) Non-menstrually related disorders.

'Asymptomatic' patients are self-explanatory, but the remainder of the terms are now described in turn.

## Physiological premenstrual changes

They are of the same timing and character as PMS, but they are of insufficient severity to disrupt the patient's normal functioning and do not require specific treatment.

## Primary PMS

The cyclical recurrence of severe symptoms in the luteal phase which resolve completely by the end of menstruation. There should be a symptom-free week between the menstruation and the time of ovulation. Symptoms must have occurred in at least four of the six previous cycles.

## Secondary PMS

These women have underlying psychological problems as well as a cyclical disorder. They are differentiated by a partial rather than a complete resolution of symptoms following menstruation. Although symptoms remain they should significantly improve by the end of menstruation and this improvement should be sustained for at least one week.

## Psychiatric disorder wrongly attributed to PMS

The similarity between the symptoms of depression and those of PMS may cause

245

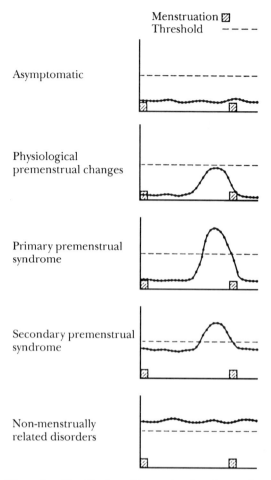

Menstruation ▨
Threshold ― ― ― ―

Asymptomatic

Physiological
premenstrual changes

Primary premenstrual
syndrome

Secondary premenstrual
syndrome

Non-menstrually
related disorders

**Figure 1**   *Classification of premenstrual symptomatology*

confusion between the two. The failure of symptoms to disappear or improve following menstruation identifies this group. They should undergo psychiatric assessment and relevant treatment.

## AETIOLOGY

Theories abound as to factors that operate in PMS, but none has been scientifically substantiated. It appears unlikely that a simple biochemical or neuroendocrine factor will be found responsible and it is expected that the cause of PMS will finally be explained by the interaction of gonadal steroids with the neurotransmitter, neuroendocrine and circadian systems that control mood behaviour

and cognition. Natural ovarian activity, however, appears to be essential as it is evident that PMS closely relates to the changes of the menstrual cycle.

The present consensus points to the *normal* ovarian cycle being the trigger for events in the central nervous system and other target tissues. The symptoms are thought to be caused by increased responsiveness of the tissues to the hormonal changes of the normal cycle, particularly to the high concentrations of progesterone that occur during the luteal phase. This may be mediated by a deficiency of neurotransmitters such as serotonin or endorphins.

### Ovarian hormones

Abnormal ovarian hormone production is an attractive theory, as PMS symptoms by definition occur in the luteal phase of the menstrual cycle and abate when cyclical ovarian activity is absent. The syndrome does not occur preceding puberty, during pregnancy and following menopause. A putative role for ovarian steroids in the aetiology of PMS is also suggested by analogous mood changes associated with oral contraceptive use (Kane 1976) and post-menopausal hormone replacement therapy (Hammarback *et al.* 1985). There is also a paucity of symptoms in spontaneous anovular cycles (Hammarback, Ekholm and Backstrom 1991). Further support for this hypothesis is derived from studies demonstrating the elimination of premenstrual symptoms during gonadotrophin releasing hormone (GnRH)-agonist treatment, which dramatically reduces circulating ovarian steroid levels (Muse *et al.* 1984; Hammarback and Backstrom 1988). There is currently no consensus of opinion based on studies that attempt to correlate PMS symptoms with specific changes in oestrogen or progesterone levels (Backstrom and Mattsson 1975; O'Brien 1987; Rubinow *et al.* 1988; Hammarback, Damber and Backstrom 1989).

### Oestrogens

Oestrogens have a positive effect on the biosynthesis, uptake and turnover of monoamines and opioids (Shoupe and Lobo 1985) in the central nervous system, which is consistent with an antidepressant effect. Some women taking the oestrogen receptor blocker clomiphene citrate report lability of mood or depression (Reid 1988). These findings suggest that oestrogen withdrawal or deficiency may be involved in this syndrome. This is supported by the fact that women only rarely experience PMS symptoms midcycle, when oestrogen levels peak.

## Progesterone deficiency

This has been a popular theory as a cause for PMS. The symptoms appear to depend on ovulation and follow the pattern of progesterone produced by the corpus luteum. However, there are no consistent findings in luteal-phase progesterone in women with PMS, with some investigators reporting decreased levels (Backstrom and Cartensen 1974; Smith 1976; Munday, Brush and Taylor 1977), others increased levels (Hammarback, Damber and Backstrom 1989) and a majority finding no difference (Backstrom and Mattsson 1975; Rubinow *et al.* 1988). The finest argument against the belief that low progesterone levels cause PMS symptoms is the fact that progesterone levels are lowest in the first half of the cycle, when symptoms are absent (Shoupe 1991).

There are no studies which validate the benefits of progesterone therapy. Moreover, luteal-phase administration of low-dose mifepristone (RU 486), the progesterone antagonist, which provides effective progesterone receptor blockade, does not significantly reduce the physical or behavioural manifestations of PMS (Chan *et al.* 1994).

Experimental research shows that women who complained of PMS prior to hysterectomy and bilateral salpingo-oophorectomy do not re-develop symptoms when they receive continuous oestrogen therapy. They do, however, acquire well-defined symptoms when given progesterone or progestogens (Henshaw *et al.* 1993) (Figure 2). The finding of this study suggests that progesterone is the key component in the genesis of PMS.

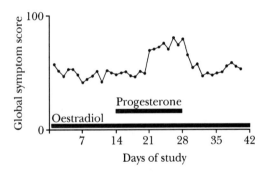

**Figure 2** *Symptom scores for premenstrual syndrome in women who have had hysterectomy and bilateral oophorectomy and require hormone replacement therapy. During oestrogen-only therapy they have no symptoms. When progesterone is added experimentally symptoms recur. (Adapted from Henshaw, C., O'Brien, P. M. S., Foreman, D. et al. (1993) An experimental model for PMS. Neurophsychopharmacology 9(25), 713, with permission of Elsevier Science Ltd)*

## Neuroendocrine response

Ovarian steroid hormones act within the central nervous system at various levels, although the details of this interaction are not fully understood at the present time. They can influence neurotransmitter synthesis, release, re-uptake enzymatic inactivation and also the sensitivity of presynaptic and postsynaptic receptors. They can act directly on nerve membranes, affecting excitability, couple to second messenger systems within the cell and exert influence through genomic action (Pearlstein 1995). The most convincing neuroendocrine hypothesis relates to serotonergic and opioid mechanisms, but catecholamines, encephalins, monoamines, γ-amino-butyric acid and prostaglandins could presumably be involved (Backstrom 1992).

Abnormally low levels of β-endorphin have been shown in luteal phase of women with PMS, but not in asymptomatic controls (Chuong *et al.* 1985) (Figure 3). Modulation of β-endorphin concentration by the endorphin inhibitor naltrexone reduces PMS-like symptoms (Chuong 1988).

Deficiency of vitamin $B_6$ (pyridoxine) may be important as it is a cofactor in the final step in the synthesis of serotonin and dopamine from tryptophan. However, no convincing data have yet demonstrated abnormalities either of brain amine synthesis or deficiency of cofactors like vitamin $B_6$.

Reduced serotonergic activity seems to be important in affective disorders, and abnormalities in whole blood serotonin, and serotonin platelet uptake have been demonstrated throughout the cycle in women with PMS (Ashby *et al.* 1988; Rapkin 1992; Steege *et al.* 1992).

Several controlled clinical trials have demonstrated that the serotonin-enhancing drugs fluoxetine (Stone, Pearlstein and Brown 1991; Menkes *et al.* 1992; 1993; Figure 4) and clomipramine (Sundblad *et al.* 1992) are effective in relieving premenstrual symptoms in severely affected women.

It the explanation for PMS is neuroendocrine, it becomes much easier to explain why exogenous factors such as environment, dietary intake and underlying psychological status can also influence the manifestation of PMS.

## Prolactin

The role of prolactin in PMS has been investigated by many research groups, perhaps because it is a so-called stress hormone which also stimulates the breast and promotes sodium, potassium and water retention. However, it has *not* been clearly demonstrated to undergo cyclical change in the normal menstrual cycle, *nor* do women with PMS demonstrate elevated blood levels. Moreover, women with hyperprolactinaemia do *not* report PMS-like symptoms. Therapeutic studies of bromocriptine have failed to demonstrate any significant effect on symptoms, with the notable exception of cyclical mastalgia. Hence, the general role of prolactin in the aetiology of PMS now seems doubtful (O'Brien and Symonds 1982).

## Prostaglandins and essential fatty acids

The widespread nature of prostaglandins throughout the body makes them principal candidates to play an aetiological role in PMS. No precise explanation associating fatty acid synthesis have been demonstrated in a study by Brush and colleagues (1984), but these findings

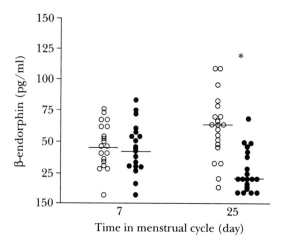

**Figure 3** β-endorphin levels in premenstrual syndrome (PMS) (●) compared to controls (○). The PMS group is significantly different from controls on day 25 (P < 0.0001). Bars indicate the median. (Reproduced with permission of Chuong, C. J., Coulam, C. B., Kao, P. C. et al. (1985) Neuropeptide levels in premenstrual syndrome. Fertil Steril 44(6), 760–5, with permission of the American Society of Human Reproduction [formerly the American Fertility Society])

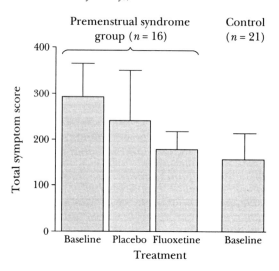

**Figure 4** Premenstrual syndrome (PMS) symptom assessment score (mean and standard deviation) after three months each of baseline (pretreatment), placebo and serotonin re-uptake inhibitor (fluoxetine, 20 mg daily) treatment. Patients whose PMS symptoms are predominantly psychological experience significant relief following treatment with fluoxetine. *P < 0.05 compared with baseline. **P < 0.01 compared with placebo. (Reproduced from Menkes, D. B., Taghavi, E., Mason, P. A. et al. (1992) Fluoxetine's spectrum of action in premenstrual syndrome. BMJ 305, 346–7, with permission of the BMJ Publishing Group)

have not been replicated by others (O'Brien and Massil 1990).

Both prostaglandin inhibitors and precursors have been alleged to relieve PMS. *In vitro* studies have demonstrated interactions at a cellular level between polyunsaturated essential fatty acids and the receptor activity of oestrogen, progesterone, angiotensin II and β-endorphins. Interaction with angiotensin II, essential fatty acids and different prostaglandins has also been shown *in vivo*. Faulty prostaglandin metabolism may give rise to a breakdown in this equilibrium, allowing exaggerated response to normal circulating levels of these different hormone systems.

### Endocrine effects on fluid and electrolytes

Many studies have been taken to address the role of sodium and water retention in PMS, but recent research has discounted a causative link. Although many women develop abdominal distension and premenstrual bloatedness as a symptom, it frequently occurs without increasing body weight, total exchangeable body sodium, total body water, extracellular fluid volume or plasma volume (Hussain 1993). This finding also brings into question the use of diuretics in PMS. It seems more likely that the symptoms of bloatedness may have a large perceived component or, alternatively, it is possible that these symptoms are associated with gaseous gut distension and gut hypotonia due to progesterone-induced relaxation of the smooth muscle in either the small or large intestine, or both.

### Summary

Factors other than the differences in the levels of specific hormones must be important in the aetiology of PMS. The return of symptoms in some women who take progestogen as part of hormone replacement therapy may be further evidence of a differential response to cyclical progesterone. Despite receiving identical dosage of sex steroid only certain women show recurrence of PMS, suggesting that symptoms depend on a differential response to a similar level of ovarian steroids. Ablation of ovarian cycle by bilateral oophorectomy (Casson *et al.*

1990) and suppression of ovaries with danazol and GnRH analogues (Muse 1992) reliably cure PMS by eliminating the ovarian trigger, while serotonergic drugs probably treat premenstrual syndrome by modulating the neuroendocrine response to the ovary (Rapkin 1992).

## SYMPTOMS

Symptoms of PMS are similar to, but more severe than, the normal premenstrual symptoms and they are of sufficient severity to disrupt work and family relations. Broad categories include affective alterations, somatic and behavioural changes and food cravings. Over a hundred different symptoms have been recorded in the literature, but none are specific to this syndrome. The American Psychiatric Association's *Diagnostic and Statistical Manual of Mental Disorders* (DSM-IV) defines diagnostic criteria for the severe form of PMS, or premenstrual dysphoric disorder (PDD). The emphasis of this definition is on dysphoric mood as the core symptom, hence the terminology is restricted.

Loss of control of emotions and behaviour are probably the most distressing features of PMS. The list of psychological symptoms is long and includes aggression, irritability, anxiety, tension, depression, anger and mood swings. Extreme clumsiness, inability to perform normal tasks, unexplained crying and poor concentration may also be distressing. Some women feel that during the premenstrual phase of the cycle they totally lose control, which may lead to criminal acts including arson, baby battering, suicide and murder.

The key physical symptoms are abdominal bloating, a feeling of weight increase, swelling of the breasts and premenstrual mastalgia. Acne, headache and migraine are also common. Premenstrual pelvic pain is common and must be distinguished from premenstrual pain of endometriosis.

It is the timing, not the specific character of symptoms which is critical to the diagnosis of PMS. When assessing a patient it is important to ascertain the relationship of menstruation on the symptoms and the consequences of the symptoms to the patient's life.

## DIAGNOSIS

There are no biochemical markers that identify the syndrome. The diagnosis is based on history and self-assessment questionnaires. Prospective daily ratings of symptoms are required to substantiate a patient's history using a PMS calendar. This should be kept for a minimum of two, but ideally for three cycles (Johnson 1992). However, the information provided is limited. In the near future computerised recording of symptoms (on a linear visual analogue scale) and data storage and analysis will be possible using a simple patient-operated hand held computer device (PMS Symptometrics).

A wide variety of tools has been devised to measure the cyclical component of PMS symptoms. The Moos' menstrual distress questionnaire (1985), specific linear visual analogue scales (Faratian *et al.* 1984), the Calendar of Premenstrual Experience (COPE), developed at the University of San Diego, the Prospective Record of the Impact and Severity of Menstrual (PRISM) Symptoms (Reid 1988) and the Premenstrual Assessment Form (PAF) (Halbreich *et al.* 1982).

It is possible to quantify the contribution of underlying psychopathology using established psychiatric questionnaires. The simplest of these is the General Health Questionnaire (Goldberg and Hillier 1979), completed in the *follicular* phase of the menstrual cycle. What should be obtained by the second clinic visit is information regarding the timing and character of the symptoms, the degree of underlying psychopathology and the extent to which the problem disrupts the patient's normal functioning. In difficult cases the patient may either require psychiatric assessment or a *goserelin test*.

Goserelin, a GnRH agonist analogue, is given as a depot at exactly 28-day intervals to eliminate cyclical ovarian activity for three months. Symptoms are rated during goserelin therapy and by the third month the response can be assessed. Complete elimination of symptoms suggests that they are entirely dependent on ovarian activity, and the diagnosis is one of primary PMS. If the symptoms continue into the third month then an underlying psychiatric disorder should

be suspected. The goserelin test is also valuable if a hysterectomy is to be performed and the patient is also being considered for bilateral oophorectomy for her PMS.

## MANAGEMENT

No single approach to treat PMS has consistently been successful. As women present with heterogeneous symptoms, management approaches must be designed on an individual basis. Only a small percentage of women with premenstrual syndrome seek medical help. Hallman (1986) estimates that only 7.5% of women with PMS feel they need to see a physician. Alleviating anxiety and rationalising symptoms are important aspects of treatment.

The reason for the apparent efficacy of so many methods is the high placebo effect, up to 89% in double-blind studies (Mattsson and von Schoultz 1974), although the generally agreed figure is nearer 50%. Any therapeutic study where placebo is omitted must be interpreted with caution.

Drug therapy or surgical treatment is unnecessary for most patients. Patients with physiological symptoms may need no more than reassurance and counselling.

Endocrine manipulation or surgical techniques can be justified when a patient is grossly incapacitated by PMS. However, treatment methods considered appropriate for women with moderate symptoms have been evaluated less precisely in clinical trials and these patients appear the most difficult to manage.

### Non-pharmacological treatment

A large number of non-medical interventions has been suggested and may be all that is required in mild cases. As general health and prevailing levels of stress may contribute to a patient's symptoms, it is possible that measures to improve these are of value. These cover dietary adaptations, exercise, hypnosis, yoga, acupuncture and meditation. Although anecdotal success is reported with lifestyle modifications, few controlled studies have been undertaken to evaluate these techniques. Two placebo-controlled studies suggest that relaxation techniques are helpful (Goodale, Domar and Benson 1990; Morse *et al.* 1991). A controlled study of ear, hand and foot reflexology suggested a positive benefit (Oleson and Flocco 1993). Regular carbohydrate meals have been advocated enthusiastically, aiming to combat hypoglycaemia, although hypoglycaemia has never been demonstrated in PMS (Kleijnen, Ter Reit and Knipschild 1990).

Two of the most popular treatment options involve taking vitamin B6 or evening primrose oil.

## Vitamin B6 (pyridoxine)

Dietary interventions such as vitamin B6, calcium and magnesium may be based on logical hypotheses since some are cofactors in the synthesis of neurotransmitters such as serotonin and dopamine (Rapkin 1992). There have now been several studies, some of which have demonstrated superiority over placebo, while others have refuted this (Kleijnen, Ter Reit and Knipschild 1990; Johnson 1992). Vitamin B6 is usually given cyclically in a dosage of 60–100 mg per day. Higher dosages have been reported to have significant neurological adverse effects.

## Evening primrose oil

Evening primrose oil has been shown in several studies to be effective in premenstrual mastalgia (Pye *et al.* 1985). However, studies on general premenstrual syndrome show non-significant trends in favour of its use compared to placebo (Khoo, Munro and Battistutta 1990; O'Brien and Massil 1990).

Gamolenic acid (GLA, tradename Efamast) is the essential fatty acid in evening primrose oil. Women with severe cyclical mastalgia appear to have low levels of immediate metabolites of GLA (Horrobin 1990). It is not clear whether this is due to an inadequate intake or abnormal metabolism. Efamast produces a progressive improvement in breast pain with maximum benefit after four months therapy. However, up to six to eight capsules (500 mg/day) may have to be used for a good response.

## Drug therapy

Claims have been made for a wide variety of treatments, but drugs should only be resorted to when non-pharmacological methods fail.

### Non-hormonal drugs

*Psychotropic drugs.* In theory, these drugs are most useful in secondary PMS, where PMS coexists with underlying depression. Selective serotonin re-uptake inhibitors (SSRI), such as fluoxetine and paroxetine, are currently being assessed and used. Four double-blind studies with fluoxetine (20 mg/day) demonstrated impressive efficacy and a relative lack of side effects (Stone, Pearlstein and Brown 1991; Menkes *et al.* 1992; Wood *et al.* 1992; Steiner *et al.* 1995). They can be recommended in the early management of appropriate patients. Two open, long-term studies have indicated beneficial effects of fluoxetine over an extended period of time (Elks 1993; Pearlstein and Stone 1994). Clomipramine has also been found to be effective in double-blind trials in doses of 25–75 mg/day (Goodale, Domar and Benson 1990; Rapkin 1992; Sundblad *et al.* 1992; Wood *et al.* 1992). Sertraline has been evaluated in 184 women in a multicentre comparison with placebo and preliminary results confirm that it is superior (Yonkers *et al.* 1995). Double-blind studies suggest that alprazolam (Smith *et al.* 1987; Harrison, Endicott and Nee 1990; Freeman *et al.* 1995) and buspirone (Rickels, Freeman and Sondheimer 1989) taken only in the luteal phase may be helpful. Patients may experience sedation and reduced libido.

*Diuretics.* Extensive claims have been made for the efficacy of diuretics for both physical and psychological symptoms of PMS, but this enthusiasm has been based on uncontrolled observations. They are useful only in the group of women who have appreciable weight gain in the luteal phase of the cycle. Women with bloatedness and even severe abdominal distension without weight gain cannot be retaining fluid and cannot be helped with diuretics. Hence, there is significant risk to diuretic therapy and no rational basis for their use. There is a small group of women who experience true water retention as one of their symptoms and diuretics should be reserved for them. When diuretics are necessary (symptoms associated with measured weight gain), the use of aldosterone antagonist (e.g. spironolactone) should reduce the risk of idiopathic oedema (Hellberg, Claesson and Nilsson 1991).

### Hormonal treatment

In the absence of a proven endocrine imbalance, or deficiency, the use of hormones for replacement has little logic. However, the rationale for the use of hormones is either to disrupt the patient's endogenous cycle or to completely suppress it. Progesterone, progestogens, oral contraceptive pill, danazol, oestrogens (as implants or patches) and GnRH agonist analogues have now been used extensively.

The latter four are used when normal ovarian function, rather than a hormonal imbalance, is the cyclical trigger for the neuroendocrine events within the CNS.

*Progesterone and progestogens.* The use of such agents is the best known and most controversial form of therapy and, despite the lack of scientific support, progesterone therapy continues to have many advocates. Its use to treat PMS has been on the basis of progesterone deficiency (Dalton 1984). This premise appears paradoxical given the putative mechanisms of PMS. Several randomised, double-blind, placebo-controlled trials have now been conducted and reviewed and they indicate an overall lack of efficacy (Freeman *et al.* 1990). Cyclical and depot medroxyprogesterone acetate have been used clinically, but there are no adequate efficacy studies (Hellberg, Claesson and Nilsson 1991). A large, randomised, double-blind, placebo-controlled study has definitively confirmed the

increasing evidence that progesterone vaginal suppository therapy has no therapeutic effect over placebo treatment for PMS (Freeman *et al.* 1990).

*Oral contraceptive pill.* The pill, by suppressing ovulation, should reduce symptoms, but a new endocrine cyclicity appears during the pill-free interval (Walker and Bancroft 1990) and when the combined oral contraceptive is given the response is unpredictable. Both the monophasic and triphasic pill have been found to be equally ineffective (Backstrom 1992).

A logical approach would be to give continuous combined oral contraceptive treatment which would abolish the ovarian cycle. There are no published studies using this approach and in practice it appears unsuccessful. Some of the side effects of the pill are similar to premenstrual symptoms and these may develop for the first time on oral contraception.

*Danazol.* Well conducted trials have shown that danazol is effective in dosages of 100–400 mg/day in divided doses (Derzko 1990; Halbreich, Rojansky and Palter 1991). Suppression of ovulation and menstruation (achieved by 400 mg in 90% of patients) abolish the symptoms (Deeny, Hawthorn and McKay Hart 1991), but masculinising side effects are more common with higher doses and long-term use. Monitoring of lipid levels will be required if long-term use is considered.

Recent assessment of danazol when given during the luteal phase shows that, while it relieves cyclical mastalgia, no beneficial effects are seen for any other PMS symptoms (Abukhalil and O'Brien, unpublished data).

*Oestrogen implants.* Oestrogen implants (50–100 mg) show sustained improvement when compared to placebo. In a study of 50 patients who received implants and cyclical progestogens (Watson *et al.* 1990), new premenstrual symptoms developed in 58%. Sixteen per cent had a hysterectomy mainly because of progestogenic side effects and bleeding.

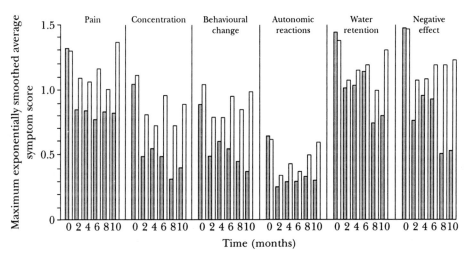

**Figure 5** *Effect of oestradiol implant and norethisterone (empty bars) on premenstrual syndrome (PMS) symptoms compared to placebo (dark bars). The placebo effect is seen initially but the continued response is only seen during active therapy (Reproduced from Magos, A. L., Brincat, M. and Studd, J. W. W. (1986) Treatment of premenstrual syndrome by subcutaneous oestradiol implants and cyclical oral norethisterone: placebo-controlled study. BMJ 292, 1629–33, with permission of the BMJ Publishing Group)*

Changing the type of progesterone to suit individual patients or reducing the dose may minimise these symptoms.

In an earlier study, 68 women with clear-cut premenstrual symptoms (Magos, Brincat and Studd 1986; Figure 5) were included in a well conducted, placebo-controlled trial. Thirty-three of these received an implant of 100 mg oestradiol plus 5 mg of norethisterone for seven days of the cycle. Another 35 received a placebo for both implant and norethisterone. Treatment showed high response rates in both groups. However, the effects of placebo treatment decreased after a short interval, while that of active implant and norethisterone was maintained throughout the study. Tachyphylaxis may be a problem with long-term implant use, especially if the 100 mg dose is used.

*Oestrogen patches.* Oestrogen patches release 100–200 µg of oestradiol. Significant improvement in symptoms was noted in a study of 40 women (Watson *et al.* 1989) who received 100 mg patches every third day. They also received cyclical norethisterone. Side effects included breast tenderness, skin reaction and migraine. To avoid the progestogenic side effects several workers have now used patches in just the luteal phase. Both patches and implants are effective in young as well as perimenopausal women with severe symptoms.

In future, studies will be published where continuous oestrogen is given in combination with the levonorgestrel intrauterine system (e.g. Mirena; Pharmacia-Leiras, Milton Keynes, Buckinghamshire) to protect the endometrium, thus minimising the regeneration of PMS caused by systemic oral progesterones, as systemic levels with this approach are extremely low.

*GnRH agonist analogues.* The use of GnRH agonist analogues is the most reliable means available to suppress ovarian function medically. They act by creating a reversible pseudo-menopause. These drugs are licensed for use in prostatic cancer, endometriosis and infertility. In endometriosis, cessation of therapy is followed by the return of menstruation, but not usually the endometriosis. In the management of PMS the symptoms return immediately on discontinuation of treatment (Hussain *et al.* 1992) (Figure 6).

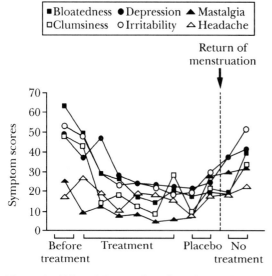

**Figure 6** *Effect of the gonadotrophin releasing hormone analogue buserelin on premenstrual symptoms. Symptoms are significantly reduced during ovarian cycle suppression but recur during the last cycle of placebo therapy following probable ovulation and prior to return of the first period. (Adapted from Hussain, S. Y., Massil, J. H., Matta, W. H. et al. (1992) Buserelin in premenstrual syndrome. Gynecol Endocrinol 6, 57–64, with permission of the Parthenon Publishing Group)*

Nasal preparations (buserelin and nafarelin) give less precise suppression of the cycle and symptoms are often exacerbated during the initial stimulation phase. The depot preparation goserelin is the most reliable and predictable as its use is independent of patient compliance (Muse 1992). However, adverse effects in the short-term (flushes), medium-term (vaginal atrophy) and long-term (osteoporosis and cardiovascular disease) preclude their universal or long-term use (Hussain *et al.* 1992). These agents can be used in severely affected patients for a six-month respite from symptoms and as a diagnostic test to distinguish the proportion of symptoms due to underlying psychopathology from those actually due to the ovarian cycle. They may also be used to test the potential value of bilateral oophorectomy in patients who are to undergo pelvic surgery. For instance, if a woman is to undergo hysterectomy for fibroids and she also has severe PMS, then removal or conservation or ovaries must also be considered; per-

forming the goserelin test will assist in this decision.

In cases of severe PMS it may be appropriate to give goserelin and to protect the skeleton with 'add-back' therapy. If this is given with conventional hormone replacement therapy (Mortola, Girton and Fischer 1991; Leather *et al.* 1993), the symptoms of PMS will recur in many women. A prospective, placebo-controlled trial using depot leuprorelin with 'add-back' oestrogen and progesterone was effective in treating premenstrual symptoms with progressive improvement over a 12-month period (Mezrow *et al.* 1994). The therapy prevented lipid changes while adequately protecting the endometrium. The drop in bone density was not found to be statistically significant.

## Surgical treatment

This is probably the only permanent cure for premenstrual syndrome, but is appropriate for only a few severely affected women. Bilateral oophorectomy and hysterectomy is curative (Casson *et al.* 1990) and has a particular role when a hysterectomy is planned for another indication, such as menorrhagia. Hypo-oestrogenic side effects can then be prevented by unopposed oestrogen, without the need for cyclical progestogen. Symptoms persist after hysterectomy alone, although one study showed that symptoms were reduced without bilateral oophorectomy (Metcalf *et al.* 1991). This may be the result of steroid changes which occur even when the ovaries are conserved. The results of one uncontrolled study support the use of endometrial ablation (Lefler and Lefler 1992); logically this should not be effective because ovarian activity persists. In addition, there are documented cases where PMS persists following the procedure.

## CONCLUSION

Premenstrual syndrome is a constellation of symptoms that occurs during normal ovarian cycles and possibly exclusively in ovulatory cycles. The aim is to provide the simplest and most effective treatment, but a patient's charac-

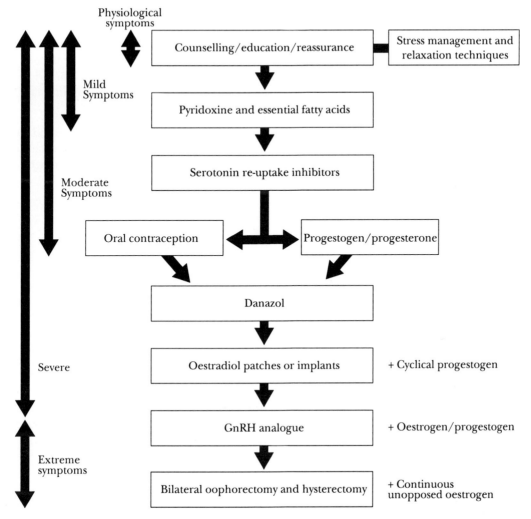

**Figure 7** *Hierarchical approach to the management of premenstrual syndrome. (Reproduced from O'Brien, P. M. S. (1993) Helping women with premenstrual syndrome. BMJ **307**, 1417–5, with permission of the BMJ Publishing Group)*

teristics will influence a clinician's choice. Figure 7 summarises the management options are available to treat women with PMS.

(1) It is best to start with non-pharmacological methods, using drugs only if these methods fail.

(2) When symptoms are predominantly psychological or the patient has secondary PMS, serotonergic drugs may provide the most benefit.

(3) The majority of patients do not require hormone therapy, although danazol or

oestrogen patches may be tried in individual patients.

(4) Age and proximity to menopause favour the use of oestrogens.

(5) If the woman wishes to become pregnant ovulation cannot be suppressed and also the risk of teratogenesis (e.g. masculinisation of female fetus with danazol) should be taken into account.

(6) Those wishing to avoid pregnancy may opt for a trial of combined oral contraceptives. In addition, women should be made aware

that most of the techniques used to treat PMS are *not* effective contraceptives.

(7) Oestrogen implants and GnRH analogues may occasionally be used for severely affected patients but they should only be used in units where there is particular interest in the PMS.

(8) Severe PMS will, in practical terms, be defined as failure to respond to non-invasive methods. More aggressive methods will be needed for women who do not respond to the non-hormonal and non-surgical techniques.

(9) The management of premenstrual syndrome induced by hormone replacement is difficult. Tibolone or combined continuous hormone replacement may be tried in the first place.

(10) Cyclical mastalgia should be treated with evening primrose oil in the first place, and then cyclical or continuous danazol or bromocriptine if that fails.

# References

American Psychiatric Association (1994) *Diagnostic and Statistical Manual of Mental Disorders,* 4th edn, pp. 714–18. Washington, DC: American Psychiatric Association

Ashby, C. R. Jr, Carr, L. A., Cook, C. L., Steptoe, M. M. and Franks, D. D. (1988) Alteration of platelet serotonergic mechanisms and monoamine oxidase activity in premenstrual syndrome. *Biol Psychiatry* 24, 225–33

Backstrom, T. (1992) Neuroendocrinology of premenstrual syndrome. *Clin Obstet Gynecol* 35, 612–28

Backstrom, T. and Cartensen, H. (1974) Estrogen and progesterone in plasma in relation to premenstrual tension. *J Steroid Biochem* 5, 257–60

Backstrom, T. and Mattsson, T. (1975) Correlation of symptoms in premenstrual tension to oestrogen and progesterone concentrations in blood plasma. *Neuropsychobiology* 1, 80–6

Brush, M. G., Watson, S. J., Horrobin, D. F. and Manku, M. S. (1984) Abnormal essential fatty acid levels in plasma of women with premenstrual syndrome. *Am J Obstet Gynecol* 150, 363–6

Casson, P., Hahn, P. M., van Vugt, D. A. and Reid, R. L. (1990) Lasting response to ovariectomy in severe intractable premenstrual syndrome. *Am J Obstet Gynecol* 162, 99–105

Chan, A. F., Morotola, J. F., Wood, S. H. and Yen, S. S. C. (1994) Persistence of premenstrual syndrome during low-dose administration of progesterone antagonist RU 486. *Obstet Gynecol* 84, 1001–5

Chuong, C. J. (1988) Clinical trial of naltrexone in premenstrual syndrome. *Obstet Gynecol* 72, 332–6

Chuong, C. J., Coulam, C. B., Kao, P. C., Bergstalh, E. J. and Go, V. L. W. (1985) Neuropeptide levels in premenstrual syndrome. *Fertil Steril* 44(6), 760–5

Dalton, K. (1984) *The Premenstrual Syndrome and Progesterone Therapy,* 2nd edn. London: William Heineman Medical Books Ltd.

Deeny, M., Hawthorn, R. and McKay Hart, D. (1991) Low dose danazol treatment of the premenstrual syndrome. *Postgrad Med J* 67, 450–4

Derzko, C. M. (1990) Role of danazol in relieving the premenstrual syndrome. *J Reprod Med* 35 (Suppl. 1), 97–102

Elks, M. L. (1993) Open trial of fluoxetine therapy for premenstrual syndrome. *South Med J* 86, 503–7

Faratian, B., Gaspar, A., O'Brien, P. M. S. *et al.* (1984) Premenstrual syndrome: weight, abdominal size and perceived body image. *Am J Obstet Gynecol* 150, 200–4

Freeman, E., Rickels, K., Sondheimer, S. J. and Polansky, M. (1990) Ineffectiveness of progesterone supporitory treatment for premenstrual syndrome. *J Am Med Assoc* **264**, 349–53

Freeman, E. W., Rickels, K., Sondheimer, S. J. and Polansky, M. (1995) A double-blind trial of oral progesterone, alprazolam, and placebo in treatment of severe premenstrual syndrome. *J Am Med Assoc* **274**, 51–7

Goldberg, D. P. and Hillier, V. (1979) A scaled version of the General Health Questionnaire. *Psychological Med* **9**, 139–45

Goodale, I. L., Domar, A. D. and Benson, H. (1990) Alleviation of premenstrual syndrome with relaxation response. *Obstet Gynecol* **75**, 649–55

Halbreich, U., Endicott, J., Schacht, S. and Nee J. (1982) The diversity of premenstrual changes as reflected in the Premenstrual Assessment Form. *Acta Psychiatr Scand* **68**, 125–30

Halbreich, U., Rojansky, N. and Palter, S. (1991) Elimination of ovarian and menstrual cyclicity (with danazol) improves dysphoric premenstrual syndrome. *Fertil Steril* **56**, 1066

Hallman, J. (1986) The premenstrual syndrome — an equivalent of depression? *Acta Psychiatr Scand* **73**, 403–11

Hammarback, S. and Backstrom, T. (1988) Induced anovulation as treatment of premenstrual tension syndrome: a double-blind cross-over study with GnRH-agonist versus placebo. *Acta Obstet Gynecol Scand* **67**, 159–66

Hammarback, S., Backstrom, T., Holst, J., von Schoultz, B. and Lyrenas, S. (1985) Cyclical mood changes as in the premenstrual tension syndrome during sequential estrogen–progestogen postmenopausal replacement therapy. *Acta Obstet Gynecol Scand* **64**, 393–7

Hammarback, S., Damber, J.-E. and Backstrom, T. (1989) Relationship between symptom severity and hormone changes in women with premenstrual syndrome. *J Clin Endocrinol Metab* **68**, 125–30

Hammarback, S., Ekholm, U.-B. and Backstrom, T. (1991) Spontaneous anovulation causing disappearance of cyclical symptoms in women with premenstrual syndrome. *Acta Endocrinol (Copenh)* **125**, 132–7

Harrison, W. M., Endicott, J. and Nee, J. (1990) Treatment of premenstrual dysphoria with alprazolam: a controlled study. *Arch Gen Psychiatry* **47**, 270–5

Hellberg, D., Claesson, B. and Nilsson, S. (1991) Premenstrual tension: a placebo-controlled efficacy study with spironolactone and medroxyprogesterone acetate. *Int J Obstet Gynecol* **34**, 243–8

Henshaw, C., O'Brien, P. M. S., Foreman, D., Belcher, J. and Cox, J. (1993) An experimental model for PMS. *Neuropsychopharmacology* **9**(25), 713

Horrobin, D. F. (1990) γ-Linolenic acid: an intermediate in essential fatty acid metabolism with potential as an ethical pharmaceutical and as a food. *Rev Contemp Pharmacotherapy* **1**, 1–45

Hussain, S. Y. (1993) The compartmental distribution of fluid and electrolytes in relation to the symptomatology of the ovarian cycle and premenstrual syndrome, *PhD thesis*, University of London

Hussain, S. Y., Massil, J. H., Matta, W. H., Shaw, R. W. and O'Brien, P. M. S. (1992) Buserelin in premenstrual syndrome. *Gynecol Endocrinol* **6**, 57–64

Johnson, S. (1992) Clinician's approach to the diagnosis and management of premenstrual syndrome. *Clin Obstet Gynecol* **35**, 649–57

Kane, F. J. (1976) Evaluation of emotional reactions of oral contraceptive use. *Am J Obstet Gynecol* **126**, 968–72

Khoo, S. K., Munro, C. and Battistutta, D. (1990) Evening primrose oil and treatment of premenstrual syndrome. *Med J Australia* **153**, 189–92

Kleijnen, J., Ter Reit, G. and Knipschild, P. (1990) Vitamin B6 in the treatment of the premenstrual syndrome — a review. *Br J Obstet Gynaecol* **97**, 847–52

Leather, A. T., Studd, J. W. W., Watson, N. R. and Holland, E. F. (1993) The prevention of bone loss in young women treated with GnRH analogues with 'add-back' estrogen therapy. *Obstet Gynecol* **82**, 104–7

Lefler, H. T. and Lefler, C. F. (1992) Endometrial ablation. Improvement in PMS related to the decrease in bleeding. *J Reprod Med* **37**, 596–8

Logue, A. M. and Moos, R. H. (1986) Perimenstrual symptoms; prevalence and risk factors. *Psychosom Med* **48**, 388–414

Magos, A. L., Brincat, M. and Studd, J. W. W. (1986) Treatment of the premenstrual syndrome by subcutaneous oestradiol implants and cyclical oral norethisterone: placebo-controlled study. *BMJ* **292**, 1629–33

Mattsson, B. and von Schoultz, B. (1974) A comparison between lithium, placebo and a diuretic in premenstrual tension. *Acta Psychiatr Scand* **255** (Suppl.), 75–84

Menkes, D. B., Taghavi, E., Mason, P. A., Spears, G. F. S. and Howard, R. C. (1992) Fluoxetine treatment of severe premenstrual syndrome. *BMJ* **305**, 346–7

Menkes, D. B., Taghavi, E., Mason, P. A. and Howard R. C. (1993) Fluoxetine's spectrum of action in premenstrual syndrome. *Int Clin Psychopharmacol* **8**, 95–102

Metcalf, M. G., Livesley, J. H., Wells, J. E. *et al.* (1991) Premenstrual syndrome in hysterectomized women: mood and physical symptom cyclicity. *J Psychosom Res* **35**, 555–67

Mezrow, G., Sharpe, D., Spicer, D. *et al.* (1994) Depot leuprolide acetate with estrogen and progestin add-back for long term treatment of premenstrual syndrome. *Fertil Steril* **62**, 932–7

Moos, R. (1985) *Premenstrual Symptoms: A Manual and Overview of Research with the Menstrual Distress Questionnaire.* Palo Alto, CA: Department of Psychiatry and Behavioural Sciences, Standford University School of Medicine

Morse, C. A., Dennerstein, L., Farrell, E. and Varnavides, K. A. (1991) Comparison of hormone therapy, coping skills training, and relaxation for the relief of premenstrual syndrome. *J Behav Med* **14**, 469–89

Mortola, J. F., Girton, L. and Fischer, U. (1991) Successful treatment of severe premenstrual syndrome by combined use of gonadotrophin releasing hormone agonist and estrogen/progestin. *J Clin Endocrinol Metab* **71**, 252A–F

Munday, M., Brush, M. G. and Taylor, R. W. (1977) Progesterone and aldosterone levels in premenstrual syndrome. *J Endocrinol* **73**, 21–5

Muse, K. (1992) Hormonal manipulation in the treatment of premenstrual syndrome. *Clin Obstet Gynecol* **35**, 658–66

Muse, K., Cetel, N., Futterman, L. and Yen, S. S. C. (1984) The premenstrual syndrome. Effects of 'medical ovariectomy'. *N Engl J Med* **311**, 1345–9

O'Brien, P. M. S. (1987) *Premenstrual Syndrome.* Oxford: Blackwell Scientific Publications

O'Brien, P. M. S. (1993) Helping women with premenstrual syndrome. *BMJ* **307**, 1471–5

O'Brien, P. M. S. and Massil, H. (1990) 'Premenstrual syndrome: clinical studies on essential fatty acids' in: D. F. Horrobin (Ed.). *Omega-6-essential fatty acids: pathology and roles in clinical medicine*, pp. 523–45. New York: Wiley/Liss

O'Brien, P. M. S., Selby, C. and Symonds, E. M. (1980) Progesterone, fluid and electrolytes in premenstrual syndrome. *BMJ* **i**, 1161–3

O'Brien, P. M. S. and Symonds, E. M. (1982) Prolactin levels in the premenstrual syndrome. *Br J Obstet Gynaecol* **89**, 306–8

Oleson, T. and Flocco, W. (1993) Randomised control study of premenstrual symptoms treated with ear, hand and foot reflexology. *Obstet Gynecol* **82**, 906–11

Pearlstein, T. B. (1995) Hormones and depression. What are the facts about premenstrual syndrome, menopause, and hormone replacement therapy? *Am J Obstet Gynecol* **175** (2), 646–53

Pearlstein, T. B. and Stone, A. B. (1994) Long-term fluoxetine treatment of the late luteal phase dysphoric disorder. *J Clin Psychiatry* **55**, 332–5

Pye, J. K., Mansel, R. E. and Hughes, L. E. (1985) Clinical experience of drug treatments for mastalgia. *Lancet* **ii**, 373–7

Rapkin, A. J. (1992) The role of serotonin in premenstrual syndrome. *Clin Obstet Gynecol* **35**, 629–36

Reid, R. L. and Yen, S. S. C. (1981) Premenstrual syndrome. *Am J Obstet Gynecol* **139**, 85–104

Reid, R. L. (1988) 'Etiology: medical theories' in: W. R. Keye Jr (Ed.). *The Premenstrual Syndrome*, pp. 66–93. Philadelphia: W. B. Saunders

Rickels, K., Freeman, E. and Sondheimer, S. (1989) Buspirone in the treatment of premenstrual syndrome [Letter]. *Lancet* **i**, 777

Rubinow, D. R., Hoban, C., Grover, G. N. *et al.* (1988) Changes in plasma hormones across the menstrual cycle in patients with menstrually related mood disorder and in control subjects. *Am J Obstet Gynecol* **158**, 5–11

Shoupe, D. and Lobo, R. A. (1985) The effects of estrogen and progestin on endogenous opioid activity in oophorectomized women. *J Clin Endocrinol Metab* **60**, 178

Shoupe, D. (1991) 'The premenstrual syndrome' in: D. R. Mishell Jr, V. Davajar and R. A. Lobo (Eds.). *Infertility, Contraception and Reproductive Endocrinology*, 3rd edn, pp. 503–17. Boston: Blackwell Scientific Publications

Smith, S. L. (1976) The menstrual cycle and mood disturbances. *Clin Obstet Gynecol* **19**, 391–7

Smith, S., Rinehart, J. S., Ruddock, V. E. and Schiff, I. (1987) Treatment of premenstrual syndrome with alprazolam: results of a double-blind, placebo-controlled, randomized crossover clinical trial. *Obstet Gynecol* **70**, 37–43

Steege, J. F., Stout, A. L., Knight, D. L. and Nemeroff, C. B. (1992) Reduced platelet tritium-labelled imipramine blinding sites in women with premenstrual syndrome. *Am J Obstet Gynecol* **167**, 168–72

Steiner, M., Steinberg, S., Stewart, D. *et al.* (1995) Fluoxetine in the treatment of premenstrual dysphoria. *N Engl J Med* **332**, 1529–34

Stone, A. B., Pearlstein, T. B. and Brown, W. A. (1991) Fluoxetine in the treatment of late luteal phase dysphoric disorder. *J Clin Psychiatry* **52**, 290–3

Sunblad, C., Modigh, K., Andersch, B. and Eriksson, E. (1992) Clomipramine effectively reduces premenstrual irritability and dysphoria: a placebo-controlled trial. *Acta Psychiatr Scand* **85**, 39–47

Walker, A. and Bancroft, J. (1990) Relationship between premenstrual symptoms and oral contraceptive use. *Psychosom Med* **52**, 86–96

Watson, N. R., Studd, J. W. W., Savvas, M., Garnett, T. and Baber, R. J. (1989) Treatment of severe premenstrual syndrome with oestradiol patches and cyclical oral norethisterone. *Lancet* **ii**, 730–2

Watson, N. R., Studd, J. W. W., Savvas, M. and Baber, R. J. (1990) The long-term effects of oestradiol implant therapy for treatment of premenstrual syndrome. *Gynecol Endocrinol* **4**, 99–107

Wood, S. H., Mortola, J. F., Chan, Y. F., Moosazadeh, F. and Yen, S. S. (1992) Treatment of premenstrual syndrome with fluoxetine; a double blind, placebo controlled, cross over study. *Obstet Gynecol* **80**, 339–44

Woods, N. F., Most, A. and Dery, G. K. (1982) Prevalence of perimenstrual symptoms. *Am J Public Health* **72**, 1257–64

Yonkers, K. A., Halbreich, U., Freeman, E. W., Brown, C. S. and Pearlstein, T. B. (1995) Efficacy of sertraline for treatment of premenstrual dysphoric disorder [Abstract], presented at the *148th Annual Meeting of the American Psychiatric Association*, May 1995

# 26

# Advances in vulval cancer

*John B. Murdoch*

The management of vulval cancer has developed over many years in a logical fashion in response to improved understanding of the usually predictable natural history of the disease. Squamous carcinoma is characterised by a long history of vulval discomfort and irritation followed by the development of an invasive lesion which may be neglected by the patient. The tumour invades locally and in the majority of cases metastasises embolically to the superficial and deep inguinofemoral nodes followed sequentially by pelvic nodal spread and systemic disease. Direct spread from the vulva to pelvic lymph nodes is sufficiently uncommon to have little impact on treatment strategies.

It is true that overall cure rates have changed little. The Halsteadean approach demanded by early workers (Basset 1912; Taussig 1940; Way 1960) was highly effective, achieving optimum cure rates, but at considerable cost to the patient in physical and psychosexual morbidity. The gold standards defined by consistent application of traditional radical vulvectomy and *en bloc* inguinofemoral node dissection with selective pelvic node dissection provides 94.3% five-year survival in node-negative patients and 62.5% five-year survival in node-positive patients in one large British series (Monaghan 1987). Modern intra-operative and postoperative care allows a 96% 'operability' rate in achieving these results.

As with breast carcinoma, the main advances in vulval carcinoma have been aimed at minimising treatment morbidity while maintaining cure rates. It is imperative to realise that in pursuit of more conservative management, locoregional disease control must be com-promised. Historically, the first major departure from *en bloc* dissection to become established in clinical practice was the triple-incision radical vulvectomy (TIV) technique. This was first described in detail by Byron, Mishell and Yonemoto (1965), but became fully established in more recent large series (Hacker *et al.* 1981; Grimshaw, Murdoch and Monaghan 1993). The embolic nature of early metastasis was confirmed in practice when only three of 200 patients in these series developed skin-bridge metastases. The benefits of TIV are primary closure in all cases and primary healing in 65%, with a mean hospitalisation of 18 days in the primary healing group and 30 days after wound breakdown (Grimshaw, Murdoch and Monaghan 1993). Furthermore, in the latter series, the corrected survival for stage I tumours was 96.7% and 85% for stage II tumours, indicating preservation of acceptable cure rates.

Triple-incision radical vulvectomy not only reduces morbidity while maintaining cure rates, it is also important because it introduces the concept of separating the groin node dissection from the management of the central tumour. This allows individual management at each site, leading to a plethora of management options (Table 1).

## CENTRAL TUMOUR MANAGEMENT

Standard management of central tumours with *en bloc* and TIV surgery demands removal of all vulval skin and dissection down to the deep perineal fascia. This results in extensive scarring with distortion of body image and loss of coital

261

**Table 1**  *Management options for vulval cancer*

*Tumour surgery:*
  radical wide local excision
  radical hemivulvectomy
  radical vulvectomy (triple incision)
  radical vulvectomy (butterfly/*en bloc*)
  radical anovulvectomy
  exenteration

*Node surgery:*
  ipsilateral complete groin dissection
  bilateral complete groin dissection
  no surgery

*Radiotherapy and chemotherapy:*
  adjuvant groin and pelvic radiotherapy
  primary prophylactic groin radiotherapy
  salvage tumour radiotherapy
  combination chemoradiation therapy (using
    5-fluorouracil)

satisfaction. These effects have been considered a necessary price in the pursuit of local disease control and this remains the case in neglected large lesions. However, the same may not be the case for T1 lesions (< 2 cm diameter) and smaller T2 lesions (> 2 cm diameter). There has been a clear shift in emphasis away from radical removal of the vulva towards an appreciation that the critical factor in success is the excision margin around the tumour itself. This requires excision of a 2 cm margin of healthy vulva around the tumour and dissection to the deep perineal fascia. A wide margin is necessary to minimise local recurrence. Heaps *et al.* (1990) defined a surgical resection margin of 8 mm on formalin-fixed tissues as an important watershed in the risk of local recurrence. This equates to approximately 12 mm in the fresh specimen. The fate of the rest of the vulva is to some extent irrelevant. How much vulval epithelium is removed radically is dictated by the size and site of the cancer. Where there is adjacent vulval dystrophy, surgery can be tailored to superficial excision of epithelium, so long as radicality is maintained around the tumour.

This technique demands careful preoperative mapping of lesions, ideally in my view, with the aid of a colposcope. This may include colpo-

scopic examination of the anal canal (Ogunbiyi *et al.* 1994), although this remains controversial. The Sheffield group has demonstrated a correlation between vulval neoplasia, anal intraepithelial neoplasia and anal carcinoma. However, the suggestion that anal intraepithelial neoplasia should be excised to prevent later development of carcinoma is contentious as the treatment has a high-morbidity profile and anal cancer remains rare.

Postoperatively, lifelong detailed follow-up is required, particularly in young women with unstable lower genital tract field changes (Kelley *et al.* 1992). This approach has been reported by the MD Anderson group in a series of 76 patients (Burke *et al.* 1995). In tumours invading to a depth of > 1 mm, the authors performed radical wide excisions with a 2 cm lateral margin of healthy tissue and dissection to the deep perineal fascia. There were 33 T1 (< 2 cm) and 42 T2 (> 2 cm) tumours. Only eight patients had some degree of breakdown of the vulval wound. Seven patients were node positive after superficial node dissection. Actuarial survival at four years for the whole group was 81%. Nine women developed new or recurrent disease, five of whom had preinvasive lesions only at recurrence. Of the four patients (5%) who developed further invasive lesions, only one recurred at the site of the previous surgery and in this case it recurred at multiple sites on the vulva. All four patients were salvaged by further surgery and local radiotherapy. In a review which compared a radical vulvectomy series of 376 cases with stage I tumours, Piura *et al.* (1993) reported 39 vulval recurrences (10%), of which 27 occurred in stage I or II disease. Hacker and Van der Velden (1993) reviewed the literature comparing radicality and local recurrence showing that recurrence rates for T1 tumours were 7.2% when locally excised versus 6.3% after radical vulvectomy (*P* = 0.85).

It would seem that radical wide excision fulfils the requirements for an advance in management with reduced morbidity and maintained cure rates. This will of course only be sustained when applied to the wider community if the following basic rules are applied:

(1) Preoperative mapping is detailed;

(2) Peritumour radicality is maintained; and

(3) Follow-up is meticulous and extended over many years.

The reduction in extent of skin removal and separation of the groin dissection from that of the central disease has greatly reduced post-operative in-patient stays. Mean postoperative stays are now 18 days for TIV (Grimshaw, Murdoch and Monaghan 1993) and 10 days for radical wide excision (Burke *et al.* 1995)

A second consideration in the extent of vulval excision is the ease with which plastic reconstruction can be achieved. Primary closure of large vulval defects is usually feasible with mobilisation of vulval remnants and by pulling the vagina down, but this produces a wound under some tension which heals with loss of vulval architecture. Although split-skin grafts can be used, they act as little more than biological dressings, providing no bulk and leaving disfiguring results. Myocutaneous flaps can be raised, but these are extensive procedures on top of already radical assaults on an often aged patient. Scarring is extensive and the skin island on gracilis flaps is notorious for failure. Finally, myocutaneous flaps are too bulky in most cases. The author has adopted an intermediate and highly successful technique of raising rotational skin and subcutaneous tissue flaps from the media aspect of the upper thigh and buttock. These flaps are approximately 10 cm long, 5 cm wide and 2 cm deep. Raised bilaterally they admirably fill a radical vulvectomy defect with no tension and heal to preserve the architecture of the vulva. The cosmetic effect is most successful when seen from the front, so that the patient, when viewing herself standing in front of a mirror, will find that she has retained much of the familiar vulval shape. The only problematic cases that the author has encountered concerned two women, one very obese and one very thin, whose donor site scars were under tension and broke down. The flaps themselves have been universally successful and have become part of the surgical routine.

## MANAGEMENT OF LOCALLY ADVANCED DISEASE

Tumours encroaching on the distal urethra are managed quite simply by including up to 10 mm of the distal urethra in the resection without loss of urinary continence. More extensive tumours involving the upper urethra, bladder or rectum may require exenterative surgery (Cavanagh and Shepherd 1982). The key factor in survival is the presence of lymph node metastases. In node-positive patients, the outlook is bleak and the use of such extensive surgery as a palliative procedure must be questioned. Locoregional control in node-negative patients can be excellent, but careful selection of patients is essential as many will be in poor condition. A second group consists of patients with stage III and IV vulval disease and local extension to the anus only, with or without nodal spread. Current options comprise surgery or chemoradiation therapy. Effective radical surgery requires the formation of an end colostomy. Not surprisingly, resection of all or part of the anal sphincter results in faecal incontinence (Hoffman *et al.* 1989). Surgery can involve exenteration or abdominoperineal resection. An alternative approach with reduced morbidity and high cure rates was suggested by Grimshaw, Aswad and Monaghan (1991) using a two-stage radical anovulvectomy. In this procedure, the formation of an end colostomy is followed two weeks later by an *en bloc* or triple-incision radical vulvectomy and bilateral ileofemoral node dissection in which the excision is carried behind the anus to radically excise all tumour tissue. The rectal stump is retained as a mucous fistula. This approach achieved an 80% five-year survival in cases with stage III disease, but none of the women with stage IV disease survived. The patients with stage IV disease were catagorised as such due to bilateral groin node involvement. This emphasises the dismal outlook for patients with advanced local *and* systemic disease. Even so, as a primary palliative surgical procedure, the morbidity is lower than for primary exenteration. The main problems with the technique for survivors are occasional troublesome mucoid discharge from the rectal stump, stump prolapse and interference by the rectal stump with successful reconstructive surgery.

All surgical techniques that deal with the problems of anal involvement demand sacrifice of the anal sphincter. Traditionally, radiotherapy has been considered a second best option in management of vulval carcinoma due to the sensitivity of the normal vulva to radiation damage and relatively low rates of local control (Slevin and Pointon 1989). As a result, in the United Kingdom primary radiotherapy has been reserved for patients unfit for radical surgery.

The revolution in management of primary anal carcinoma in the last decade has, however, prompted reappraisal of radiotherapy for control of vulval disease encroaching on the anal canal. There has been a major shift away from abdominoperineal resection as the primary therapy for anal carcinoma towards primary radiotherapy with or without synchronous chemotherapy (Pinter, Worthover and Nicholls 1989). In a large series of patients treated with radiotherapy alone, Schlienger *et al.* (1989) report a five-year survival of 73.3% in node-negative patients and a 36.1% five-year survival in node-positive patients, with a 55% rate of preservation of anal function. An alternative therapy combining radiotherapy and chemosensitisation using 5-fluorourcil (5FU) and mitomycin C was developed by Nigro, Vaitkevicius and Considine (1974). In a non-randomised, comparative study of radiotherapy alone, radiotherapy plus 5FU and mitomycin C, and radiotherapy with just 5FU, Cummings *et al.* (1991) reported cause-specific survivals of 68%, 76% and 64% respectively, again with preservation of anal function in 88% of patients.

The prospect of anal preservation with disease control in cases with stage III and IV cancer has prompted the study of these regimens in vulval carcinoma. Rotmensch *et al.* (1990) reported on 13 patients treated by radiotherapy alone in which 50 Gy was delivered to the vulva and 45 Gy to the vaginal and pelvic nodes. There was a disappointing 45% five-year survival, but a promising 62.5% sphincter preservation rate. Alternatively, Whitaker *et al.* (1990) used a modification of the Nigro regi-

men in a pilot study of 12 patients and reported three successful treatments, five local failures, two deaths from distant metastases and two deaths after palliative therapy alone. In a study of combined bleomycin and irradiation, Scheistroen and Trope (1993) found that 17 out of 20 patients relapsed and died with a median survival of eight months.

More recently, it has become clear that 5FU is the key component of the combination. The St Bartholomews/Marsden group has reported (in abstract form only to date) a 36% complete response with chemoradiation for locally advanced disease and similar survival (26%) with primary radical and exenterative surgery (28%) in a non-randomised comparison of the two options. At the 1995 meeting of the International Gynaecological Cancer Society, Thomas presented data on 16 patients with advanced or centrally located early disease who were treated with 5FU and 58–70 Gy radiation therapy. Fourteen of 16 patients remained disease-free after a median follow-up of four years. Four patients required salvage surgery.

These promising results must be viewed with caution. Direct comparisons with primary surgery are difficult, not least because there is no control for nodal status (the single most important variable for survival). The application of chemoradiation in this site and this population is difficult, with significant problems associated with moist desquamation. The vital questions yet to be adequately answered in this debate are:

(1) In node-negative patients, does chemoradiation offer equivalent local control and survival to sphincter-sacrificing surgery?

(2) In node-positive patients, can palliative local control be achieved with acceptable treatment-related morbidity where sphincter sacrificing surgery may not be indicated in view of the dismal prognosis?

## LYMPH NODE MANAGEMENT

The standard therapy remains complete extirpation of the superficial inguinal and deep femoral node groups.

In the two studies of TIV using complete node dissection there were no isolated groin recurrences. This is important as groin recurrence usually results in death. In the series described by Hacker *et al.* (1981) pelvic node dissection was used selectively, but this was not the case for the Gateshead series (Grimshaw, Murdoch and Monaghan 1993), which reflects the doubt concerning the benefit of such extensive dissection in the likely presence of systemic disease. Further light was shed on the issue by the American Gynecological Oncology Group (GOG) study randomising groin node-positive patients to pelvic and groin radiotherapy versus pelvic node dissection. The study (Homesley *et al.* 1986) demonstrated a clear survival advantage (68% versus 54%, $P = 0.03$) in the radiotherapy group with no difference in morbidity. Importantly, the survival gain lay in prevention of groin metastases rather than control of pelvic disease, indicating that once the disease has passed the inguinal ligament it is systemic cancer for which there is no effective response. Homesley *et al.* (1986) further indicated that adjuvant radiotherapy was useful in the presence of two or more positive nodes.

The GOG then took the next logical step by initiating a randomised study of groin dissection versus groin irradiation in patients with clinically non-suspicious groin nodes (Stehman *et al.* 1992). The study suggested that 60 Gy to the groin was insufficient to prevent groin recurrence. Patients who had complete groin dissection had longer progression-free intervals ($P = 0.03$) and survival ($P = 0.04$). However, there are two major flaws in this study:

(1) The study was closed prematurely raising the possibility of methodological failure; and

(2) More importantly, there are data to suggest that primary prophylactic groin radiotherapy failed because the wrong technique was used.

Koh *et al.* (1993) studied pretreatment groin computer tomography scans in 50 patients to determine the distance of the femoral vessels beneath the skin; they found a mean of 6.1 cm (range 2.0–18.5 cm). Re-calculating the failures in the GOG study where the protocol stipulated a treatment depth of 3 cm they showed that all failures received potential tumour doses below 47 Gy, with three patients being underdosed by over 30%. This view was supported in a retrospective comparison of 23 patients receiving inguinofemoral irradiation and 25 patients receiving complete inguinofemoral node dissection (Petereit *et al.* 1993). In this study, 4, 6 or 10 M photons were used with opposed fields to ensure 50 Gy was applied to the node bearing tissue. The groin recurrence rate was similar and the authors reported that 80% of irradiated patients were hospitalised for less than two weeks compared to 80% of the surgical patients who were hospitalised for more than two weeks. It should be remembered, of course, that this was a non-randomised, retrospective study with insufficient power to show a difference in recurrence and the surgical patients underwent inappropriate *en bloc* resection with very high (72%) groin wound separation rates. If modern surgical techniques were used, the short-term morbidity would have been much less. The only true comparable morbidity (and the only reason for attempting to avoid node surgery) is long-term lower limb lymphoedema. In this study, four out of 25 surgical patients and two out of 23 irradiated patients were reported to suffer this complication.

Lymphoedema has been variously reported to affect 13–65% of survivors and represents the major long-term physical sequela of treatment. In keeping with the philosophy of minimising morbidity and maintaining cure rates, Wharton, Gallagher and Rutledge (1974) reviewed their data and identified 10 patients who had primary tumours < 2 cm in diameter with < 5 mm invasion and had no evidence of node metastases. Their suggestion that node dissection could be omitted in this group was met by a vigorous response from other workers and the consensus view is that the node-positivity rate in this group of patients ranges from 7% to 34% (Hacker and Van der Velden 1993). The clinical assessment of groin nodes is notoriously unreliable, with errors of 25% both ways (i.e. overestimation of node-positivity in 25% and underestimation of node-positivity in a further 25% of cases). As a result, DiSaia, Creasman and Rich (1979) suggested an alternative strategy in a report on 20 patients in whom a superficial inguinal node dissection with frozen-section analysis was used as a screening test for node positivity. Full groin dissection was reserved for node-positive patients. This study, of course, proved little as the expected prevalence of node positivity in the study group was too low and the numbers too few to test the hypothesis. The GOG, however, responded by studying the concept further. Unfortunately, the issue was prejudged and a formal randomised trial of superficial node dissection versus formal complete node dissection was replaced by a one-armed observational study. The study design became further flawed when no provision was made to record data on the superficial node-positive patients (true positives), thereby preventing assessment of the performance of the screening test. Fortunately, the results were sufficiently robust to overcome these difficulties. There were nine groin recurrences with five deaths related to groin recurrences (Stehman *et al.* 1992). Historical controls suggested there should be none and these results are compatible with failure of the strategy to achieve its aims. Furthermore, the evidence for reduced morbidity when deep femoral dissection is not performed is weak. It, therefore, seems clear that superficial node dissection has no role to play in this condition.

Despite this, the technique continues to be used. Burke *et al.* (1995) offered superficial node dissection to the 76 patients who had radical wide excision of their T1 or T2 tumours. Seven true positives were identified, but four false negatives subsequently appeared (i.e. a sensitivity of only 46%). This is unacceptable, given that one out of seven true positives died compared to three out of four false negatives.

Until techniques are developed and carefully validated which allow selective node biopsy or less invasive identification of node-positive patients, it will remain mandatory to perform complete groin node dissections. There would appear to be no acceptable watershed for lesions > 1 mm deep (Table 2). Indeed, Podczaski *et al.* (1990) recorded groin recurrence and death in

two patients with maximum depth of disease of 1.5 mm and 2 mm. In addition, there are two case reports of metastatic disease in early invasive cancers which were less than 1 mm deep. Clearly, clinicians must choose a point at which relative morbidity is balanced in the light of their own clinical experience. This requires rapport between the experienced surgeon and his knowledgable histopathologist. The author's current preference is to avoid groin dissection in patients with disease < 1 mm deep and to offer complete groin dissection to all others.

The prevention of groin recurrence has been given paramount importance. This is correct in that groin recurrence is difficult to treat and usually fatal. Prophylactic groin dissection, however, means that a high proportion of patients with clinically impalpable nodes are overtreated. Using the experience of Burke *et al.* (1995), 85% of patients with T1 and T2 had, in retrospect, 'unnecessary' groin therapy. It is noteworthy that prophylactic node dissection is not favoured in the management of many non-gynaecological skin cancers. There has never been a prospective, randomised, controlled trial comparing prophylactic node dissection versus observation and deferred treatment of node positives in vulval cancer. Relevant end-points would include global morbidity, local control rates and survival rates. It is likely that such a trial would not find broad support among gynaecologists until more accurate identification of histologically positive, clinically node-negative patients is possible.

**Table 2**  *Node positivity according to depth of invasion of primary squamous vulval cancer. (Reproduced from Hacker and Van der Valden 1993\* with permission of Wiley-Liss Inc., a subsidiary of John Wiley & Sons Inc.)*

| Depth of invasion (mm) | Cases (n) | Positive nodes (%) |
| --- | --- | --- |
| < 1 | 163 | 0 |
| 1–2 | 145 | 7.7 |
| 2–3 | 131 | 8.3 |
| 3–5 | 101 | 26.7 |
| > 5 | 38 | 34.2 |

*Hackner, N. F. and Van der Valden J. (1993) Conservative management of early vulval cancer. *Cancer* **71**, 1673–7

The final lesson from both the TIV series and more extensive perusal of the literature (Hacker and Van der Valden 1993) suggests that, for T1 (< 2 cm diameter) lateral tumours, the incidence of contralateral node positivity in the absence of ipsilateral node positivity is less than 1%. In these circumstances it is reasonable, therefore, to perform a unilateral complete groin dissection with the proviso that subsequent detection of node metastases on histopathological examination will require either a second operation on the contralateral groin or possibly adjuvant bilateral groin radiotherapy, so long as an appropriate technique is used (Grimshaw, Murdoch and Monaghan 1993).

## MANAGEMENT OF RECURRENT DISEASE

The critical factor in determining the likely outcome in patients with recurrence of vulval disease is the site of recurrence. In a large, surgically treated series (Piura *et al* 1993), 63% of patients whose disease recurred on the vulva alone were salvaged by radical wide local excision, and death from disease was more than three times as likely with recurrence outside the vulva. This reflects the absence of effective therapy for systemic disease.

For this reason, patients with vulval recurrence after radical wide excision are usually salvaged by further excision with radiotherapy as required. They are closely monitored, recurrences are small and intervention occurs before systemic disease develops. The prognosis for patients with large local recurrence and systemic disease remains dismal (P. Blake, personal communication).

## MANAGEMENT OF MALIGNANT MELANOMA OF THE VULVA

Malignant melanoma of the vulva is a rare disease. It accounts for approximately 5% of vulval cancers and is second in frequency to squamous carcinoma. Thus, with 800 cancers appearing in England and Wales each year, only 40 new malignant melanomas will be reported per annum. Traditionally, gynaecologists have treated the disease in a similar manner to squamous cancer using radical vulvectomy and bilateral groin dissection. Based on scant data this management is still suggested (Monaghan 1990; Aziz and McGarth 1995). Other authorities acknowledge the argument for conservative treatment but do not give clear advice (Krupp 1992).

It seems clear in reading these authors that the prognosis for the patient is entirely dependent on the unpredictable natural history of the disease. Early blood-borne spread means that at least 50% of recurrences will be distant. There is little evidence to suggest that the extent of the surgery has any impact on outcome. This could be because either there is no such impact or the data are too few to demonstrate an effect. A prospective, clinicopathological study of primary malignant melanoma of the vulva conducted by the GOG included patients treated by at least modified radical vulvectomy with optional groin node dissection (Phillips *et al.* 1994). In the study, 34 patients had radical hemivulvectomy, 37 had radical vulvectomy and 56 had groin node dissection. Independent predictors of groin node status were capillary lymphatic space involvement and centrally sited lesions. Recurrence correlated with depth of invasion. The authors concluded that vulval melanoma had the same natural history as melanoma sited elsewhere. Logic, therefore, demands that we should turn to the wider literature on nongenital melanoma for guidance.

Diagnosis of lesions should be by excision rather than incision biopsy, allowing full histopathological measurements (Ball and Thomas 1995). Lesions < 0.76 mm thick have a very low risk of recurrence following an excision biopsy with normal margins. In a large study, Milton, Shaw and McCarthy (1985) found an overall local recurrence rate of 7.6%. With excision margins < 2 cm, lesions < 1 mm recurred in only 2% of cases. Narrow margins in thicker tumours resulted in increased recurrence peaking at 21% in lesions > 3 mm thick. Thick tumours were prospectively randomised to 2-cm or 4-cm excision margins in one North American study with no difference in survival being detected (Balch *et al.* 1993). There is no evidence that excising deeper tissues has any impact on survival (Kenady, Brown and McBride 1982).

From this, it can be concluded that in the absence of a clear survival advantage, radical vulval surgery cannot be justified in the management of vulval melanoma. A margin of 1–2 cm is sufficient for thin lesions. A greater, as yet undefined margin < 4 cm is sufficient for thicker lesions.

The role of prophylactic node dissection in clinically node-negative patients is controversial, but the consensus view with lower limb lesions is that this is not justified (Scott and McKay 1993). The justification for prophylactic node dissection is the hope that occult metastases will be removed. A prospective, randomised, controlled trial of lower limb melanoma comparing immediate 'prophylactic' node dissection and deferred node dissection in clinically recurrent node disease failed to show any survival advantage (Veronesi et al. 1982). In contrast to this, there is good evidence for improved locoregional control in the event of clinically overt node metastasis (Kissen et al. 1987). Survival is unaffected. However, the extent of the node dissection required is controversial.

Thus, extrapolating to the vulva, it is apparent that in the absence of good evidence to the contrary, the management of vulval malignant melanoma should comprise wide excision with groin node surgery reserved for clinically apparent nodal metastatic disease.

## MANAGEMENT OF LYMPHOEDEMA

Lymphoedema is a chronic, long-term and debilitating, but not life-threatening, complication of radical female lower genital tract surgery and radiotherapy. The incidence varies from 13% to 65% (Zafar, Paterson and Murdoch 1995) treatment is often inadequate or unavailable. While the primary mechanism of lymphoedema is either surgical occlusion or fibroids of the main limb lymphatic trunks after radiotherapy, predisposing factors include heart failure, hypoproteinaemia, prolonged immobilisation, prolonged dependency of the leg, secondary lymphangitis or recurrent pelvic disease. Once established, the protein-rich lymphoedema fluid induces fibrosis and further stagnation due to obstructed microlymphatics (Foldi and Casley Smith 1978). Patients who avoid lymphoedema have efficient collateral superficial lymphatic channels.

The diagnosis of lymphoedema is primarily clinical. Contrast lymphangiography is commonly used, but it adds little new information and may actually worsen the condition via inflammation of microlymphatics by contrast medium and the introduction of infection.

The incidence of lymphoedema can, in certain circumstances, be reduced by adoption of ipsilateral rather than bilateral lymphadenectomy. There are few data to suggest that superficial lymph node dissection markedly reduces the incidence of lymphoedema. Improved targeting of patients who need lymphadenectomy is not yet available. Surgical remedies for established lymphoedema have been disappointing. In the meantime, the most productive strategies include advice on avoiding long periods of dependency of limbs, treatment of bruises, scratches and superficial skin infections (including fungal infections), and therapy of aggravating factors such as diabetes, cardiac failure and hypoproteinaemia. Specific treatment involves the use of four-quadrant, physical, decongestive massage to stimulate superficial collateral lymphatic activity, containment bandaging and graduated containment garments. Pneumatic devices are commonly advocated, but often fail as they achieve only short-term benefit. Foldi, Foldi and Clodius (1989) suggest that they are only useful in conjunction with massage which opens lymphatics to receive and distribute lymph into the trunk.

## CONCLUSION

For the reader of an article on advances in vulval cancer, much depends on the starting point of that individual. The traditional radical vulvectomy with inguinofemoral and pelvic node dissection practiced by Way and his contemporaries should have been universally abandoned. Some will be using the modified butterfly technique which succeeded it. This technique is increasingly hard to justify given the associated morbidity. Radical local surgery tailored to the requirements of the individual tumour is the crucial element for success. Prolonged follow-up is important to monitor preserved potentially unstable vulval skin. Simple reconstruction to promote healing and preserve vulval architecture should be routine.

Inguinofemoral node dissection falls into two categories:

(1) *Therapeutic dissection* with adjuvant radiotherapy, the use of which is not disputed;

(2) *Prophylactic node dissection* in clinically node-negative patients, which is current standard practice in all cases with invasion > 1 mm.

This, however, means that a large percentage of women are subjected to (in retrospect) unnecessary surgery with its attendant morbidity. Intellectually, the dilemma suggests that a trial addressing the global morbidity and mortality associated with this practice is necessary. Such a trial is, however, difficult to reconcile with current clinical opinion and practice. As an alternative, better methods of diagnosis of subclinical metastatic disease are needed.

From an unpromising start, radiotherapy (usually combined with chemotherapy) is beginning to establish a place in vulval cancer management. The data available to make proper judgements are fragmentary. This is typical of vulval cancer research. In the era of evidence-based medicine, clinicians should practice standard treatment until quality evidence points to change rather than adopting

**Table 3**  *The vulval cancer team*

*Medical:*
  gynaecological oncologist
  specialist clinical oncologist
  specialist histopathologist
  plastic surgeon

*Paramedical:*
  psychosexual counsellor
  lymphoedema therapist
  experienced nurses
  stomatherapist

the latest fashion uncritically. In a rare cancer, this requires a large multicentre study, ideally randomised, but at least by collated observation. Practitioners who perform occasional radical surgery do not participate in such studies. The only way to generate the power to make sustained progress is via centralisation with commitment in these centres to participation in studies. Centralisation is also necessary on economic and clinical grounds. The modern care of genital tract cancer is multidisciplinary (Table 3) and teamwork like this is not viable in units seeing occasional cases. The objections offered to centralisation usually take the form of protest that unfit, elderly women will not travel to the centre. Some will not, but most will. It seems inappropriate to deny optimum care to many on these grounds alone. The future of vulval cancer management lies in centralised care, with individualised management based on quality evidence from multicentre study of specific questions.

# References

Aziz, A. I. and McGarth, J. (1995) Malignant melanoma of the vulva. *Contemp Rev Obstet Gynaecol* **7**, 101–5

Balch, C. M., Urist, M. M., Karakousis *et al.* (1993) Efficacy of 2 cm surgical margins for intermediate thickness melanoma; effect on recurrence and survival rates. *Surgery* **218** (3), 615–18

Ball, A. S. and Thomas, J. (1995) Surgical management of malignant melanoma. *Aust NZ J Surg* **55**, 225–8

Basset, A. (1912) Traitement chiurgical operatoire de l'epitheliomaprimitif due clitoris indications–technique–resultats. *Rev Chir* **46**, 546

Burke, T. W., Levenbach, C., Coleman, R. L. *et al.* (1995) Surgical therapy of T1 and T2 vulvar carcinoma: further experience with radical wide extension and selective inguinal lymphadenectomy. *Gynecol Oncol* **57**, 215–20

Byron, R. L., Mishell, D. R. and Yonemoto, R. H. (1965) The surgical treatment of invasive carcinoma of the vulva. *Surg Gynecol Obstet* **121**, 1243–51

Cascinetti, N., Preda, F., Vagliai, M. *et al.* (1983) Metastatic spread of stage I melanoma of the skin. *Tumori* **69**, 449–54

Cavanagh, D. and Shepherd, J. H. (1982) The place of pelvic exenteration in the primary management of advanced carcinoma of the vulva. *Gynecol Oncol* **13**, 318–22

Cummings, B. I., Keane, T. J., O'Sullivan, B., Wong, C. S. and Catton, C. N. (1991) Epidermoid anal cancer: treatment by radiation alone or by radiation and 5-fluorouracil with and without mitomycin C. *Int J Radiat Oncol Biol Phys* **21**(5), 1115–25

DiSaia, P. J., Creasman, W. T. and Rich, W. M. (1979) An alternative approach to early cancer of the vulva. *Am J Obstet Gynecol* **133**, 825–30

Foldi, E., Foldi, M. and Clodius, L. (1989) The lymphoedema chaos: a lancet. *Am J Plastic Surg* **22**, 505–15

Foldi, M. and Casley Smith, J. R. (1978) 'The roles of lymphatics and the cells on high protein odemas' in: *Molecular Aspects of Medicine*, p. 77. Oxford: Pergamon Press

Grimshaw, R. N., Aswad, S. G. and Monaghan, J. M. (1991) The role of anovulvectomy in locally advanced carcinoma of the vulva involving the perianal or anal skin. *Gynecol Oncol* **35**, 215–18

Grimshaw, R. N., Murdoch, J. B. and Monaghan, J. M. (1993) Radical vulvectomy and bilateral inguinal femoral lymphadenectomy through separate incisions. Experience with 100 cases. *Int J Gynecol Cancer* **3**, 18–23

Hacker, N. F., Leuchter, R. S., Berek, J. S. and Castaldo, T. W. (1981) Radical vulvectomy and bilateral inguinal lymphadenectomy through separate groin incisions. *Obstet Gynecol* **58**, 574–9

Hacker, N. F. and Van der Velden, J. (1993) Conservative management of early vulva cancer. *Cancer* **71**, 1637–7

Heaps, J. M, Yao, S. F., Montz, F. J. *et al.* (1990) Surgical–pathological variables predictive of local recurrence in squamous cell carcinoma of the vulva. *Gynecol Oncol* **38**, 309–14

Hoffman, M. S., Roberts, W. S., LaPolla, J. P., Fiorica, J. V. and Cavanagh, D. (1989) Carcinoma of the vulva involving the perianal or anal skin. *Gynecol Oncol* **35**, 215–18

Homesley, H. D., Bundy, B. N., Sedlis, A. and Adlock, L. (1986) Radiation therapy versus pelvic node resection for carcinoma of the vulva with positive groin nodes. *Obstet Gynecol* **68**(6), 733–740

Kelley, J. L., Burke, T. W., Tornos, C. *et al.* (1992) Minimally invasive vulvar carcinoma: an indication for conservative surgical therapy. *Gynecol Oncol* **44**, 240–4

Kenady, D. E., Brown, B. W. and McBride, C. M. (1982) Excision of underlying fascia with a primary malignant melanoma; effect on recurrence and survival rates. *Surgery* **92**, 615–18

Kissen, M. W., Simpson, D. A., Easton, D. *et al.* (1987) Prognostic factors related to survival and groin recurrence following therapeutic lymph node dissection for lower limb malignant melanoma. *Br J Surg* **74**, 1023–6

Koh, W-S., Chiu, M., Stelzer, K. J. *et al.* (1993) Femoral vessel depth and the implications for groin node radiation. *Int J Radiat Oncol Biol Phys* **27**(4), 969–74

Krupp, P. J. (1992) in: Coppleson, M. (Ed.). *Gynecologic Oncology*, 2nd edn, Chapter 27, pp. 489–90. Edinburgh: Churchill Livingstone

Milton, G. W., Shaw, H. M. and McCarthy, W. H. (1985) Resection margins for melanoma. *Aust NZ J Surg* **55**, 225–8

Monaghan, J. M. (1987) Vulvar carcinoma: the case for individualisation of treatment. *Bailliére's Clin Obstet Gynaecol* **1**(2), 263–76

Monaghan, J. M. (1990) in: J. H. Shepherd and J. M. Monaghan (Eds.). *Clinical Gynaecological Oncology*, 2nd edn, p. 143. Oxford: Blackwell Science Ltd

Nigro, N. D., Vaitkevicius, V.K. and Considine, B. (1974) Combined therapy for cancer of the anal canal. A preliminary report. *Dis Colon Rectum* **27**, 354–6

Ogunbiyi, O. A., Scholefeld, J. H., Robertson, G. et al. (1994) Anal human virus infection and squamous norplasia in patients with invasive cancer. *Obstet Gynecol* **83**, 212–16

Petereit, D. G., Mehta, M. P., Buchler, D. A. and Kinsella, T. J. (1993) Inguinofemoral radiation of NO, N1 vulvar cancer may be equivalent to lymphadenectomy if proper radiation. *Int J Radiat Oncol Biol Phys* **27**(4), 963– 7

Phillips, G. I., Bundy, B. N., Okagaki, T., Kucera, P. R. and Stenham, F. B. (1994) Malignant melanoma of the vulva treated by radical hemivulvectomy. A prospective study of the Gynecologic Oncology Group. *Cancer* **73**, 2626–32

Pintor, M. P., Northover, J. M. A. and Nicholls, R. J. (1989) Squamous cell carcinoma of the anus at one hospital from 1948 to 1984. *Br J Surg* **76**, 806–10

Piura, B., Masotina, A., Murdoch, J. B. et al. (1993) Recurrent squamous cell carcinoma of the vulva: a study of 73 cases. *Gynecol Oncol* **48**(2), 189–95

Podczaski, E., Sexton, M., Kaminski, P. et al. (1990) Recurrent carcinoma of the vulva after conservative treatment for 'microinvasive' disease. *Gynecol Oncol* **39**, 65–8

Rotmensch, J., Rubin, S. J., Sutton, H. G. et al. (1990) Preoperative radiotherapy followed by radical vulvectomy with inguinal lymphadenectomy for advanced vulvar carcinomas. *Gynecol Oncol* **36**, 181–4

Scheistroen, M. and Trope, C. (1993) Combined bleomycin and irradiation in preoperative treatment of advanced squamous cell carcinoma vulva. *Acta Oncol* **36**, 181–4

Schlienger, M., Krzisch, C., Pene, F. et al. (1989) Epidermoid carcinoma of the anal canal: treatment results and prognostic variables in a series of 242 cases. *Int J Rad Oncol Biol Physics* **17**(6), 1141–51

Scott, R. N. and McKay, A. J. (1993). Elective lymph node dissection in management of malignant melanoma. *Br J Surg* **80**, 284–8

Slevin, N. J. and Pointon, R. C. S. (1989) Radical radiotherapy for carcinoma of the vulva. *Br J Radiol* **62**, 145–7

Stehman, F. B., Bundy, B. N., Dvoretsky, P. M. and Creasman, W. T. (1992) Early stage 1 carcinoma of the vulva treated with ipsilateral superficial inguinal lymphadenectomy and modified radical hemivulvectomy: a prospective study of the Gynecologic Oncology Group. *Obstet Gynecol* **79**(4), 490–7

Stehman, F. B., Bundy, B. N., Thomas, G. et al. (1992) Groin dissection versus groin radiation in carcinoma of the vulva: a Gynaecological Oncology Group Study. *Int J Radiat Oncol Biol Phys* **24**(2), 389–96

Taussig, F. J. (1940) Cancer of the vulva. An analysis of 155 cases (1911–1940). *Am J Obstet Gynecol* **40**, 764–79

Veronesi, U., Adams, J., Bandiera, D. C. et al. (1982) Delayed regional lymph node dissection in stage I melanoma of the skin of the lower extremities. *Cancer* **49**, 2420–30

Way, S. (1960) Carcinoma of the vulva. *Am J Obstet Gynecol* **79**, 692–8

Wharton, J. T., Gallager, S. and Rutledge, F. N. (1974) Microinvasive carcinoma of the vulva. *Am J Obstet Gynecol* **118**(2), 159–62

Whitaker, S. J., Kirkbridge, P., Arnott, S. J., Hudson, C. N. and Shepherd, J. H. (1990) A pilot study of chemoradiotherapy in advanced carcinoma of the vulva. *Br J Obstet Gynaecol* **97**, 436–42

Zafar, N., Paterson, M. E. L. and Murdoch, J. B. (1995) Lymphoedema complicating radical therapy for gynaecological cancer. *Obstet Gynaecol Today* **6**(2), 9–10

# 27

# Cervical carcinoma

*Sean Kehoe and Mahmood Shafi*

On a worldwide basis, cervical carcinoma is the most common gynaecological tumour and is responsible for 500,000 cases annually. Most women (75%) in developed countries present with early stage disease, while 75% of those in underdeveloped countries present with advanced disease. The overall five-year survival is approximately 60% (Petterson 1991). Prevention by cytological screening can reduce mortality as indicated by the recent figures in the United Kingdom. This has shown a fall in annual deaths from over 2000 in the 1980s to under 1400 in 1993–1994, which is partly due to the cytological screening programme (see Figure 1) (Sasieni, Cuzick and Farmery 1995). Indeed, the programme continues to improve with 85.7% of target population screened at least once in the previous five years. The management of cervical cancer consists primarily of surgery and/or radiotherapy, although chemotherapy can also play a role.

## PRESENTATION

Classically, cervical carcinoma is associated with postcoital bleeding, although any abnormal vaginal bleeding/offensive discharge should raise the suspicion of malignancy. Abnormal vaginal bleeding in pregnancy may also be due to a cervical cancer and the cervix should be inspected. Occult disease tends to be first encountered during cytological screening and is subsequently confirmed by histology, while patients with more advanced disease involving local structures present with ureteric obstruction fistulae, renal failure, pain and weight loss.

## DIAGNOSIS

A full history and clinical examination is required. Careful inspection of the cervix will often reveal abnormalities which are suspicious of, or are obviously, malignant. At colposcopy abnormal vasculature and severe acetowhite changes are suggestive of early invasive disease (Figures 2 and 3). All cases of suspected malignancy must be confirmed by histology (Figure 4).

## STAGING

The purposes of staging are to:

(1) Aid the clinician in planning treatment;

(2) Give some indication of prognosis;

(3) Assist in evaluation of results of treatment;

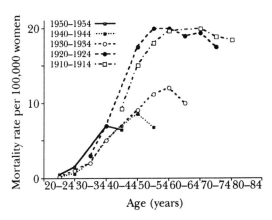

**Figure 1** *The age-specific mortality rates by birth cohort in England and Wales between 1950 and 1994. (Reproduced from Sasieni, P., Cuzick, J. and Farmery, E. (1995) Accelerated decline in cervical mortality in England and Wales. Lancet **346**, 1566–7, with permission from the Lancet Ltd)*

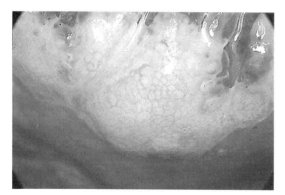

**Figure 2** *Acetowhite changes consistent with cervical intraepithelial neoplasia and mosaic vascular pattern*

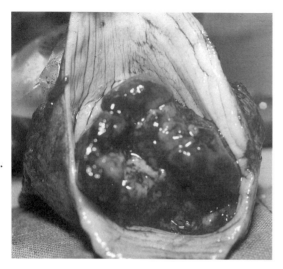

**Figure 3** *Surgical specimen showing bulky cervical carcinoma with clear excision margins*

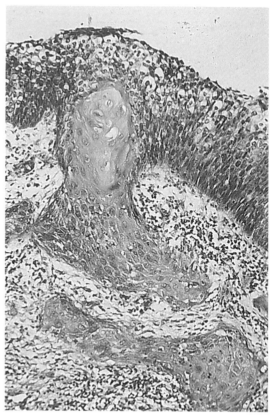

**Figure 4** *Cervical intraepithelial neoplasia (CIN) 3 with focus of early invasion*

(4) Facilitate exchange of information between treatment centres; and

(5) Contribute to the continuing investigation of human cancer.

Of these the first must be the most important reason. Examination under anaesthesia, cystoscopy, sigmoidoscopy, chest X-ray, intravenous urogram and relevant tissue biopsies are procedures allowed for staging. A combined rectovaginal examination is imperative for adequate assessment of the parametrial tissues. Other investigations such as computerised axial tomography (CAT) or magnetic resonance imaging (MRI) scans can be helpful, but presently do not form part of the staging process. Recently, staging has been modified and this primarily affects early disease (Table 1).

## HISTOLOGY

While the majority of tumours are squamous (85–90%), between 5–10% are adenocarcinomas. Rarer histological types include clear cell, small cell, lymphomas and sarcomas.

## MANAGEMENT

### Surgery

*Limited procedure*

The objective of surgery is to excise the malignancy with adequate clear margins. Therefore, the extent of surgery depends on the tumour volume. If disease is very localised (stage IA1) a cone biopsy may suffice. Obviously, the biopsy

**Table 1**  *FIGO staging of cervical carcinoma*

| | |
|---|---|
| *Stage I:* | The carcinoma is strictly confined to the cervix (extension to the corpus should be disregarded) |
| stage IA | Invasive cancer identified only microscopically. Invasion is limited to measured stromal invasion with a maximum depth of 5 mm and no wider than 7 mm |
| stage IA1 | Measured invasion of stroma no greater than 3 mm in depth and no wider than 7 mm |
| stage IA2 | Measured invasion of stroma greater than 4 mm and no greater than 5 mm in depth and no wider than 7 mm |
| stage IB | Clinical lesions confined to the cervix or preclinical lesions greater than IA all gross lesions, even with superficial invasion |
| stage IB1 | Clinical lesions no greater than 4 cm in size |
| stage IB2 | Clinical lesions greater than 4 cm in size |
| *Stage II:* | The carcinoma extends beyond the cervix, but has not extended on to the pelvic side wall. The carcinoma involves the vagina, but not as far as the lower one-third |
| stage IIA | No obvious parametrial involvement |
| stage IIB | Obvious parametrial involvement |
| *Stage III:* | The carcinoma has extended to the pelvic wall. On rectal examination here is no cancer free space between the tumour and the pelvic wall. The tumour involves the lower one-third of the vagina. All cases with hydronephrosis or non-functioning kidney should be included, unless they are known to be due to other cause |
| stage IIIA | No extension on to the pelvic wall, but involvement of the lower one-third of the vagina |
| stage IIIB | Extension on to the pelvic wall or hydronephrosis or non-functioning kidney |
| *Stage IV:* | The carcinoma has extended beyond the true pelvis or has clinically involved the mucosa of the bladder or the rectum |
| stage IVA | Spread of the growth to adjacent organs |
| stage IVB | Spread to distant organs |

confirms both disease stage and adequacy of management in this case. The biopsy may be performed by a diathermy loop excision (LLETZ) or knife cone. Both are acceptable, although the knife cone has the advantage of facilitating histological assessment by avoiding diathermy artefact at the edges of the specimen. Alternatively, stage IA1 may be treated by a simple hysterectomy. Pelvic nodal involvement in this stage is rare (< 1%). An exception to the rule of conservatism is stage IA1 adenocarcinomas. In this case, it is recognised that 'skip' lesions occur, so while margins may be clear on the cone, this does not exclude the presence of further disease above the level of biopsy. A greater understanding of this disease's natural history may in the future permit more conservative interventions.

## More radical hysterectomy

Beyond this, the standard operation is a Wertheim's hysterectomy. This is performed up to stage IIA. The major differences between this and a simple hysterectomy are ligation of the uterine arteries at their origin, identification of the ureter to its bladder insertion, excision of paracervical tissue and vaginal cuff along with pelvic lymphadenectomy. Para-aortic node sampling is not routinely performed, but should happen if more advanced or bulky disease is present with a suspicion of either pelvic or para-aortic node secondaries.

Occasionally, disease spread will be more extensive than detected at examination under anaesthesia. Obvious involvement of other intra-abdominal organs or para-aortic nodes should be managed by appropriate sampling, and disease distribution noted. The planned hysterectomy should be abandoned. There is some evidence suggesting that excision of large positive nodes may enhance survival as radiotherapy often fails to eliminate disease in masses > 5 cm in diameter (Hacker, Wain and Nicklin 1995). Properly randomised studies are needed to confirm whether any benefit truely exists.

One scenario to be avoided is the 'failed hysterectomy' (i.e. a subtotal hysterectomy). This does not benefit the patient, makes adjuvant radiotherapy more difficult and increases morbidity. Therefore, the parametrial tissues should be palpated at laparotomy. If doubt still exists as to the parametrial tumour extension, the relevant tissues planes should be dissected and the area inspected. The operation should be abandoned if it is judged that surgery is impossible. Embarking on the hysterectomy prior to assessing parametrial spread is often the reason for a subtotal hysterectomy.

### Oophorectomy

In peri- or postmenopausal women routine bilateral oophorectomy (BSO) is recommended and many would advocate BSO in women over 40 years. In the younger patient and in those with squamous carcinomas, where ovarian secondaries are rare, the ovaries can be preserved. However, with adenocarcinomas between 1.7% (Sutton *et al.* 1992) and 5.3% (Aida *et al.* 1992) of stage IB carcinomas will have metastases in the ovaries so some consider routine BSO appropriate. Similarly, in patients considered to be at high risk of needing adjuvant radiotherapy, BSO can be performed. Although it is possible to transpose the ovaries out of the radiation field, this does not guarantee continued function or lack of radiation damage (Feeney *et al.* 1995). It should also be remembered that 3–7% of patients will return with ovarian problems requiring surgical intervention (Parker *et al.* 1993; Feeney *et al.* 1995). The psychological distress caused to the patient with residual ovarian problems must be considered and appropriate counselling and advice is important.

### Hormonal replacement therapy

There is no indication that hormone replacement therapy (HRT) influences survival in patients treated for cervical cancer. There is a theoretical possibility that HRT may adversely influence growth/recurrence of some adenocarcinomas, although this is not evidence based. Even so, there is no fixed rule and each case must be dealt with separately. If survival prospects are poor and menopausal symptoms are interfering with the patient's quality of life, then withholding HRT may not be appropriate.

### During pregnancy

This is rare, only occurring in approximately one in 10,000 pregnancies. The general consensus is to manage the disease in a similar manner to a non-pregnant patient. Embarking on cone biopsy is more difficult due to increased blood supply, and a wedge biopsy may be an easier alternative. In early pregnancy, a Wertheim's procedure can be performed without a need to undertake a termination. If the pregnancy is at a stage where the fetus is viable, then a Wertheim's which includes a Caesarean should be performed. The general rule is that a six-week interval from diagnosis to intervention is acceptable, which means that delay can be considered in those from 22–23 weeks pregnancy with a good chance of fetal viability. Such suggestions are not strict because the disease stage and, indeed, the patient's wishes, must be taken into account. It would seem that outcome is comparable to non-pregnant patients, whichever approach is taken (Duggan *et al.* 1993).

### Fertility preservation

As already discussed earlier in this chapter, a loop cone biopsy may suffice and permit retention of fertility for stage IA1 squamous carcinomas. Another procedure which can be undertaken is a radical trachelectomy, but only once it is confirmed that the pelvic nodes are negative. This entails excision of the cervix with the application of a prophylactic cerclage at the isthmus to prevent abortion. Unfortunately, the series reported is small and their follow-up short (Dargent and Mathevet 1995). Successful pregnancies to term have been achieved, but a proper evaluation of this approach is required before any recommendations can be made. Until such time, the authors cannot confidently advocate the procedure as part of routine care. Even so, in exceptionally rare cases it may be an option for consideration.

## Laparoscopic procedures

The increased enthusiasm for minimal access surgery has inevitably resulted in their use to perform Wertheim's hysterectomies or modifications such as the Schauta procedure (Dargent and Mathevet 1995). In expert hands such procedures are feasible. However, comparative studies between the laparoscopic approach and standard operations have not been undertaken and while the techniques are well described in the literature, it should be noted than many patients treated laparoscopically are exposed to preoperative caesium (Canis *et al.* 1995). This not only confounds the reliability of the results, but ignores a major objective of surgery in avoiding radiotherapy and reducing problems of sexual dysfunction in a proportion of patients. Interestingly, the main advantages of earlier discharge from hospital do not seem to be obvious as the average hospital stay is approximately 7 days. The question to answer is not 'can we do this procedure laparoscopically', but 'should we be doing this procedure laparoscopically'.

## Radiotherapy

Radiotherapy forms the primary intervention for patients with advanced inoperable disease, patients deemed unsuitable for surgery because of concomitant medical conditions, or in situations where surgical expertise is not available. It is also given as adjuvant therapy in those with positive lymph nodes, a tumour close to excision margins or a tumour with a high-risk of recurrence (Thomas and Stehman 1994).

Planned combinations of radiotherapy and surgery are not advocated as this increases morbidity with no attendant gain in cure, or survival rates. As a general rule, external beam therapy delivers 45 Gy to point 'A' which, with the addition of intracavitary brachytherapy, gives a total dose to point 'A' of around 75 Gy. However, the use of modern after-loading techniques with the Selectron reduces both the patient morbidity and exposure of staff.

There are no controlled studies showing improved survival with postoperative pelvic radiation following radical surgery in the presence of positive pelvic nodes. Multiple reports do suggest that, although it does not significantly impact on survival, it does improve pelvic control rates, especially in those considered at high risk of central relapse. Most centres use primary radiation therapy for lesions > 3–4 cm in diameter. Some continue to use primary surgery and most are then given adjuvant pelvic radiation therapy. However, not only are there no data to support that this latter approach gives better control of central disease than radiation therapy alone, but the attendant morbidity may be higher when surgery and radiotherapy are used together.

Extending the field of radiotherapy to include treatment of positive para-aortic lymph nodes is also performed. Again, controlled studies have not been performed, but the available data does suggest some improvement in survival, although at the expense of increased morbidity (Rutledge 1988). Further investigation is required in this area.

## Chemotherapy

Agents with known cytotoxic activity in cervical carcinoma include platinum compounds (cisplatin or carboplatin), bleomycin, ifosfamide, mitomcyin C and vincristine. Clinical trials employing these and other agents indicate higher response rates (up to 60% or more) associated with platinum-containing regimens, with single agent cisplatin and ifosfamide being most effective (Sausville and Young 1986; Young 1987; Thigpen, Lambuth and Vance 1992). Whether survival is enhanced by chemoradiotherapy is presently unknown.

## Follow-up

Routine follow-up of patients normally consists of hospital visits every three to four months for the first three years and then six-monthly thereafter, up to five years. Most (90%) of patients relapse within three years of the initial diagnosis. Manifestations of relapse can be vaginal bleeding/discharge, renal failure, bone pain or a palpable mass in the vaginal vault on examination. Over 80% of patients will have symptoms associated with relapse (Tinga *et al.* 1992).

As part of clinical examination on follow-up, the supraclavicular nodes should be palpated as this is a recognised site for recurrence. A vaginal and rectal examination is also required. Patients exposed to radiotherapy may have radiation effects resulting in a 'frozen pelvis' making clinical examination difficult. In such cases CAT/MRI scans are helpful.

## Vault smears

In cases where cervical intraepithelial neoplasia was present at the resection edges, there is a risk of residual preinvasive disease at the vaginal vault. These patients should undergo vault smears at six and 12 months postoperatively and, if these are negative, three-yearly smears are performed. Whether such screening prevents vault carcinoma or impacts on outcome is unknown. It may be justified by using the premise for cervical screening.

Routine vault smears for all patients is advocated by some. Their value is questionable. Prior radiotherapy can give false-positive results or make smears uninterpretable. The impact of routine vault or cervical smears on patient outcome has not been addressed adequately, and are often negative in the presence of recurrent disease (Cary *et al.* 1992).

## Recurrent disease

Intervention cannot be contemplated without histological evidence of recurrence. For example, ureteric obstruction in most cases is caused by recurrent disease, although in a proportion of patients is due to benign retroperitoneal fibrosis secondary to radiotherapy (Parliament *et al.* 1989). Central recurrences are most common and easily biopsied vaginally. Occasionally, a laparotomy may be required to obtain a tissue specimen.

### Surgery

Exenterative procedures aim to cure women with recurrent cervical carcinoma, although these are only suitable in selected patients. Symptoms of sciatica, leg oedema, ureteric obstruction or obvious distant metastases are contraindications to such operations. It is also important to ensure that the patient can psychologically cope with the consequences of surgery. The most radical procedure results in excision of the vagina, bladder and rectum with a colostomy and urinary ileal conduit. Even with available reconstructive surgery, some patients may not consider this acceptable for their quality of life. The importance of counselling cannot be overemphasised.

Other surgical procedures may be possible with preservation of organs, depending on tumour involvement. The bowel and rectum are preserved in anterior, and bladder in posterior, exenterations. It is imperative that extrapelvic disease is excluded prior to surgery. Preoperative evaluation should include a chest X-ray, intravenous urogram and ultrasound of the abdomen and pelvis and relevant blood tests to rule out distant disease. Today, most would also use CAT or MRI scans in preoperative evaluation. Although these investigations may indicate localised pelvic disease, at operation the first step is sampling of the para-aortic nodes, which are sent for frozen section. If these prove positive, then the operation should be abandoned. The patient should be made aware of this possibility, along with the fact that there is a significant morbidity and mortality (5–10%). With properly selected patients, a five year survival of up to 50% is achievable, which is excellent considering this is treating recurrent disease. Poorer outcome is associated with older patients (greater than 69 years), recurrent tumour within three years, persistent primary tumour and positive resection margins (Shepherd *et al.* 1994).

### Radiotherapy

Patients with relapsed disease who have previously completed a full course of radiotherapy are usually not suitable for further therapy. In patients who have not previously completed a full course or have a long time interval from primary exposure, repeated radiotherapy can achieve reasonable response rates (Prempree *et al.* 1984). Successful outcome with radiotherapy in previously treated patients is reported, although this is confined to highly selected cases (Russell *et al.* 1987). It does have a role in alleviating metastatic bone pain or bleeding from a vaginal vault recurrences.

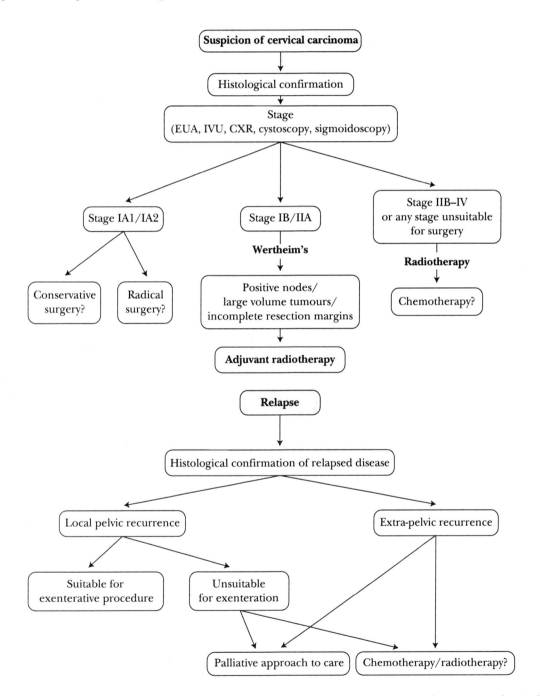

**Figure 5** *A flow chart showing the management options available to a woman presenting with a suspicion of cervical carcinoma. EUA, examination under anaesthesia; IVU, intravenous urogram; CXR, chest X-ray*

## Chemotherapy

The choice of agents has already been mentioned. Failure to respond to an initial course of chemotherapy, particularly platin- or ifosfamide-containing regimens, means there is little chance of achieving any response by changing to other agents. A palliative approach to care is then appropriate, although any novel agents should be considered and discussed with the patient.

## Palliation

Palliative care is an active rather than passive process. The primary objective is to relieve or control any symptoms affecting the patient's quality of life, while maintaining the patient's dignity. Vaginal vault tumours can cause distress through bleeding or malodorous discharge. Metronidazole can reduce the odour, and hydrogen peroxide packs or radiotherapy any bleeding. Pain caused by bone secondaries may be alleviated by radiotherapy, although neuralgic pain analgesics (tablets or local anaesthetic blocks) and steroids are helpful. Diversionary procedures should be considered for those with vesicovaginal or rectovaginal fistulae. Occasionally, non-intervention is best, as in some patients presenting with renal failure. The use of percutaneous nephrostomies to overcome this problem must be carefully considered as it may prevent a humane form of death (Kehoe *et al.* 1993).

## SUMMARY

It is welcome to see that death from cervical carcinoma is decreasing in England and Wales, and that the cervical cytology programme is having an effect. Even so, the disease incidence is static, and correct management important. Unresolved issues include surgery in those with a high risk of adjuvant radiotherapy versus radiotherapy alone, surgical debulking of large nodes and the benefits of chemotherapy. Also the use of laparoscopic procedures requires defining, although the onus for this is with those who advocate such operations. The present management of cervical carcinoma is depicted in Figure 5.

As many patients require therapy beyond surgery, the multidisciplinary team approach is important. The implementation of the Calman report in cancer services should eventually ensure that all patients are treated in hospitals where such expert teams are available (Department of Health 1995). As indicated by research into other cancers, this will hopefully further improve survival patterns.

# References

Aida, H., Kodama, S., Aoki, Y. *et al.* (1992) The study of ovarian metastases in uterine cancer. *Acta Obstet Gynecol Jpn* **44**, 315–322.

Canis, M., Mage, G., Pouly, J. L. *et al.* (1995) Laparoscopic radical hysterectomy for cervical cancer. *Bailliére's Clin Obstet Gynaecol* **9**(4), 675–81

Cary, A., Free, K. E., Wright, R. G. and Shield, P. W. (1992) Carcinoma of the cervix – recurrences in Queensland 1982–1986. *Int J Gynecol Cancer* **2**, 207–14

Dargent, D. and Mathevet, P. (1995) Schauta's vaginal hystetectomy combined with laparoscopic lymphadenectomy. *Bailliére's Clin Obstet Gynaecol* **9**(4), 691–701

Department of Health (1995) *A Policy Framework for Commissioning Cancer Services. Guidance for Purchasers and Providers of Cancer Services*, EL ('95) 51. London: Department of Health

Duggan, B., Muderspach, L. I., Roman, L. D. *et al.* (1993) Cervical cancer in pregnancy: reporting on planned delayed therapy. *Obstet Gynecol* **82**, 598–602

Feeney, D. D., Moore, D. H., Look, K. Y., Stehman, F. B. and Sutton, G. B. (1995) The fate of ovaries after radical hysterectomy and ovarian transposition. *Gynecol Oncol* **56**, 3–7.

Hacker, N. F., Wain, G. V. and Nicklin, J. L. (1995) Resection of bulky positive lymph nodes in patients with cervical carcinoma. *Int J Gynecol Cancer* **5**, 250–6

Kehoe, S., Luesley, D., Budden, J. and Earl, H. (1993) Percutaneous nephrostomies in women with cervical cancer. *Br J Obstet Gynaecol* **100**, 283–4

Parker, M., Bosscher, J., Barnhill, D. and Park, R. (1993) Ovarian management during radical hysterectomy in the pre-menopausal patient. *Obstet Gynecol* **82**, 187–90

Parliament, M., Genest, P., Girard, A., Berig, L. and Prefontaine, M. (1989) Obstructive uropathy following radiation therapy for carcinoma of the cervix. *Gynecol Oncol* **33**, 237–40

Petterson, F. (Ed.) (1991) Annual report on the results of treatment in gynecological cancer. *Int J Gynecol Obstet* **21**, 27–130

Prempree, T., Amornmarn, R., Villasanta, U., Kwon, T. and Scott, R. M. (1984) Retreatment of very late recurrent invasive squamous cell carcinoma of the cervix with irradiation. *Cancer* **54**, 1950–5

Russell, A. H., Koh, W.-J., Markette, K. *et al.* (1987) Radical reirradiation for recurrent or second primary carcinoma of the female reproductive tract. *Gynecol Oncol* **27**, 226–32

Rutledge, F. N. (1988) Management of para-aortic nodal metastases from carcinoma of the cervix. *Baillière's Clin Obstet Gynaecol* **2**(4), 921–31

Sasieni, P., Cuzick, J. and Farmery, E. (1995) Accelerated decline in cervical cancer mortality in England and Wales. *Lancet* **346**, 1566–7

Sausville, E. A. and Young, R. C. (1986) 'Gynecologic malignancies' in: Pindeo, H. M. and Chabner, B. A. (Eds.). *Cancer Chemotherapy Annual 8*, pp. 442–445. Amsterdam: Elsevier Science Publishers BV

Shepherd, J. H., Ngan, H. Y. S., Neven, P. *et al.* (1994) Multivariate analysis of factors affecting survival in pelvic exenteration. *Int J Gynecol Cancer* **4**, 361–70

Sutton, G. P., Bundy, B. N., Delgado, G. *et al.* (1992) Ovarian metastases in stage IB carcinoma of the cervix: a Gynecologic Oncology Group study. *Am J Obstet Gynecol* **166**, 50–3

Thigpen, T., Lambuth, B. W. and Vance, R. B. (1992) The role of ifosfamide in gynecologic cancer. *Semin Oncol* **19** (Suppl. 1), 30–4

Thomas, G. M. and Stehman, F. B. (1994) Early invasive disease: risk assessment and management. *Semin Oncol* **21**, 17–24

Tinga, D. J., Bouma, J., Boonstra, H. and Aaldres, J. G. (1992) Symptomatology, localization and treatment of recurrent cervical carcinoma. *Int J Gynecol Cancer* **2**, 179–88

Young, R. C. (1987) 'Gynecologic malignancies' in: Pindeo, H. M., Longo, D. L. and Chabner, B. A. (Eds.). *Cancer Chemotherapy and Biological Response Modifiers*, Annual 9. Amsterdam: Elsevier Science Publishers BV

# 28

# The first trimester of pregnancy: new developments and current controversies

*James R. Scott*

The first trimester of pregnancy has received relatively little attention until recently. Measures to prevent early pregnancy wastage and to assess the effectiveness of diagnostic tests and treatment regimens were previously poorly investigated or largely ignored. However, the molecular events responsible for successful implantation and growth of the conceptus are presently under intense investigation. Moreover, with modern sonographic techniques it is now possible to view the conceptus very early in pregnancy. Embryonic heart motion can be detected with vaginal ultrasound by six weeks' gestation. When embryonic or fetal viability is confirmed during the first trimester, the chance of a live birth is greater than 95% (van Leewan, Branch and Scott 1993).

## SPORADIC EARLY PREGNANCY LOSS

Early pregnancy loss is the most common complication of human pregnancy, and up to 75% of pregnancies never advance past the first trimester (Boklage 1990). Most of these losses are unrecognised and occur before or with the expected next menses (Wilcox *et al.* 1988). About 15–20% are spontaneous abortions (miscarriages) or ectopic pregnancies diagnosed after clinical recognition of pregnancy. In the United States alone, at least one million of the six million pregnancies each year are lost in the first trimester (Carson and Buster 1993; Fraser,

Grimes and Schultz 1993). These losses occur at the rate of 114 cases every hour and result in substantial physical pain, grief, medical expense and absenteeism.

The majority of single sporadic spontaneous abortions are due to non-repetitive intrinsic defects in the developing conceptus (e.g. genetic abnormalities and defective implantation or placentation). Types of early pregnancy loss include *anembryonic* pregnancy (gestational sac with failure of a detectable embryo to develop), *embryonic* loss (fertilisation through the ninth postmenstrual week of gestation), and *fetal* death (> 10 postmenstrual weeks of gestation). Early sonographic detection of fetal abnormalities is also a promising new area as evidenced by nuchal translucency as a marker for chromosome abnormality (Nicolaides *et al.* 1992).

Most otherwise healthy women do not need an extensive evaluation because of one miscarriage, but all patients deserve explanation, sympathy and emotional support. It is often comforting to couples when they understand the favourable prognosis for future pregnancies. Approximately 80–90% of women with a single spontaneous abortion will deliver a viable live infant in the next pregnancy (Boue, Boue and Lazar 1975; Regan 1988). The likelihood of a successful pregnancy is highest if the woman has previously had one or more live births, and it is modestly reduced in women over the age of 35 years.

## RECURRENT EARLY PREGNANCY LOSS

Up to 5% of all couples attempting pregnancy suffer two consecutive miscarriages, 1% experience three or more consecutive miscarriages, and 1% experience three or more consecutive losses (Coulam 1991). Many controversies surrounding first-trimester pregnancy events involve potential immunological aspects of recurrent miscarriage. Uncertainties regarding aetiology and prevention are two reasons that recurrent pregnancy loss (RPL) remains a particularly frustrating problem for both physicians and patients. Although RPL has been well publicised in the news media and lay press (Beck and Wickelgren 1988; Brody 1992), some articles are misleading and encourage couples to seek unproven diagnostic tests and treatments. Recommendations in the medical literature are also conflicting and have done little to clarify the situation.

### Evaluation

It is generally agreed that a work-up is indicated in most patients after three consecutive miscarriages and in some women over 35 years with one to two miscarriages. Classically, maternal genetic, anatomical and hormonal factors have been most frequently implicated. Even these are coming under closer scrutiny because treatments advocated are empirical, have not been submitted to controlled trials, and are not totally successful. The evidence for infections, unrecognised diabetes, toxic agents or psychological trauma as significant aetiological factors is even more tenuous.

A variety of new diagnostic tests for RPL are continually being proposed to replace those that have been disproved and discarded over the years. It is usually claimed that the abnormal test is associated with a higher risk for early pregnancy loss. Those in vogue at present include antithyroid antibodies (Stagnero-Green *et al.* 1990), elevated follicular phase luteinising hormone (LH) levels (Regan, Owen and Jacobs 1990), circulating maternal embryotoxic factor (Hill *et al.* 1992)

and abnormal CD lymphocyte subset ratios such as elevated CD56+ levels (Coulam *et al.* 1995). It is beyond the scope of this chapter to critically analyse each assay, but the mechanism of pregnancy loss and potential relationship to each of these expensive laboratory assays remains largely theoretical. Until effective treatments are identified and proven by properly designed studies, these screening tests have little utility in the routine evaluation of patients with RPL.

### Autoimmune

Antiphospholipid syndrome (APS) has been recognised as a proven cause of RPL for about a decade (Silver and Branch 1994). Approximately 5% of women with RPL have lupus anticoagulant (LA), anticardiolipin (aCL), or both. Low levels of immunoglobulin (Ig)G aCL or IgM aCL often represent non-specific binding and are of questionable significance (Silver *et al.* 1996). There is little evidence that autoantibodies other than LA or aCL contribute to the diagnosis or management of patients with autoimmune RPL (Ober *et al.* 1993; Cowchock and Fort 1994).

The most important finding in these patients is the high rate of late first- or second-trimester death of a fetus determined to have cardiac activity, and 30–40% of the pregnancy losses occur after 13 weeks' gestation (Branch and Scott 1992). Patients with high levels of antiphospholipid antibodies or a history of prior fetal death are at the greatest risk of another fetal loss.

Clear-cut therapeutic recommendations are difficult because of differences in inclusion criteria between studies and the lack of controlled trials. At present, heparin with low-dose aspirin appears to be the most effective and safest treatment (Cowchock *et al.* 1992; Kutteh 1996). Concomitant use of corticosteroids and heparin is not recommended, because this combination has not been shown to be better than either alone in achieving a live birth, and severe osteoporosis with fractures has occurred in women with this combination regimen (Branch and Scott 1991). The use of high-dose intravenous immunoglobulin (IVIG) has also generated interest, due to anecdotal reports of successful pregnancy outcomes with lowered aPL levels, but no controlled trials have been performed (Scott *et al.* 1988; Spinnato *et al.* 1995).

## Unexplained

The majority of recurrent miscarriage patients have no discernable cause uncovered with a standard evaluation. With this in mind, reproductive immunologists have long suggested that allogeneic factors play a role in pregnancy loss based largely on experimental animal models. Not all evidence favours an alloimmune pathogenesis for recurrent miscarriage, and extrapolation from animal models to the human situation can be misleading because of interspecies endocrine, immunological, anatomical and reproductive differences. Since the mechanisms that allow a mother to tolerate her semi-allogeneic conceptus are incompletely understood, it is still difficult to assess to what extent immunological factors are responsible for reproductive failure.

Early reports proposed that HLA compatibility between couples, the absence of maternal leucocytotoxic antibodies or the absence of maternal blocking antibodies were related to recurrent pregnancy loss. The importance of these factors has not been substantiated, and these expensive tests are no longer clinically indicated (Scott, Rote and Branch 1987; Smith and Cowchock 1988; Coulam 1992). Investigators are focusing on local decidual/trophoblast immunosuppressive factors, but currently there are no practical clinical tests available for these.

Although an alloimmune mechanism has yet to be unequivocally identified, a number of medical centres around the world offer leucocyte immunisation regimens as treatment for RPL. The most popular regimen involves maternal immunisation with husband's leucocytes. The efficacy of this treatment has often been questioned, because of the reasonable chance for a successful pregnancy even without treatment (Scott 1989).

When data from prospective randomised trials were combined in a recent meta-analysis, there appeared to be a slight benefit to leucocyte immunisation (Figure 1). The live birth

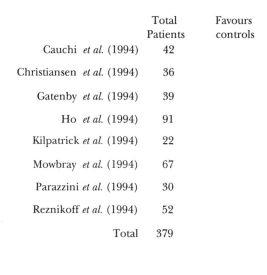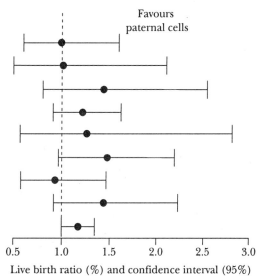

**Figure 1** *Live birth rates following paternal cell immunisation in prospective randomised trials. These results are from analysis of individual data sheets for each patient obtained from each investigator. (Reproduced from Scott, J. R. and Branch, D. W. (1994) Potential factors and immunotherapy in recurrent miscarriage.* Clin Obstet Gynecol *37, 761–7, with permission of J. B. Lippincott Co.)*

rates were 68% for immunised versus 61% for control patients (Scott *et al.* 1994). To put this into perspective clinically, 13 patients have to be immunised to achieve one additional live birth. Moreover, calculation of the overall success rate and whether treatment is statistically better than no treatment depends on how the meta-analysis is performed (Jeng, Scott and Burmeister 1995). Due to the questionable efficacy as well as risks and costs with immunotherapy, it seems most appropriate to conduct this treatment as part of ongoing research protocols.

Intravenous immune globulin has been proposed as an alternative therapy in patients with unexplained pregnancy loss. The results of three controlled trials are conflicting and not dramatically different than leucocyte immunisation (Mueller-Eckhardt for the German RSA/IVIG Group 1994; Christiansen *et al.* 1995; Coulam *et al.* 1995). Due to the equivocal results and high cost, IVIG offers little apparent advantage over paternal cell immunisation.

## THE FUTURE

Effective treatment awaits better knowledge of the underlying pathophysiology of unexplained RPL. Preliminary studies using molecular genetic techniques suggest that the total genetic contribution to pregnancy loss has been under-estimated (McDonough 1985). As yet undefined subchromosomal genetic abnormalities may interfere with early embryonic and fetal development in the human as has been shown in animals (Figure 2). If there is a subset of women with alloimmune-related RPL, a specific assay to diagnose this condition and a reliable method to determine which patients will and will *not* benefit from immunotherapy are urgently needed.

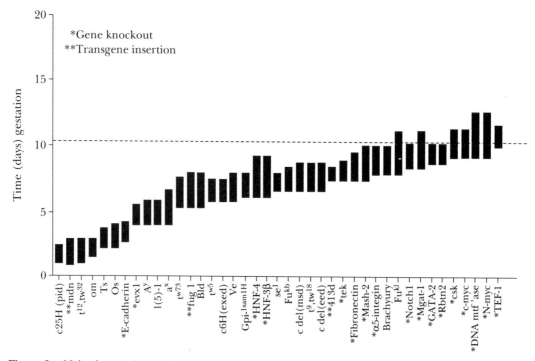

**Figure 2** *Molecular genetic mutations responsible for embryonic and fetal deaths in mice. (Based on a figure appearing in Copp 1995)*

# References

Beck, M. and Wickelgren, I. (1988) Miscarriages. *Newsweek* **Aug. 15**, 46–52

Boklage, C. E. (1990) Survival probability of human conceptions from fertilization to term. *Int J Fertil* **35**, 189–94

Boue, J., Boue, A. and Lazar, P. (1975) Retrospective and prospective epidemiological studies of 1500 karyotyped spontaneous human abortions. *Teratology* **12**, 11–26

Branch, D. W. and Scott, J. R. (1991) 'Clinical implications of anti-phospholipid antibodies: the Utah experience', in: E. N. Harris, T. Exner, G. R. Hughes *et al.* (Eds.). *Phospholipid-binding Antibodies*, pp. 335–46. Boca Raton, CRC Press

Branch, D. W. and Scott, J. R. (1992) 'Immunological aspects of pregnancy loss: Alloimmune and autoimmune considerations', in: E. A. Reece, J. C. Hobbins, J. C. Mahoney *et al.* (Eds.). *Medicine of the Fetus and its Mother*, pp. 217–33. Philadelphia, J. B. Lippincott Co.

Brody, J. (1992) Researchers discover new therapies to avert repeated miscarriages. *New York Times (medical science)* **Dec. 15**

Carson, S. A. and Buster, J. E. (1993) Ectopic pregnancy. *N Engl J Med* **329**, 1174–81

Christiansen, O. B., Mathiesen, O., Husth, M. *et al.* (1995) Placebo-controlled trial of treatment of unexplained secondary recurrent spontaneous abortions and recurrent late spontaneous abortions with i.v. immunoglobulin. *Hum Reprod* **10**, 2690–5

Copp, A. J. (1995) Death before birth: clues from gene knockouts and mutations. *Trends Genet* **11**, 87–93

Coulam, C. B. (1991) Epidemiology of recurrent spontaneous abortion. *Am J Reprod Immunol* **26**, 23–7

Coulam, C. B. (1992) Immunologic tests in the evaluation of reproductive disorders: a critical review. *Am J Obstet Gynecol* **167**, 1844–51

Coulam, C. B., Goodman, C., Roussev, R. G. *et al.* (1995) Systemic CD56+ cells can predict pregnancy outcome. *Am J Reprod Immunol* **33**, 40–6

Coulam, C. B., Krysa, L., Stern, J. *et al.* (1995) Intravenous immunoglobulin for treatment of recurrent pregnancy loss. *Am J Reprod Immunol* **34**, 333–7

Cowchock, F. S. and Fort, J. G. (1994) Can tests for IgA, IgG or IgM antibodies to cardiolipin or phosphatidylserine substitute for lupus anticoagulant assays in screening for antiphospholipid antibodies? *Autoimmunity* **17**, 119–22

Cowchock, F. S., Reece, E. A., Balaban, E. *et al.* (1992) Repeated fetal losses associated with antiphospholipid antibodies: a collaborative randomized trial comparing prednisone with low-dose heparin treatment. *Am J Obstet Gynecol* **166**, 1787–98

Fraser, E. J., Grimes, D. A. and Schultz, K. F. (1993) Immunization for recurrent spontaneous abortion: a review and meta-analysis. *Obstet Gynecol* **82**, 854–9

Hill, J. A., Polgar, K., Harlow, B. L. *et al.* (1992) Evidence of embryo and trophoblast toxic cellular immune response(s) in women with recurrent spontaneous abortion. *Am J Obstet Gynecol* **166**, 1044–52

Jeng, G. T., Scott, J. R., Burmeister, J. F. (1995) A comparison of meta-analytic results using literature vs individual patient data: paternal cell immunization for recurrent miscarriage. *J Am Med Assoc* **274**, 830–4

Kutteh, W. H. (1996) Antiphospholipid antibody-associated recurrent pregnancy loss: treatment with heparin and low dose aspirin is superior to low-dose aspirin alone. *Am J Obstet Gynecol* **174**, 1589–9

McDonough, P. G. (1985) Repeated first-trimester pregnancy loss: evaluation and management. *Am J Obstet Gynecol* **153**, 1–6

Mueller-Eckhardt, G. for the German RSA/IVIG Group (1994) Intravenous immunoglobulin for treatment of recurrent pregnancy loss. *Br J Obstet Gynaecol* **101**, 1072–7

Nicolaides, K. H., Azar, G., Byrne, D. *et al.* (1992) Fetal nuchal translucency: ultrasound screening for chromosomal defects in first trimester of pregnancy. *Br Med J* **303**, 867–9

Ober, C., Karrison, T., Harlow, L. *et al.* (1993) Autoantibodies and pregnancy history in a healthy population. *Am J Obstet Gynecol* **169**, 143–7

Regan, L. (1988) 'A prospective study of spontaneous abortion' in: R. W. Beard and F. Sharp (Eds.). *Early Pregnancy Loss,* pp. 23–37. London: Springer-Verlag

Regan, L., Owen, E. and Jacobs H. S. (1990) Hypersecretion of luteinizing hormone, infertility, and miscarriage. *Lancet* **336**, 1141–4

Scott, J. R. (1989) 'Habitual abortion — recommendations for a reasonable approach to an enigmatic problem' in: M. Soules (Ed.). *Controversies in Reproductive Endocrinology and Infertility,* pp. 95–106. New York: Elsevier

Scott, J. R. and Branch, D. W. (1994) Potential factors and immunotherapy in recurrent miscarriage. *Clin Obstet Gynecol* **37**, 761–7

Scott, J. R., Branch, D. W., Kochenour, N. K. *et al.* (1988) Intravenous immune globulin treatment of pregnant patients with recurrent pregnancy loss due to antiphospholipid antibodies and Rh disease. *Am J Obstet Gynecol* **159**, 1055–7

Scott, J. R., Chalmers, I., Jeng, G. T. *et al.* (1994) Worldwide collaborative observational study and meta-analysis on allogeneic leukocyte immunotherapy for recurrent spontaneous abortion. *Am J Reprod Immunol* **32**, 55–72

Scott, J. R., Rote, N. S. and Branch, D. W. (1987) Immunologic aspects of recurrent abortion and fetal death. *Obstet Gynecol* **70**, 645–56

Silver, R. M. and Branch, D. W. (1994) Recurrent miscarriage: autoimmune considerations. *Clin Obstet Gynecol* **37**, 745–60

Silver, R. M., Porter, T. F., Greenhill, A. E. *et al.* (1996) Anticardiolipin antibodies: clinical consequences of 'low titers'. *Am J Obstet Gynecol* **87**, 494–500

Smith, J. B. and Cowchock, F. S. (1988) Immunological studies in recurrent spontaneous abortion: effects of immunization of women with paternal mononuclear cells on lymphocytotoxic and mixed lymphocyte blocking antibodies and correlation with sharing of HLA and pregnancy outcome. *J Reprod Immunol* **14**, 99–113

Spinnato, J. A., Clark, A. L., Pierangeli, S. S. *et al.* (1995) Intravenous immunoglobulin therapy for the antiphospholipid syndrome in pregnancy. *Am J Obstet Gynecol* **172**, 690–4

Stagnero-Green, A., Roman, S. H., Cobin, R. H. *et al.* (1990) Detection of at-risk pregnancy by means of a highly sensitive assay for thyroid autoantibodies. *J Am Med Assoc* **264**, 1422–5

van Leeuwan, I., Branch, D. W. and Scott, J. R. (1993) First trimester ultrasound findings in women with a history of recurrent pregnancy loss. *Am J Obstet Gynecol* **168**, 111–14

Wilcox, A. J., Weinberg, C.R., O'Connor, J. F. *et al.* (1988) Incidence of early loss of pregnancy. *N Engl J Med* **319**, 189–94

# 29

# First trimester fetal nuchal translucency screening

*Pranav P. Pandya and Sarah Bower*

First trimester nuchal translucency screening is the most recent method of screening for trisomy 21. It is based on the finding that increased fetal nuchal translucency in the first trimester is associated with an increased risk of aneuploidy, and particularly fetal trisomy. The non-invasive nature of this method and its application in the first trimester make it an attractive screening option.

## METHODS OF SCREENING

Screening for fetal trisomy 21 was introduced in the early 1970s, when laboratory techniques were developed for determining fetal karyotype. Initially, screening was based on maternal age and the 'high-risk' women who were offered amniocentesis were aged 37 years or more. This group constituted approximately 5% of the pregnant population, but contributed only 20–30% of the chromosomally abnormal babies. Not surprisingly, screening on the basis of maternal age has not resulted in a substantial fall in the proportion of infants born with these conditions (Cuckle, Nanchahal and Wald 1991).

In the late 1980s a new method of screening was introduced that takes into account not only maternal age, but also the concentration of various fetoplacental products in the maternal circulation. At 16 weeks of gestation the median maternal serum concentrations of α-fetoprotein, oestriol and chorionic gonadotrophin (total, free α- and free β-hCG) in trisomy 21 pregnancies are sufficiently different from the median in normal pregnancies to allow the use of combinations of some or all of these substances to select a 'high-risk' group. This method of screening is proving to be more effective than maternal age alone and for the same rate of invasive testing (about 5%) it can identify 48–69% of the fetuses with Down's syndrome (Haddow *et al.* 1992; Phillips *et al.* 1992; Wald *et al.* 1992a; Spencer and Carpenter 1993).

An alternative or complementary method of screening is ultrasound examination in the first trimester of pregnancy. Increased fetal nuchal translucency thickness at 10–14 weeks of gestation is a common phenotypic expression of trisomies 21, 18 and 13, Turner's syndrome and triploidy (Nicolaides *et al.* 1992a). Nuchal translucency measurement is emerging as an important potential screening marker. It compares favourably with existing screening methods and has been reported to detect more than 80% of affected fetuses for a false-positive rate of about 5% when used in combination with maternal age (Pandya *et al.* 1995a). However, much of these data have been collected in high-risk women and by the same group. Thus, there remains some uncertainty over the utility of this test in general obstetric practice and some question whether these excellent results will be reproduced consistently by other countries. If nuchal translucency is to be introduced as part of routine practice, it is important that the test is shown to achieve comparable results in centres with different resources and experience.

## CHROMOSOMAL DEFECTS, MATERNAL AGE AND GESTATION

Estimates of risks of trisomy 21 for each maternal age first became available in the late 1980s, they were derived from the data of surveys in live births and are routinely used in antenatal clinics to counsel individual women (Cuckle, Wald and Thompson 1987; Hecht & Hook 1994). While such data provide information about the risk of delivering a baby with trisomy 21, they do not accurately reflect the prevalence of trisomy 21, or other chromosomal defects, at the gestation of antenatal screening. To determine the significance of a given ultrasonographic marker for any chromosomal abnormality, it is essential to know the prevalence of the abnormality at the gestation under study, based on the maternal age of the population that is examined.

Snijders, Sebire and Nicolaides (1995) combined data from studies on first trimester chorion villus sampling and midtrimester amniocentesis to estimate the risk for trisomies 21, 18 and 13 in relation to maternal age and gestation. In addition, the data provided information about the rate of intrauterine lethality for different chromosomal defects (Table 1). Hence, for trisomy 21 the rate of intrauterine lethality between 16 weeks and 40 weeks is 32% and between 12 and 40 weeks is 41%.

## ABNORMAL NUCHAL FLUID

During the second and third trimesters of pregnancy, abnormal accumulation of fluid behind the fetal neck can be classified as nuchal cystic hygromas, which are associated with Turner's syndrome (Chervenak *et al.* 1983), and nuchal oedema, which has a diverse aetiology including trisomies, cardiovascular and pulmonary defects, skeletal dysplasias, congenital infection and metabolic and haematological disorders (Nicolaides *et al.* 1992b). Furthermore, the chromosomally normal fetuses had a very poor prognosis because in many cases there was an underlying skeletal dysplasia, genetic syndrome or cardiac defect (Nicolaides *et al.* 1992b).

### Nuchal translucency

In the first trimester abnormal accumulation of nuchal fluid is referred to as nuchal translucency. Although in some studies the condition was defined as multiseptated, thin-walled cystic mass (cystic hygroma) similar to that seen in the second trimester (Cullen *et al.* 1990; Shulman *et al.* 1992; Suchet, van der Westhuizen and Labatte 1992; Johnson *et al.* 1993; Nadel, Bromley and Benacerraf 1993; Trauffer *et al.* 1994), in others the term was used loosely to include nuchal thickening or oedema (Szabo and Gellen 1990; Schulte-Vallentin and Schindler 1992; van Zalen-Sprock, van Vugt and van Geijn 1992). However, the term translucency is preferable because this is the ultrasonographic feature that is observed (Figure 1). In the second trimester the nuchal translucency usually resolves, but in a few cases it evolves

**Table 1** *Estimates for the rate of spontaneous loss in fetuses with various chromosomal defects. (Reproduced from Snijders, Sebire and Nicolaides 1995\* with permission of S. Karger AG)*

| | Estimated loss rate (%) | |
| --- | --- | --- |
| *Chromosomal defect* | *From 12 weeks to 40 weeks* | *From 16 weeks to 40 weeks* |
| Trisomy 21 | 41 | 32 |
| Trisomy 18 | 86 | 74 |
| Trisomy 13 | 82 | 71 |
| Turner's syndrome | 75 | 52 |
| 47,XXX | 5 | 3 |
| 47,XXY | 5 | 3 |
| 47,XYY | 5 | 3 |
| Triploidy | > 99 | > 99 |

\*Snijders, R. J. M., Sebire, N. J. and Nicolaides, K. H. (1995) Maternal age and gestational age specific risk for chromosomal defects. *Fetal Diagn Ther* **10**, 356–67 into either second trimester oedema or cystic hygromata.

Hyett, Moscoso and Nicolaides (1995a; 1995b; 1995c) reported on the pathological examination of the fetal heart and great arteries in chromosomally abnormal fetuses with increased nuchal translucency at 10–14 weeks' gestation. After suction termination of pregnancy the heart and great arteries were identified, fixed with paraformaldehyde, and examined using a stepwise microdissection method and scanning electron microscopy. The most common cardiac lesions seen in fetuses affected by trisomy 21 were atrioventricular or ventricular septal defects (Hyett, Moscoso and Nicolaides 1995b), whereas trisomy 18 was associated with ventricular septal defects and polyvalvular abnormalities (Hyett, Moscoso and Nicolaides 1995b). In addition, the aortic isthmus was significantly narrower than in normal fetuses and the degree of narrowing of the isthmus was significantly greater in fetuses with high nuchal translucency thickness (Hyett, Moscoso and Nicolaides 1995c). It could therefore be postulated that narrowing of the aortic isthmus may be one of the underlying mechanisms for increased nuchal translucency.

## MEASUREMENT OF NUCHAL TRANSLUCENCY

### Technique

Transabdominal ultrasound examination is performed to obtain a sagittal section of the fetus for measurement of fetal crown–rump length. The maximum thickness of the subcutaneous translucency between the skin and the soft tissue overlying the cervical spine is measured (Nicolaides *et al.* 1992a). Care is taken to distinguish between fetal skin and amnion, because at this gestation both structures appear as thin membranes (Figure 1). This is achieved by waiting for spontaneous fetal movement away from the amniotic membrane. Alternatively, the fetus is bounced off the amnion by asking the mother to cough and/or by tapping the maternal abdomen.

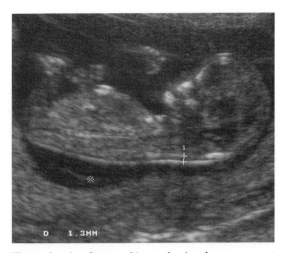

**Figure 1**  *An ultrasound image showing the measurement of the fetal nuchal translucency. The amnion can be seen as a separate membrane from the fetal skin*

## Repeatability

A potential criticism of screening by ultrasound is that scanning requires not only highly skilled operators, but it is also prone to operator variability. Roberts *et al.* (1995) reported poor reproducibility of measurement of fetal nuchal translucency thickness. They took a 3-mm cut-off to identify high- and low-risk groups and demonstrated that by repeating the measurement with the same operator or a different operator, 17.5% and 18.8% of translucency measurements would be reclassified as normal or abnormal, respectively. In a prospective study to assess the repeatability of measurement at 10–14 weeks' gestation, the translucency was measured by two of four operators in 200 pregnant women (Pandya *et al.* 1995b). The repeatability was unrelated to the size of the nuchal translucency and when the mean of two measurements was used, the 95% confidence interval for the intraobserver and interobserver repeatability was less than 0.54 mm and 0.62 mm, respectively. A large part of the variation in measurements was accounted for by the placement of the callipers rather than the generation of the image. It was therefore suggested that the mean of at least two good measurements should be used. Digital image processing and automation of calliper placement should reduce the differences in measurement. Braithwaite and Economides (1995) used transabdominal and transvaginal ultrasound to measure nuchal translucency; by combining the scanning modes they were able to measure the nuchal translucency in all cases, and reported repeatability coefficients of 0.4 mm and 0.2 mm, respectively. In general they found a good correlation between the two methods, but a significant, although small, over-measurement was observed with the transabdominal technique. They recommend the transvaginal route for measurements of nuchal translucency in a screening programme for chromosome abnormalities, or at least when a prior measurement by the transabdominal route is close to the threshold level.

### Increase with gestational age

Nuchal translucency thickness has been shown to increase with crown–rump length (Pajkrt et al. 1995; Pandya et al. 1995a). Therefore, it is important to take gestation into account when determining whether a given measurement is increased.

## NUCHAL TRANSLUCENCY AND CHROMOSOMAL DEFECTS

### Observational and high-risk studies

In the early 1990s several reports of small series in high-risk pregnancies demonstrated a possible association between increased nuchal translucency and chromosomal defects (Table 2). Although the mean prevalence of chromosomal defects in 20 series involving a total of 1698 patients was 29%, there were large differences between the studies with the prevalence ranging from 19% to 88%. This variation in results presumably reflects the differences in the maternal age distribution of the populations examined and differences in the definition of minimum thickness of the abnormal translucency (ranging from 2 mm to 10 mm).

Subsequently, a series of screening studies in high-risk pregnancies were carried out. These involved measurement of nuchal translucency thickness immediately before fetal karyotyping, mainly for advanced maternal age. Nicolaides, Brizot and Snijders (1994) reported on a series of 1273 pregnancies; the nuchal translucency was ≥ 2.5 mm in 84% of the fetuses with trisomy 21 and 4.5% of the chromosomally normal fetuses. Similar findings were obtained in an additional four studies of pregnancies undergoing first-trimester fetal karyotyping (Table 3). However, in a study by Brambati et al. (1995) involving 1819 pregnancies at eight to 15 weeks' gestation, nuchal translucency thickness of ≥ 3 mm identified only 30% of the chromosomally abnormal fetuses (no data were provided specifically for trisomy 21) and the false-positive rate was 3.2%. In this series approximately 47% of the measurements were made at eight to 10 weeks, at a gestation where chorion villus sampling is no longer considered to be safe.

An additional finding of the screening studies in high-risk populations was that the prevalence of chromosomal defects increased with both the fetal nuchal translucency and maternal age (Nicolaides et al. 1994; Pandya et al. 1994; Pandya et al. 1995c). Pandya et al. (1995c) observed, in a study of 1015 pregnancies with increased fetal nuchal translucency thickness at 10–14 weeks' gestation, the number of trisomies 21, 18 and 13 in fetuses with translucencies of 3 mm, 4 mm, 5 mm and ≥ 6 mm was approximately threefold, 18-fold, 28-fold and 36-fold higher than the respective number expected on the basis of maternal age (Figure 2); the incidence of Turner's syndrome and triploidy was ninefold and eightfold higher, but the incidence of other sex chromosome aneuploidies was similar to that expected.

### Screening studies in unselected populations

A common criticism of ultrasound is that the so-called 'markers' of chromosomal abnormality are initially reported in referral centres and are subsequently not substantiated by others. In addition, the population studied is usually high risk, such as women undergoing fetal karyotyping, and therefore not representative of the general population.

**Table 2** Summary of reported series on first-trimester fetal nuchal translucency providing data on the presence of associated chromosomal defects. In some series the translucency is merely referred to as cystic hygroma (CH) and no data on thickness is given

| Author | Gestation (weeks) | Size nuchal translucency (mm) | n | Total n | Total % | Trisomy 21 | Trisomy 18 | Trisomy 13 | 45,X | Other |
|---|---|---|---|---|---|---|---|---|---|---|
| Johnson et al. (1993) | 10–14 | ≥ 2.0 | 68 | 41 | 60 | 16 | 9 | 2 | 9 | 5 |
| Hewitt (1993) | 10–14 | ≥ 2.0 | 29 | 12 | 41 | 5 | 3 | 1 | 2 | 1 |
| Shulman et al. (1992) | 10–13 | ≥ 2.5 | 32 | 15 | 47 | 4 | 4 | 3 | 4 | — |
| Nicolaides et al. (1992a; 1994) | 10–13 | ≥ 3.0 | 88 | 33 | 38 | 21 | 8 | 2 | — | 2 |
| Pandya et al. (1994; 1995c) | 10–13 | ≥ 3.0 | 1015 | 193 | 19 | 101 | 51 | 13 | 14 | 15 |
| Szabo and Gellen (1990) | 11–12 | ≥ 3.0 | 8 | 7 | 88 | 7 | — | — | — | — |
| Wilson, Venir and Faquharson (1992) | 8–11 | ≥ 3.0 | 14 | 3 | 21 | — | — | — | — | — |
| Ville et al. (1992) | 9–14 | ≥ 3.0 | 29 | 8 | 28 | 4 | 3 | 1 | 1 | 2 |
| Trauffer et al. (1994) | 10–14 | ≥ 3.0 | 43 | 21 | 49 | 9 | 4 | 1 | 4 | 3 |
| Brambati et al. (1995) | 8–15 | ≥ 3.0 | 70 | 13 | 19 | ? | ? | ? | ? | ? |
| Comas et al. (1995) | 9–13 | ≥ 3.0 | 51 | 9 | 18 | 4 | 4 | — | — | 1 |
| Szabo, Gellen and Szemere (1995) | 9–12 | ≥ 3.0 | 96 | 43 | 45 | 28 | 10 | — | 2 | 3 |
| Nadel, Bromley and Benacerraf (1993) | 10–15 | ≥ 4.0 | 63 | 43 | 68 | 15 | 15 | 1 | 10 | 2 |
| Savoldelli et al. (1993) | 9–12 | ≥ 4.0 | 24 | 19 | 79 | 15 | 2 | 1 | 1 | — |
| Shulte-Vallentin and Schindler (1992) | 10–14 | ≥ 4.0 | 8 | 7 | 88 | 7 | — | — | — | — |
| van Zalen-Sprock, van Vugt and van Geijn (1992) | 10–14 | ≥ 4.0 | 18 | 5 | 28 | 3 | 1 | — | 1 | 1 |
| Cullen et al. (1990) | 11–13 | ≥ 6.0 | 29 | 15 | 52 | 6 | 2 | — | 4 | 3 |
| Suchet, van der Westhuizen and Labatte (1992) | 8–14 | ≥ 10.0 | 13 | 8 | 62 | — | — | — | 7 | 1 |
| Total | 8–15 | | 1698 | 495 | 29 | 245 | 116 | 25 | 59 | 39 |

**Table 3** *The sensitivity and false-positive rate of screening with fetal nuchal translucency ≥ 3 mm and ≥ 4 mm in six high-risk screening studies*

| Author | Gestation (weeks) | n | Trisomy 21 | Nuchal translucency ≥ 3 mm | | Nuchal translucency ≥ 4 mm | |
|---|---|---|---|---|---|---|---|
| | | | | Sensitivity (%) | False positive (%) | Sensitivity (%) | False positive (%) |
| Shulte-Vallentin and Schindler (1992) | 10–14 | 632 | 7 | — | — | 100 | 0.2 |
| Salvodelli *et al.* (1993) | 9–12 | 1400 | 28 | — | — | 53.6 | 0.4 |
| Nicolaides *et al.* (1994a) | 10–14 | 1273 | 25 | 84.0 | 4.5 | 60.0 | 1.0 |
| Comas *et al.* (1995) | 9–13 | 481 | 7 | 57.1 | 9.5 | 57.1 | 0.7 |
| Szabo, Gellen and Szemere (1995) | 9–12 | 3380 | 31 | 90.0 | 1.6 | 67.7 | 0.4 |
| Total | | 7166 | 98 | 84.1 | 3.0 | 63.3 | 0.5 |

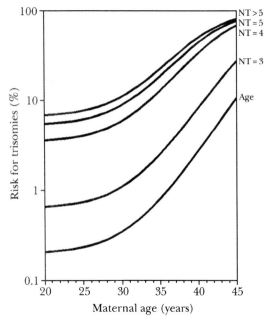

**Figure 2** *Semilogarithmic graph illustrating estimated risks for fetal trisomies 21, 18 or 13 at 10–14 weeks' gestation on the basis of maternal age alone and maternal age with fetal nuchal translucency thickness of 3 mm, 4 mm, 5 mm and > 5 mm*

older and, as a result, during 1993 two of 11 fetuses with Down's syndrome were detected prenatally. Nuchal translucency screening was implemented without the need for increasing the number of staff or the equipment. Women with fetal translucency ≥ 2.5 mm were offered fetal karyotyping. In addition, women aged 35 years or older were offered amniocentesis at 16 weeks' gestation. The data of the first five months after the introduction of the new policy were analysed following completion of the pregnancies. During this period 74% of women delivering in the two hospitals attended for first-trimester scanning and the nuchal translucency was successfully measured in all these pregnancies. The translucency was raised in 3.6% of cases and the total percentage of invasive procedures was 5.1%. All four cases of Down's syndrome (three with increased nuchal translucency and three with a maternal age of 42 years) that occurred in this period were diagnosed prenatally.

Bewley *et al.* (1995) reported a prospective observational screening study of 1368 women with singleton pregnancies attending University College Hospital, London, for routine antenatal care at eight to 14 weeks' gestation. The measurements were made transabdominally in 1127 cases, giving a failure rate of 18%. The translucency was ≥ 3 mm in 6% of all cases and in one out of three cases with trisomy 21. All five cases of fetal aneuploidy (trisomy 21 *n* = 3, trisomy 18 *n* = 2) occurred in women who

Thus, studies in low-risk or unselected obstetric populations are important.

Pandya *et al.* (1995d) reported the introduction of nuchal translucency screening in two units providing routine antenatal care. Prior to the onset of nuchal translucency scanning, the policy of these hospitals was to offer amniocentesis to women aged 35 years or were 39 years of age or older. An increased miscarriage rate was reported in those with an increased nuchal translucency measurement, although this was not statistically significant, and it was suggested that increased nuchal translucency may preferentially identify those fetuses destined to miscarry.

Bower *et al.* (1996) combined the data from three separate studies, including that of Bewley *et al.* (1995), in an attempt to assess the efficacy of the test in an unselected obstetric population. All of the studies were prospective, but two were observational and one interventional. Measurements were attempted in 2849 pregnancies at eight to 14 weeks' gestation and achieved in 2566, giving a failure rate of 9.9%. Nuchal translucency measurement was ≥ 3 mm in 6.6% and in five out of 11 cases of trisomy 21, two out of three cases of trisomy 18 and in one case of Turner's syndrome. The maternal age was over 38 years in 13 out of 15 women with aneuploid fetuses and all cases of aneuploidy were detected antenatally — except one child with trisomy 21, born to a 31-year-old mother, which was diagnosed postnatally.

Hafner, Schuchter and Phillip (1995) successfully screened 1972 women with transabdominal ultrasound at 10–13 weeks when attending for routine antenatal care at a National Health Service hospital in Vienna. The nuchal translucency thickness was ≥ 2.5 mm in 1.3% of the cases and in eight out of 11 chromosomally abnormal fetuses, including two of the four with trisomy 21. All cases of chromosome abnormality were detected antenatally, either by karyotyping for increased nuchal translucency, maternal age or positive biochemistry testing.

Pandya *et al.* (1995a) reported a multicentre screening study at 10–14 weeks' gestation involving 20,804 pregnancies, including 164 cases of chromosomal abnormalities. The study suggested that nuchal translucency increases with crown–rump length and proposed a model to calculate the risk of trisomy 21 by multiplying the *a priori* risk (based on maternal and gestational age) by a likelihood ratio, which depended on the degree of deviation in nuchal translucency from the normal median. Using this new model it was suggested that 78% of fetuses with trisomy 21 could be detected if invasive testing is offered to 5% of the population.

In an expanded series of 42,619 completed pregnancies involving 20 centres the sensitivity for trisomy 21 was 76% for 5% false-positive rate (Nicolaides *et al.* 1996). If the patients examined at the Harris Birthright Research Centre for Fetal Medicine, London, are excluded, on the assumption that these patients are high risk on the basis of maternal age (24% of the women were at least 37 years old) and that they were seen in a referral centre, there were a remaining 22,076 pregnancies screened. In this unselected population the detection rate for trisomy 21 was 84% for an invasive karyotyping rate of 6% (Nicolaides *et al.* 1996).

## NUCHAL TRANSLUCENCY AND MATERNAL SERUM BIOCHEMISTRY

In trisomy 21 pregnancies during the first trimester of pregnancy the maternal serum concentration of free β-hCG is higher and pregnancy associated plasma protein-A (PAPP-A) is lower than in chromosomally normal pregnancies (Ozturk *et al.* 1990; Wald *et al.* 1992b; Aitkin *et al.* 1993; Brambati *et al.* 1993; Bersinger *et al.* 1994; Brizot *et al.* 1994; Macintosh *et al.* 1994). Pregnancy-specific β-1 glycoprotein (SP1) and α-fetoprotein do not provide useful distinctions between affected and normal pregnancies (Brizot *et al.* 1995a).

Studies examining the relationship between maternal serum PAPP-A or free β-hCG concentrations and fetal nuchal translucency thickness have demonstrated no significant association between biochemistry and ultrasound findings in either the chromosomally normal or the trisomy 21 pregnancies (Brizot *et al.* 1994; Brizot *et al.* 1995b). Therefore, maternal serum PAPP-A, free β-hCG and fetal nuchal translucency can be combined in calculating the risk for fetal trisomies. In a study of 2529 pregnancies at 10–14 weeks' gestation it was estimated that inclusion of maternal serum free β-hCG with maternal age and fetal nuchal translucency thickness can improve the sensitivity of screening for trisomy 21 by about 5% (Noble *et al.* 1996).

## NUCHAL TRANSLUCENCY AND SPONTANEOUS PREGNANCY LOSS

The obvious advantage of screening for chromosomal defects in the first trimester of pregnancy is that it allows earlier prenatal diagnosis and safer and less traumatic termination of pregnancy for those who choose this option. However, many chromosomally abnormal fetuses will be lost before viability and it is possible that earlier screening is simply identifying those pregnancies destined to miscarry. The same criticism could also be levelled at second trimester biochemical screening because, although approximately 41% of affected fetuses die between 12 weeks', gestation and term (Snijders *et al.* 1995), it is estimated that 32% are lost between 16 weeks' gestation and term (Snijders *et al.* 1995).

Most studies have been interventional and so it is difficult to assess the relationship between nuchal translucency and fetal lethality.

### Interventional studies

In a recent study of six fetuses with increased nuchal translucency and trisomy 21, where the parents chose to continue with the pregnancy, the translucency resolved in five of the cases in the second trimester and in one it evolved into nuchal oedema (Pandya *et al.* 1995e). All six pregnancies resulted in live births, suggesting that increased nuchal translucency does not necessarily identify those trisomic fetuses that are destined to die *in utero*. An alternative method for assessing the detection rate is to calculate the expected number of babies born with trisomy 21 from the age distribution of the population screened and to compare this with the observed number of trisomy 21 births. From the Fetal Medicine Foundation, London, multicentre study of 42,619 pregnancies, correcting for the higher prevalence of trisomy 21 at 10–14 weeks' gestation, it was estimated that the reduction in live-birth prevalence of trisomy 21 was by at least 80% (Nicolaides *et al.* 1996).

### Observational studies

Bewley *et al.* (1995) reported that there was an increased miscarriage rate in those fetuses with increased nuchal translucency (two out of 70 versus 18 out of 1057), but this was not statistically significant. However, Bower *et al.* (1996) did not reproduce this finding and found no difference in miscarriage rate in those with and without increased nuchal translucency (two out of 169 versus 35 out of 2397). None of the chromosomally abnormal fetuses miscarried, although 13 out of 15 pregnancies were interrupted in the second trimester following prenatal diagnosis by screening methods already in place. Further large non-interventional studies would be required to answer this question accurately.

## MULTIPLE PREGNANCIES

Screening for chromosomal defects in multiple pregnancies is complicated for several reasons:

(1) Screening by maternal serum biochemistry is not applicable;

(2) Invasive testing may produce uncertain results or may be associated with higher risks of miscarriage; and

(3) Fetuses may be discordant for an abnormality.

In multiple pregnancies when one of the fetuses is found to have a chromosomal abnormality and the other is normal, the parents may choose to have selective termination of pregnancy. In such cases, the presence of a sonographically detectable marker ensures the correct identification of the abnormal twin. Furthermore, a recent multicentre study has demonstrated that embryo reduction before 16 weeks' gestation is associated with a much lower risk of miscarriage (5.4%) than selective termination after 16 weeks (14.4%) (Evans *et al.* 1994). Therefore, a test which will identify the fetus as high risk in the first trimester will allow selection of the appropriate diagnostic technique, so that selective fetocide can be performed more safely before 16 weeks.

Pandya *et al.* (1995f) examined the nuchal translucency thickness of each fetus in eight twin pregnancies where karyotyping at 10–14 weeks of gestation demonstrated that at least one of the fetuses was chromosomally abnormal. Eight fetuses had trisomy 21 and two had trisomy 18. The nuchal translucency thickness was more than 2.5 mm in nine (90%) of the trisomic fetuses and in one of the chromosomally normal ones.

## CHROMOSOMALLY NORMAL FETUSES

In two studies examining a total of 32 chromosomally normal fetuses with increased nuchal translucency ( ≥ 2 mm) there were four terminations of pregnancy (three because of progressive hydrops and one because of amnion dysruption sequence), one intrauterine death in a fetus with obstructive uropathy, one spontaneous abortion and 26 live births. Of these 26, 23 were healthy, two had non-specific dysmorphic features and one had Noonan's syndrome (Johnson *et al.* 1993; Trauffer *et al.* 1994).

Shulman *et al.* (1994) reported on 32 chromosomally normal fetuses with increased nuchal translucency ( ≥ 2.5 mm). In one case there were persistent hygromas that were successfully repaired at birth and in the other 31 cases the translucency resolved by 20 weeks' gestation and all babies were healthy at birth. The follow-up examination at 12 months demonstrated normal growth and development in all infants.

Pandya *et al.* (1994; 1995c) reported on the outcome of 565 chromosomally normal fetuses with nuchal translucency of 3–9 mm. The prevalence of structural defects, mainly cardiac, diaphragmatic, renal and abdominal wall was approximately 4%, which is higher than would be expected in an unselected population. Additionally, fetuses with increased translucency, as with nuchal oedema in later pregnancy, may be at increased risk of rare genetic syndromes such as Stickler syndrome, Smith–Lemli–Opitz syndrome, Jarco Levine's syndrome or arthrogryposis (Hyett, Moscoso and Nicolaides 1995; Hyett *et al.* 1996). The overall survival, taking into account perinatal deaths and termination of pregnancy for fetal defects, decreased with increasing nuchal translucency thickness from 97% for 3 mm to 53% for ≥ 5 mm (Pandya *et al.* 1995c).

## CONCLUSION

Increased fetal nuchal translucency is associated with an increased rate of aneuploidy and is clearly a very promising new screening test. It also identifies fetuses at risk of other fetal defects and perinatal death. However, much of the data have been collected in high-risk populations. Its role in screening unselected or 'low-risk' obstetric populations is at present being evaluated. Impressive detection rates of about 80% for trisomy 21 have been reported in studies co-ordinated by the same group (Pandya *et al.* 1995a; Pandya *et al.* 1995d; Nicolaides *et al.* 1996), but two smaller studies by different groups (Hafner, Schuchter and Phillip 1995; Bower *et al.* 1996) have reported detection rates of 50% for trisomy 21. It now requires further large studies to be undertaken by different centres to assess whether these results are reproducible. It is important for the test to be evaluated in unselected obstetric populations and for staff performing the test to be properly trained and their results subject to regular audit.

For those women that want antenatal screening, a test that allows the option of early investigation and diagnosis before the end of the first trimester is very appealing. The future may lie in the combination of ultrasound screening by nuchal translucency measurement and serum screening by biochemical markers, but this requires further evaluation.

# References

Aitken, D. A., McCaw, G., Crossley, J. A. *et al.* (1993) First-trimester biochemical screening for fetal chromosome abnormalities and neural tube defects. *Prenat Diagn* **13**, 681–9

Bersinger, N. A., Brizot, M. L., Johnson, A. *et al.* (1994) First trimester maternal serum pregnancy-associated plasma protein A and pregnancy-specific β1-glycoprotein in fetal trisomies. *Br J Obstet Gynaecol* **101**, 970–4

Bewley, S., Roberts, L. J., Mackinson, A.-M. and Rodeck, C. H. (1995) First trimester fetal nuchal translucency: problems with screening the general population 2. *Br J Obstet Gynaecol* **102**, 386–8

Bower, S., Chitty, L., Bewley, S. *et al.* (1996) First trimester nuchal translucency screening of the general obstetric population: data from three centres (submitted)

Braithwaite, J. M. and Economides, D. L. (1995) The measurement of nuchal translucency with transabdominal and transvaginal sonography — success rates, repeatability and levels of agreement. *Br J Radiology* **68**, 720–3

Brambati, B., Macintosh, M. C. M., Teisner, B. *et al.* (1993) Low maternal serum level of pregnancy associated plasma protein (PAPP-A) in the first trimester in association with abnormal fetal karyotype. *Br J Obstet Gynaecol* **100**, 324–6

Brambati, B., Cislaghi, C., Tului, L. *et al.* (1995) First-trimester Down's syndrome screening using nuchal translucency: a prospective study. *Ultrasound Obstet Gynecol* **5**, 9–14

Brizot, M. L., Snijders, R. J. M., Bersinger, N. A., Kuhn, P. and Nicolaides, K. H. (1994) Maternal serum pregnancy associated placental protein A and fetal nuchal translucency thickness for the prediction of fetal trisomies in early pregnancy. *Obstet Gynecol* **84**, 918–22

Brizot, M. L., Kuhn, P., Bersinger, N. A., Snijders, R. J. M. and Nicolaides, K. H. (1995a) First trimester maternal serum α-fetoprotein in fetal trisomies. *Br J Obstet Gynaecol* **102**, 31–4

Brizot, M. L., Snijders, R. J. M., Butler, J., Bersinger, N. A. and Nicolaides, K. H. (1995b) Maternal serum hCG and fetal nuchal translucency thickness for the prediction of fetal trisomies in the first trimester of pregnancy. *Br J Obstet Gynaecol* **102**, 127–32

Chervenak, F. A., Isaacson, G., Blakemore, K. J. *et al.* (1983) Fetal cystic hygroma: cause and natural history. *N Engl J Med* **309**, 822–5

Comas, C., Martinez, J. M., Ojuel, J. *et al.* (1995) First-trimester nuchal edema as a marker of aneuploidy. *Ultrasound Obstet Gynecol* **5**, 26–9

Cuckle, H. S., Wald, N. J. and Thompson, S. G. (1987) Estimating a woman's risk of having a pregnancy associated with Down's syndrome using her age and serum α-fetoprotein level. *Br J Obstet Gynaecol* **94**, 387–402

Cuckle, H. S., Nanchahal, K. and Wald, N. J. (1991) Birth prevalence of Down's syndrome in England and Wales. *Prenat Diagn* **11**, 29–34

Cullen, M. T., Gabrielli, S., Green, J. J. *et al.* (1990) Diagnosis and significance of cystic hygroma in the first trimester. *Prenat Diagn* **10**, 643–51

Evans, M. I., Goldberg, J. D., Dommergues, M. *et al.* (1994) Efficacy of second-trimester selective termination for fetal abnormalities: international collaborative experience among the world's largest centers. *Am J Obstet Gynecol* **171**, 90–4

Haddow, J. E., Palomaki, G. E., Knight, G. J. *et al.* (1992) Prenatal screening for Down's syndrome with use of maternal serum markers. *N Engl J Med* **327**, 588–93

Hafner, E., Schuchter, K. and Phillip, K. (1995) Screening for chromosomal abnormalities in an unselected population by fetal nuchal translucency. *Ultrasound Obstet Gynecol* **6**, 330–3

Hecht, C. A. and Hook, E. B. (1994) The imprecision in rates of Down's syndrome by 1-year maternal age intervals: a critical analysis of rates used in biochemical screening. *Prenat Diagn* **14**, 729–38

Hewitt, B. (1993) Nuchal translucency in the first trimester. *Aust NZ J Obstet Gynaecol* **33**, 389–91

Hyett, J. A., Clayton, P. T., Moscoso, G. and Nicolaides, K. H. (1995) Increased first trimester nuchal translucency as a prenatal manifestation of Smith–Lemli–Opitz syndrome. *Am J Med Genet* **58**, 374–6

Hyett, J. A., Moscoso, G. and Nicolaides, K. H. (1995a) First trimester nuchal translucency and cardiac septal defects in fetuses with trisomy 21. *Am J Obstet Gynecol* **172**, 1411–13

Hyett, J. A., Moscoso, G. and Nicolaides, K. H. (1995b) Cardiac defects in trisomy 18 fetuses affected by increased first trimester nuchal translucency. *Fetal Diagn Ther* **10**, 381–6

Hyett, J. A., Moscoso, G. and Nicolaides, K. H. (1995c) Increased nuchal translucency in trisomy 21 fetuses: relation to narrowing of aortic isthmus. *Hum Reprod* **10**, 3049–51

Hyett, J. A., Moscoso, G., Papapanagiotou, G., Perdu, M. and Nicolaides, K. H. (1996) Abnormalities of the heart and great vessels in chromosomally normal fetuses with increased nuchal translucency thickness at 10–13 weeks' gestation. *Ultrasound Obstet Gynecol* **7**, 245–50

Johnson, M. P., Johnson, A., Holzgreve, W. *et al.* (1993) First-trimester simple hygroma: cause and outcome. *Am J Obstet Gynecol* **168**, 156–61

Macintosh, M. C., Iles, R., Teisner, B. *et al.* (1994) Maternal serum human chorionic gonadotrophin and pregnancy-associated plasma protein A, markers for fetal Down's syndrome at 8–14 weeks. *Prenat Diagn* **14**, 203–8

Nadel, A., Bromley, B. and Benacerraf, B. R. (1993) Nuchal thickening or cystic hygromas in first- and early second-trimester fetuses: prognosis and outcome. *Obstet Gynecol* **82**, 43–8

Nicolaides, K. H., Azar, G., Byrne, D., Mansur, C. and Marks, K. (1992a) Fetal nuchal translucency: ultrasound screening for chromosomal defects in first trimester of pregnancy. *BMJ* **304**, 867–9

Nicolaides, K. H., Azar, G., Snijders, R. J. M. and Gosden, C. M. (1992b) Fetal nuchal edema: associated malformations and chromosomal defects. *Fetal Diagn Ther* **7**, 123–31

Nicolaides, K. H., Brizot, M. L. and Snijders, R. J. M. (1994) Fetal nuchal translucency: ultrasound screening for fetal trisomy in the first trimester of pregnancy. *Br J Obstet Gynaecol* **101**, 782–6

Nicolaides, K. H., Sebire, N. J., Snijders, R. J. M. and Johnson, S. (1996) Down's syndrome screening in the UK (letter). *Lancet* **347**, 906–7

Noble, P. L., Abraha, H. D., Snijders, R. J. M., Sherwood, R. and Nicolaides, K. H. (1996) Screening for trisomy 21 in the first trimester of pregnancy: maternal serum free β-hCG and fetal nuchal translucency thickness. *Ultrasound Obstet Gynecol* **6**, 390–5

Ozturk, M., Milunsky, A., Brambati, B. *et al.* (1990) Abnormal maternal serum levels of human chorionic gonadotropin free subunits in trisomy 18. *Am J Med Genet* **36**, 480–3

Pajkrt, E., Bilardo, C. M., Van Lith, J. M., Mol, B. W. and Bleker, O. P. (1995) Nuchal translucency measurement in normal fetuses. *Obstet Gynecol* **86**, 994–7

Pandya, P. P., Brizot, M. L., Kuhn, P., Snijders, R. J. M. and Nicolaides, K. H. (1994) First trimester fetal nuchal translucency thickness and risk for trisomies. *Obstet Gynecol* **84**, 420–3

Pandya, P. P., Altman, D. G., Brizot, M. L., Pettersen, H. and Nicolaides, K. H. (1995b) Reproducibility of measurement of fetal nuchal translucency thickness at 10–14 weeks' gestation. *Ultrasound Obstet Gynecol* **5**, 334–7

Pandya, P. P., Goldberg, H., Walton, B. *et al.* (1995d) The implementation of first trimester scanning at 10–13 weeks' gestation and the measurement of fetal nuchal translucency thickness in two maternity units. *Ultrasound Obstet Gynecol* 5, 20–5

Pandya, P. P., Hilbert, F., Snijders, R. J. M. and Nicolaides, K. H. (1995f) Nuchal translucency thickness and crown–rump length in twin pregnancies with chromosomally abnormal fetuses. *J Ultrasound Med* 14, 565–8

Pandya, P. P., Kondylios, A., Hilbert, L., Snijders, R. J. M. and Nicolaides, K. H. (1995c) Chromosomal defects and outcome in 1,015 fetuses with increased nuchal translucency. *Ultrasound Obstet Gynecol* 5, 15–19

Pandya, P. P., Snijders, R. J. M., Johnson, S. J., Brizot, M. and Nicolaides, K. H. (1995a) Screening for fetal trisomies by maternal age and fetal nuchal translucency thickness at 10–14 weeks of gestation. *Br J Obstet Gynaecol* 102, 957–62

Pandya, P. P., Snijders, R. J. M., Johnson, S. and Nicolaides, K. H. (1995e) Natural history of trisomy 21 fetuses with fetal nuchal translucency. *Ultrasound Obstet Gynecol* 5, 381–3

Phillips, O. P., Elias, S., Shulman, L. P. *et al.* (1992) Maternal serum screening for fetal Down syndrome in women less than 35 years of age using α-fetoprotein, hCG, and unconjugated estriol: a prospective 2-year study. *Obstet Gynecol* 80, 353–8

Roberts, L. J., Bewley, S., Mackinson, A.M. and Rodeck, C. H. (1995) First trimester fetal nuchal translucency: problems with screening the general population 1. *Br J Obstet Gynaecol* 102, 381–5

Savoldelli, G., Binkert, F., Achermann, J. and Schmid, W. (1993) Ultrasound screening for chromosomal anomalies in the first trimester of pregnancy. *Prenat Diagn* 13, 513–18

Schulte-Vallentin, M. and Schindler, H. (1992) Non-echogenic nuchal oedema as a marker in trisomy 21 screening. *Lancet* 339, 1053

Shulman, L. P., Emerson, D., Felker, R. *et al.* (1992) High frequency of cytogenetic abnormalities with cystic hygroma diagnosed in the first trimester. *Obstet Gynecol* 80, 80–2

Shulman, L. P., Emerson, D. S., Grevengood, C. *et al.* (1994) Clinical course and outcome of fetuses with isolated cystic nuchal lesions and normal karyotypes detected in the first trimester. *Am J Obstet Gynecol* 171, 1278–81

Snijders, R. J. M., Sebire, N. J. and Nicolaides, K. H. (1995) Maternal age and gestational age specific risk for chromosomal defects. *Fetal Diagn Ther* 10, 356–67

Spencer, K. and Carpenter, P. (1993) Prospective study of prenatal screening for Down's syndrome with free β-human chorionic gonadotrophin. *BMJ* 307, 764–9

Suchet, I. B., van der Westhuizen, N. G. and Labatte, M. F. (1992) Fetal cystic hygromas: further insights into their natural history. *Can Assoc Radiol J* 6, 420–4

Szabo, J. and Gellen, J. (1990) Nuchal fluid accumulation in trisomy-21 detected by vaginosonography in first trimester. *Lancet* 336, 1133

Szabo, J., Gellen, J. and Szemere, G. (1995) First trimester ultrasound screening for fetal aneuploides in women over and less than 35 years of age. *Ultrasound Obstet Gynecol* 5, 161–3

Trauffer, M. L., Anderson, C. E., Johnson, A. *et al.* (1994) The natural history of euploid pregnancies with first-trimester cystic hygromas. *Am J Obstet Gynecol* 170, 1279–84

van Zalen-Sprock, M. M., van Vugt, J. M. G. and van Geijn, H. P. (1992) First-trimester diagnosis of cystic hygroma — course and outcome. *Am J Obstet Gynecol* 167, 94–8

Ville, Y., Lalondrelle, C., Doumerc, S. *et al.* (1992) First trimester diagnosis of nuchal anomalies: significance and fetal outcome. *Ultrasound Obstet Gynecol* 2, 314–16

Wald, N. J., Kennard, A., Densem, J. W. *et al.* (1992a) Antenatal Maternal Serum Screening for Down's syndrome: results of a demonstration project. *BMJ* 305, 391–4

Wald, N. J., Stone, R., Cuckle, H. S. *et al.* (1992b) First trimester concentrations of pregnancy associated plasma protein A and placental protein 14 in Down's syndrome. *BMJ* **305**, 28

Wilson, R. D., Venir, N. and Faquharson, D. F. (1992) Fetal nuchal fluid – physiological or pathological? – in pregnancies less than 17 menstrual weeks. *Prenat Diagn* **12**, 755–63

# 30

# Transabdominal cervicoisthmic cerclage

*Sarah Flint and Donald Gibb*

Cervical incompetence (weakness) is one of the causes of second trimester pregnancy loss and is usually treated with transvaginal cervical cerclage. It is important to consider carefully the alternative diagnoses before this is done. Transabdominal cervicoisthmic cerclage (TCC) was first described by Benson and Durfee in 1965 and subsequently several groups have reported results with various modifications of selection criteria and technique. The place of TCC in the management of cervical incompetence is considered and the authors' most recent data presented with a review of literature.

## DIFFERENTIAL DIAGNOSIS IN MIDTRIMESTER LOSS

Cervical incompetence is classically described as painless dilatation of the cervix leading to rupture of the membranes and pregnancy loss in the midtrimester. Other causes of second-trimester miscarriage include multiple pregnancy, vaginal bleeding, fetal abnormalities (i.e. intrauterine death) anatomical abnormalities of the uterus and infection. In reviews of the causes of miscarriage there may be little distinction drawn between those relating to the first and those relating to the second trimester (Rai, Clifford and Regan 1996). While there are many studies of the causes of first-trimester miscarriage, there are few publications specifically addressing the causes of miscarriage in the second trimester. Gaillard *et al.* (1993) investigated the causes of miscarriage in 422 second-trimester losses and concluded that fetal abnormality, vaginal bleeding, cervical incompetence and genital tract infection accounted for the major-

ity of cases. Based upon the history, cervical incompetence was thought to be the cause in 8.7% of cases in this study.

There is increasing evidence for the role of infection, in the form of bacterial vaginosis, in preterm delivery and second-trimester miscarriage. Bacterial vaginosis detected in the first trimester is a risk factor for preterm delivery and second-trimester miscarriage (Hay *et al.* 1994) and treatment may reduce the risk of preterm delivery (Hauth *et al.* 1995). There may be an autoimmune explanation for a significant proportion of recurrent first- and second-trimester miscarriages. Antiphospholipid antibodies (APA) are detected in only 2% of women with no history of miscarriage but in 15% of women with recurrent miscarriage (Rai *et al.* 1995). The prevalence of APA has not been reported in a trimester-specific analysis of recurrent miscarriage.

## CERVICAL INCOMPETENCE (WEAKNESS)

Reference to conditions consistent with cervical incompetence may be found in literature from the nineteenth century, but the phrase 'cervical incompetence' was first proposed by Lash and Lash in 1950, in a report on the reconstruction of a non-pregnant cervix. Shirodkar described his technique in 1955 and MacDonald described the simpler purse-string suture in 1957. Both originally applied the technique in an emergency situation when the cervix was already opening.

The diagnosis of cervical incompetence is difficult and this is reflected in differing indications for cervical cerclage (Medical Research Council/Royal College of Obstetricians and Gynaecologists Working Party 1993). The diagnosis is usually based upon the past obstetric history and clinical examination of the cervix. Between pregnancies the passage of a Hegar dilator (size 8 or greater) with ease (Lash and Lash 1950), hysterosalpingography (Jeffcoate and Wilson 1956), the Foley catheter traction technique (Bergman and Svenerund 1957) and cervical resistance studies (Anthony, Calder and MacNaughton 1981) have been used. In recent years transvaginal ultrasound of the cervix in pregnancy has been proposed to guide the decision of cervical cerclage. Ultrasound imaging of the cervix provides a more objective assessment of the cervix than digital examination. Transvaginal ultrasound has advantages over transabdominal ultrasound in that it is not limited by maternal obesity and may be performed with an empty bladder. It has been demonstrated that bladder filling affects measurements of cervical length and dilatation of the internal os in pregnancy (Okitsu *et al.* 1992).

In patients with a clinical diagnosis of cervical incompetence, the cervix is significantly shorter than in controls (Brook *et al.* 1981; Podobnik, Bulic and Smiljanic 1988). There is substantial evidence that a short cervix is a risk factor for preterm delivery with the risk being inversely related to the cervical length (Anderson *et al.* 1990; Iams *et al.* 1996). It has therefore been suggested that transvaginal ultrasound should be used to guide the decision to insert a cervical cerclage. However, as dynamic changes may occur between examinations, it has been suggested that cervical cerclage should be recommended in patients with a strong history of cervical incompetence. Where the diagnosis is less clear, transvaginal ultrasound surveillance may be used to guide the decision for cerclage (Romero, Gomez and Sepulveda 1992).

Once the diagnosis of cervical incompetence has been made, the traditional management is the insertion of a transvaginal cervical cerclage. Due to the difficulty in diagnosis cervical incompetence has probably been overdiagnosed in the past. This may partly explain the disappointing results in studies of this technique. Lazar *et*

*al.* (1984) and Rush *et al.* (1984) were unable to demonstrate benefit of cervical cerclage in randomised, controlled trials. In the Medical Research Council and Royal College of Obstetricians and Gynaecologists multicentre randomised study (1993) patients were eligible for entry when their obstetricians were uncertain as to whether to insert a cervical suture, thus selecting a heterogeneous group of women. The other aspects of their antenatal care were not standardised, although clinicians were asked to minimise the use of tocolytics and bed rest. Furthermore, while this study demonstrated a modest beneficial effect of cervical cerclage, its use was associated with increased intervention as judged by admission to hospital, induction of labour and Caesarean section, and puerperal pyrexia. In the subgroup who had three or more midtrimester miscarriages cerclage was beneficial.

Comparison of suture techniques in the literature is inconclusive. The authors undertook a survey of British obstetricians and found that the majority used a MacDonald technique using Mersilene tape. Those clinicians who had been practising the longest were more likely to use a Shirodkar technique. This suggests that the choice of suture may be at least partly affected by an obstetrician's experience and training. In the Medical Research Council and Royal College of Obstetricians and Gynaecologists study (1993), the type of cerclage was not prespecified and, in 74% of cases where the information was available, a purse string (MacDonald) suture was used. There was no clear difference between the techniques, although these findings must be interpreted with caution as the trial was not designed to make this comparison and the number of cases with Shirodkar cerclage is small. Harger (1980) retrospectively reviewed 251 cervical cerclage procedures and found similar success rates and morbidity with MacDonald and Shirodkar procedures.

## TRANSABDOMINAL APPROACH

A few patients cannot be treated with a transvaginal cervical cerclage because their cervices are too short, scarred or lacerated. This may be due to previous vaginal cerclage or following extensive conisation of the cervix. The transabdominal approach was first described in 1965 (Benson and Durfee 1965). Subsequently, several reports have confirmed that in a highly selected group of women there is an improved outcome after the procedure. The indications for TCC are anatomical abnormalities of the cervix (e.g. scarring, deep lacerations or extreme shortening) and previous failed vaginal cerclage.

## Patients and methods

Between 1 January 1984 and 31 March 1996, TCC was performed on 56 occasions in 54 women. Many of these patients were referrals often from a distance. The indication for TCC was previous midtrimester pregnancy loss or early preterm delivery in all but three women; these three had undergone extensive conisation of the cervix without previous pregnancy loss. The primary indication for offering TCC rather than a transvaginal approach was the absence of vaginal cervix due to previous surgery and previous failed vaginal cerclage. In many cases the women had been advised to give up trying to have a child. Prepregnancy counselling in the form of personal consultation and written information sheet was offered whenever possible. The decision to proceed was based upon history and clinical examination. Towards the end of the series, transvaginal ultrasound measurements of cervical length and internal os dilatation were also performed. Strict selection criteria were applied before recommending the procedure.

Patients were asked to confirm their pregnancy as soon as possible and were seen at eight to nine weeks' gestation for ultrasound scanning and further discussion. Vaginal swabs were taken to detect genital tract infection and, if necessary, specific treatment was given. All women were given prophylactic erythromycin and clotrimazole pessaries. Erythromycin was chosen because of its action against organisms such as *Chlamydia* and *Ureaplasma*. The procedure was scheduled for 11 weeks' gestation. An ultrasound scan was performed shortly before the operation to confirm fetal viability, detect major abnormality and measure nuchal translucency (Nicolaides, Brizot and Snijders 1994).

## Surgical technique

A transverse suprapubic incision is suitable in most cases, although a longitudinal incision may be preferred when difficult surgical access is anticipated. The fold of uterovesical peritoneum is divided and the bladder and paravesical tissues reflected to expose the supravaginal cervix. The uterine vessels are displaced laterally, opening the paracervical connective tissue space. The lower portion of the isthmus at the level of the internal os is palpated between thumb and finger with the uterus in the palm of the hand. Three anatomical features are identified to locate the site of suture insertion: the widening of the cervix into the soft isthmus, the uterine vessel passing longitudinally and the point of insertion of the uterosacral ligaments into the uterus. The suture material used is 5-mm wide Mersilene tape with round-bodied needles on each end (RS22 Ethicon). The needle is passed anteroposteriorly through the paracervical tissues immediately adjacent to the cervix superior to the insertion of the uterosacral ligaments, taking care to avoid the uterine vessels (Figure 1). This is done on both sides.

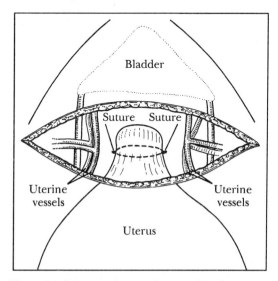

**Figure 1** *Schematic diagram showing where the suture is placed during a transabdominal cervicoisthmic cerclage operations*

The band of suture material is adjusted to ensure that it lies flush on the anterior aspect of the cervicoisthmic region before being tied posteriorly. The suture therefore lies in a extraperitoneal position anteriorly and in a intraperitoneal posteriorly (Figure 2). The free ends of the suture are trimmed and secured with a non-absorbable suture and placed in the pouch of Douglas to aid access via posterior colpotomy, if this becomes necessary.

Postoperatively, prophylactic hormones or tocolytics were not used. With the increasing evidence regarding the association between genital tract infection and preterm delivery, intraoperative and postoperative antibiotics were used.

Subsequent antenatal care was planned on an individual basis, although all included serial ultrasound scans. Some patients chose antenatal admission due to anxiety relating to previous pregnancy losses. Delivery was planned by elective Caesarean section at 38 weeks' gestation. If the couple wished to consider a further pregnancy the suture was left in place, otherwise it was removed during the Caesarean section. If complications arose prior to 24 weeks' gestation the suture was removed by posterior colpotomy and vaginal miscarriage followed.

## Results

Sixty-six pregnancies following TCC are reported. The adverse outcomes are shown in Table 1. One immediate postoperative loss occurred in a woman with fibroid uterus which was difficult to manipulate. The suture was successfully inserted, but the fetus was in the vagina at the end of the procedure. The placenta and membranes were aspirated, leaving the suture in place. She conceived again, but the membranes ruptured at 20 weeks' gestation. The stitch was removed by posterior colpotomy and miscarriage occurred. In another woman who had an early miscarriage, the membranes ruptured three days after the procedure at 13 weeks' gestation. In the third case, a miscarriage occurred 10 days after the procedure; this had been performed on the insistence of the couple, despite vaginal bleeding having occurred in the first trimester. The uterus was evacuated through the intact suture and she has since had another pregnancy with a successful

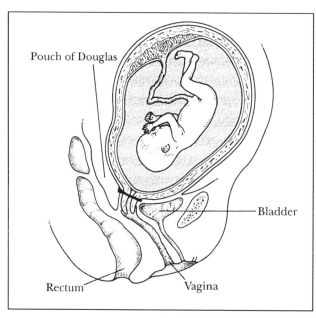

**Figure 2**  *Schematic diagram of the longitudinal view through a pregnant woman showing the position of the suture after transabdominal cervicoisthmic operation*

outcome. In a fourth case, a successful outcome after TCC and delivery by Caesarean section with the suture in place, was followed by an 11-week miscarriage, with evacuation of products of conception while the suture remained.

Three patients had a midtrimester pregnancy loss. One patient had TCC in a twin pregnancy: the membranes ruptured at 20 weeks' gestation. In another case, membrane rupture occurred four weeks after the procedure and, in the third, intrauterine death occurred at 20 weeks' gestation: uterine blood flow had not been affected.

**Table 1**  *Adverse outcome following transabdominal cervicoisthmic cerclage*

| Outcome* | Number |
|---|---|
| Miscarriage before 14 weeks' gestation | 4 |
| Loss 14–24 weeks' gestation | 3 |
| Preterm delivery and neonatal death | 2 |
| Intrauterine death | 1 |
| Total | 10 |

*Three women have had a living child subsequently

**Table 2**  *Outcome in 54 women following transabdominal cervicoisthmic cerclage (TCC)*

| Outcome | Number |
|---|---|
| No living child | 7 |
| Preterm delivery and survival | 4* |
| One term delivery | 34** |
| Two term deliveries | 9*** |

*Includes one set of quadruplets; **includes one set of twins; ***includes one woman who has had TCC twice followed by term delivery

This patient conceived again and had a second TCC with successful outcome (case A).

One patient in her first pregnancy, conceived by *in vitro* fertilisation, and having had previous extensive cervical surgery, had an intrauterine death at 26 weeks' gestation associated with severe pre-eclampsia.

The results before and after TCC are shown in Tables 2 and 3. Seven women do not have a living child. Premature deliveries occurred at 24, 31, 31 and 34 weeks' gestation: one delivery at 31 weeks' gestation was of quadruplets. All these babies survived.

No case suffered immediate maternal complications after the operation. Blood transfusion was not required in any case. The only significant long-term complication was one recto-uterine fistula. This occurred eight years after a successful pregnancy where the suture was left in place at delivery. The fistula was repaired successfully with full recovery.

**Specific cases**

Three cases deserve special mention.

*Case A*

Case A was referred by another consultant after having one living child and seven pregnancy losses, six with vaginal cerclage in place. Her cervix had become badly lacerated. When she presented to the authors she was 42 years old. Transabdominal cervicoisthmic cerclage was considered appropriate and was inserted without difficulty. She declined invasive prenatal diagnosis. When she attended for the 20 week

**Table 3**  *Outcome before and after transabdominal cervicoisthmic cerclage (TCC)*

| Outcome | Before TCC | After TCC |
|---|---|---|
| Term delivery | 10 | 52 |
| Miscarriage before 14 weeks' gestation | 36 | 4 |
| Midtrimester miscarriage | 152 | 3 |
| Premature delivery with neonatal death or stillbirth | 13 | 3 |
| Premature delivery with neonatal survival | 6 | 4 |
| Total number of pregnancies | 217 | 66 |
| Fetal survival (%) | 7.4 | 84.8 |
| beyond first trimester | (8.8) | (90.3) |

ultrasound scan intrauterine fetal death was diagnosed. After appropriate counselling general anaesthesia was administered. A posterior colpotomy was performed and the knot of the stitch was located in the pouch of the Douglas. It was cut and removed. Prostaglandin treatment resulted in vaginal miscarriage. Two years later, at the age of 44 years, she again presented pregnant. She became the first patient on record to have the procedure a second time. Again declining invasive prenatal diagnosis she carried that pregnancy to term. She has now had the suture removed!

### Case B

Case B had the procedure at the age of 38 years after numerous difficult pregnancies with only one successful outcome. She had second-trimester biochemical screening for Down's syndrome which was reported to be negative. She declined invasive prenatal diagnosis. A healthy girl was delivered by Caesarean section at term, who was subsequently diagnosed as having Down's syndrome. During the Caesarean section she had requested that the suture be removed, although she did not want tubal ligation. The baby was operated on at the age of six months because of congenital heart defect and died under anaesthesia. This was very traumatic for the couple, but three years later they proposed to try again for a child. At the age of 41 years she conceived again and became the second patient to have a second insertion of TCC. She carried this pregnancy successfully to term with the birth of a healthy baby.

### Case C

Case C was referred having lost five previous pregnancies. In three of these, transvaginal cervical cerclage had been placed. In one instance a silastic tube had been used. On the basis of previous failed cerclage, although the cervix appeared anatomically normal, a TCC was inserted. At 20 weeks' gestation the membranes ruptured. The suture was removed by posterior colpotomy. The uterus was evacuated with difficulty using high doses of prostaglandin and oxytocin over 48 hours. This patient has since had a term pregnancy with no cerclage! Either she did not have cervical weakness originally or the surgical procedures on her cervix had led to therapeutic fibrosis.

## DISCUSSION

The results from the authors' series of 66 pregnancies show a fetal survival rate of 90%, which compares favourably with the other series published (Table 4). These studies consistently produce an impressive success rate which may reflect the careful selection of patients for TCC and the higher anatomical placement of the suture. As described earlier in the chapter, the indications for TCC are anatomical defects in the cervix and previous failed vaginal cerclage, which is likely to produce a more homogeneous

**Table 4** *Cumulative results of transabdominal cervicoisthmic cerclage (TCC)*

| Publication | No. of patients | Fetal survival before TCC | Fetal survival after TCC |
|---|---|---|---|
| Benson and Durfee (1965) | 10 | 11 | 82 |
| Watkins (1972) | 2 | 55 | 100 |
| Mahran (1978) | 10 | 10 | 70 |
| Olsen and Tobiassen (1982) | 17 | 12 | 88 |
| Novy (1982) | 16 | 24 | 95 |
| Wallenberg and Lotgering (1987) | 14 | 16 | 94 |
| Herron and Parer (1988) | 8 | 15 | 85 |
| van Dongen and Nijhuis (1991) | 14 | 30 | 94 |
| Novy (1991) | 20 | 20 | 90 |
| Cammarano, Herron and Parer (1995) | 23 | 18 | 93 |
| Flint and Gibb (this series) | 54 | 9 | 90 |

group of women than those who receive transvaginal cerclage.

There are several disadvantages of TCC. There is a need for two abdominal operations during one pregnancy with the potential complications relating to the procedures themselves and to the anaesthetic. There is a risk of haemorrhage when the operative field is so vascular which has prompted the suggestion that TCC should be performed as an interval procedure. There have been occasional reports of excessive bleeding during this procedure (Novy 1991, Herron and Parer 1988; van Dongen and Nijhuis 1991), but in all our cases estimated blood loss was less than 400 ml and blood transfusion has not been necessary in any of the cases. There is no study comparing the use of TCC in the non-pregnant state with those inserted in pregnancy, although a review of the literature has shown that over 80% are inserted between 10 and 14 weeks' gestation, at a time when the risk of spontaneous first-trimester miscarriage has passed but the uterus may be manipulated more easily, the posterior broad ligament visualised on either side without difficulty. From the author's own experience, manipulation of the uterus may be difficult after this gestation. One recent case was referred late and insertion failed for this reason. This patient experienced a subsequent midtrimester miscarriage. Theoretically, delivery by Caesarean section could be avoided by removal of the suture by posterior colpotomy to allow vaginal delivery, but none of the patients have elected for this management.

When a complication arises prior to fetal viability, the suture may be removed by posterior colpotomy. To facilitate this, the suture is tied posteriorly. As TCC is likely to be performed in a referral centre, when the patient returns to the local hospital it is important that effective communication occurs between clinicians to ensure correct management (even when staff are unfamiliar with the procedure).

Other complications which have occasionally been associated with TCC include intrauterine death, growth retardation, preterm premature rupture of the membranes, placenta abruption and suture migration (Novy 1982; Novy 1991; Gibb and Salaria 1995).

## CONCLUSION

Transabdominal cervicoisthmic cerclage may be considered for women with previous history of recurrent second-trimester miscarriage or early preterm delivery with anatomical defects of the cervix and previous failed vaginal cerclage. The successful pregnancy rate following this procedure is consistently in the region of 85–95%.

# References

Andersen, H. F., Nugent, C. E., Wanty, S. D. and Hayashi, R. H. (1990) Prediction of risk for preterm delivery by ultrasonographic measurement of cervical length. *Am J Obstet Gynecol* **163**, 859–67

Anthony, G. S., Calder, A. A. and MacNaughton, M. (1981) Cervical resistance studies in patients with previous spontaneous midtrimester abortion. *Br J Obstet Gynaecol* **89**, 1046–9

Benson, R. C. and Durfee, R. B. (1965) Transabdominal cervicouterine cerclage during pregnancy for the treatment of cervical incompetency. *Obstet Gynecol* **25**, 145–55

Bergman, P. and Svenerund, A. (1957) Traction test for demonstrating incompetency of the internal os of the cervix. *Int J Fertil* **2**, 163

Brook, I., Feingold, M., Schwatz, A. and Zakut, H. (1981) Ultrasonography in the diagnosis of cervical incompetence in pregnancy — a new diagnostic approach. *Br J Obstet Gynaecol* **88**, 640–3

Cammarano, C. L., Herron, M. A. and Parer, J. T. (1995) Validity of indications for transabdominal cervicoisthmic cerclage incompetence. *Am J Obstet Gynecol* **172**, 1871–5

Gaillard, D. A., Paradis, P., Vallemand, A. *et al.* (1993) Spontaneous abortion during the second trimester of gestation. *Arch Pathol Lab Med* **117**, 1022–6

Gibb, D. M. F. and Salaria, D. A. (1995) Transabdominal cervicoisthmic cerclage in the management of recurrent second trimester miscarriage and preterm delivery. *Br J Obstet Gyneacol* **102**, 802–6

Harger, J. H. (1980) Comparison of success and morbidity in cervical cerclage procedures. *Obstet Gynecol* **56**, 543–8

Hauth, J. C., Goldenberg, R. L., Andrews, W. W., DuBard, M. B. and Copper, R. L. (1995) Reduced incidence of preterm delivery with metronidazole and erythromycin in women with bacterial vaginosis. *N Engl J Med* **333**, 1732–6

Hay, P. E., Lamont, R. F., Taylor-Robinson, D. *et al.* (1994) Abnormal bacterial colonisation of the genital tract and subsequent preterm delivery and late miscarriage. *BMJ* **308**, 295–8

Herron, M. A. and Parer, J. T. (1988) Transabdominal cerclage for fetal wastage due to cervical incompetence. *Obstet Gynecol* **71**, 865–8

Iams, J. D., Goldenberg, R. L., Meis, P. J. *et al.* (1996) The length of the cervix and the risk of spontaneous premature delivery. *N Engl J Med* **334**, 567–72

Jeffcoate, T. N. and Wilson, J. K. (1956) Uterine causes of abortion and premature labour. *NY State J Med* **56**, 680

Lash, A. F. and Lash, S. R. (1950) Habitual abortion: the incompetence internal os of the cervix. *Am J Obstet Gynecol* **59**, 68–76

Lazar, P., Gueguen, S., Dreyfus, J. *et al.* (1984) Multicentre controlled trial of cervical cerclage in women at moderate risk of preterm delivery. *Br J Obstet Gynaecol* **91**, 731–5

Mahran, M. (1978) Transabdominal cerclage during pregnancy. A modified technique. *Obstet Gynecol* **52** 502–6

McDonald, I. A. (1957) Suture of the cervix for inevitable miscarriage. *J Obstet Gynaecol Br Emp* **64**, 346–50

Medical Research Council/Royal College of Obstetricians and Gynaecologists Working Party on Cervical Cerclage (1993) Final report of the Medical Research Council/Royal College of Obstetricians and Gynaecologists multicentre randomised trial of cervical cerclage. *Br J Obstet Gynaecol* **100**, 516–23

Nicolaides, K., Brizot, M. and Snijders, R. (1994) Fetal nuchal translucency thickness: ultrasound screening for fetal trisomy in the first trimester of pregnancy. *Br J Obstet Gynaecol* **101**, 782–6

Novy, M. J. (1982) Transabdominal cervicoisthmic cerclage for the management of repetitive abortion and premature delivery. *Am J Obstet Gynecol* **143**, 44–54

Novy, M. J (1991) Transabdominal cervicoisthmic cerclage: a reappraisal 25 years after its introduction. *Am J Obstet Gynecol* **164**, 1635–42

Okitsu, O., Mimura, T., Nakayama, T. and Aono, T. (1992) Early prediction of preterm delivery by transvaginal ultrasonography. *Ultrasound Obstet Gynecol* **2**, 402–9

Olsen, S. and Tobiassen, T. (1982) Transabdominal isthmic cerclage for the treatment of incompetent cervix. *Acta Obstet Gynecol Scand* **61**, 473–5

Podobnik, M., Bulic, M. and Smiljanic, N. (1988) Ultrasonography in the detection of cervical incompetency. *J Clin Ultrasound* **13**, 383–91

Rai, R., Clifford, K. and Regan, L. (1996) The modern preventative treatment of recurrent miscarriage. *Br J Obstet Gynaecol* **103**, 106–10

Rai, R. S., Regan L., Cliiford K. *et al.* (1995) Antiphospholipid antibodies and à$_2$ glycoprotein I in 500 women with recurrent miscarriage: results of a comprehensive screening approach. *Hum Reprod* **10**, 2001–5

Romero, R., Gomez, R. and Sepulveda, W. (1992) The uterine cervix, ultrasound and prematurity. *Ultrasound Obstet Gynecol* **2**, 385–8

Rush, R. W., Isaacs, S., McPherson, *et al.* (1984) A randomised controlled trial of cervical cerclage in women at high risk of spontaneous preterm delivery. *Br J Obstet Gynaecol* **91**, 731–5

Shirodkar, V. N. (1955) A new method of operative treatment for habitual abortion in the second trimester of pregnancy. *Antiseptic J* **52**, 299–300

van Dongen, P. W. J. and Nijhuis, J. G. (1991) Transabdominal cerclage. *Eur J Obstet Gynecol Reprod Biol* **41**, 97–104

Wallenburg, H. C. and Lotgering, F. K. (1987) Transabdominal cerclage for closure of the incompetent cervix. *Eur J Obstet Reprod Biol* **25**, 121–9

Watkins, R. A. (1972) Transabdominal cervico-uterine suture. *Aust NZ J Obstet Gynecol* **12**, 62–4

# 31

# Pre-eclampsia: the role
# of the vascular endothelium

*Andrea J. Wilkinson, Janet R. Ashworth and Philip N. Baker*

Although pre-eclampsia was first described over 100 years ago, one of the difficulties in writing a review about it is the problem surrounding its definition (Nelson, Zuspan and Mulligan 1966; World Health Organisation 1987; Davey and MacGillivray 1988; Redman and Jeffries 1988; Gifford, August and Chelsey 1990; Perry and Beevers 1994). The variety of names for the syndrome of hypertension peculiar to pregnancy associated with proteinuria, thrombocytopenia, hyperuricaemia and compromised renal and hepatic function emphasises the confusion surrounding the condition. Diseases can be diagnosed, but syndromes can only be recognised (Redman and Roberts 1993), and pre-eclampsia is a clinical syndrome which is recognised by clinical signs. As no feature is consistently present, the absence of a particular sign can never exclude the syndrome. In clinical practice, hypertension and proteinuria are easy to detect, and so are emphasised in definitions of the disease.

Pre-eclampsia is a misnomer, as eclampsia is not always preceded by the pre-eclampsia syndrome, and pre-eclampsia does not necessarily lead to eclampsia (Douglas and Redman 1994). It is becoming increasingly clear that pre-eclampsia is a disease of separate aetiology from early essential hypertension and from hypertension of renal origin, both of which may present as hypertension in pregnancy (Chelsey 1980). Although central to the diagnosis of pre-eclampsia, hypertension is now regarded as a secondary effect of the primary pathogenesis and should be considered as part of a spectrum of disease, which includes the HELLP syndrome (haemolysis, elevated liver enzymes and low platelet count) and intrauterine growth retardation, which are not characterised by hypertension.

As the debate continues, for the purpose of this review, pre-eclampsia will be defined as a clinical syndrome in which a previously normotensive woman (with no pre-existing renal disease and after 20 completed weeks' gestation), develops a blood pressure of at least 140/90 mmHg on two occasions separated by at least four hours, in the presence of proteinuria of at least 0.3 g/l in a 24-hour collection of urine (in the absence of an urinary tract infection), both of which resolve by the sixth week postpartum (Davey and MacGillivray 1988). Pregnancy-induced hypertension (PIH) will be defined as the onset of hypertension in a previously normotensive woman of at least 140/90 mmHg on two occasions separated by at least four hours, after 20 completed weeks' gestation, which is not associated with significant proteinuria.

## PATHOGENESIS OF PRE-ECLAMPSIA

### Genetic

The familial nature of pre-eclampsia was first recognised over a century ago (Elliot 1873). Population studies show that the susceptibility to eclampsia is highly heritable and that a single recessive gene may be responsible (Chelsey and Cooper 1986; Arnigrimsson *et al.* 1990).

Association between pre-eclampsia and particular gene variants have been made (Ward *et al.* 1993). However, discordance between monozygotic twin sisters shows that maternal genotype cannot be the only determining factor (Thornton and Sampson 1990). The fetal genotype has been shown to play a role, with an association between pre-eclampsia and trisomy 13 (Thornton and Sampson 1990) and an excess of male fetuses in pregnancies complicated by pre-eclampsia (James 1993). The interaction between maternal and fetal genotypes in pre-eclampsia may mimic that seen in recurrent miscarriage (which appears to have an association with eclampsia), and is characterised by an increased incidence of histocompatibity locus A (HLA) antigen sharing between maternal and paternal genotypes (Cooper *et al.* 1988).

## Immunological

Pre-eclampsia is a disorder of first pregnancies, but the protective effect of multiparity may be lost after a change of partner (Feeney and Scott 1980). This has led to an immunologically mediated pathogenesis for pre-eclampsia to be proposed. Initially, a widespread disturbance of the immune system was suggested, with various hypotheses regarding the stimulation of lymphocytes and platelets by circulating immune complexes. One hypothesis suggested that circulating immune complexes may stimulate lymphocytes and platelets to release inflammatory mediators (Petrucco 1981; Massobrio *et al.* 1985). Another is that transport of trophoblastic cells leads to maternal antigenic overload and deposition of immune complexes in target organs (Petrucco 1981). However, the evidence for a widespread disturbance in immune function in pre-eclampsia is contradictory, and changes in immunoglobulin and complement do not precede the onset of clinical disease (Cooper, Baker and Milton 1995). Recently, it has been suggested that the immune mechanism operates at a local level (i.e. the placenta) rather than a widespread immune activation. In the first trimester, the decidua is primarily an immune tissue containing many cells of bone marrow origin, including macrophages, T cells and large granular lymphocytes (Starkey, Sargent and Redman 1988). The subpopulation of cytotrophoblast cells that invade the uterus express a unique class 1 HLA antigen of the non-classical HLA-G locus (Ellis, Palmer and McMichael 1990; Kovats *et al.* 1990), which is thought to confer resistance to natural killer cell activity in the first-trimester decidua (Yoke 1994). At present there is no direct evidence that abnormal recognition of this antigen occurs in pre-eclampsia.

## Placental

Pre-eclampsia is uniquely a disease of pregnancy and, as such, must be mediated by one of the products of conception or changed uterine environment. Pre-eclampsia has been reported in women with abdominal pregnancies (Roberts and Redman 1993), so a uterine cause is unlikely. The presence of a fetus is not a prerequisite for pre-eclampsia, as it may occur, and indeed is more common, in molar pregnancies (Newman and Eddy 1988).

Placental tissue must be present for pre-eclampsia to develop. The placenta is further implicated in the pathogenesis of pre-eclampsia, by virtue of the fact that pre-eclampsia occurs more commonly in conditions characterised by hyperplacentosis (e.g. multiple pregnancy, hydatidiform mole and non-immune hydrops). The placenta in pre-eclampsia is characterised by a failure of the trophoblast to invade the spiral arteries of the inner-third of the myometrium. Studying the spiral arteries throughout their course, from their origin at the radial arteries, through the myometrium and decidua, the arteries from normotensive pregnant women are found to increase in diameter by four- to sixfold compared with the non-pregnant state. The endothelium, internal elastic lamina and smooth muscle layer is replaced by trophoblast and amorphous fibrin-containing matrix. These changes extend from the intervillous space to the inner-third of the myometrium (Brosens, Robertson and Dixon 1972; Sheppard and Bonnar 1974). In contrast, in women with pre-eclampsia, the spiral artery dilatation is only 40% of that seen in normal pregnancy; the portion of the spiral artery within the myometrium is not invaded by trophoblast and is essentially unaltered from the non-pregnant state. A similar lack of adaptation to pregnancy is also present in up to half of the decidual portions of the spiral arteries (Brosens, Robertson and Dixon 1972; Sheppard and Bonnar 1974; Khong *et al.* 1986). Furthermore, some of the spiral arteries in women with pre-eclampsia demonstrate lesions of acute atherosis, consisting of fibrinoid deposition in the vessel wall and foam cell accumulation in the intima, leading to total or partial vessel occlusion (Kitzmiller and Benirschke 1973). The fetal–maternal interface is the placental syncytiotrophoblast, a multi-nucleate true syncytium with an extensive microvillus brush border, which is in direct contact with maternal blood. In pre-eclampsia the microvilli are abnormally shaped, with focal areas of necrosis (Jones and Fox 1980). This necrosis may explain the greatly increased trophoblast deportation characteristic of pre-eclampsia (Chua *et al.* 1991). Similar changes can be induced by culturing normal placental villi under hypoxic conditions (MacLennan, Sharp and Shaw 1972).

Trophoblastic invasion is associated with a modulation in the distribution of adhesion molecules, increased expression of HLA-G antigen and activity of a type IV collagenase (Cooper, Baker and Milton 1995). Pre-eclampsia is associated with abnormal adhesion molecule expression by trophoblast cells, which retain adhesion molecules that are normally only expressed by villus stem cells and proximal cytotrophoblast cells (Zhou *et al.* 1993). The end result of this abnormal trophoblast invasion is an inadequate development of the uteroplacental blood supply, increased resistance in the placental vascular bed and, consequently, diminished fetal perfusion. Animal studies in which blood flow to the uterus and placenta are reduced produces a condition similar to pre-eclampsia (Combs *et al.* 1993). The role of the endothelium in the translation of the fetoplacental pathology to the pathophysiological features of the clinical syndrome will now be discussed.

## THE ENDOTHELIUM IN PRE-ECLAMPSIA

The vascular endothelium in a healthy woman weighs approximately 1.5 kg (Henderson 1991). Endothelial cells are not an inert barrier between the intra- and extravascular compartments, which allow the transfer of nutrients, waste products, regulatory molecules and phagocytic cells across the basement membrane, but have sophisticated metabolic and secretory functions relevant to pregnancy homeostasis.

Pathophysiological changes associated with pre-eclampsia include increased sensitivity to pressor agents, reduced plasma volume and activation of the coagulation cascade. Many of these changes precede the onset of the hypertension and can be explained by alteration of normal endothelial function.

### Pressor sensitivity

The vasoconstriction of pre-eclampsia is probably secondary to increased sensitivity to normally circulating pressor agents. Serial infusions of the potent vasoconstrictor angiotensin II in normotensive primigravidae by Gant, Daley and Chand (1973), showed a progressive decrease in the sensitivity to angiotensin II throughout the first two trimesters. In women who subsequently developed pre-eclampsia, this resistance to the pressor effects of angiotensin II was gradually lost from 18 weeks' gestation, such that by 32 weeks' gestation these women were more sensitive to angiotensin II than non-pregnant women (Gant, Daley and Chand 1973). A similar increase in sensitivity to other infused vasopressors (e.g. adrenaline, noradrenaline and vasopressin) has also been demonstrated (Talledo, Chelsey and Zuspan 1968).

### Endothelial derived vasorelaxation

Normal endothelial cells modify the contractile response of adjacent smooth muscle cells (Furchgott and Zawadski 1980) by the secretion of vasoconstrictors (e.g. endothelin) and the vasorelaxants (e.g. nitric oxide [NO], prostacyclin [PGI$_2$] and a hyper-polarising factor). The net vasoactive effect of the endothelium is to contribute a basal level of vasodilatation to vascular tone and to limit the effect of various vasoconstrictors and neurogenic stimuli. The endothelium is also exposed to changes in shear stress, which occur secondary to changes in blood flow, and this may be the most important stimulus for NO release (Pohl *et al.* 1986). Many endogenous vasoactive substances (e.g. histamine, bradykinin, serotonin and adenine nucleotides) have been shown to increase the production of NO (Morris, Eaton and Gekker 1996).

Nitric oxide is an inorganic free radical with a wide range of biological activity which was recently comprehensively reviewed in relation to pregnancy and pre-eclampsia (Morris, Eaton and Dekker 1996). It is released by endothelial cells and binds to the heme component of soluble guanylate cyclase in adjacent smooth muscle cells. This increases cyclic guanosine monophosphate (cGMP) production, which activates phosphokinase and reduces the intracellular calcium concentration, resulting in relaxation of perivascular smooth muscle, and hence vasodilatation. Nitric oxide reduces platelet sensitivity to proaggregatory agents, thus inhibiting platelet aggregation. It also functions as a neurotransmitter and has a role in the pathogenesis of septic shock and chronic hypertension. Nitric oxide is synthesised from the essential amino acid L-arginine by a cytosolic enzyme nitric oxide synthase (NOS). Three isoforms of NOS have been identified. Two isoforms, endothelial (eNOS) and neuronal are constitutive, that is, they are always present. The inducible isoform is mainly found in the macrophage and is produced in response to infection, bacterial endotoxin, exotoxin or cytokines. The constitutive forms are activated by calcium influx into the cell, whereas the inducible form is relatively calcium independent. The endothelial isoform of this enzyme (eNOS) is found in both large and small vessel endothelium, platelets, endocardium, myocardium and vascular smooth muscle cells. The production of NO requires molecular oxygen and at least four cofactors and is inhibited by L-arginine analogues, flavoprotein binders and calmodulin binders. As NOS activity is oxygen dependent, a reduction in oxygen saturation reduces NO synthesis. Endothelial nitric oxide synthase activity is stimulated by serotonin and bradykinin, which are released during platelet activation and, hence, prevent excessive platelet aggregation and adhesion.

Nitric oxide synthesis is increased in pregnancy, reflected in the increased urinary excretion of nitrate, the stable NO metabolite (Conrad, Joffe and Kruszyna 1993). Nitric oxide synthase has been localised to the syncytiotrophoblast cell layer in the human placenta, with both calcium-dependent and independent NOS activity in placental villi and basal plate, but minimal activity in the placental bed (Morris *et al.* 1993). Although the majority of this (94%) is constitutive eNOS, messenger RNA for inducible NOS has been shown to be present in placentae (Morris *et al.* 1993).

Different groups have suggested that the increased sensitivity to vasopressors seen in pre-eclampsia could be explained by a decreased production of NO. Unfortunately, data regarding levels of plasma and urinary nitrites are conflicting. This may be accounted for by differences in disease definitions, methods used, a lack of dietary control and the use of random, rather than 24-hour urine collections (Baker, Davidge and Roberts 1995).

## Coagulation

Normal vascular endothelial cells resist platelet aggregation and coagulation in several ways. First, endothelial cells secrete prostacyclin (PGI$_2$), a potent vasodilator and inhibitor of platelet aggregation. Other anticoagulant molecules (e.g. thrombomodulin and heparin sulphate) are synthesised and secreted onto the luminal surface of endothelial cells. Protein C, a potent circulating anticoagulant, also requires endothelial cells for its cell-dependent activation. Endothelial cells modulate fibrinolysis by synthesising plasminogen activators and inhibitors. Hence, local control of coagulation is exerted by endothelial cells (Colman *et al.* 1994).

The coagulation cascade is activated in pre-eclampsia and changes may predate clinical recognition of the disease by several weeks (de Boer *et al.* 1989). Although clinical disseminated intravascular coagulation is only evident in 20% of women with severe pre-eclampsia, even in mild disease, activation of the coagulation cascade can be demonstrated (Redman, Bonnar and Beilin 1978). Pre-eclampsia is associated with alteration in prostaglandin metabolism (Fitzgerald *et al.* 1987; Myatt 1987). Prostacyclin is the major prostanoid produced by endothelial cells. In pre-eclampsia, the intravascular production of $PGI_2$ and the concentration of $PGI_2$ in both blood and urine is decreased. Thromboxane is also present in the endothelium, particularly in uterine vessels, and pre-eclampsia is associated with an increase in the thromboxane : $PGI_2$ ratio (Wang *et al.* 1991). Loss of the vasodilatory and anticoagulant effects of $PGI_2$ would explain the increased sensitivity to pressor agents and activation of the coagulation cascade.

Platelet activation is a physiological feature of healthy pregnancy (Fay, Hughes and Farron 1983) and is exaggerated in pre-eclampsia (Whigham *et al.* 1978). Platelet consumption is shown by a progressive thrombocytopenia and an increase in platelet size (Redman, Bonnar and Beilin 1978). In pre-eclampsia, platelets are more prone to adhere to the endothelium, releasing $\alpha$ and dense granules. Thromboxane and serotonin released from activated platelets cause platelet aggregation and induce fibrin formation. The increased level of serotonin induces further activation and may also amplify the vasoconstrictor action of catecholamines and angiotensin II (Middelkoop *et al.* 1993).

Antithrombin II, a serine protease inhibitor, which is active against thrombin, factor $X_a$ and factor VII is decreased in pre-eclampsia, and its product thrombin–antithrombin III complex is increased. These changes occur prior to the onset of the clinical syndrome. There is an increase in the thrombin–antithrombin ratio in normal pregnancy and this is significantly exaggerated in pre-eclampsia (deBoer *et al.* 1989). These changes of endothelial function can be explained by endothelial activation.

## ENDOTHELIAL ACTIVATION

The concept of endothelial cell activation was first proposed in the 1960s when morphological changes were noted in postcapillary venules of inflamed tissues. The endothelial cells were noted to be swollen and ultrastructural examination showed increased biosynthetic organelles (e.g. endoplasmic reticulum and Golgi apparatus). Willms-Kretschner, Flax and Cotran (1967) referred to this as activation, implying a functional consequence to the altered morphology. In the 1970s, this dynamic view of the endothelium was replaced by a model in which the endothelial role was thought to be passive, and activation was dismissed as a morphological manifestation of a response to injury. In the early 1980s, Pober and colleagues showed that rather than causing sublethal injury and subsequent dysfunction, $\gamma$-interferon (IFN$\gamma$), a cytokine (a soluble factor produced by activated T lymphocytes) caused endothelial cells to express new molecules and biological functions. Hence, the term endothelial cell activation was redefined in cell biological terms (Pober 1988).

Endothelial activation has been defined as 'quantitative changes in the level of expression of specific gene products (i.e. proteins) that endow endothelial cells with new capacities that cumulatively allow endothelial cells to perform new functions' (Pober 1988).

It is thought that endothelial cell activation normally plays a beneficial role in host defences by promoting the development of cell-mediated immune reactions. However, it has been proposed that endothelial activation can also contribute to disease processes.

Activated endothelial cells are recognised by the expression of adhesion molecules on their cell surface. Endothelial leucocyte adhesion molecule (ELAM)-1 serves to bind polymorphonuclear leucocytes and is not present on unstimulated endothelial cells, but is transiently induced by numerous cytokines. Other adhesion molecules, such as intercellular adhesion molecule (ICAM)-1, also show increased expression. As well as producing alterations in adhesion molecule expression, cytokines can alter endothelial cell morphology producing membrane, cytoskeletal and matrix organisation. Two cytokines, tumour necrosis factor (TNF) and IFNγ cause cells to become plump and retract, producing intercellular gaps. These changes are reversed on cytokine withdrawal (Pober 1988).

## Endothelial cell activation in pre-eclampsia

Weiss and Dexter first speculated that pre-eclampsia was an endothelial disease in the 1940s (Ferris 1991). However, it is only recently that the hypothesis has gained credence after being advocated by Roberts et al. (1989). There is now substantial evidence for endothelial dysfunction in pre-eclampsia. Morphological evidence of endothelial cell activation is provided by the characteristic renal lesion of pre-eclampsia, which is not seen in any other hypertensive disorder, called glomerular endotheliosis. Electron microscopic examination of renal biopsies have shown the changes to be in the glomerular endothelial cells, which are swollen with electron dense cytoplasmic inclusions that may occlude the capillary lumen (McCartney 1969). Examination of renal biopsies from a series of nulliparous women with pre-eclampsia showed approximately 80% to have glomerular endotheliosis (Spargo, Lichtig and Luger 1976). This change may be due to direct endothelial cell damage or secondary to hypoperfusion.

In pre-eclampsia, extensive ultrastructural endothelial injury has also been found in placental bed specimens (Shanklin and Sibai 1989), with changes in the spiral arteries termed 'acute atherosis'. The increased capillary permeability seen in pre-eclampsia is consistent with alterations to normal vascular endothelium (Brown, Zammit and Lowe 1989).

In vitro studies suggest that exposure to a factor in the maternal plasma, or sera, exerts an effect on cultured endothelial cells (Roberts et al. 1992). Serum from women with pre-eclampsia exerts a greater cytotoxic effect on cultured endothelial cells (Rodgers, Taylor and Roberts 1988; Tsukimori et al. 1992) and a greater mitogenic effect on cultured fibroblasts (Musci et al. 1988) than serum from normotensive pregnant women. These alterations in cell function occur without increased lactate dehydrogenase release (a marker of cell viability), which shows that the changes are due to activation rather than cell death (Baker, Davidge and Roberts 1995).

Biochemical evidence of endothelial cell activation in pre-eclampsia includes levels of von Willebrand's factor (factor VII-related antigen) (Redman, Bonnar and Beilin 1978), fibronectin, cellular fibronectin (Roberts, Taylor and Goldfien 1991) and thrombomodulin. There is also a selective increase in the soluble cell adhesion marker (VCAM)-1 (Lyall et al. 1994). Endothelial cells exposed to plasma from women with pre-eclampsia show increased production of platelet-derived growth factor-B (PDGF-B) (Taylor et al. 1991). In addition to representing markers of endothelial cell activation, the increased release of fibronectin and PDGF-B may have a role in the pathogenesis of pre-eclampsia. Platelet-derived growth factor-B is a potent mitogen and may mediate the mesangial hypertrophy and hyperplasia associated with glomerular endotheliosis. Increased cellular fibronectin on the surface of endothelial cells increases platelet aggregation and activation.

Pre-eclampsia is associated with an alteration in prostaglandin metabolism (Fitzgerald et al. 1987; Myatt 1987), with a decrease in the $PGI_2$ : thromboxane ratio. Paradoxically, sera from women with pre-eclampsia initially stimulates $PGI_2$ production by endothelial cells cultured in vitro (relative to sera from normotensive pregnant subjects), and this is followed by a relative reduction in $PGI_2$ production over 24–48 hours (Figure 1) (Baker, Davidge and Roberts 1995). These changes are not seen in prostaglandin $E_2$ production, suggesting the differential effect of chronic exposure to plasma from women with pre-eclampsia may be specific to $PGI_2$ production.

Various mechanisms have been proposed for this alteration in $PGI_2$ metabolism. Lipid peroxidation, the oxidative conversion of unsaturated fatty acids to lipid peroxides, occurs in all cells and lipid peroxides are physiological activators of prostaglandin endoperoxide synthase (Lands

1985). However, as lipid peroxide levels become pathologically high, PGI₂ synthase is specifically impaired. Lipid peroxidation products have been shown to be elevated in women with pre-eclampsia which may inhibit PGI₂ synthase and explain the diminution in PGI₂ production.

Alternatively, the differential effect could be due to the modulatory effect of NO on prostaglandin production. Under different conditions, NO may activate or inhibit the enzyme cyclo-oxygenase, a key regulatory enzyme in prostaglandin synthesis. Inhibition of NOS reduces production of both NO and prostaglandins in bovine endothelial cells, suggesting that NO acts to increase cyclo-oxygenase activity. Conversely, increasing endogenous NO production in endothelial cell culture results in an increase in ecosanoid production. This has been shown to be the result of activation of prostaglandin H synthase (Davidge *et al.* 1995). The mechanism of activation is not understood. However, prostaglandin synthase II requires a hydroperoxide initiator for activity and it is proposed that NO, as an oxidising radical, could alter the activity of the enzyme. Bovine endothelial cells exposed to sera from women with pre-eclampsia show increased NO production which may contribute to the initial elevation in prostaglandin synthesis (Baker, Davidge and Roberts 1995).

An unexpected finding was that plasma from women with pre-eclampsia increases NO production and NOS activity in cultured microvascular endothelial cells, when the opposite result might be expected (Figure 2). However, it is dangerous to extrapolate this result to the situation *in vivo* as the experiments were performed in the absence of shearing stress, a known potent stimulator of NO production. In addition, an endothelial monolayer *in vivo* is modulated by paracrine signals from adjacent cells, especially smooth muscle cells. If the increased NO production in endothelial cells is a true reflection of the changes that occur *in vivo*, the increased levels of NO may mediate vascular endothelial damage by combining with oxygen and oxygen radicals to form peroxynitrate, a chemical oxidant which results in oxidative endothelial damage. Alternatively, increased

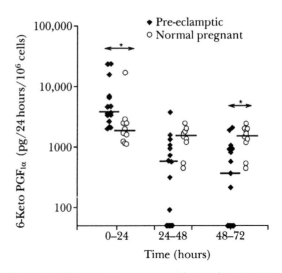

**Figure 1** *The sera from women with pre-eclampsia initially stimulates prostacyclin (PGI₁α) production* in vitro. *There is then a relative decline in PGI₁α production over the next 24–48 hours. (Reproduced from Baker, P. N., Davidge, S. T. and Roberts, J. M. (1996). Plasma of pre-eclamptic women stimulates and then inhibits endothelial prostacyclin.* Hypertension **27**, *56–61 with permission of The American Heart Association)*

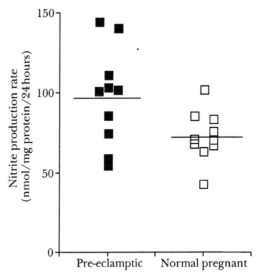

**Figure 2** *Nitrate production by endothelial cells exposed to plasma from patients with pre-eclampsia and from normal pregnant women. (Reproduced from Baker, P. N., Davidge, S. T. and Roberts, J. M. (1995) Plasma from women with pre-eclampsia and increases in endothelial cell nitric oxide production.* Hypertension **26**, *244–8, with permission of The American Heart Association)*

NO production in pre-eclampsia may reflect a compensatory mechanism to counteract the vasospasm associated with the disorder.

## Oxidative stress and pre-eclampsia

Pre-eclampsia has been proposed as a disease of antioxidant inadequacy, appearing when the normal antioxidant equilibrium is upset (Hubel *et al.* 1989). The antioxidant equilibrium is normally maintained by antioxidants such as vitamin E in the plasma and cell membrane, glutathione peroxidase, constitutive and inducible superoxide dismutase and catalase intracellularly, and caeruloplasmin extracellularly.

Lipid peroxides are produced as a result of decreased antioxidant activities. In human pregnancies the concentration of plasma lipid peroxides increases as pregnancy progresses and levels are significantly higher in hypertensive pregnancies (Wickens *et al.* 1981). This is supported by the presence of burr cells or echinocytes in peripheral blood (Weinstein 1982), which are comparable to those produced *in vitro* under peroxidising conditions. Deficiencies in known antioxidants, such as vitamin E and selenium, are associated with increased incidence of pre-eclampsia (Lu *et al.* 1990; Wang *et al.* 1991). The acute atherosis of pre-eclampsia resembles the atherogenic process in other arteries, in which a progressive deposition of lipid peroxide is associated with antibody directed against certain antigenic components, such as malondialdehyde-lysine (Stark 1993). Antibody and complement have been demonstrated where there are lipid-containing macrophages.

## Nature of the activating factor

Our current understanding of pre-eclampsia is that deficient trophoblast invasion in the first trimester signals the development of endothelial activation later in pregnancy and produces the clinical features of the syndrome.

A current hypothesis is that poor placentation is the result of a genetic predisposition, which is mediated via trophoblast cells and immunologically active decidual cells. The shallow endovascular trophoblast invasion results in a deficient uteroplacental blood supply. The resultant reduction in placental perfusion and relative placental hypoxia releases an agent into the circulation which activates endothelial cells throughout the body. Speculative contenders for the active agent in the plasma of women with pre-eclampsia which causes endothelial activation include antibodies, cytokines, syncytiotrophoblast microvillus membranes and lipid peroxides.

Antiphospholipid antibodies are associated with a syndrome of thrombosis, recurrent fetal loss and thrombocytopenia and have been shown to cause activation of cultured endothelial cells *in vitro* (Simantov *et al.* 1995). Anti-endothelial antibodies have been demonstrated in the blood of women with pre-eclampsia and these increase with the severity of the disease (Rappaport *et al.* 1990). The effect of sera on endothelial cells is significantly decreased by 48 hours postpartum, which fits the rapid clinical resolution postpartum. However, the long half-life of immunoglobulin would preclude this as a possible mediator.

Lipid peroxides disrupt cell membranes and other cell components and induce smooth muscle contraction. Hubel *et al.* (1989) hypothesised that the hypoxic placenta produces increased levels of lipid peroxides with subsequent endothelial damage. The induction of enzymes by lipid peroxides would also explain some of the biochemical abnormalities of pre-eclampsia.

Syncytiotrophoblast microvillus membranes have been shown to specifically disrupt and suppress proliferation of endothelial cells (Smarason *et al.* 1993) and trophoblast deportation has been shown to be increased in pre-eclampsia.

Cytokines and growth factors are popular candidates for the plasma mediator (Roberts and Redman 1993). They have a short half-life, are mitogenic, and several other stigmata of pathological cytokine activity are recognisable in pre-eclampsia (Stark 1993). Women with liver damage in pregnancy show two sets of tissue changes that might be interpreted as severe cytokine-induced abnormality. Light microscopy of patchy and irregular hepatic haemorrhages shows no remarkable features. However, electron microscopy shows the mitochondria to be swollen and distorted, which is the first intracellular effect of the potent cytokine TNF. In acute fatty liver, intracellular collections of fat globules are present. Tumour necrosis factor is known to greatly increase hepatic synthesis of both fatty acid and triglycerides and may mediate these lipid accumulations, which are not exported from malfunctioning cells (Stark 1993). Women with pre-eclampsia also show other milder features of an acute phase state, probably mediated by cytokines. These include increased caeruloplasmin concentration, activation of the complement cascade and increased activity of circulating monocytes (Stark 1993).

Recently, attention has focused on the growth factor, vascular endothelial factor (VEGF), a specific growth factor for vascular endothelium. It causes an increase in cytosolic calcium concentration and von Willebrand's factor release from cultured endothelial cells (Brock, Dvorak and Senger 1991) and promotes increased capillary permeability. The factor (VEGF) has been shown to be produced by trophoblast cells throughout pregnancy (Jackson *et al.* 1994) and its expression is greatly increased by hypoxia (Minchenko *et al.* 1994).

Certainly, VEGF levels are increased in the plasma of women with pre-eclampsia (Baker *et al.* 1995). Furthermore, VEGF has homology to, and forms heterodimers with, another growth factor, placental growth factor (PlGF). Placental growth factor also modulates the interaction of VEGF with its receptor (Thomas 1996). This interaction between VEGF and PlGF is typical of all cytokines, and may well reflect the fact that a single mediator is not responsible for the endothelial activation, but that the interaction of several factors influences the degree of endothelial activation and the timing of its onset.

The multisystem features of pre-eclampsia can be explained by the concept of endothelial activation. *In vitro* work has shown altered function of cultured endothelial cells when incubated with plasma from women with pre-eclampsia. Although the circulating factor(s) have not been identified, cytokines and lipid peroxides are likely candidates. Difficulties in extrapolating this work to the *in vivo* situation, results from the complex nature of the paracrine control mechanism between endothelial and vascular smooth muscle cells.

# References

Arnigrimsson, R., Bjornsson, S., Geirsson, R. T. *et al.* (1990) Genetic and familial disposition to eclampsia and pre-eclampsia in a defined population. *Br J Obstet Gynaecol* **93**, 898–908

Baker, P. N., Davidge, S. T. and Roberts, J. M. (1995) Plasma from women with pre-eclampsia increases endothelial cell nitric oxide production. *Hypertension* **26**, 244–8

Baker, P. N., Davidge, S. T. and Roberts, J. M. (1996) Plasma of pre-eclamptic women stimulates and then inhibits endothelial prostacyclin. *Hypertension* **27**, 56–61

Baker, P. N., Krasnow, J., Roberts, J. M. and Yeo, K.-T. (1995) Elevated serum levels of vascular endothelial growth factor in patients with pre-eclampsia. *Obstet Gynecol* **86**, 815–21

Brock, T. A., Dvorak, H. F. and Senger, D. R. (1991) Tumor secreted vascular permeability factor increases cytosolic $Ca^{2+}$ and von Willebrand factor release in human endothelial cells. *Am J Pathol* **138**, 213–21

Brosens, I. A., Robertson, W. B. and Dixon, H. G. (1972) The role of the spiral arteries in the pathogenesis of pre-eclampsia. *Obstet Gynecol Annu* **1**, 177–91

Brown, M. A., Zammit, V. C. and Lowe, S. A. (1989) Capillary permeability and extracellular fluid volumes in pregnancy induced hypertension. *Clin Sci* **77**, 599–604

Chelsey, I. C. (1980) Hypertension in pregnancy; definitions, familial factor and remote prognosis. *Kidney Int* **18**, 234–40

Chelsey, I. C. and Cooper, D. W. (1986) Genetics of hypertension in pregnancy: possible single gene control of pre-eclampsia in the descendants of eclamptic women. *Br J Obstet Gynaecol* **93**, 898–908

Chua, S., Wilkins, T., Sargent, I. and Redman, E. (1991) Trophoblast deportation in pre-eclamptic pregnancy. *Br J Obstet Gynaecol* **98**, 973–79

Colman, R. W., Marder, V. J., Salzman, E. W. and Hirsch, J. (1994) 'Overview of haemostasis' in: R. W. Colman, V. J. Marder, E. W. Salzman and J. Hirsch (Eds.). *Hemostatsis and Thrombosis. Basic Principles and Clinical Practice*, pp. 3–18. Philadelphia: Lippincott

Combs, C. A., Katz, M. A., Kitzmiller, J. A. and Brescia, R. J. (1993) Experimental pre-eclampsia produced by chronic constriction of the lower aorta, validation with longitudinal blood pressure measurements in conscious rhesus monkeys. *Am J Obstet Gynecol* **169**, 215–23

Conrad, K. P., Joffe, G. M. and Kruszyna, H. (1993) Identification of increased nitric oxide biosynthesis during pregnancy in rats. *FASAB J* **7**, 566–71

Cooper, D. W., Hill, A., Chelsey, I. and Bryans, C. I. (1988) Genetic control of susceptibility to eclampsia and miscarriage. *Br J Obstet Gynaecol* **95**, 644–53

Cooper, J. C., Baker, P. N. and Milton, P. J. (1995) 'Pre-eclampsia, current theories of pathogenesis' in: R. Asch and J. Studd (Eds.). *Progress in Reproductive Medicine*, Vol. 2, pp. 165–76. Edinburgh: Churchill Livingstone

Davey, D. A. and MacGillivray, I. (1988) The classification and definition of pre-eclampsia. *Am J Obstet Gynecol* **158**, 892–8

Davidge, S. T., Baker, P. N., McLaughlin, M. K. and Roberts, J. M. (1995) Nitric oxide produced by endothelial cells increases production of ecosanoids through activation of prostaglandin H synthase. *Circulation Res* **77**, 274–83

deBoer, K., Tencarte, J. W., Sturk, A., Bonn, J. J. I. and Treffers, P. E. (1989) Enhanced thrombin generation in normal and hypertensive pregnancy. *Am J Obstet Gynecol* **160** 95–100

Douglas, K. A. and Redman, C. W. G. (1994) Eclampsia in the United Kingdom. *BMJ* **309**, 1395–4000

Elliot, G. T. (1873) Case 120: puerperal eclampsia in the eighth month: extraordinary family history, in: *Obstetric Clinic*, pp. 291–3. New York: Appleton

Ellis, S. A., Palmer, M. S. and McMichael, A. (1990) Human trophoblasts and the choriocarcinoma cell line Be Wo express a truncated HLA class 1 molecule. *J Immunol* **144**, 731–5

Fay, R. A., Hughes, A. O. and Farron, N. T. (1983) Platelets in pregnancy – hyperdestruction in pregnancy. *Obstet Gynecol* **61**, 238–40

Feeney, J. G. and Scott, J. S. (1980) Pre-eclampsia and changed paternity. *Eur J Obstet Gynecol Reprod Biol* **11**, 35–8

Ferris, T. F. (1991) Pregnancy, pre-eclampsia and the endothelial cell. *N Engl J Med* **25**, 1439–42

Fitzgerald, D. J., Entman, W. S., Mulloyk, K. and Fitzgerald, G. A. (1987) Decreased prostacyclin biosynthesis preceding the clinical manifestation of pregnancy induced hypertension. *Circulation* **75**, 956–63

Furchgott, R. F. and Zawadski, J. V. (1980) The obligatory role of endothelial cells in the relaxation of smooth muscle by acetylcholine. *Nature* **288**, 373–6

Gant, N. F., Daley, G. L. and Chand, S. (1973) A study of angiotensin II pressor response throughout primigravid pregnancy. *J Clin Invest* **52**, 2682–9

Gifford, R. W., August, P. and Chelsey, I. C. (1990) National high blood pressure education program working group report on high blood pressure in pregnancy. *Am J Obstet Gynecol* **163**, 1691–1712

Henderson, A. H. (1991) Endothelium in control. *Br Heart J* **65**, 116–25

Hubel, C. A., Roberts, J. M., Taylor, R. N. *et al.* (1989) Lipid peroxidation in pregnancy: new perspectives on pre-eclampsia. *Am J Obstet Gynecol* **161**, 1025–34

Jackson, M. R., Carney, E. W., Lye, S. J. and Ritchie, J. W. K. (1994) Localisation of two angiogenic growth factors (PDECGF and VEGF) in human placentae throughout gestation. *Placenta* **15**, 341–53

James, W. H. (1993) Sex ratios in the families of women ascertained by a toxaemic pregnancy. *Br Obstet Gynaecol* **100**, 1151

Jones, C. I. and Fox, H. (1980) An ultra-structural and ultrahistochemical study of the human placenta in maternal pre-eclampsia. *Placenta* **1** 61–76

Khong, T. Y., de Wolf, F., Robertson, W. B. and Brosens, I. A. (1986) Inadequate maternal vascular response to placentation in pregnancies complicated by pre-eclampsia and small for gestational age infants. *Br J Obstet Gynaecol* **93** 1049–59

Kitzmiller, J. I. and Benirschke, K. (1973) Immunofluorescent study of placental bed vessels in pre-eclampsia. *Am J Obstet Gynecol* **115**, 248–51

Kovats, S., Main, E. K., Librach, C. *et al.* (1990) A class 1 antigen, HLA-G expressed in human trophoblasts. *Science* **248**, 220–3

Lands, W. E. M. (1985) Interactions of lipid peroxides with eicosanoid biosynthesis. *J Free Rad Biol Med* **1**, 97–101

Lu, B., Zhang, S. W., Huang, B., Liu, W. and Li, C. F. (1990) Changes in selenium in patients with pregnancy-induced hypertension. *Chin J Obstet Gynaecol* **25**, 323–7

Lyall, F., Greer, I. A., Boswell, F. B. *et al.* (1994) The cell adhesion molecule VCAM-1 is selectively elevated in the sera of pre-eclampsia. *Br J Obstet Gynaecol* **101**, 485–7

MacLennan, A. H., Sharp, F. and Shaw, J. D. (1972) The ultrastructure of human trophoblast in spontaneous and induced hypoxia using a system of organ culture. *J Obstet Gynaecol Br Commonw* **79**, 113–21

Massobrio, M., Benedetto, C., Bertini, E., Tetta, C. and Carnussi, G. (1985) Immune complexes in normal and pre-eclamptic pregnancies. *Am J Obstet Gynecol* **152**, 578–83

McCartney, C. P. (1969) The acute hypertensive disorders of pregnancy, classified by renal histology. *Gynaecologia* **167**, 214–20

Middelkoop, C. M., Dekker, G. A., Kraayenbrink, A. A. and Popp-Snijders, C. (1993) Platelet poor plasma serotonin in normal and pre-eclamptic pregnancy. *Clin Chem* **39**, 1675–8

Minchenko, A., Bauer, T., Salceda, S. and Caro, J. (1994) Hypoxic stimulation of vascular endothelial growth factor expression *in vitro* and *in vivo*. *Lab Invest* **71**, 374–9

Morris, N. H., Eaton, B. M. and Dekker, G. (1996) Nitric oxide, the endothelium, pregnancy and pre-eclampsia. *Br J Obstet Gynaecol* **103**, 4–15

Morris, N. H., Sooranna, S. R., Eaton, B. M. and Steer, P. I. (1993) NO synthase activity in placental bed and tissues from normotensive pregnant women. *Lancet* **342**, 679–80

Musci, J. M., Roberts, J. M., Rodgers, G. M. and Taylor, R. N. (1988) Mitogenic activity is increased in the sera of pre-eclamptic women prior to delivery. *Am J Obstet Gynecol* **159**, 1146–51

Myatt, L. (1987) 'Eicosanoids and blood pressure regulation' in: F. Sharp and E. Symonds (Eds.). *Hypertension in Pregnancy. Proceedings of the 16th Study Group of the Royal College of Obstetricians and Gynaecologists*, pp. 167–82. New York: Perinatology Press

Nelson, G. H., Zuspan, F. P., Mulligan, I. T. (1966) Defects of lipid metabolism in toxaemia of pregnancy. *Am J Obstet Gynecol* **194**, 310–315

Newman, R. and Eddy, G. L. (1988) Associations of eclampsia with hydatidiform mole: case report and review of the literature. *Obstet Gynecol Surv* **43**, 185–90

Perry, I. J. and Beevers, D. G. (1994) The definition of pre-eclampsia. *Br J Obstet Gynaecol* **101**, 587–91

Petrucco, O. (1981) 'Aetiology of pre-eclampsia' in: J. Studd (Ed.). *Progress in Obstetrics and Gynaecology*, pp. 51–69. Edinburgh: Churchill Livingstone

Pober, J. S. (1988) Cytokine-mediated activation of vascular endothelium. *Am J Pathol* **133**(3), 426–33

Pohl, U., Holtz, J., Buse, R. and Bassenge, E. (1986) The crucial role of the endothelium in the vasodilator response to increased flow. *Hypertension* **8** 37–44

Rappaport, V., Hirata, G., Yap, H. K. and Jordan, S. C. (1990) Antivascular endothelial cell antibodies in severe pre-eclampsia. *Am J Obstet Gynecol* **162**, 138–46

Redman, C. W. G. and Jefferies, M. (1988) Revised definition of pre-eclampsia. *Lancet* **ii**, 809–12

Redman, C. W. G. and Roberts, J. M. (1993) Management of pre-eclampsia. *Lancet* **341**, 1451–4

Redman, C. W. G., Bonnar, J. and Beilin L. (1978) Early platelet consumption in pre-eclampsia. *BMJ* **i**, 467–9

Roberts, I. M. and Redman, C. W. G. (1993) Pre-eclampsia: more than just pregnancy-induced hypertension. *Lancet* **341**, 1447–54

Roberts, J. M., Edep, M. E., Goldfien, A. and Taylor, R. N. (1992) Sera from pre-eclamptic women specifically activate human umbilical vein endothelial cells *in vitro*: morphological and biochemical evidence. *Am J Reprod Immunol* **27**, 101–8

Roberts, J. M., Taylor, R. N. and Goldfien, A. (1991) Clinical and biochemical evidence of endothelial cell dysfunction in the pregnancy syndrome pre-eclampsia. *Am J Hypertens* **4**, 700–8

Roberts, J. M., Taylor, R. N., Musci, T. J. *et al.* (1989) Pre-eclampsia: an endothelial cell disorder. *Am J Obstet Gynecol* **161**, 1200–4

Rodgers, G. M., Taylor, R. N. and Roberts, J. M. (1988) Pre-eclampsia is associated with a serum factor cytotoxic to human endothelial cells. *Am J Obstet Gynecol* **159**, 908–14

Shanklin, D. R. and Sibai, B. M. (1989) Ultrastructural aspects of pre-eclampsia. *Am J Obstet Gynecol* **161**, 735–41

Sheppard, B. I. and Bonnar, J. (1974) The ultrastructure of the arterial supply of the human placenta in early and late pregnancy. *J Obstet Gynaecol Br Commonw* **81**, 487–511

Simantov, R., LaSala, J. M., Lo, S. K. *et al.* (1995) Activation of cultured endothelial cells by anti-phospholipid antibodies. *J Clin Invest* **96**, 2211–19

Smarason, A. K., Sargent, I. L., Starkey, P. M. and Redman, C. W. G. (1993) The effect of placental syncytiotrophoblast microvillous membranes from normal and pre-eclamptic women on the growth of endothelial cells *in vitro*. *Br J Obstet Gynaecol* **100**, 943–9

Spargo, B. H., Lichtig, E. and Luger, A. M. (1976) 'The renal lesion in pre-eclampsia: examination by light-, electron, and immunofluorescent-microscopy' in: M. D. Lindheimer, A. I. Katz and F. P. Zuspan (Eds.). *Hypertension in Pregnancy,* New York: Wiley

Stark, J. M. (1993) Pre-eclampsia and cytokine induced oxidative stress. *Br J Obstet Gynaecol* **100**, 105–9

Starkey, P. M., Sargent, I. I. and Redman, C. W. G. (1988) Cell populations in human early pregnancy decidua characterisation and isolation of large granular lymphocytes by flow cytometry. *Immunology* **65**, 129–34

Talledo, O. E., Chelsey, I. C. and Zuspan, F. P. (1968) Renin–angiotensin system in normal and toxaemic pregnancies III. Differential sensitivity to angiotensin II and norepinephrine in toxaemia of pregnancy. *Am J Obstet Gynecol* **100** 218–21

Taylor, RN., Musci, T. I., Rodgers, G. M. and Roberts, J. M. (1991) Pre-eclamptic sera stimulate increased platelet derived growth factor nRNA and protein expression by cultured endothelial cells. *Am J Reprod Immunol* **25**, 105–8

Thomas, K. A. (1996) Vascular endothelial growth factor, a potent and selective angiogenic agent. *J Biol Chem* **271**(2), 603–6

Thornton, J. G. and Sampson, J. (1990) Genetics of pre-eclampsia. *Lancet* 336, 1319–20

Tsukimori, Y., Maeda, H., Singu, M. *et al.* (1992) The possible role of endothelial cells in hypertensive disorders during pregnancy. *Obstet Gynecol* **80**, 229–33

Wang, Y., Walsh, S. W., Guo, J. and Zhang, J. (1991) The imbalance between thromboxane and prostacyclin in pre-eclampsia is associated with an imbalance between lipid peroxides and vitamin E in maternal blood. *Am J Obstet Gynecol* **165**, 1695–700

Ward, K., Hata, A., Jeunemaitre, X. *et al.* (1993) A molecular variant of angiotensinogen associated with pre-eclampsia. *Nature Genet* **4**, 59–61

Weinstein, L. (1982) Syndrome of haemolysis, elevated liver enzymes and low platelet count: a severe consequence of hypertension in pregnancy. *Am J Obstet Gynecol* **142**, 159–67

Whigham, K. A. E., Howie, P. W., Drummond, A. H. and Prentice, C. R. M. (1978) Abnormal platelet function in pre-eclampsia. *Br J Obstet Gynaecol* **85**, 28

Wickens, D., Wlins, M. H., Lunec, J., Ball, G. and Dormandy, T. L. (1981) Free radical oxidation (peroxidation) products in normal and abnormal pregnancy. *Am J Clin Biochem* **18**, 158–62

Willms-Kretschmer, K., Flax, M. H. and Cotran, R. S. (1967) The fine structure of the vascular response in hapten specific delayed hypersensitivity and contact dermatitis. *Lab Invest* **17**, 334–49

World Health Organisation (1987) *The Hypertensive Disorders of Pregnancy*, Technical Report Series, Vol. 758. Geneva: World Health Organisation

Yoke, Y. W. (1994) 'Trophoblast growth, migration and immunological significance' in: R. H. T. Ward, S. K. Smith and D. Donnai (Eds.). *Early Fetal Growth and Development*, pp. 145–51. London: RCOG Press

Zhou, T., Damsky, C. H., Chiu, K., Roberts, J. M. and Fisher, S. J. (1993) Pre-eclampsia is associated with abnormal expression of adhesion molecules by invasive cytotrophoblasts. *J Clin Invest* **91**, 950–60

# 32

# Fibroids and pregnancy

*Peter A. Greenwood*

Fibroids or fibromyomas are the most common benign tumour affecting the female uterus. They may be solitary or multiple and each individual fibroid seems to arise from a single original smooth muscle cell (Townsend *et al.* 1970); this cell divides repeatedly to form a whorled sphere.

Many figures have been quoted regarding the prevalence of fibroids. It is clear that they become more prevalent with age and are more common in the Negroid races, with a 3–7:1 ratio compared to Caucasians (Buttram and Reiter 1981). Any prevalence figure is, therefore, heavily dependent on age and racial mix. A commonly quoted rate is that 20% of all women of reproductive age have one or more fibroids (West 1992).

A further confounding factor for prevalence is the investigative definition of a fibroid. Most figures will be based on fibroids of greater than 2 cm in diameter, as this is a reasonable minimum size that can be diagnosed using ultrasound scanning. It is easier to find and diagnose small fibroids histologically on the hysterectomy or postmortem specimen than by using current imaging methods.

Fibroids are certainly rare before the menarche and their prevalence increases up to the menopause, when regression may occur in size but not numbers (as long as no minimum size is defined).

Early reports of fibroids mainly relate to massive tumours (Myerscough 1982), as good quality diagnostic imaging in the non-bony (soft) pelvis is a relatively recent development. Overwhelming suspicion of fibroids was often present preoperatively, but definitive diagnosis had to wait for histological analysis of the hysterectomy specimen. Some cases were not diagnosed until the uterus was submitted to the pathologist and occasionally pregnant uteri were suspected to be massive fibroids (and vice versa). The author was present as a medical student, in 1978, when an intended abdominal hysterectomy for a fibroid uterus became a pregnancy of 22 weeks' gestation diagnosed by laparotomy. There were, perhaps, extenuating circumstances in that case and the patient (aged 41 years), although parous, was adamant that she had not suspected pregnancy preoperatively. Occasionally, fibroids were diagnosed as a result of acute complications, such as haemorrhage, torsion, prolapse of a submucous fibroid through the cervical canal, or the classical red degeneration first described in 1899 by Gebhard (Faulkner 1947).

The presence of fibroids in the pregnant uterus historically presented a major challenge to the clinician, as diagnosis was based on clinical examination. The existence of many other causes for a pelvic/abdominal tumour in pregnancy led to many fascinating case reports before ultrasound was used (Myerscough 1982). Fibroids in the first and second trimester have been thought to be ovarian tumours, bicornuate horns or ectopic pregnancies and, in the third trimester, the head of a second twin (a cause of a second stage lasting for years rather than minutes!). The complications of pregnancy ascribed to fibroids 50 years ago were no different to those described more recently, but the incidence was skewed by the reporting of cases with relatively large fibroids.

With the introduction of ultrasound scanning and, over the past 15 years, the more widespread use of nuclear magnetic resonance (NMR) imaging, ease of diagnosis has improved. An additional factor is the more frequent use of laparoscopy in the investigation of women. This easier diagnosis has, without doubt, inflated more recent prevalence figures, and has probably led to fibroids being blamed for more cases of menorrhagia and dysmenorrhoea than is their due.

The presence of uterine fibroids may be a negative factor for fertility in individual cases, depending on their site and size. This will be partly due to the increase in the average age of the 'fibroid' group, due to increasing prevalence of fibroids with age, but this can be taken into account using a correction factor. A fibroid uterus will certainly lead to an excess of pregnancy complications (Phelan 1995), but its presence does not necessarily mean that it is responsible for antepartum complications that arise; a rigorous approach must be taken to achieve the appropriate diagnosis.

## CURRENT DIAGNOSIS AND MONITORING

Most fibroids associated with pregnancy are diagnosed during the pregnancy. This is because, for women in the United Kingdom, the first ultrasound scan of the pelvic contents generally occurs when dating a pregnancy. The likelihood of detection is increased if the fibroid is > 2 cm in diameter.

In a substantial minority of cases fibroids are identified prior to pregnancy. This group will include:

(1) Subfertile women where investigations have included an ultrasound scan or laparoscopy;

(2) Women with pelvic symptoms such as pain or menorrhagia where ultrasound investigation has been carried out; and

(3) Women identified through screening programmes for cervical abnormality, where a bimanual examination is carried out at the same time. This latter examination would detect fibroids identifiable on clinical grounds.

## Ultrasound

The ultrasound scan is the mainstay of diagnosis and follow-up of fibroids in pregnancy. The specificity of the investigation depends upon the size, site and acoustic structure of the fibroid, quality of the ultrasound equipment, obesity of the patient and whether the presence of fibroids is sought by the operator. The more widespread use of vaginal ultrasound probes in early pregnancy may lead to increased diagnosis (Mayer and Shipilov 1995). In pregnant patients where significant doubt exists as to the nature of a pelvic mass, an NMR scan should be considered in order to avoid unnecessary operative intervention.

Ease of diagnosis is influenced by the relationship between the fibroid and the uterine body. The fibroid may be intramural, submucosal or subserosal. The suspicion would be that intramural fibroids are the most difficult to diagnose in pregnancy as the uterine wall itself hypertrophes and the fibroid is not distorting a tissue fluid interface. Therefore, a small fibroid in the body of the uterus with similar echogenicity to uterine wall could be easily missed. The further monitoring of the fibroid during pregnancy is an area of debate. Small fibroids (< 2 cm) may not be visible in late pregnancy and the frequency of further ultrasound scans will need to be influenced by past obstetric history, subfertility, symptomatology, size and site of the fibroid, and associated obstetric factors.

The ability of ultrasound to discriminate between a fibroid and the normal wall relies on an often subtle difference in echogenicity. The fibroid tissue is typically muscular so that echogenicity is similar to uterine wall. The rounded nature of the lesion may lead to concentration of attention on that area, allowing firm diagnosis. Some fibroids have a high fibre to muscle ratio which, being significantly different to uterine wall, makes diagnosis easier; other fibroids may by calcified.

The larger the fibroid, the greater the distortion of the normal outline of the uterus. Cystic spaces may be present where past degeneration has occurred. There is good correlation between ultrasound and laparoscopy in diagnosing fibroids > 2 cm in diameter, but smaller fibroids are often missed by one or both methods. Colour-flow Doppler during ultrasound may help in discrimination, as the fibroid is surrounded by a 'halo' of supplying vessels. There have been recent reports on the monitoring of fibroids' vascularity and size with colour-flow Doppler during the course of down-regulation treatment with luteinising hormone releasing hormone (LHRH) agonist (Creighton *et al.* 1994), and this investigation could be of use in pregnancy.

There may be confusion with an ovarian fibroma where the ovaries have not been separately identified. This difficulty in locating the ovaries separately on an ultrasound scan becomes more pronounced in pregnancy, leading to diagnostic uncertainty which may only be clarified through NMR scanning or laparotomy.

The diagnosis of submucous fibroids may be eased by the application of sonohysterography using normal saline (Hoetzinger 1991) or by the well-tried techniques of X-ray hysterosalpingography or hysteroscopy. Sonohysterography creates an artificial interface between uterine tissue and fluid, a situation replicated naturally by the early pregnancy sac. An alternative interface can be created with the highly echogenic substance Echovist (Schering AG, Berlin, Germany), which has already been introduced into clinical practice for ultrasound hysterosalpingograms (Deichert et al. 1989). None of these techniques is applicable to, or feasible in, pregnancy.

Three-dimensional ultrasound has an uncertain place in the assessment of fibroids. Certainly, three-dimensional ultrasound is not appropriate as a screening technique, but once fibroids have been identified, it may offer additional information on spatial relationships by computer tomography (CT) of the image. It is, however, clear that NMR scanning gives a good assessment of the size, location and anatomical relationships in all cases diagnosed by ultrasound.

## Nuclear magnetic resonance imaging

This is the most accurate imaging technique for the detection and siting of fibroids. Fibroids as small as 0.5 cm can be detected. Although T1 weighted images have a similar appearance to uterine muscle, T2 weighting gives excellent contrast — with the fibroid showing as very dark compared to the background myometrium. Short T1 inversion recovery images have high contrast but poor specificity and increased signal to noise ratios.

The cost and claustrophobia of NMR leads to its infrequent use in pregnancy, although the images obtained are good. One problem is the prolonged image capture time, as fetal movement may occur. In a study looking at adnexal masses, pancuronium was administered intramuscularly to the fetus through an amniocentesis needle in order to cause temporary paralysis (Angtuaco *et al.* 1992). One milligram of Glucagon intramuscularly may also improve the quality of images by inhibiting maternal bowel action.

Nuclear magnetic resonance scanning cannot distinguish malignant degeneration (which is fortunately rare) from other forms of degeneration; however, torsion and red degeneration can be identified by an increase in whiteness on T1 imaging (Hamlin *et al.* 1985).

The major value of NMR in pregnancy is to reduce the need for antepartum surgical intervention. Where ultrasound is certain that a parauterine mass is fibroid, ultrasound monitoring of growth is appropriate; however, if ultrasound is inconclusive an NMR scan will normally be the definitive investigation.

There is also a place for NMR in selected cases to assess the feasibility of vaginal delivery. This particularly applies to cases where the fibroid is posterior and, hence, difficult to visualise by transabdominal ultrasound. The NMR scan will give a precise indication as to the relationship between the fetal head, fibroid and bony pelvis. Fibroids seen in the first trimester on ultrasound are often not located by this technique in the third trimester due to the bulk of fetomaternal tissue. They can, in a posterior pelvic position, be an unexpected cause of cephalopelvic disproportion, even when relatively small.

## PRECONCEPTUAL EFFECTS OF FIBROIDS

There have been no population-based studies on the incidence of fibroids and subsequent fertility. The absence of a fibroid at the time of screening will not exclude the presence of a fibroid by the time pregnancy occurs. Studies relating fibroids to subfertility often assume cause and effect, but no study has randomised patients to myomectomy or conservative follow-up. Certainly, myomectomy by laparoscopy or laparotomy can lead to subfertility due to the formation of pelvic adhesions, and later pregnancy complications may result from a weakened and scarred uterine wall (Hutchins 1995).

The more plausible mechanisms by which fibroids may reduce fertility are dependent on the site of the fibroid. They may:

(1) Interfere with egg, sperm or embryo transport/migration; or

(2) Interfere with embryo implantation and early development.

Fibroids can mechanically obstruct the cervical canal or cornual portion of the Fallopian tube. The size of a subserosal fibroid could distort the course of the Fallopian tube ostium, making the mechanics of fertilisation and ovum pick-up more difficult. It is not easy to confirm or refute these possibilities; they rest on logical expectation, rather than a specific basis. Cases such as these are also relatively unusual, so that any randomised trial between myomectomy and conservative management would need to be multicentred.

If a fibroid is in such a position at the cornua of the uterus that it completely blocks the Fallopian tube, it is clear that this is a form of tubal infertility. There are case reports of successful restoration of tubal patency in Fallopian tubes affected by cornual fibroids through treatment with LHRH agonist (Gardner and Shaw 1989; Ben-Ami, Battino and Shalev 1993). A similar outcome was reported by the author of this chapter (1995), although unilateral patency already existed, so that the influence of the treatment on subsequent pregnancy is uncertain.

The second effect of fibroids on fertility is through submucosal position. Again, there is a strong logical basis for the effect proposed (i.e. that embryo implantation is made more difficult and early growth of the pregnancy is more precarious, resulting in an increase in the miscarriage rate). There is, however, a spectrum of opinion as to how aggressively to deal with fibroids in this situation. Certainly, hysteroscopic resection without proven subfertility, or before a first pregnancy, would not be typically advised in the United Kingdom. There has been no satisfactory randomised trial of conservative versus surgical management in this area. The miscarriage rate for fibroids at any site is 7% (Phelan 1995), which is close to the quoted rate for miscarriage in 'normal' circumstances.

The reduction of fertility caused by a submucosal fibroid has not been satisfactorily quantified (and quantification would be difficult due to the heterogeneity of the fibroid site, size and composition). There has to be strong suspicion that fibroids cause subfertility from a simple comparison of prevalence figures. Thomas (1992) is confident that fibroids occur in 25–30% of women, but Phelan (1995) quotes the incidence of fibroids in pregnancy as 0.09–3.69%. Clearly, such a gross mismatch in figures must mean either that fibroids are a highly significant cause of subfertility or that there is significant failure to recognise or detect fibroids in pregnancy. There is certainly a need for a definitive longitudinal, population-based study of fibroids and subsequent fertility and pregnancy outcome.

## COMPLICATIONS OF FIBROIDS IN PREGNANCY

Fibroids affecting the pregnant uterus may cause a variety of complications and make other pregnancy-associated problems more likely. These complications may be due to the position and size of the fibroid in relation to the uterine wall, or to the special features of the fibroid. Fibroids may also increase in size during pregnancy.

The positional effects of fibroids mainly relate to those in a submucosal site. These may cause problems with implantation, development and longevity of the pregnancy. In a small number of cases the fibroid occupies a significant proportion of the pelvic cavity and, as a result, affects the function of surrounding organs and the possibility of vaginal delivery.

## Submucosal fibroids

Reference has already been made to the possible increase in the miscarriage rate with the presence of a submucosal fibroid. This is believed to occur due to the proportion of the uterine cavity which is occupied by an abnormal growth. It is known that the endometrium overlying a fibroid is thinner than normal endometrium during the menstrual cycle (Hunt and Wallach 1974). Implantations of the embryo on this suboptimal area would be expected to lead to poorer placental invasion and maternal vascular support (although it is more likely that the embryo will implant on adjacent normal endometrium). This may lead to an increase in the early miscarriage rate. A large submucous fibroid occupying a greater proportion of the cavity surface should increase the likelihood of miscarriage. A small submucous fibroid may well have a minimal adverse effect on early pregnancy. It is not known whether a fibroid can adversely influence the endometrium which is neither overlying nor immediately adjacent to it. Individual clinical experience of fibroids of various size and site, and the assessment of these cases, has not reached such a stage of analysis that these issues can be clarified.

If a fibroid-affected pregnancy ends in miscarriage, there is an increase in the chance of retained products of conception, because tissue can be trapped above the fibroid which bulges into the cavity. Curettage by suction or sharp curette may need to be prolonged in order to remove such tissue.

At the end of a successful pregnancy submucosal fibroids are associated with an increased chance of retained placenta because:

(1) The placenta villi may have invaded the surface of the fibroid; and

(2) The distortion of the cavity makes it more difficult for the placenta to be expelled by the uterine contraction.

Again, the rate of retained products following vaginal delivery would be increased. Retention of such products would lead to a greater chance of postpartum endometritis; this was a severe complication in the pre-antibiotic era, as the fibroid could become an ulcerated, necrotic mass secondary to thrombosis or rupture of the supplying vessels (Myerscough 1982). Postpartum haemorrhage is more common due to a combination of the following factors:

(1) The greater difficulty for the uterus to contract as a unit;

(2) The increase in retained placenta and products; and

(3) The consequent increase in uterine infection.

Other rarer complications associated with submucosal fibroids are:

(1) Abruption;

(2) Premature rupture of membranes;

(3) Premature labour; and

(4) Pressure effects on the fetus.

Some authorities believe that antepartum haemorrhage is also more common where the placenta is implanted over a fibroid (Muram, Gillieson and Walters 1980).

Abruption is believed to be a complication that may be more common in the fibroid uterus if the placental bed is covering the fibroid. Abruption itself is an unusual pregnancy outcome and the evidence for an increased risk due to fibroids is largely anecdotal. It is possible that the presence of fibroids and the known problems with fibroid-associated pain results in an increase in the rate of '? abruption' in these cases in the third trimester.

An increase in the rate of premature rupture of membranes has been reported, but an explanation of this risk is difficult to find. The increased chance of premature labour is slight and thought to be secondary to the fibroid, compromising the normal expansion of the uterus. There have been a few reports of fetal limb abnormalities due to pressure from fibroids during pregnancy (Graham *et al.* 1980).

## Malpresentation

This may be due to a fibroid which is submucosal, intramural or subserosal. The essential feature is that the fibroid occupies an obstructive position in the bony pelvis and continues to do so throughout pregnancy. A large fibroid will prevent any possibility of longitudinal fetal presentation, whereas a small fibroid may prevent engagement of the fetal head or lead to relative cephalopelvic disproportion in labour. The outcome of these various scenarios is that Caesarean section is necessary to ensure delivery of a healthy fetus (Figure 1).

Where a fibroid is subserosal or pedunculated, it is possible for it to be lifted free of the

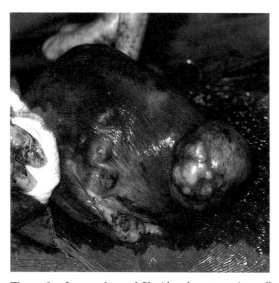

**Figure 1**  *Large subserosal fibroid on lower posterior wall of uterus during a lower-segment Caesarean section at 38 weeks' gestation*

pelvis as uterine growth progresses. A submucosal or intramural fibroid in the lower part of the uterus, or a cervical fibroid, are in such positions that they will remain in the obstructive position despite uterine growth.

Fibroids in the cavity of the bony pelvis may also cause the problems more typically associated with large fibroids in the non-pregnant uterus. They may interfere with the function of surrounding organs. Incarceration of the fibroid uterus may cause constipation and severe backache, or urinary retention, and, in extreme, very rare cases, hydronephrosis (Myerscough 1982).

## Red degeneration (necrobiosis), torsion and rupture

Red degeneration is a descriptive term applied to a symptom complex associated with fibroids in pregnancy. It is unusual to obtain histological confirmation of the diagnosis, due to the acknowledged risks of myomectomy to the ongoing pregnancy. If myomectomy is performed, the fibroid has a typical 'raw beefsteak' appearance on section. This is due to cystic change and engorgement of the tumour.

Although red degeneration typically occurs in the second trimester of pregnancy, it has also been reported in women with uterine fibroids at the time of the menopause and also in women treated with LHRH agonist to induce a medical menopause and shrinkage of fibroids (Vollenhoven, Lawrence and Healy 1990).

The symptoms of red degeneration are pain and tenderness localised to the fibroid, low-grade fever and a raised white cell count. As there are other unusual causes of similar symptoms in pregnancy, it is important not to be led to the obvious diagnosis by the known presence of a fibromyoma, without considering alternative diagnoses such as appendicitis. Ultrasound may demonstrate an increase in cystic spaces in the fibroid, or a significant increase in fibroid dimensions. The changes in blood flow, as assessed by Doppler studies, have not yet led to precise diagnostic criteria. The management of the condition is largely one of pain control.

Occasionally, premature labour may threaten, necessitating treatment with tocolytics and, very rarely, surgical intervention may be necessary in the second trimester.

Torsion of a pedunculated subserous fibroid may occur and the clinical picture is similar to red degeneration. In such cases conservative management is appropriate. Subserosal fibroids occasionally have sizeable engorged veins coursing over the surface. Rupture of such a vein is very rare, but is a reported cause of intraperitoneal haemorrhage in pregnancy, necessitating laparotomy (Myerscough 1982). The symptoms associated with this rare complication are those of intraperitoneal haemorrhage, with peritonism and, possibly, hypovolaemic shock and fetal distress.

## FIBROID GROWTH IN PREGNANCY

It was believed for many years that fibroids increased in size during pregnancy, because fibroids are sensitive to the increasing oestrogen concentration present in pregnancy and hence grow. It has only been since the widespread use of ultrasound in pregnancy that this supposition could be investigated. Data from studies by Lev Toaff, Coleman and Arger (1987) and Aharoni et al. (1988) suggest that, on average, there is no overall change in fibroid size during pregnancy. Such studies are, however, flawed by the paucity of data from the first trimester and preconceptual periods. Limited data from the follow-up of patients with large fibroids (Greenwood 1995), where diagnosis of fibroids was made preconceptually or early in the first trimester, suggest that there is a consistent growth in early pregnancy, and size stabilisation in the second trimester, with no significant size changes through to term. In the postnatal period there tends to be diminution in size of large fibroids to the prepregnant size. These findings are consistent with the known sensitivity of fibroids to oestrogen and progesterone, levels of which rise steeply in early pregnancy and fall rapidly in the postpartum period. It also fits with the data reported by many workers that fibroids tend to shrink if oestrogen levels fall to menopausal

levels following administration of LHRH agonists (West et al. 1987).

A further factor which has compromised ultrasound studies in fibroid growth in pregnancy has been the problem of fibroid visualisation as pregnancy progresses. Where the fibroid is large, visualisation is not a problem; however, in studies where the fibroids may be as small as 2 cm in diameter, it is not uncommon for the fibroid to be 'lost' in the third trimester. This problem is demonstrated in the postpartum period by the Aharoni study (1988), where of the 13 women scanned postnatally, the fibroid which had been studied during the pregnancy was only visualised in five cases.

The best way to clarify the question of fibroid growth in pregnancy would be to carry out a longitudinal study starting preconceptually and ending postnatally, with images obtained by NMR. This modality is more accurate than ultrasound in identifying and assessing fibroid location and size.

## TREATMENT

### Medical

Medical treatment of fibroids in pregnancy is largely a question of the relief of the pain that may arise when a fibroid undergoes red degeneration or simply becomes more sensitive and tender. Consideration will also be given as to whether there are any treatment options available for the medical control of fibroid growth.

The development of fibroid associated pain must be managed on an individual basis. Minor pain and tenderness may be controlled with paracetamol, but red degeneration can cause severe pain and morphiates are often required. These latter drugs are best given in the form of oral morphine sulphate in a slow-release preparation. The dose is given twice a day and increased until satisfactory pain control is achieved without undue side affects. Careful consideration must be given to the length of treatment. The pain of red degeneration usually resolves over seven to 14 days, so the medication can be progressively withdrawn as the pain recedes.

There have been reports of the analgesic benefits of prostaglandin synthetase inhibitors in the control of fibroid-associated pain (Dildy *et al.* 1992). However, risk to the fetus of premature closure of the ductus arteriosus secondary to the use of such drugs must be considered. Long-acting epidural analgesia has also been tried. It is obviously important to monitor patients closely when they are having such strong analgesia. The pain of a degenerating fibroid does not preclude other serious complications of pregnancy and these may be masked by the depth of analgesia achieved. Pain of abruption, the rupture of a scarred uterus and of appendicitis may all be suppressed and there may also be delay in diagnosing the onset of premature labour.

Many drugs have been used to try to shrink fibroids in the non-pregnant uterus. Progestogens and oestrogens promote the growth of fibroids, whereas mifepristone, gestrinone and danazol all lead to a reduction in fibroid size. None of these agents can be safely used in pregnancy. Luteinising hormone releasing hormone agonists are the most widely used agents for inducing a medical menopause, resulting in a shrinkage of fibroids secondary to hypooestrogenism. These drugs would be ineffective in pregnancy as the fetoplacental unit is the major source of oestrogens and progestogens. It may be that LHRH agonist would have a direct effect on fibroids as they contain receptors to the polypeptide (Wiznitzer *et al.* 1988), but their use in pregnancy would not seem appropriate.

Fibroids are normally relatively quiescent during pregnancy and complications tend to occur only for a short period. The short-term effect of any of these drugs on fibroid size is limited and such agents are all contraindicated in pregnancy; however, they may be used preconceptually to reduce the size of fibroids, but as the fibroids so treated tend to regain their original dimensions over the six months following treatment, the overall benefits are limited (Williams and Shaw 1990).

## Surgical

There is no place for surgical management of fibroids in pregnancy (independent of delivery), except in extreme circumstances. Intraperitoneal haemorrhage due to rupture of a vein on the surface of the fibroid would be one such circumstance. Red degeneration should always, initially, be managed conservatively.

Myomectomy in pregnancy is fraught with risk, unless the fibroid is pedunculated and the pedicle is narrow. The removal of a fibroid from an intramural or subserosal site exposes a hyperaemic vascular bed and the problems of achieving haemostasis are likely to lead to the need to deliver the fetus and, on occasion, proceed to hysterectomy. Laparoscopic treatment, either by suture, laser, diathermy or myolysis, similarly has no place in management.

Caesarean section is approximately twice as likely where the uterus is affected by fibroids than in a 'normal' pregnancy. Some of these cases will be due to pelvic obstruction by the fibroid (Figure 1), while others will be due to a combination of factors which may include concerns about past subfertility and maternal age.

A preoperative ultrasound scan of the uterus or, in ideal circumstances, an NMR scan, may be extremely useful in the preoperative work-up of the individual case. The Caesarean section must aim to avoid the sites of subserosal, intramural and submucosal fibroids in order to minimise the risks of excessive bleeding. If there is a fibroid in the anterior wall of the lower segment, then a classical incision would be appropriate (Figure 2). The presence of multiple fibroids may lead to a situation where it is impossible to avoid all fibroids and in such cases (as well as a substantial proportion of the less challenging ones), it is best to warn the patient that hysterectomy may become necessary if bleeding at Caesarean section cannot be otherwise controlled. Fundal fibroids or fibroids in the posterior wall of the uterus should cause no intraoperative problems.

Pedunculated fibroids found at Caesarean section may be opportunistically removed if the pedicle is narrow, but otherwise the elective

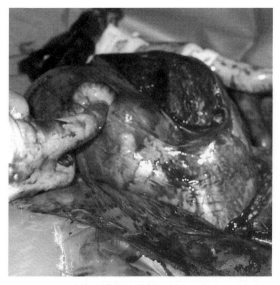

**Figure 2** *Multiple fibroids in anterior body and lower segment of uterus during a classical Caesarean section at 37 weeks' gestation*

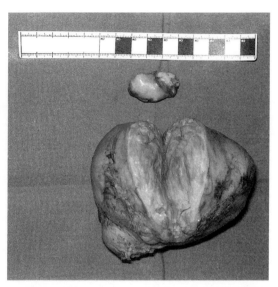

**Figure 3** *Myomectomy specimen, three months after successful pregnancy affected by red degeneration*

removal of fibroids should not be attempted at the time of Caesarean section.

Where a woman has had significant complications in pregnancy specifically related to the presence of fibroids, it is important to consider surgical removal of these prior to a further pregnancy (Figure 3). If the fibroid is largely intramural this is still best performed by laparotomy rather than using laparoscopic techniques, because laparotomy allows accurate repair of the uterine wall, which should reduce the chances of uterine rupture in a further pregnancy (Hutchins 1995). Laparoscopic removal of intramural fibroids is possible, but accurate closure of the cavity in layers is difficult and haemorrhage in the cavity may lead to a weak uterine scar. Uterine rupture has been reported in pregnancy following laparoscopic myomectomy (Harris 1992). Laparoscopic removal of pedunculated fibroids is safe and reduces recovery time compared with open surgery, and hysteroscopic removal of submucosal fibroids is certainly preferable to older surgical techniques.

## CONCLUSION

There are many uncertainties regarding the natural history and relative risks of fibroids in the preconceptual and pregnant uterus. This is inevitable, because it is only in the last 25 years that satisfactory investigative and monitoring techniques have been developed. Research in this area is also hampered by the heterogeneity of the fibroid uterus, with major variations between women with regard to site, size and number of fibroids. Most clinical decisions are taken on the basis of good sense and past experience, rather than scientific evidence. There must be a caveat against overtreatment of patients with fibroids, as it is probable that the majority of fibroids cause no significant problems during pregnancy.

Certainly, when a pregnancy is established in the fibroid uterus the clinician should 'watch, wait and listen to the patient'. Symptoms and complications must be treated conservatively in line with normal obstetric practice and, as term approaches, an assessment must be made as to the likelihood of successful vaginal delivery.

# References

Aharoni, A., Reiter, A., Golan, D., Paltiely, Y. and Sharf, M. (1988) Patterns of growth of uterine leiomyomas during pregnancy. A prospective longitudinal study. *Br J Obstet Gynaecol* **95**, 510–13

Angtuaco, T. L., Shah, H. R., Mattison, D. R. *et al.* (1992) MR imaging in high-risk obstetric patients: a valuable complement to U.S. *Radiographics* **12**, 91–109

Ben-Ami, M., Battino, S. and Shalev, E. (1993) Pregnancy following GnRH agonist therapy of uterine leiomyoma obstructing a single Fallopian tube. *Hum Reprod* **8**, 780–1

Buttram, V. C. and Reiter, R. C. (1981) Uterine leiomyomata: etiology, symptomatology and management. *Fertil Steril* **36**, 433–45

Creighton, S., Bourne, T. H., Lawton, F. G., Crayford, T. J. B., Vyas, S., Campbell, S. and Collins, W. P. (1994) Use of transvaginal ultrasonography with colour Doppler imaging to determine an appropriate treatment regimen for uterine fibroids with GnRH agoinst surgery: a preliminary study. *Ultrasound Obstet Gynecol* **4**, 494–8

Deichart, U., Schlief, R., Van de Sandt, M. and Juhnke, I. (1989) Transvaginal hysterosalpingo-contrast-sonography (HyCoSy) compared with conventional tubal diagnosis. *Hum Reprod* **4**, 418–24

Dildy, G. A., Moise, K. J., Smith, L. G., Kirshon, B. and Carpenter, R. J. (1992) Indomethacin for the treatment of symptomatic leiomyoma uteri during pregnancy. *Am J Perinatal* **9**, 185–9

Faulkner, R. L. (1947) Red degeneration of uterine myomas. *Am J Obstet Gynecol* **53**, 474–82

Gardner, R. L. and Shaw, R. W. (1989) Cornual fibroids: a conservative approach to restoring tubal patency using a gonadotrophin-releasing agonist (goserelin) with successful pregnancy. *Fertil Steril* **52**, 332–4

Graham, J. M., Miller, M. E., Stephan, M. J. and Smith, D. W. (1980) Limb reduction anomalies and early *in utero* limb compression. *J Pediatr* **96**, 1052

Greenwood, P. A. (1995) 'Large fibroids complicating pregnancy' in: the *27th British Congress of Obstetrics and Gynaecology*, Dublin, abstract 115

Hamlin, D. J., Pettersson, H., Fitzsimmons, J. *et al.* (1985) MR imaging of uterine leiomyomas and their complications. *J Comput Assist Tomogr* **9**, 902–7

Harris, W. (1992) Uterine dehiscence following laparoscopic myomectomy. *Obstet Gynecol* **80**, 545–6

Hoetzinger, H. (1991) Hysterosonography and hysterography in benign and malignant diseases of the uterus. A comparative *in vitro* study. *J Ultrasound Med* **10**, 259–63

Hunt, J. E. and Wallach, E. E. (1974) Uterine factors in infertility — an overview. *Clin Obstet Gyncol* **17**, 44–64

Hutchins, F. L. (1995) 'Abdominal myomectomy as a treatment for symptomatic uterine fibroids' in: *Obstetrics and Gynaecology Clinics of North America, December 1995. Uterine Fibroids*, pp. 781–9. Philadelphia: W. B. Saunders Co.

Lev-Toaff, A. S., Coleman, G. B., Arger, P. H. *et al.* (1987) Leiomyomas in pregnancy: sonographic study. *Radiology* **164**, 375–80

Mayer, D. P. and Shipilov, V. (1995) 'Ultrasonography and magnetic resonance imaging of uterine fibroids' in: *Obstetrics and Gynaecology Clinics of North America, December 1995. Uterine Fibroids*, pp. 667–725. Philadelphia: W. B. Saunders Co.

Muram, D., Gillieson, M. and Walters, J. H. (1980) Myomas of the uterus in pregnancy, ultrasonographic follow-up. *Am J Obstet Gynecol* **138**, 16–19

Myerscough, P. R. (1982) 'Pelvic tumours; other surgical complications in pregnancy, labour and the puerperium' in: *Munro Kerr's Operative*

*Obstetrics*, 10th edn pp. 203–27. London: Baillière Tindall

Phelan, J. P. (1995) 'Myomas and pregnancy' in: *Obstetrics and Gynaecology Clinics of North America, December 1995. Uterine Fibroids*; pp. 801–5. Philadelphia: W. B. Saunders Co.

Thomas, E. J. (1992) 'The aetiology and pathogenesis of fibroids' in: *Uterine Fibroids, Time for Review*, pp. 1–7. Carnforth, Lancashire: Parthenon Publishing Group

Townsend, D. E., Sparkes, R. S., Baluda, M. C. and McCelland, G. (1970) Unicellular histogenesis of uterine leiomyomas as determined by electrophoresis of glucose-6-phosphate dehydrogenase. *Am J Obstet Gynecol* **107**, 1168–74

Vollenhoven, B. J., Lawrence, A. S. and Healy, D. L. (1990) Uterine fibroids: a clinical review. *Br J Obstet Gynaecol* **97**, 285–98

West, C. P. (1992) 'Uterine fibroids: clinical presentation and diagnostic techniques' in: *Uterine Fibroids, Time for Review*, pp. 34–45. Carnforth, Lancashire: Parthenon Publishing Group

West, C. P., Lumsden, M. A., Lawson, S., Williamson, J. and Baird, D. T. (1987) Shrinkage of uterine fibroids during therapy with goserelin: a luteinizing hormone releasing hormone agonist administered as a monthly subcutaneous depot. *Fertil Steril* **48**, 45–51

Williams, I. A. and Shaw, R. W. (1990) Effect of Naferelin on uterine fibroids measured by ultrasound and magnetic resonance imaging. *Eur J Obstet Gynecol Reprod Biol* **34**, 111–17

Wiznitzer, A., Marback, M., Hazum, B. *et al.* (1988) Gonadotrophin releasing hormone specific binding sites in uterine leiomyomata. *Biochem Biophys Res Comm* **152**, 1326–31

# 33

# Monitoring meconium concentration in the amniotic fluid during labour

*Anne C. Deans and Peter J. Danielian*

The importance of meconium-stained amniotic fluid during labour and its association with adverse outcome has been recognised for hundreds of years. References can be found as early as 1676 as well as in the writings of Aristotle who commented on the opium-like effects seen in neonates born through meconium-stained amniotic fluid (Schulze 1925). The name meconium is derived from the Greek for poppy juice. Yet, despite modern obstetric practices, meconium aspiration syndrome (MAS) remains a significant cause of perinatal mortality and morbidity.

Surprisingly, little is known about what actually causes meconium passage. It is a mistake to assume that the factors responsible for causing the passage of meconium are necessarily the same as those that cause the fetus to aspirate meconium. Trying to correlate the presence of meconium to clinical events is difficult due to the inability to reliably detect the precise time that meconium is passed, often many hours prior to delivery, and collect relevant data at that time. In this chapter the authors review the literature on this important subject and describe how their group (under the direction of Professor P. J. Steer) has devised a method for continuously monitoring the concentration of meconium in amniotic fluid during labour using an intrauterine probe. They hope to show that there is a need for such a device in widening our understanding about the pathophysiology of meconium passage and that it has the potential to improve monitoring of the fetal condition in labour so that, in the future, preventive measures may be developed against meconium aspiration.

## INCIDENCE OF MECONIUM

Meconium is passed by the fetus into the surrounding amniotic fluid in approximately 10% of all pregnancies (Wiswell, Tuggle and Turner 1990). This may be a conservative estimate as the overall incidence of meconium-stained amniotic fluid during labour appears to be rising, with some authors reporting steadily increasing rates in excess of 26% of all deliveries (Dysart *et al.* 1991). The experience of the authors' group concurs with this because at the West London Hospital (United Kingdom) the rate rose from 17% to 20% between 1989 and 1991. Meconium passage appears to be more common in black women, even after controlling for demographic and clinical characteristics (Alexander *et al.* 1994).

The fetus will aspirate meconium in around 5% of labours where it is present in the amniotic fluid, causing or contributing to neonatal death in the form of MAS in an estimated 0.05% (i.e. 1 in 2000) of all pregnancies (Coltart, Byrne and Bates 1989; Rossi *et al.* 1989). A large literature review (Katz and Bowes 1992) combining data from 249,005 pregnancies reported a neonatal death rate of 7% in babies with MAS. Meconium aspiration syndrome was implicated in 4.5% of all deaths in a 10-year study examining the causes of perinatal mortality and morbidity (Rosenthal and Abramowsky 1988). On the basis of these figures we can expect 300 babies to die in the neonatal period every year in England and Wales (600,000 births annually) from, or in association with, MAS. Furthermore, it is probable that about one-third of the survivors of MAS will have long-term mild respiratory compromise (Anonymous 1988; Macfarlane and Heaf 1988; Swaminathan *et al.* 1989; Gupta and Anand 1991).

## WHAT IS MECONIUM?

Meconium is the intestinal contents of the fetus *in utero* and has been found to be present in the fetal gut from 10 weeks' gestation (Woods and Dolkart 1989). The main constituent is water, which makes up approximately 75% of the total weight. Around 80% of the dry weight is comprised of mucus glycoproteins which are resistant to proteolytic enzymes. Proteins (principally plasma proteins) make up a further 10% of the dry weight of meconium in a normal fetus, but may exceed 80% in a fetus with cystic fibrosis (Harries 1978). The proteins, along with mucopolysaccharides and digestive enzymes, are secreted by the fetal gut.

Bile pigments, coproporphyrinogens I and III, are found in meconium (Martin 1979). Along with biliverdin (responsible for the green colour of meconium), they are excreted as by-products of the catabolism of haemoglobin from the biliary tract into the fetal small gut from the fourth month of fetal life. In the adult biliverdin is reduced to bilirubin, but this does not happen in the fetus because it cannot synthesise secondary bile acids due to the absence of any intestinal flora (Sharp *et al.* 1971).

Steroids, such as cholesterol and its precursors, and other lipids are also present, mainly as a result of ingestion of amniotic fluid by the fetus. Copious fetal swallowing explains the high water content of meconium as well as the presence of desquamated cells (from the fetal skin and from the amnion), lanugo hair and vernix found in meconium.

## WHY IS MECONIUM PASSED *IN UTERO?*

Little is known about the mechanisms in the fetus that control gut motility and the relaxation of the internal and external anal sphincter required for the passage of meconium. In the adult, defaecation involves a complex interaction of hormonal, myogenic and neurogenic factors and it is well known that emotional stresses can produce involuntary bowel emptying while physiological stresses may produce constipation. Are there similar situations in the fetus? Unfortunately, at the present time the situation is not clear and, indeed, if the fetal gut does act in a similar way to adult gut, then hypoxia would probably result in gut stasis rather than emptying. Animal studies have shown reduced peristalsis after induction of maternal hypoxia (Becker *et al.* 1940) or have indicated that passage of meconium is a very late phenomenon after hypoxia has occurred (Emmanoulides, Townsend and Bauer 1968).

The incidence of meconium passage increases with gestational age, and in most cases is probably physiological, reflecting the increasing maturation of the neuromuscular system of the fetal gut and therefore its ability to pass meconium (Becker *et al.* 1940). It is rare to find meconium-stained amniotic fluid before 34 weeks' gestation, but the incidence reaches approximately 30% at 40 weeks' gestation and 50% at 42 weeks' gestation (Meis *et al.* 1978; Miller and Read 1981; Steer *et al.* 1989).

Meconium passage can, however, occur in the preterm fetus. One documented cause for this is fetal infection, classically with *Listeria monocytogenes,* although *Ureaplasma urealyticum* and rotaviruses have also been implicated (Romero *et al.* 1991). It has been postulated that these organisms lead to fetal enteritis which causes meconium to be passed. However, it is known that meconium in amniotic fluid predisposes to bacterial growth so the association of meconium passage with these intrauterine infections may not be causal (Florman and Teubner 1969; Hoskins *et al.* 1987). Mazor *et al.* (1995) reported that women in preterm labour had higher rates of microbial invasion of the amniotic cavity and clinical chorioamnionitis when the amniotic fluid was noted to be meconium-stained compared to those with clear amniotic fluid. Interestingly, these observations demonstrate that the musculature and intramural plexuses of the preterm fetal gut are sufficiently developed for peristalsis to occur. However, meconium passage before 34 weeks' gestation remains a rare event.

There have been two reports in the literature suggesting a role for the intestinal hormone motilin (Lucas *et al.* 1979; Mahmoud *et al.* 1988). Umbilical cord motilin levels appear to be higher in fetuses who have passed meconium before delivery, but the evidence to relate this finding to fetal heart rate abnormalities and the role of hypoxic stress is contradictory.

## MECONIUM PASSAGE AND HYPOXIA

It has been suggested for many years that fetal hypoxia leads to meconium passage, but evidence for this is largely presumptive. Early authors claiming such a link relied on subjective clinical diagnoses of fetal hypoxia and had little or no direct evidence to support their hypothesis (Desmond *et al.* 1957; Fenton and Steer 1962). With the advent of fetal blood sampling and more objective measures of hypoxia there is now plenty of evidence to suggest that meconium passage, in the absence of other signs, is not a sign of hypoxia and that infants with normal intrapartum cardiotocography have similar outcomes whether or not meconium is present (Miller *et al.* 1975; Bochner *et al.* 1987; Shaw and Clark 1988; Steer *et al.* 1989; Baker, Kilby and Murray 1992). Richey *et al.* (1995) also failed to find a correlation between markers of acute asphyxia, such as umbilical artery blood pH, lactate or hypoxathine, and the presence of meconium in otherwise normal labours but, interestingly, reported that erythropoitin levels (a possible marker for chronic hypoxia) were significantly raised.

Contrary to the above, Starks (1980) found that thick meconium-stained amniotic fluid was associated with lower fetal scalp blood pH measurements and concluded that thick meconium usually indicated fetal hypoxia or acidosis regardless of an abnormal fetal heart rate. More recently, Berkus *et al.* (1994) reported that the presence of moderate or thick meconium significantly increased the risk of needing emergency Caesarean section in labour and having an acidotic umbilical cord arterial pH. However, as Berkus *et al.* pointed out, pregnancies with increasing gestational age or decreased placental perfusion and chronic fetal hypoxia have oligohydramnios so any passage of meconium will result in thick meconium. Thus, the presence of thick meconium indicates a high-risk group with increased likelihood of abnormal fetal heart rate (FHR) tracing and acidosis, although the passage of meconium, in itself, is likely to be a physiological event. Meconium staining of the liquor does not appear to be more common in cases where the neonate is hypoxic (Naeye *et al.* 1989).

However, when fetal heart rate abnormalities are present those fetuses with meconium-stained amniotic fluid are at higher risk of being acidotic, born in poor condition and requiring resuscitation at birth (Steer *et al.* 1989).

## FETAL DAMAGE FROM MECONIUM

It is not the passage of meconium that is a risk to the fetus, but rather the aspiration of meconium that leads to a less than optimum postnatal outcome. Meconium aspiration, defined as the presence of meconium below the cords, has been reported in 21–58% births when meconium-stained fluid was present (Gregory *et al.* 1974; Dooley *et al.* 1985). Its presence in the fetal or neonatal lung can result in a spectrum of disease, ranging from mild transitory respiratory distress to severe respiratory compromise and death. Oropharyngeal suction and endotracheal intubation of the infant immediately after delivery, before the first breath (which is standard practice in most units for over 20 years) does not prevent meconium aspiration (Davis *et al.* 1985; Dooley *et al.* 1985; Mitchell *et al.* 1985; Sepkowitz 1987; Falciglia 1988; Rossi *et al.* 1989; Yeomans *et al.*, 1989; Cunningham *et al.* 1990). The conclusion is that aspiration of meconium is predominantly an antepartum (intrauterine) process.

Fetuses are capable of inhalation of amniotic fluid and meconium by either gasping or deep breathing movements. Gasping is a normal response to hypoxaemia and can be induced under experimental conditions of hypoxaemia (Dawes *et al.* 1972; Duenhoelter and Pritchard 1977; Block *et al.* 1981). In contrast, deep irregular breathing movements, more frequent as gestation advances, are very common and are not initiated by hypoxia (Dawes *et al.* 1972). Situations that induce fetal hypoxia will result in fetal gasping and would seem likely to increase the chances of meconium aspiration. Yeomans *et al.* (1989) found a significantly higher incidence of meconium below the vocal cords if the umbilical pH was < 7.20. However, while some workers have reported a strong association between aspiration of meconium and the presence of abnormal FHR tracing during labour and low cord arterial pH at birth, others have found that these measures are poor predictors of infants with meconium below the cords and those without (Starks *et al.* 1980; Dooley *et al.* 1985). This may well be a reflection of the poor specificity of cardiotocography to detect hypoxia and the use of cord artery pH values that do not represent significant acidosis, but several authors agree that a baseline tachycardia is particularly sinister in terms of increasing the risk of meconium aspiration (Hernandez *et al.* 1993). Neonates, however, do not have to have been hypoxic *in utero* to suffer from MAS.

Thick meconium has been associated with increased incidence and severity of the aspiration syndrome (Meis *et al.* 1978; Starks 1980; Mitchell *et al.* 1985; Rossi *et al.* 1989; Berkus *et al.* 1994). This may be a reflection of the fact that oligohydramnios (and therefore thick undiluted meconium) is more likely to lead to fetal hypoxia due to cord compression and, consequently, increased fetal breathing.

Meconium in the amniotic fluid may be harmful to the fetus in other ways. Meconium has been demonstrated to cause vascular necrosis and vasoconstriction in the umbilical cord after diffusion into cord vessels (Altshuler, Arizawa and Molnar-Nadasy 1992). Naeye (1995) has postulated that meconium could be responsible for initiating a transient severe vasoconstriction of the umbilical vessels which results in ischaemic brain injury to the fetus. This might not manifest as acidosis at birth if enough time had elapsed between the end of the vasoconstriction and delivery. He uses this theory to explain the findings of a large prospective study in the United States that found 14% of the risk for quadriplegic cerebral palsy was associated with meconium in the amniotic fluid, this risk being independent of other risk factors for cerebral palsy on logistic regression.

## MECONIUM ASPIRATION SYNDROME

Meconium aspiration is most conveniently defined as the presence of meconium below the vocal cords (Katz and Bowes 1992). Meconium aspiration syndrome is usually evident at, or within a few hours of, birth and encompasses a wide spectrum of disease ranging from transient respiratory distress, requiring the minimum of treatment, to severe respiratory compromise necessitating long-term ventilatory support and neonatal death. Meconium in the respiratory tract is noxious in a number of ways. If thick it blocks small airways leading to alveolar collapse in some areas of the lung and consequent hyperinflation and pneumothoraces in others. Meconium adversely affects the function of surfactant, causes cell damage and tissue necrosis, enhances bacterial growth, as well as causing a chemical pneumonitis. It may be that it can also directly cause pulmonary vasoconstriction and necrosis. In addition, in severe cases persistent pulmonary hypertension develops which is resistant to antihypertensive therapy. This, together with right-to-left shunting and persistent fetal circulation, give rise to a profound hypoxia.

A baby who aspirated meconium, but has not been hypoxic during labour, is unlikely to suffer any serious consequences — indeed, 90% will be asymptomatic (Dooley *et al.* 1985; Falciglia 1988; Rossi *et al.* 1989). It is those fetuses who have been subjected to intrauterine hypoxia who are likely to suffer from a severe form of MAS. The hypoxic insult produces pulmonary vasoreactivity and lung destruction in its own right, which is then severely exacerbated by meconium. Many of the lung abnormalities may be due to hypoxia exacerbated by the presence of meconium in the lungs causing chemical damage to the lung, inhibition of surfactant, physical obstruction of the airways and promotion of infection. The severity of the resulting respiratory disease is related more to the severity of the preceding hypoxic insult to the fetus than to the meconium itself, although the majority of severe cases of MAS occur when the meconium has been thick.

## PREVENTING MECONIUM ASPIRATION

### By increased visualisation?

In the past many obstetricians felt that the detection of meconium in the amniotic fluid merited urgent delivery. Saling (1966) advocated visualisation of the amniotic fluid using an amnioscope passed up through the cervical canal and placed against intact membranes if labour had not started 10 days after the expected date of confinement. He claimed a threefold reduction in perinatal mortality by undertaking amniotomy and fetal blood sampling if meconium was detected in this manner. Such convincing results have not been reproduced by other studies (Browne and Bernan 1968; Huntingford et al. 1968).

### By early induction?

As meconium passage is more common with advanced gestational age, it might be tempting to deduce that by inducing women before 40 weeks, this would reduce the incidence of meconium-stained amniotic fluid. Unfortunately, even though this may be the case, such a policy does not consistently reduce the incidence of meconium aspiration and, even when it does, there appears to be no effect on perinatal mortality or morbidity (Cole, Howie and Macnaughton 1975; Cardozo, Fysh and Pearce 1986; Dyson, Miller and Armstrong 1987).

### By social support and using oxytocin?

There have been two reports that suggest that social support during labour reduces the incidence of meconium staining, but in both studies the group with no support used more oxytocin compared to the group with support (Sosa et al. 1980; Klaus et al. 1986). The use of oxytocin in labour complicated by meconium staining has been associated with a higher risk of meconium aspiration (Morel et al. 1994). However, those women receiving oxytocin had significantly lower umbilical cord pH measurements, which suggests uterine hyperstimulation may have occurred with oxytocin.

### By amnioinfusion?

Amnioinfusion, the instillation of normal saline into the uterus during labour, has been proposed as a method to reduce meconium concentration and, therefore, the effects of any aspiration that occurs. There have been several reports showing that when amnioinfusion is performed in labours complicated by thick or moderate meconium-stained liquor there is an improvement in the cord arterial pH and/or base deficit, an improvement in Apgar scores, a reduction in operative deliveries for 'fetal distress', a decrease in the incidence of meconium aspiration and the need for positive pressure ventilation, and a reduction in the incidence of MAS (Sadovsky et al. 1989; Wenstrom and Parsons 1989; Strong et al. 1990; Macri et al. 1992; Uhing et al. 1993; Cialone et al. 1994). However, more recent reports have failed to demonstrate an improved perinatal outcome after amnioinfusion for thick or moderate meconium-stained liquor (Spong, Ogundipie and Ross 1994; Usta et al. 1995). Spong et al. found amnioinfusion to be of no benefit in patients where there was moderate to heavy meconium-stained liquor but no fetal heart rate abnormalities. This raises the possibility that amnioinfusion works by reducing cord compression in cases of oligohydramnios, thus alleviating variable fetal heart rate decelerations and preventing or decreasing the frequency of fetal gasping movements which occur in the presence of fetal hypercapnia or acidaemia. Usta *et al.* performed a retrospective review of 937 labours complicated by thick or moderate meconium-stained amniotic fluid, in a unit with a policy of routine amnioinfusion for such patients. They found that 141 (15%) eligible women did not receive amnioinfusion because the presence of meconium was diagnosed too late to start the procedure. In fact, over 50% of labours complicated by meconium were not suitable for amnioinfusion because of either occult meconium, imminent delivery or intervention was required for 'fetal distress'.

## CONCENTRATION OF MECONIUM IN AMNIOTIC FLUID

Traditionally, birth attendants have relied on subjective assessment to describe the concentration of meconium in amniotic fluid, using terms such as thick and thin, or a grading system I to III. Such subjective measurements correlate poorly with objective methods of assessment of meconium consistency in the clinical situation (Cialone *et al.* 1994). Visual examination of the amniotic fluid draining through the cervix may not accurately reflect the intrauterine concentration of meconium. The tight fit of the fetal head as it descends in labour may exclude observation of the amniotic fluid until after delivery. In cases of oligohydramnios no liquor may drain at all, thus masking the presence of meconium. A method of reliably detecting meconium once it has been passed in labour and objectively assessing its concentration in the amniotic fluid might be a useful clinical tool in high-risk labours.

Early suggestions that there is a characteristic appearance to meconium on ultrasonography which could be used to indicate the presence of meconium in amniotic fluid (Benacerraf, Gatter and Ginsburgh 1984) have not been substantiated by others (Sherer *et al.* 1991; Brown *et al.* 1994). The increased echogenicity is more likely to be due to vernix than meconium.

Inserting an intrauterine catheter (IUPC) and regularly aspirating samples of amniotic fluid from the intrauterine cavity for analysis is theoretically possible. Mass or nuclear magnetic resonance spectrometry can be used to charac-

terise the polysaccharide components of meconium glycoproteins (Hounsell *et al.* 1989). Liquid chromatography with ultraviolet-visible and fluorescence spectroscopy will detect the presence of zinc coproporphyrinogens I and III in meconium. Unfortunately, these measurement techniques require elaborate preparation of the sample to be analysed and are not practical for the clinical situation. An alternative is to quantify the meconium concentration by centrifuging a sample of amniotic fluid and measuring the amount of solid matter in the sample (the 'meconiumcrit') (Weitzner *et al.* 1990; Trimmer and Gilstrap 1991). However, this is not only time-consuming, but vernix and solid matter other than meconium which are present in the amniotic fluid can produce false-positive or falsely elevated results.

Although repeated samples theoretically could be obtained through aspiration of an IUPC in order to detect changes in meconium concentration during labour, the authors have found difficulty in obtaining more than a single sample during labour, presumably due to either oligohydramnios and/or blockage of the intrauterine catheter by very thick meconium (*vide infra*). This difficulty would limit the use of this method for the continuous measurement of meconium concentration in the amniotic fluid.

### Spectrophotometry

Molcho *et al.* (1986) described a spectrophotometric method for measuring meconium concentration in amniotic fluid. Fresh meconium from neonates was added to amniotic fluid (obtained at amniocentesis) in known concentrations. The absorption spectra of these samples were measured and it was found that the presence of meconium produced an absorption peak at a wavelength between 405 nm and 415 nm. The magnitude of this peak correlated with meconium concentration. Laboratory studies by our group (Danielian 1995) showed that only samples with a meconium concentration of less than 20 g/l could be assessed using the optical absorption method put forward by Molcho and co-workers (1986). As meconium concentrations increased above this amount the amniotic fluid became very turbid and rendered absorption methods based on the transmission of light difficult and inaccurate. Amniotic fluid with thick meconium staining has meconium concentrations in the region of 80 g/l. Another problem encountered was that blood can often be present in amniotic fluid. Blood also produces an absorption peak at 415 nm plus two additional peaks at 540 nm and 575 nm. The heights of the absorption peaks increase as the concentration of meconium or blood increases, so any proposed optical absorption method of measuring meconium concentration has to discriminate between blood and meconium.

Our group, instead, devised a method to measure the amount of light back-scattered in amniotic fluid contaminated with meconium (i.e. using reflectance rather than absorption of light) (Genevier *et al.* 1993). In contrast to absorption methods, the more light that is reflected the more opaque the sample, and thus the higher concentrations of meconium more likely to be encountered in clinical practice may be measured. This technique was incorporated into an intrauterine probe so that continuous measurement of the amniotic fluid throughout labour could be performed.

## The intrauterine probe

This intrauterine probe is made of polyurethane and is 400 mm long, 14 mm wide and 4 mm thick and encapsulates a 'Y'-shaped silica optical fibre bundle and an optical cell. Optical fibres are made of polymer or silica which are inert to body fluids and can therefore be introduced safely into the human body. The probe can be easily inserted through the cervix once the membranes have ruptured in a manner similar to inserting an IUPC so that it lies in the uterine cavity as shown in Figure 1. Once it is connected to its xenon light source (Figure 2), light is carried by one branch of the fibre bundle to the optical cell situated at the end of the probe where it is back-scattered by the amniotic fluid onto the other branch bringing the light back to spectrophotometric equipment. The optical cell is sited 3 cm from the tip of the probe and is seated in a specially designed cuvette which is designed to minimise any spurious reflections from its walls which could produce erroneous results. Its design also allows amniotic fluid to flow freely over the optical cell, but prevents the uterine wall or fetal skin blocking the openings.

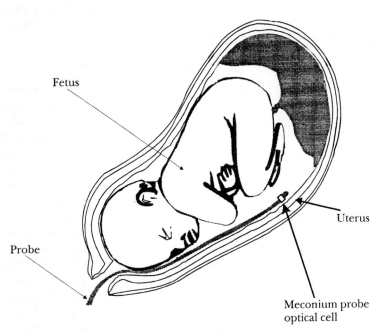

**Figure 1** *Position of the intrauterine probe inside the uterine cavity after insertion*

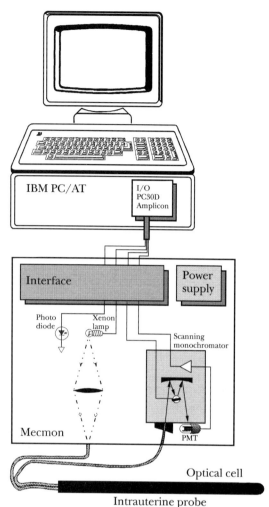

**Figure 2** *Diagram of the meconium monitoring system. (Reproduced from Genevier, E. S. G., Danielian, P. J. and Steer, P. J. (1993) Continuous meconium monitoring during labour using an intrauterine probe. Physiol Meas 14, 337–46, with permission of the Institute of Physics Publishing)*

The optical spectrum of the back-scattered light is processed by a measurement algorithm on a personal computer. Quantification of the meconium concentration is made by calculating the ratio of the amount of light back-scattered at meconium's absorption peak of between 405–415 nm and reference wavelengths of 700 nm. At 700 nm meconium absorbs little or no light so this reference wavelength compensates for the varying turbidity of meconium and amniotic fluid. The ratio increases linearly with meconium concentration. This system will measure meconium with an accuracy of ± 30% and a linearity of better than 95% (Genevier *et al.* 1993). Modification of the measurement algorithm to use an additional reference wavelength of 540 nm enables the system to distinguish between blood and meconium in the amniotic fluid. The personal computer is also linked to a fetal monitor (we use a Sonicaid Meridian, Oxford Medical, Abingdon, Oxfordshire) so that on the computer screen the FHR, intrauterine pressure and continuous meconium concentration can be displayed in graphical format.

## Occult meconium

During clinical trials the meconium probe was used in labouring women who had clear amniotic fluid draining after rupture of the membranes as well as in those with meconium staining. In four women the passage of meconium during labour was documented by measurements from the probe, although no meconium was seen to be draining *per vaginum*. In fact, the meconium was only observed clinically after delivery of the baby by the birth attendant. This detection of 'occult' meconium has important implications. Knowing that meconium is present during a labour would alter the significance placed on fetal rate abnormalities. Without this knowledge there could be suboptimal management of the labour and delivery.

## Case reports

*Case 1.* Figure 3 shows a recording from the meconium probe during a 90-minute period of a labour where initially thin, old meconium-staining of the amniotic fluid was noted. The probe recorded a meconium concentration of approximately 10 g/l and then demonstrated a sudden rise in meconium concentration to approximately 100 g/l (this was not clinically apparent to the attendant medical staff). After a further 20 minutes, a fetal tachycardia developed, complicated by late decelerations. At Caesarean section two hours later, copious thick fresh meconium was seen by the birth attendants for the first time. The baby was

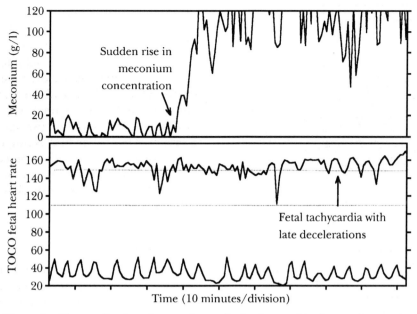

**Figure 3** *The recording from the meconium probe showing a sudden increase in meconium concentration in amniotic fluid during labour. See case 1 in text for details*

diagnosed as having mild MAS and required admission to the neonatal intensive care unit for 24 hours.

*Case 2.* Figure 4 shows a 50-minute recording from the meconium probe. Initially, the probe recorded a meconium concentration of 10–20 g/l, consistent with the thin meconium seen *per vaginum.* The patient then had an epidural top-up and seven minutes later an uncomplicated fetal tachycardia developed, although the patient never became clinically hypotensive. The probe recorded two sharp rises in meconium concentration; the first to a level of approximately 40 g/l as the fetal tachycardia developed, and the second to approximately 80 g/l after a further 10 minutes. The meconium concentration remained at this level for approximately 10 minutes, then fell slowly to a level of 20 g/l, which was maintained for the remainder of the labour. The authors' group has observed this phenomenon in two other cases and feel it lends support to the hypothesis that epidural top-up can induce mild fetal compromise (Katz and Bowes 1992).

## Meconium concentration during amnioinfusion

Monitoring the concentration of meconium in the amniotic fluid could potentially be an advantage when performing amnioinfusion. At present there is no agreement among investigators on how much fluid should be infused into the uterus during amnioinfusion or on the method of assessing the effects of such a technique on the concentration of the meconium in the amniotic fluid. There have been a wide range of protocols described for amnioinfusion which highlight the clinician's inability to assess the meconium concentration. These protocols tend to advise that a fixed amount of fluid should be infused in each case requiring amnioinfusion, although some allow for additional amounts of fluid to be infused dependent on determining the amniotic fluid index (Sadovsky *et al.* 1989; Wenstrom and Parsons 1989; Strong *et al.* 1990; Macri *et al.* 1992; Uhing *et al.* 1993; Cialone *et al.* 1994). As significant increases in intrauterine pressure have been reported with as little as 250 ml of amnioinfusion, it seems prudent to keep the amount of

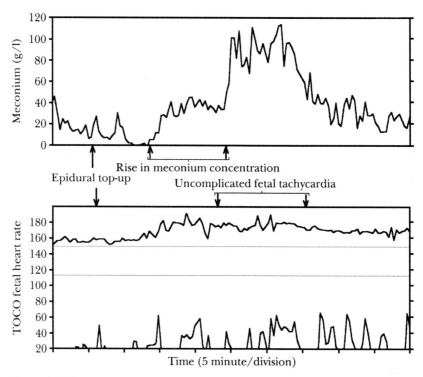

**Figure 4** *The recording from the meconium probe showing an increase in meconium concentration associated with epidural top-up. See case 2 for details*

fluid infused to the minimum required (Strong *et al.* 1990).

Figure 5 (Deans *et al.* 1995) shows the results obtained while monitoring amnioinfusion during labour. Thick, particulate meconium was noted to be draining *per vaginum* after spontaneous rupture of the membranes. After the probe was inserted readings from the probe were recorded for 20 minutes to enable baseline measurements to be obtained. During this time the meconium concentration varied between 46 and 79 g/l. This variation probably represents considerable turbulence *in utero* due to fetal movement and uterine activity. A normal saline solution which had been previously heated to 37°C was then infused by gravity flow through the amnioinfusion port of an Intrans Plus IUPC catheter in accordance with manufacturers' instructions. A total of 650 ml was infused continuously over 50 minutes until the meconium concentration was seen to fall to zero as seen on the graph in Figure 5. The probe was left *in situ* for a further 10 minutes of readings to confirm

that the meconium concentration remained below 10 g/l.

This is a simple technique that allows for assessment of the quantity of fluid that should be amnioinfused in an individual case to reduce the meconium concentration *in utero* during labour. It will also enable research to be carried out to determine the critical level of meconium concentration in amniotic fluid at which MAS occurs and allow the development of universal protocol for amnioinfusion.

## CONCLUSION

The cause of meconium passage by the fetus is still uncertain. However, fetal hypoxia appears to be an important factor in the aspiration of meconium by the fetus and the resulting morbidity and mortality from MAS. The authors' group have demonstrated a device for continuously monitoring the concentration of meconium in amniotic fluid during labour. Its

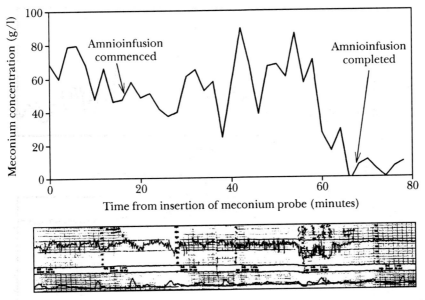

**Figure 5** *Readings obtained during continuous meconium concentration monitoring during amnioinfusion with the simultaneous cardiotocogram*

use in labour may enable us to develop a better understanding of the causes of meconium passage and mechanisms behind meconium aspiration. Work is in progress to combine this technology with an intrauterine probe that carries devices to monitor fetal heart rate, intrauterine pressure and other modalities (Allman *et al.* 1991). With such a single device to monitor the high risk fetus we may be able to be more effective at preventing MAS.

## ACKNOWLEDGEMENTS

We would like to acknowledge that all the work was done under the auspices of Professor P. J. Steer, Academic Department of Obstetrics and Gynaecology, Charing Cross and Westminster Medical School at the West London Hospital and the Chelsea and Westminster Hospital where A. C. Deans and P. J. Danielian were Research Fellows at this institution.

# References

Alexander, G. R., Hulsey, T. C., Robillard, P. Y., De Caunes, F. and Papiernik, E. (1994) Determinants of meconium-stained amniotic fluid in term pregnancies. *J Perinatol* **14**, 259–63

Allman, A. C. J., Danielian, P. J., Genevier, E. S. G. *et al.* (1991) 'New monitoring modalities by surface contact and other non-feto-invasive sensors for intrapartum use' in: *Fetal and Neonatal Measurements*, pp. 153–6. Oxford: Elsevier Science

Altshuler, G., Arizawa, M. and Molnar-Nadasy, G. (1992) Meconium induced umbilical cord vascular necrosis and ulceration: a potential link between the placenta and poor pregnancy outcome. *Obstet Gynecol* **79**, 760–6

Anonymous (1988) Lung function in children after neonatal meconium aspiration. *Lancet* **i**, 317–18

Baker, N., Kilby, M. D. and Murray, H. (1992) An assessment of the use of meconium alone as an indicator for fetal blood sampling. *Obstet Gynecol* **80**, 792–6

Becker, R. F., Windle, W. F., Barth, E. E. and Schulz, M. D. (1940) Fetal swallowing, gastrointestinal activity and defecation in amnio. *Surg Gynecol Obst* **70**, 603–14

Berkus, M. D., Langer, O., Samueloff, A. *et al.* (1994) Meconium-stained amniotic fluid: increased risk for adverse neonatal outcome. *Obstet Gynecol* **84**, 115–20.

Benacerraf, B. R., Gatter, M. A. and Ginsburgh, F. (1984) Ultrasound diagnosis of meconium-stained amniotic fluid. *Am J Obstet Gynecol* **149**, 570–2

Block, M. F., Kallenberger, D. A., Kern, J. D. and Nepveux, R. D. (1981) *In utero* meconium aspiration by the baboon fetus. *Obstet Gynecol* **57**, 37–40

Bochner, C. J., Medearis, A. L., Ross, M. G. *et al.* (1987) The role of antepartum testing in the management of postterm pregnancies with heavy meconium in early labor. *Obstet Gynecol* **69**, 903–7

Brown, D. L., Polger, M., Clark, P. K., Bromley, B. S. and Doubilet, P. M. (1994) Very echogenic amniotic fluid: ultrasonography–amniocentesis correlation. *J Ultrasound Med* **13**, 95–7

Browne, A. D. H. and Bernan, R. K. (1968) The application, value, and limitations of amnioscopy. *J Obstet Gynaecol Br Commonw* **75**, 616

Cardozo, L., Fysh, J. and Pearce, J. M. (1986) Prolonged pregnancy: the management debate. *BMJ* **293**, 1059–63

Cialone, P. R., Sherer, D. M., Ryan, R. M., Sinkin, R. A. and Abramowicz, J. S. (1994) Amnioinfusion during labor complicated by particular meconium-stained amniotic fluid decreases neonatal morbidity. *Am J Obstet Gynecol* **170**, 842–9

Cole, R. A., Howie, P. W. and Macnaughton, M. C. (1975) Elective induction of labour. A randomised prospective trial. *Lancet* **ii**, 767–70

Coltart, T. M., Byrne, D. L. and Bates, S. A.

(1989) Meconium aspiration syndrome: a 6-year retrospective study. *Br J Obstet Gynaecol* **96**, 411–14

Cunningham, A. S., Lawson, E. E., Martin, R. J. and Pildes, R. S. (1990) Tracheal suction and meconium: a proposed standard of care. *J Pediatr* **116**, 153–4

Danielian, P. J. (1995) *MD Thesis*, University of London

Davis, R. O., Philips, J. B., Harris, B. A., Wilson, E. R. and Huddleston, J. F. (1985) Fatal meconium aspiration syndrome occurring despite airway management considered appropriate. *Am J Obstet Gynecol* **151**, 731–6

Dawes, G. S., Fox, H. E., Leduc, B. M., Liggins, G. C. and Richards, R. T. (1972) Respiratory movements and rapid eye movement sleep in the fetal lamb. *J Physiol* **220**, 119–43

Deans, A. C., Genevier, E. S. G., Kivel, N. M. and Steer, P. J. (1995) 'Continuous meconium concentration monitoring using an intrauterine probe while performing amnioinfusion in labour' in: the *Proceedings of the 27th British Congress of Obstetrics and Gynaecology*, Dublin (abstract)

Desmond, M. M., Moore, J., Lindley, J. E. and Brown, C. A. (1957) Meconium staining of the amniotic fluid. *Obstet Gynecol* **9**, 91–103

Dooley, S. L., Pesavento, D. J., Depp, R. *et al.* (1985) Meconium below the vocal cords at delivery: correlation with intrapartum events. *Am J Obstet Gynecol* **153**, 767–70

Duenhoelter, J. H. and Pritchard, J. A. (1977) Fetal respiration. A review. *Am J Obstet Gynecol* **129**, 326–38

Dysart, M., Graves, B. W., Sharp, E. S. and Cotsonis, G. (1991) The incidence of meconium-stained amniotic fluid from 1980 through 1986, by year and gestational age. *J Perinatol* **11**, 245–8

Dyson, D. C., Miller, P. D. and Armstrong, M. A. (1987) Management of prolonged pregnancy: induction of labor versus antepartum fetal testing. *Am J Obstet Gynecol* **156**, 928–34

Emmanoulides, G. C., Townsend, D. E. and Bauer, R. A. (1968) Effects of single umbilical artery ligation in the lamb fetus. *Pediatrics* **42**, 919

Falciglia, H. S. (1988) Failure to prevent meconium aspiration syndrome. *Obstet Gynecol* **71**, 349–53

Fenton, A. N. and Steer, C. M. (1962) Fetal distress. *Am J Obstet Gynecol* **83**, 354–62

Florman, A. L. and Teubner, D. (1969) Enhancement of bacterial growth in amniotic fluid by meconium. *J Pediatr* **74**, 111–14

Genevier, E. S. G., Danielian, P. J. and Steer, P. J. (1993) Continuous meconium monitoring during labour using an intrauterine probe. *Physiol Meas* **14**, 337–46

Genevier, E. S. G., Danielian, P. J., Randall, N. J., Smith, R. and Steer, P. J. (1993) A method for continuous monitoring of meconium in amniotic fluid during labour. *J Biomed Eng* **15**, 229–34

Gregory, G. A., Gooding, C. A., Phibbs, R. H. and Tooley, W. H. (1974) Meconium aspiration in infants — a prospective study. *J Pediatr* **85**, 848–52

Gupta, A. K. and Anand, N. K. (1991) Wheezy baby syndrome — a possible sequelae of neonatal meconium aspiration syndrome. *Indian J Pediatr* **58**, 525–7

Harries, J. T. (1978) Meconium in health and disease. *Br Med Bull* **34**(1), 75–8

Hernandez, C., Little, B. B., Dax, J. S., Gilstrap, L. C. and Rosenfeld, C. R. (1993) Prediction of the severity of meconium aspiration syndrome. *Am J Obstet Gynecol* **169**, 61–70

Hoskins, I. A., Hemming, V. G., Johnson, T. R. B. and Winkel, C. A. (1987) Effects of alterations of zinc-to-phosphorus ratios and meconium content on group B *Streptococcus* growth in human amniotic fluid *in vitro*. *Am J Obstet Gynecol* **157**, 770–3

Hounsell, H. F., Lawson, A. M., Stoll, M. S. *et al.* (1989) Characterisation by mass spectrometry and 500-MHz proton nuclear magnetic resonance spectroscopy of penta- and hexasaccharide chains of human foetal gastrointestinal mucins (meconium glycoproteins). *Eur J Biochem* **786**, 597–610

Huntingford, P. J., Brunello, L. P., Dunstan, M. *et al.* (1968) The technique and significance of amnioscopy. *J Obstet Gynaecol Br Commonw* **75**, 610–15

Katz, V. L. and Bowes, W. A. (1992) Meconium aspiration syndrome: reflection on a murky subject. *Am J Obstet Gynecol* **166**, 171–83

Klaus, M. H., Kennell, J. H., Robertson, S. S. and Sosa, R. (1986) Effects of social support during parturition on maternal and infant morbidity. *BMJ* **293**, 585–7

Lucas, A., Christofides, N. D., Adrian, T. E., Bloom, S. R. and Aynsley-Green, A. (1979) Fetal distress, meconium, and motilin. *Lancet* **i**, 718

Macfarlane, P. I. and Heaf, D. P. (1988) Pulmonary function in children after neonatal meconium aspiration syndrome. *Arch Dis Child* **63**, 368–72

Macri, C. J., Schrimmer, D. B., Leung, A., Greenspoon, J. S. and Paul, R. H. (1992) Prophylactic amnioinfusion improves outcome of pregnancy complicated by thick meconium and oligohydramnios. *Am J Obstet Gynecol* **67**, 117–21

Mahmoud, E. L., Benirschke, K., Vaucher, Y. E. and Poitras, P. (1988) Motilin levels in term neonates who have passed meconium prior to birth. *J Pediatr Gastroenterol Nutr* **7**, 95–9

Martin, D. W. (1979) 'Porphyrins and bile pigments' in: Harper, H. A., Rodwell, V. W. and Mayes, P. A. (Eds.). *Review of Physiological Chemistry*, 17th Edn. pp. 228–44. USA: Lange Medical Publications

Mazor, M., Furman, B., Wiznitzer, A. *et al.* (1995) Maternal and perinatal outcome of patients with preterm labor and meconium-stained amniotic fluid. *Obstet Gynecol* **86**, 830–3

Meis, P. J., Hall, M., Marshall, J. R. and Hobel, C. J. (1978) Meconium passage: a new classification for risk assessment during labour. *Am J*

*Obstet Gynecol* **131**, 509–13

Miller, F. C., Sacks, D. A., Yeh, S.-Y. *et al.* (1975) Significance of meconium during labor. *Am J Obstet Gynecol* **122**, 573–80

Miller, F. C. and Read, J. A. (1981) Intrapartum assessment of the postdate fetus. *Am J Obstet Gynecol* **141**, 516–20

Mitchell, J., Schulman, H., Fleischer, A., Farmakides, G. and Nadeau, D. (1985) Meconium aspiration and fetal acidosis. *Obstet Gynecol* **65**, 352–5

Molcho, J., Leiberman, J. R., Hagay, Z. and Hagay, Y. (1986) Spectrophotometric determination of meconium concentration in amniotic fluid. *J Biomed Eng* **8**, 162–5

Morel, M. I., Anyaegbunam, A. M., Mikhail, M. S., Legorreta, A. and Whitty, J. E. (1994) Oxytocinon augmentation in arrest disorders in the presence of thick meconium: influence on neonatal outcome. *Gynecol Obstet Invest* **37**, 21–4

Naeye, R. L., Peters, E. C., Bartholomew, M. and Landis, J. R. (1989) Origins of cerebral palsy. *Am J Dis Child* **143**, 1154–61

Naeye, R. L. (1995) Can meconium in the amniotic fluid injure fetal brain? *Obstet Gynecol* **86**, 720–4

Richey, S. D., Ramin, S. M., Bawdon, R. E. *et al.* (1995) Markers of acute and chronic asphyxia in infants with meconium-stained amniotic fluid. *Am J Obstet Gynecol* **172**, 1212–5

Romero, R., Hanaoka, S., Mazor, M. *et al.* (1991) Meconium-stained amniotic fluid: a risk factor for microbial invasion of the amniotic cavity. *Am J Obstet Gynecol* **164**, 859–62

Rosenthal, N. and Abramowsky, C. R. (1988) Causes of morbidity and mortality among infants born at term. *Arch Pathol Lab Med* **112**, 178–81

Rossi, E. M., Philipson, E. H., Williams, T. G. and Kalhan, S. C. (1989) Meconium aspiration syndrome: intrapartum and neonatal attributes. *Am J Obstet Gynecol* **161**, 1106–10

Saling, E. (1966) Amnioscopy. *Clin Obstet Gynecol* **9**, 472–90

Sadovsky, Y., Amon, E., Bade, M. E. and Petrie, R. H. (1989) Prophylactic amnioinfusion during labor complicated by meconium: a preliminary report. *Am J Obstet Gynecol* **161**, 613–17

Schulze, M. (1925) The significance of the passage of meconium during labor. *Am J Obstet Gynecol* **10**, 83–8

Sepkowitz, S. (1987) Influence of the legal imperative and medical guidelines on the incidence and management of the meconium-stained newborn. *Am J Dis Child* **141**, 1124–7

Sharp, H. L., Peller, J., Carey, J. B. and Krivit, W. (1971) Primary and secondary bile acids in meconium. *Pediatr Res* **5**, 274–9

Shaw, K. and Clark, S. L. (1988) Reliability of intrapartum fetal heart rate monitoring of the postterm fetus with meconium passage. *Obstet Gynecol* **72**, 886–9

Sherer, D. M., Abramowicz, J. S., Smith, S. A. and Woods, J. R. (1991) Sonographically homogeneous echogenic amniotic fluid in detecting meconium-stained amniotic fluid. *Obstet Gynecol* **78**, 819–22

Sosa, R., Kennell, J., Klaus, M., Robertson, S. and Urrutia, J. (1980) The effect of a supportive companion on perinatal problems, length of labor, and mother–infant interaction. *N Engl J Med* **303**, 597–600

Spong, C. Y., Ogundipie, O. A. and Ross, M. G. (1994) Prophylactic amnioinfusion for meconium-stained amniotic fluid. *Am J Obstet Gynecol* **171**, 931–5

Starks, G. C. (1980) Correlation of meconium-stained amniotic fluid, early intrapartum fetal pH, and Apgar scores as predictors of perinatal outcome. *Obstet Gynecol* **56**, 604–9

Steer, P. J., Eigbe, F., Lissauer, T. J. and Beard, R. W. (1989) Interrelationships among abnormal cardiotocograms in labor, meconium staining of the amniotic fluid, arterial cord blood pH and Apgar scores. *Obstet Gynecol* **74**, 715–21

Strong, T. H., Hetzler, G., Sarno, A. P. and Paul, R. H. (1990) Prophylactic intrapartum amnioinfusion: a randomised clinical trail. *Am J Obstet Gynecol* **162**, 1370–5

Swaminathan, S., Quinn, J., Stabile, M. W. *et al.* (1989) Long-term pulmonary sequalae of meconium aspiration syndrome. *J Pediatr* **144**, 356–61

Trimmer, K. J. and Gilstrap, L. C. (1991) 'Meconiumcrit' and birth asphyxia. *Am J Obstet Gynecol* **165**, 1010–13.

Weitzner, J. S., Strassner, H. T., Rawlins, R. G., Mack, S. R. and Anderson, R. A. (1990) Objective assessment of meconium content of amniotic fluid. *Obstet Gynecol* **76**, 1143–4

Wenstrom, K. D. and Parsons, M. T. (1989) The prevention of meconium aspiration in labor using amnioinfusion. *Obstet Gynecol* **73**, 647–51

Wiswell, T. E., Tuggle, J. M. and Turner, B. S.

(1990) Meconium aspiration syndrome: have we made a difference. *Pediatrics* **85**, 715–21

Woods, J. R. and Dolkart, L. A. (1989) 'Significance of amniotic fluid meconium' in: Creasy, R. K. and Resnik, R. (Eds.). *Maternal–fetal Medicine. Principles and Practice*, 2nd Edn, pp. 404–13. Philadelphia: W.B. Saunders

Usta, I. M., Mercer, B. M., Aswad, N. K. and Sibai, B. M. (1995) The impact of a policy of amnioinfusion for meconium-stained amniotic fluid. *Obstet Gynecol* **85**, 237–41

Uhing, M. R., Bhat, R., Philobos, M. and Raju, T. N. K. (1993) Value of amnioinfusion in reducing meconium aspiration syndrome. *Am J Perinatol* **10**, 43–5

Yeomans, E. R., Gilstrap, L. C., Leveno, K. J. and Burris, J. S. (1989) Meconium in the amniotic fluid and fetal acid–base status. *Obstet Gynecol* **73**, 175–8

# 34

# Diagnosis and management of fetal distress in labour

*Gary J. Mires*

The term fetal distress which despite being widely used in obstetric practice and being a frequently cited reason for intervention in the interest of the fetus, lacks an agreed definition. The 'diagnosis' is usually inferred from a combination of fetal heart rate abnormalities, meconium staining of the liquor, abnormal blood gas parameters and an assessment of condition at birth by use of the Apgar score, all of which have poor association with long-term neurological morbidity (Sykes *et al.* 1982; Low, Galbraith and Muir 1983; Dijxhoorn, Vissen and Fidler 1986; Ruth and Raivio 1988; Dennis *et al.* 1989). In many cases these observed parameters reflect the physiological response of the fetus to the stress of labour, so if they are used as markers of fetal compromise, increased obstetric intervention in the absence of fetal benefit will result (MacDonald *et al.* 1985). Fetal distress has been defined as:

> '*A condition in which fetal physiology is so altered as to make death or permanent injury a probability within a relatively short period of time.*' (van Geijn *et al.* 1991)

In obstetric terms, therefore, the challenge of intrapartum fetal surveillance is to develop a method which has sufficient sensitivity and specificity to identify the fetus at such risk and to allow intervention before the onset of permanent damage.

## 'STRESS' VERSUS 'DISTRESS' AND 'BIRTH ASPHYXIA'

A normal fetus is well adapted to the intermittent periods of hypoxaemia/hypoxia which are frequently, if not universally, experienced during labour. Exposure to hypoxia, which is central to the concepts of fetal distress and birth asphyxia, results in a fetal response. This response may be healthy and adaptive or compromising, and the response will be modified by vulnerability (e.g. associated with small-for-gestational-age, prematurity and/or rapidity and adequacy of adaptive responses) and the degree of exposure. Initial healthy adaptive responses include:

(1) Chemoreceptor-mediated maintenance of cardiac output by increasing heart rate or a reflex parasympathetic decrease in heart rate and a simultaneous increase in myocardial contractility;

(2) Circulatory redistribution to the myocardium and brain at the expense of perfusion of other tissues; and

(3) Anaerobic glycolysis.

Further oxygen deprivation or lack of ability to mount the adaptive responses as a consequence of vulnerability will result in compromising responses. Among these are hypotension and heart failure, leading to decreased cardiac output and a consequent further reduction in tissue perfusion which could include the heart and brain. In addition, a cascade of cytotoxic processes resulting from the inadequate production of adenosine triphosphate (ATP) to meet cellular requirements will be initiated. These include:

(1) An accumulation of lactate and development of severe acidosis;

(2) The formation of neurotoxic levels of excitatory amino acids;

(3) The production of oxygen-free radicals; and

(4) The leakage of potassium and accumulation of calcium ions.

The ultimate consequence of this sequence of events is cell death. None of the clinically observed signs of 'fetal distress' is known to relate directly to these cellular events and, as mentioned earlier in this chapter, may coincidentally represent healthy adaptive responses.

As with the term 'fetal distress', there is some lack of agreement concerning the definition of 'birth asphyxia'. Indeed, some have suggested that it should be dropped from clinical practice in favour of terms referring to clinically observable events (Blair 1993). Exposure to hypoxia (as mentioned above) will result in a response and ultimately an outcome. The outcome, which will again be modified by severity of exposure, individual vulnerability and ability to mount an appropriate adaptive response, may be normal, temporary or permanent impairment, or death. The American College of Obstetricians and Gynecologists suggests that a neonate who has had severe hypoxia close to delivery resulting in hypoxic ischaemic encephalopathy (HIE) will show evidence of an umbilical arterial acidaemia (pH < 7.0), low Apgar score (< 3 for > 5 minutes), abnormal neurological signs in the neonatal period and evidence of hypoxic organ damage. They state that acidaemia alone, although indicative of hypoxia, is insufficient proof that injury has occurred. In support of this, Dennis et al. (1989) failed to demonstrate an association between acidosis and subsequent developmental outcome. He suggested that, paradoxically, it may be fetuses who are unable to mount the appropriate response to hypoxia by utilising anaerobic metabolism, and who do not therefore develop an acidosis, who may be at greater risk of neurological damage than those who do become acidotic.

The lack of agreement in the definition of the terms 'fetal distress' and 'birth asphyxia', the poor association between current short-term measures of outcome and subsequent neurodevelopment, as well as the apparently small contribution made by intrapartum events to neonatal encephalopathy (Adamson, Alessandri and Badawi 1995) and cerebral palsy (Nelson 1988), make the evaluation of new methods of intrapartum surveillance difficult. It is against this background that the remainder of this chapter will consider current methods of intrapartum fetal assessment in association with new developments in this field.

## CURRENT METHODS OF INTRAPARTUM FETAL SURVEILLANCE

### Fetal heart rate monitoring

Continuous fetal heart rate and uterine contraction monitoring, which is called cardiotocography (CTG), has been in widespread clinical use for over 25 years. Despite this, its role remains uncertain in so far as the predictive value of an abnormal pattern is low, although the chance of the fetus being acidotic is greater with increasingly abnormal patterns (Beard et al. 1971). The obstetrician can, however, gain reassurance from a normal trace (Zuspan et al. 1979). Knowledge about the control of the fetal heart rate remains limited, and many of the problems with the use of this technique in labour relate to a poor understanding of the various observed changes.

Evidence from randomised trials of electronic fetal monitoring (EFM) alone versus intermittent auscultation of the fetal heart, suggest that its use leads to significantly increased obsteric intervention (i.e. Caesarean section) without an improvement in neonatal outcome in both the short term (based on Apgar scores, admission to the special care baby unit [SCBU] and neonatal seizures) and the long term (based on Bayley scores at nine months of age) (Table 1, Grant 1993a). In a further analysis of randomised trial data considering the use of EFM and fetal scalp blood sampling (FBS) versus intermittent auscultation, Caesarean section was again significantly more common in the EFM + FBS group. There was no benefit in intensive monitoring in terms of Apgar scores, admission to SCBU and perinatal death. There was, however, a significant reduction in seizure rate in the EFM + FBS group (Table 2). This reduced risk of seizures was limited to labours that were induced or augmented with oxytocin

and/or were prolonged. This did not equate, however, with a reduction in cases of cerebral palsy. On the basis that the prevention of neonatal seizures is considered important enough in their own right there is, therefore, some support for the use of EFM with FBS in cases where labour is induced, augmented or prolonged. In other 'physiological' labours the current evidence suggests no benefit of EFS + FBS over regular appropriately timed intermittent auscultation of the fetal heart (Grant 1993b).

## Fetal blood sampling

The use of FBS as an adjunct to EFM to reduce intervention based on an abnormal fetal heart

**Table 1** *Electronic fetal monitoring (EFM) alone versus intermittent auscultation in labour. (Reproduced from the three trials reviewed by Grant 1993a\* with permission of Update Software)*

| Parameter measured | Odds ratio | 95% CI |
|---|---|---|
| All Caesarean sections (CS) | 2.70 | 1.92–3.81 |
| CS due to fetal distress | 4.14 | 2.29–7.51 |
| CS due to failure to progress | 2.00 | 1.32–3.03 |
| Apgar score < 4 at 1 minute | 0.99 | 0.51–1.94 |
| Admission to SCBU | 1.03 | 0.76–1.38 |
| Neonatal seizures | 0.80 | 0.21–2.95 |
| Low Bayley mental development index | 2.80 | 0.69–11.34 |
| Low Bayley psychomotor index | 1.82 | 0.63–5.31 |

\*Grant, A. M. (1993a) 'EFM alone *vs.* intermittent ausculation in labour' in: M. W. Enkin, M. J. N. C. Kierse, M. J. Renfrew and J. P. Nelson (Eds.). *The Cochrane Pregnancy and Childbirth Database.* Oxford: Update Software

**Table 2** *Electronic fetal monitoring and scalp sampling versus intermittent auscultation in labour. (Reproduced from the six trials reviewed by Grant 1993b\* with permission of Update Software)*

| Parameter measures | Odds ratio | 95% CI |
|---|---|---|
| All Caesarean sections (CS) | 1.29 | 1.08–1.54 |
| CS for fetal distress | 1.98 | 1.33–2.94 |
| CS for failure to progress | 1.19 | 0.93–1.52 |
| Operative vaginal delivery | 1.31 | 1.18–1.46 |
| Apgar < 4 at 1 minute | 1.04 | 0.78–1.40 |
| Admission to SCBU | 1.00 | 0.90–1.12 |
| Neonatal seizures | 0.49 | 0.29–0.82 |
| Cerebral palsy (CP) | 1.79 | 0.98–3.28 |
| CP after neonatal seizure | 1.00 | 0.20–4.98 |
| Low Bayley mental development index | 2.14 | 0.97–4.71 |
| Low Bayley psychomotor index | 1.72 | 0.94–3.15 |

\*Grant, A. M. (1993b) 'EFM and scalp sampling *vs.* intermittent ausculation in labour' in: M. W. Enkin, M. J. N. C. Kierse, M. J. Renfrew and J. P. Nelson (Eds.). *The Cochrane Pregnancy and Childbirth Database.* Oxford: Update Software pattern has been discussed above. However, in a survey by Wheble *et al.* (1989), only 50% of consultant units in the United Kingdom practised FBS. In addition, while the validity of the scalp capillary measurements has been questioned because the head is compressed and caput and moulding ensue (O'Connor, Hytten and Zanelli 1979), reassurance can again be gained from a normal value. A pH value of < 7.20 has become accepted as indicating fetal compromise but, although 30% of such infants are depressed at birth, most are vigorous and show no short- or long-term sequelae (Tucker and Hauth 1990). Severe metabolic acidaemia is, however, associated with an increased incidence of neonatal seizures and hypotonia.

## Meconium staining of liquor

Although approximately 20% of fetuses will pass meconium during labour, particularly in post-date pregnancies (Steer *et al.* 1989), it is heavy fresh meconium that is associated with severe or repeated stress (Meis *et al.* 1978). There is also an association between meconium staining and fetuses that are small-for-gestational-age (Steer *et al.* 1989). Its presence is an indication for EFM and, in conjunction with abnormalities in the fetal heart rate pattern, it is an indication for FBS (Miller *et al.* 1975). However, its presence has not been correlated with adverse neurological sequelae (Nelson and Ellenberg 1984; Dijxhoorn, Visser and Fiddler 1986).

## SCREENING FOR 'FETAL DISTRESS'

### Risk factors

Clinical risk factors for fetal compromise during labour includes small-for-gestational-age fetuses in whom the pH is more likely to fall during labour (Lin *et al.* 1980; Steer *et al.* 1989) with earlier and more rapid acid–base decompensation (Pearson 1975). In addition, depleted cardiac glycogen leads to an inability to mount the appropriate physiological response and, hence, increases the vulnerability of these fetuses (Rooth 1973). Prematurity itself does not appear to be associated with an increased likelihood of acidosis at delivery, with the distribution of umbilical arterial pH being similar in both preterm and term infants (Ramin *et al.* 1989; Dickson *et al.* 1992). The lower Apgar scores observed in preterm neonates (Perkins and Papile 1985) can be attributed to their immaturity, which reduces their ability to display normal newborn activities, including respiratory effort and muscular tone (Catlin *et al.* 1986).

## Umbilical Doppler

The benefit of Doppler umbilical artery flow velocity waveform (UAFVW) recordings in the antenatal assessment of fetal wellbeing in high-risk pregnancies is well documented (Cameron *et al.* 1988; Gudmundsson and Marsal 1988; Gundmundsson and Marsal 1989; Trudinger, Giles and Cook 1995). In addition, it has been suggested that UAFVW may be more sensitive than fetal heart rate monitoring for the detection of fetal distress in late pregnancy, and that UAFVW changes precede fetal heart rate changes (Trudinger *et al.* 1986). In small-for-gestational-age (SGA) fetuses an abnormal antenatal Doppler UAFVW has also been associated with an increased risk of fetal distress (late decelerations) in labour (Dempster *et al.* 1988).

As a labour-admission screening test for subsequent fetal distress UAFVW is less clear. In a study by Somerset, Murrills and Wheeler (1993), there was a 12-fold increase in the rate of emergency Caesarean section for fetal distress (95% confidence interval [CI] 4.9–29) among women with an elevated systolic/diastolic ratio. The positive predictive value was 31%, with a sensitivity of 50% and specificity of 94%. However, in a study by Gudmundsson *et al.* (1991) there was no association between abnormal UAFVW and abnormal fetal heart rate patterns, low Apgar scores or operative delivery for fetal distress. Furthermore, Chan *et al.* (1994) suggested that the test was a poor predictor of adverse outcome in an unselected population.

## Admission cardiotocography

The labour admission of CTG is performed in many obstetric units as a screening test for fetal distress. The hypothesis for its use is that the functional stress of labour may show early changes in fetal heart rate patterns in fetuses at risk of compromise, allowing early appropriate intervention. Despite its clinical use, there have been no randomised trials to evaluate the labour admission CTG. In a large observational study by Ingemarsson (1993), which involved 12,020 tests, a non-reactive admission test was associated with signs of fetal distress before and after birth. These signs included meconium staining of the liquor, increased Caesarean section rate, increased umbilical artery acidosis and low Apgar scores. Pello *et al.* (1988) also reported an increased operative delivery for fetal distress and acidosis at birth when the admission test was non-reactive. Somerset, Murrills and Wheeler (1993) reported a 25% positive predictive value, with a sensitivity of 67% and a specificity of 91%, for fetal distress when the admission CTG was performed within six hours of delivery. The author is currently embarking on a randomised trial to evaluate the admission CTG.

## NEW DEVELOPMENTS IN INTRAPARTUM FETAL SURVEILLANCE

### The fetal ECG

In a search for improved methods of intrapartum surveillance, attention has turned to the fetal ECG (FECG) to see if more information than the R–R interval to calculate fetal heart rate could be obtained. Initial difficulties with the quality of the signal and in methods of signal processing and analysis have now largely been overcome. Moreover, the use of the technique as an adjunct to the CTG in clinical practice has been evaluated in randomised trials.

Work performed by Rosen and Kjellmer (1975) in exteriorised fetal lambs and guinea pigs in whom hypoxia and acidemia were induced, produced changes in the ST-segment and T-wave, with a progressive increase in T-wave height. These changes occurred before signs of cardiovascular failure (Rosen, Hokegard and Kjellmer 1976). The changes observed in the ST- segment and, in particular, elevation of the T/QRS ratio, were correlated with anaerobic metabolism of myocardial glycogen stores (Rosen and Isaksson 1976; Greene *et al.* 1982). If there is an imbalance between myocardial oxygen supply and demand, then anaerobic metabolism occurs as a healthy adaptive response and an elevation in ST waveform height is observed (Greene 1987). In hypoxaemic, growth-retarded guinea pigs ST depression and negative T-waves were observed, while ST elevation was seen in normally grown litter mates (Widmark *et al.* 1991). These growth-retarded fetuses have lower catecholamine levels, depleted myocardial glycogen stores and, during hypoxia, have ineffective anaerobic metabolism. They, therefore, suffer directly from lack of oxygen in the deeper myocardial layers (endocardium) before the superficial layers (epicardium), thus altering the sequence of repolarisation to produce a negative ST-segment (Figure 1).

In addition to the changes observed in the ST-segment of the FECG, both animal and human studies have demonstrated that the normal negative relationship between the fetal heart rate and the PR interval of the ECG becomes positive during fetal acidosis (Pardi *et al.*

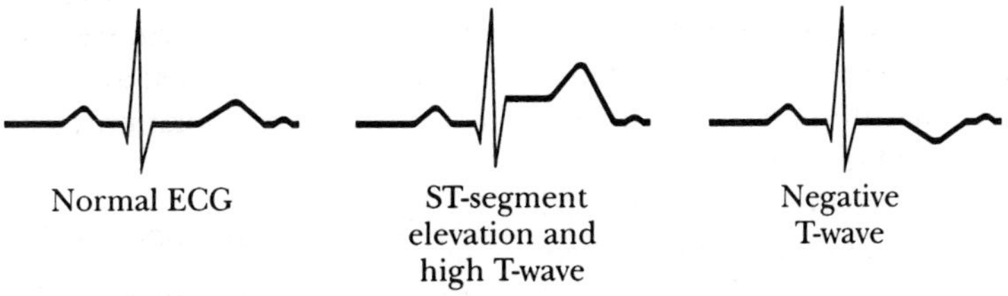

Normal ECG        ST-segment elevation and high T-wave        Negative T-wave

**Figure 1**   *The fetal ECG and changes associated with hypoxia*

1974; Murray 1986). This relationship (conduction index) can be intermittently positive for short periods of time without adverse effect, but a positive conductive index for greater than 20 minutes is associated with an increased risk of fetal compromise (Murray 1992; Mohajer *et al.* 1994).

The FECG therefore offers a means by which myocardial adaptation to hypoxia might be identified. In a randomised trial of the CTG alone versus ST waveform plus CTG for intrapartum monitoring in over 2400 high-risk cases, Westgate *et al.* (1993) demonstrated a 46% reduction in operative deliveries for fetal distress ($P < 0.001$, odds ratio [OR] 1.85, 95% CI 1.35–2.66), and a trend of less metabolic acidosis and fewer low five-minute Apgar scores in the FECG + CTG arm. In a similar randomised trial in 214 high-risk labours, using the conduction index (van Wijngaarden *et al.* 1996), a significant reduction in the number of cases having fetal blood samples (FBS) in the FECG + EFM arm was observed (RR EFM alone 3.53, $P < 0.01$, 95% CI 1.39–8.95). This was without an observed increase in adverse fetal outcome. The FBSs performed in the EFM alone group were less likely to be abnormal (pH < 7.25) than those performed in the FECG + EFM group. In addition, there was a trend towards more infants with an umbilical pH < 7.15 at birth being unsuspected and more instrumental deliveries for presumed fetal distress being performed in the EFM alone than in the FECG + EFM group. The use of the FECG in conjunction with the CTG appears, therefore, to result in less intervention without apparent fetal compromise.

## Pulse oximetry

Pulse oximetry has revolutionised anaesthetic and neonatal practice, and new technology has now made it possible to apply this technique to the fetus to measure oxygen saturation ($SaO_2$) continuously throughout labour. Pulse oximeters measure the colour of pulsotile blood. Devices similar to those used in adult and neonatal monitoring, but specifically modified for intrapartum use, have been calibrated using fetal lambs (Jongsma *et al.* 1991) and validated

in human cross-sectional studies (McNamara *et al.* 1992). However, the close correlation between oximetry and cord blood oxygenation has not been reproduced, and there is no correlation between an intermittent oximetry reading and the pH of FBS (Johnson *et al.* 1994). Gardosi, Schram and Symonds (1991) failed to obtain readings in 44 of 105 labours, and recognised the problems and limitations of this method. They conclude, however, that this technique may become an adjunct to the CTG, in so far as it can offer reassurance of fetal wellbeing non-invasively if a normal and stable $SaO_2$ baseline is obtained especially in the presence of a questionable CTG, and may reduce the need for FBS. It may also be useful in assessing fetal reserve with a low baseline $SaO_2$ at the start of labour, and recognise potential fetal compromise by a falling $SaO_2$ during labour. Johnson *et al.* (1994) do admit that the technique is still experimental and there is insufficient data to support its use as a replacement for FBS as a discriminator for an abnormal fetal heart trace. To date, there have been no randomised trials to evaluate its use in clinical practice.

## Continuous fetal transcutaneous (tc) $pO_2/pCO_2$ monitoring

This technique remains very much a research tool to obtain continuous information about blood gases in the fetus during labour and delivery. Currently, there are no transducers with a sufficiently high specificity to reflect central $pO_2$ during birth (Huch 1993). A transducer is required which remains stable for a sufficiently long time, is easy to attach to the fetal scalp and is not influenced by local changes in the skin/transducer relationship. Current transducers provide great research potential if their limitations are appreciated, but are not suitable for routine clinical practice. Problems involved with both $tcpCO_2$ measurements concern diffusion, limitations posed by peripheral perfusion, the 'tonsure' effect (O'Conner, Hytten and Zanelli 1979), formation of caput succedaneum (Lofgren and Jacobson 1977) and also interindividual differences in capillary blood flow restriction (Huch 1993). When using this technique, however, it has been demonstrated that late decelerations and severe variable decelerations are associated with hypoxaemia (Huch *et al.* 1977) and tcpO$_2$ changes with contractions, but not to a significant degree (Schneider *et al.* 1980). The tcpCO$_2$ has been demonstrated to correlate with pCO$_2$ in both capillary and umbilical arterial blood samples (Hansen *et al.* 1984; Thomsen and Weber 1984).

## Continuous tissue pH measurements

In a similar manner to the tcpO$_2$ and tcpCO$_2$ monitoring just discussed, there is presently no tissue pH electrode which is accurate, easy to use and of proven benefit to the mother and fetus. As a result, this method has only been used in research protocols. For example, the Kontron–Roche electrode developed by Stamm *et al.* (1974) is difficult to apply, resulting in a high rate of unsuccessful monitorings (Nickleson and Weber 1991), is expensive and, because of the sterilising procedure, has a short life span. In addition, its use requires a skin incision with the subsequent risk of infection. Newer developments include the fibre optic pH electrode which has a higher successful monitoring rate (80% according to Hochberg *et al.* 1988) and the PVC electrode. A good correlation has been demonstrated using this technique between tissue pH and umbilical artery pH (Nickelson and Weber 1991), and Young, Katz and Wilson (1980) have demonstrated associations between tissue pH and CTG patterns. That is, pH was normal with accelerations and moderate bradycardia, but a decreased pH was observed in 20–25% of cases of early and variable decelerations, 93% of cases of late decelerations, 60% of cases with a fetal tachycardia and 36% of cases with reduced variability. Weber and Nickelson (1993) suggest the need for randomised trials of this technique as an adjunct to CTG before the technology is used in routine clinical practice.

## Near infrared spectroscopy (NIRS)

This technique was first described by Josbis (1977), and is capable of proving, in a non-invasive fashion, continuous data about cerebral oxygenation. It is dependent on the fact that biological tissue is relatively transparent to light in the near infrared region of the spectrum, and that the tissue contains chromophores whose light absorbing properties vary with oxygenation. Within the fetal brain these chromophores include oxy- and deoxyhaemoglobin and cytochrome oxidase. Preliminary work has demonstrated that near infrared spectroscopy has great potential for studying in a continuous fashion previously inaccessible physiological parameters of brain oxygenation during labour (Wyatt and Peebles 1993). Again large appropriately designed trials are required before near infrared spectroscopy is considered for introduction into routine clinical practice.

## MANAGEMENT OF 'FETAL DISTRESS' IN LABOUR

### Interpretation of fetal heart rate patterns

The current 'gold standard' of intrapartum fetal assessment is the CTG. The limitations of this technique have been described, but are likely to be confounded by inappropriate interpretation which may result from poor education. One obvious solution to this problem is to improve education, but another is the development of computerised analysis and intelligent systems. The former considers the CTG in isolation and identifies abnormal CTG features, whereas the latter incorporates with the CTG interpretation other factors which the experienced clinician will use to determine the most appropriate management (e.g. obstetric history and risk factors, events in labour, progress of labour and scalp blood samples). Keith *et al.* (1995) performed a multicentre comparative study of experts and an intelligent computer system for managing labour using the CTG. They found the systems performance was indistinguishable from the experts in 50 cases examined, but was more consistent. Further evaluation of this system is required to establish whether the introduction of this system into the labour ward will at least do no harm.

## Fetal 'resuscitation'

Current 'first aid' measures when fetal distress is suspected include a change in maternal position, particularly to avoid aortocaval compression, stopping exogenous oxytocin administration, the use of β-sympathomimetics and the administration of oxygen.

A change in maternal position may have a beneficial effect when a fetal bradycardia is associated with aortocaval compression. The dorsal position during the second stage of labour has been demonstrated to result in a fall in umbilical arterial pH and elevated $pCO_2$ levels (Johnstone, Abdelmago and Harouny 1987).

Hyperstimulation with exogenous oxytocin will result in fetal hypoxia and CTG abnormalities. A rapid improvement is often observed with cessation of oxytocin, and a single dose of a β-agonist (e.g. ritodrine) may relax the uterus sufficiently to reduce cord compression or increase uteroplacental blood flow (Shekerloo, Mendez-Bauerl and Freese 1989). In a randomised trial, Patriarco et al. (1987) demonstrated an improvement in the fetal heart rate pattern in women treated with terbutaline who were diagnosed as having fetal distress based on CTG abnormalities. At birth, terbutaline-treated babies were less likely to be acidotic and tended to have higher Apgar scores.

A negative effect on intervillous blood flow has been postulated by Jouppila et al. (1983) when maternal inhalation of oxygen is used, thus questioning the value of this technique. In addition, only small increases of fetal arterial $pO_2$ are observed, even when 100% oxygen is inhaled by the mother (van Geijn et al. 1991).

Amnioinfusion using saline or Ringer's lactate has been described as a method of preventing or relieving umbilical cord compression during labour (Miyazaki and Navarez 1985), or preventing meconium aspiration (Wenstrom and Parsons 1989). Evidence from randomised trials suggests that amnioinfusion appears to be effective in relieving or preventing fetal heart rate decelerations, reducing operative delivery rates for fetal distress diagnosed on this basis and reducing the incidence of postpartum endometritis (Table 3; Hofmeyr 1993a). When used in cases complicated by meconium-stained liquor, there was a marked reduction in Caesarean section for fetal distress and meconium aspiration syndrome (Table 4; Hofmeyr 1993b).

## CONCLUSIONS

The journey through the maternal pelvis has been described as being one of the most hazardous most of us ever make, but it is usually well tolerated. This latter fact is important to remember, as much of the technology discussed above to assess fetal wellbeing during labour is not appropriate or desirable in all cases, and it often results in increased obstetric intervention with no fetal benefit. Current methods of assessing the condition of the fetus during labour are poorly predictive for those fetuses who are genuinely compromised and who might benefit

**Table 3** *Amnioinfusion in intrapartum cord compression diagnosed by electronic fetal monitoring (EFM). (Reproduced from the five trials reviewed by Hofmeyr 1993a\* with permission of Update Software)*

| Effect on: | Odds ratio | 95% CI |
|---|---|---|
| Persistent variable decelerations | 0.21 | 0.12–0.36 |
| Caesarean section for fetal distress | 0.31 | 0.20–0.47 |
| Caesarean section overall | 0.48 | 0.34–0.69 |
| Forceps/vacuum for fetal distress | 0.47 | 0.24–0.91 |
| Apgar score < 7 at 1 minute | 0.28 | 0.18–0.44 |
| Cord arterial pH < 7.20 | 0.44 | 0.27–0.73 |
| Postpartum endometritis | 0.47 | 0.24–0.91 |

\*Hofmeyr, G. J. (1993a) 'Amnionfusion in intrapartum umbilical cord compression' in: M. W. Enkin, M. J. N. C. Kierse, M. J. Renfrew and J. P. Nelson (Eds.). *The Cochrane Pregnancy and Childbirth Database.* Oxford: Update Software

**Table 4** *Amnioinfusion for meconium-stained liquor in labour. (Reproduced from the five trials reviewed by Hofmeyr 1993b\* with permission of Update Software)*

| Effect on: | Odds ratio | 95% CI |
|---|---|---|
| Heavy meconium staining | 0.09 | 0.02–0.32 |
| Caesarean section for fetal distress | 0.21 | 0.11–0.41 |
| Caesarean section overall | 0.47 | 0.28–0.80 |
| 5 minute Apgar < 7 | 0.25 | 0.08–0.77 |
| Umbilical arterial pH < 7.20 | 0.25 | 0.14–0.43 |
| Meconium below vocal cords | 0.14 | 0.09–0.21 |
| Meconium aspiration syndrome | 0.20 | 0.08–0.47 |
| Neonatal ventilation | 0.24 | 0.07–0.90 |

*Hofmeyr, G. J. (1993b) 'Amnioinfusion for meconium stained liquor in labour' in: M. W. Enkin, M. J. N. C. Kierse, M. J. Renfrew and J. P. Nelson (Eds.). *The Cochrane Pregnancy and Childbirth Database.* Oxford: Update Software

from intervention aimed at preventing permanent damage or death. This is set against a background of difficulty in evaluating new methods of intrapartum assessment because of lack of agreement about the definition of terms such as 'fetal distress' and 'birth asphyxia'. In addition, there is a lack of suitable end-points against which to evaluate new methods, as current end-point assessment of neonatal condition by Apgar scores or umbilical blood gas data is poorly predictive of long-term neurodevelopment. Neither technique may provide an adjunct to the currently available methods to reduce the unecessary intervention, but some require evaluation by properly designed randomised trials with adequate neurodevelopment follow-up prior to introduction into clinical practice. Others require improvements in technology, and in this respect remain research tools which provide great opportunities to obtain physiological data to improve our knowledge and understanding of previously inaccesible parameters, but at the present time remain a long way from being clinically useful tools.

# References

Adamson, S. J., Alessandri, L. M. and Badawi, N. (1995) Predictors of neonatal encephalopathy in full term infants. *BMJ* **311**, 598–602

American College of Obstetricians and Gynecologists (1991) *Utility of Umbilical Cord Blood Acid Base Assessment.* American College of Obstetricians and Gynaecologists

Beard, R. W., Filshie, G. M., Knight, C. A. and Roberts, G. M. (1971) The significance of the changes in the continuous fetal heart rate in the first stage of labour. *J Obstet Gynaecol Br Commonw* **78**, 865–81

Blair, E. (1993) A research definition for 'birth asphyxia'? *Dev Med Child Neurol* **35**, 449–55

Cameron, A. D., Nicholson, S. F., Nimrod, C. A., Harder, J. R. and Davis, D. M. (1988) Doppler waveforms in the fetal aorta and umbilical artery in patients with hypertension in pregnancy. *Am J Obstet Gynecol* **158**, 339–45

Catlin, E. A., Carpenter, M. W., Brann, B. S. *et al.* (1986) The Apgar score revisited: influence of gestational age. *J Pediatr* **109**, 865–8

Chan, G. Y., Lam, C., Lam, Y. H. *et al.* (1994) Umbilical artery Doppler velocimetry compared with fetal heart monitoring as a labour admission test. *Eur J Obstet Gynecol Reprod Biol* **54**, 1–6

Dempster, J., Mires, G. J., Taylor, D. J. and Patel, N. B. (1988) Fetal umbilical artery flow velocity waveforms: prediction of SGA infants and late decelerations in labour. *Eur J Obstet Gynecol Reprod Biol* **29**, 21–5

Dennis, J., Johnson, A., Mutch, L., Yudkin, P. and Johnson, P. (1989) Acid-base status at birth and neurodevelopmental outcome at four and one-half years. *Am J Obstet Gynecol* **161**, 213–20

Dickson, J. E., Eriksen, N. L., Meyer, B. A. and Parisi, V. M. (1992) The effect of preterm birth on umbilical cord blood gases. *Obstet Gynecol* **79**, 575–8

Dijxhoorn, M. J., Visser, G. and Fiddler, J. J. (1986) Apgar score, meconium and acidaemia at birth in relation to neonatal and neurological morbidity in term infants. *Br J Obstet Gynaecol* **93**, 217–22

Gardosi, J. O., Schram, C. M. and Symonds, M. E. (1991) Adaptation of pulse oximetry for fetal monitoring during labour. *Lancet* **337**, 1265–7

Grant, A. M. (1993a) 'EFM alone *vs.* intermittent auscultation in labour' in: M. W. Enkin, M. J. N. C. Kierse, M. J. Renfrew and J. P. Neilson (Eds.). *The Cochrane Pregnancy and Childbirth Database*, Oxford: Update Software

Grant, A. M. (1993b) 'EFM and scalp sampling *vs.* intermittient auscultation labour' in: M. W. Enkin, M. J. N. C. Keirse, M. J. Renfrew and J. P. Neilson (Eds.). *The Cochrane Pregnancy and Childbirth Database*. Oxford: Update Software

Greene, K. R. (1987) The ECG waveform. *Baillieres Clin Obstet Gynaecol* **1** (1), 131–55

Greene, K. R., Dawes, G. S., Lilja, H. *et al.* (1982) Changes in the ST waveform of the fetal ECG with hypoxemia. *Am J Obstet Gynecol* **144**, 950–8

Gudmundsson, S. and Marsal, K. (1988) Ultrasound Doppler evaluation of uteroplacental and fetoplacental circulation in pre eclampsia. *Arch Gynecol Obstet* **243**, 196–206

Gudmundsson, S. and Marsal, K. (1989) Umbilical and uteroplacental blood flow velocity waveforms in pregnancies with fetal growth retardation. *Eur J Obstet Gynecol Reprod Biol* **27**, 187–96

Gudmundsson, S., Marsal, K., Kwok, H. H., Vengadasalam, D. and Ratnam, S. S. (1991) Umbilical artery Doppler velocimetry as a labour admission test. *Obstet Gynecol* **77**, 10–16

Hansen, P. K., Thomsen, S. G., Secher, N. J. and Weber, T. (1984) Transcutaneous carbon dioxide measurements in the fetus during labour. *Am J Obstet Gynecol* **150**, 47–51

Hochberg, H. M., Roby, P. V., Snell, H. M. *et al.* (1988) Continuous intrapartum fetal scalp tissue pH and ECG monitoring by fiberoptic probe. *J Perinat Med* **16** (suppl. 1) 71–86

Hofmeyr, G. J. (1993a) 'Amnioinfusion in intrapartum umbilical cord compression' in: M. W. Enkin, M. J. N. C. Keirse, M. J. Refrew and J. P. Neilson (Eds.). *The Cochrane Pregnancy and Childbirth Database*. Oxford: Update Software

Hofmeyr G. J. (1993b) 'Amnioinfusion for meconium stained liquor in labour' in: M. W. Enkin, M. J. N. C. Keirse, M. J. Refrew and J. P. Neilson (Eds.). *The Cochrane Pregnancy and Childbirth Database*. Oxford: Update Software

Huch, A. (1993) 'Fetal tcPO$_2$ and tcPCO$_2$ monitoring: an unsolved problem for clinical routine' in: J. A. D. Spencer and R. H. T. Ward (Eds.). *Intrapartum Fetal Surveillance*, pp. 295–307 London: RCOG Press

Huch, A., Huch, R., Schneider, H. *et al.* (1977) Continuous transcutaneous monitoring of fetal oxygen tension during labour. *Br J Obstet Gynaecol* **84**, S1 1–39

Ingemarsson, I. (1993) 'Elecronic fetal monitoring as a screening test' in: J. A. D. Spencer and R. H. T. Ward (Eds.). *Intrapartum Fetal Surveillance*, pp. 45–52. London: RCOG Press

Johnson, N., Johnson, V. A., McNamara, H. *et al.* (1994) Fetal pulse oximetry: new method of monitoring the fetus. *Aust NZ J Obstet Gynaecol* **34**, 428–33

Johnstone, F. D., Abdelmago, M. S. and Harouny, A. K. (1987) Maternal posture in the second stage and fetal acid base status. *Br J Obstet Gynaecol* **94**, 753–7

Jongsma, H. W., Crevels, J., Menssen, J. J. M. *et al.* (1991) 'Applications of transmission pulse oximetry in fetal lambs'. in: H. N. Lafebar, J. G. Aarnoudse and H. W. Jongsma (Eds.). *Fetal and Neonatal Physiological Measurements*, pp. 123–28. Excerpta Medica

Josbis, F. F. (1977) Non-invasive infrared monitoring of cerebral and myocardial sufficiency and circulatory parameters. *Science* **198**, 1265–7

Jouppila, P., Kirkinen, P., Koivvla, A. *et al.* (1983) The influence of maternal oxygen inhalation on human placenta and umbilical venous blood flow. *Eur J Obstet Gynecol Reprod Biol* **16**, 151–6

Keith, R. D. F., Beckley, S., Garibaldi, J. M. *et al.* (1995) A multicentre comparative study of 17 experts and an intelligent computer system for managing labour using the cardiotocogram. *Br J Obstet Gynaecol* **102**, 688–700

Lin, C. C., Moawad, A. H., Rosenow, P. J. and River, P. (1980) Acid-base characteristics of fetuses with intrauterine growth retardation during labour and delivery. *Am J Obstet Gynecol* **137**, 553–9

Lofgren, O. and Jacobson, L. (1977) Monitoring of transcutaneous pO2 in the fetus and mother during normal labour. *J Perinat Med* **6**, 252–9

Low, J. A., Galbraith, R. S. and Muir, D. W. (1983) Intrapartum fetal hypoxia: a study of long-term morbidity. *Am J Obstet Gynecol* **145**, 129–34

MacDonald, D., Grant, A., Sheridan-Pereira, M., Baylan, P. and Chalmers, I. (1985) Dublin randomised control trial of antepartum FHR monitoring. *Am J Obstet Gynecol* **152**, 524–39

Malcus, P., Gudmundsson, S., Marsal, K. *et al.* (1991) Umbilical artery Doppler velocimetry as a labour admission test. *Obstet Gynecol* **77**, 10–16

McNamara, H., Chung, D. C., Liford, R. *et al.* (1992) Do fetal pulse oximetry readings at delivery correlate with cord blood oxygenation and acidaemia? *Br J Obstet Gynaecol* **99**, 735–8

Meis, P. J., Hall, M., Marshall, J. R. and Hobel, C. J. (1978) Meconium passage: a new classification of risk assessment during labour. *Am J Obstet Gynecol* **131**, 569–73

Miller, F. C., Sacks, D. A., Yeh, S. Y. *et al.* (1975) Significance of meconium during labour. *Am J Obstet Gynecol* **122**, 573–80

Miyazaki, F. S. and Nevarez, F. (1985) Saline amnioinfusion for relief of repetitive variable decelerations: a prospective randomised trial. *Am J Obstet Gynecol* **153**, 301–6

Mohajer, M. P., Sahota, D. S., Reed, N. N. *et al.* (1994) Cumulative changes in the fetal ECG and biochemical indices of fetal hypoxia. *Eur J Obstet Gynecol Reprod Biol* **55**, 63–70

Murray, H. G. (1986) The fetal ECG: current clinical developments in Nottingham. *J Perinat Med* **14**, 399–404

Murray, H. G. (1992) Evaluation of the fetal ECG. MD Thesis, University of Nottingham

Nelson, K. B. (1988) What proportion of cerebral palsy is related to birth asphyxia. *J Pediatr* **112**, 572–4

Nelson, K. B. and Ellenberg, J. H. (1984) Obstetric complications and risk factors for cerebral palsy or seizure disorders. *J Am Med Assoc* **251**, 1843–8

Nickleson, C. and Weber, T. (1991) The current status of intrapartum continuous fetal tissue pH measurements. *J Perinat Med* **19**, 87–92

O'Connor, M. C. and Hytten, F. E. (1979) Measurement of fetal transcutaneous oxygen tension: problems and potential. *Br J Obstet Gynaecol* **86**, 948–53

O'Connor, M. C., Hytten, F. E. and Zanelli, G. D. (1979) Is the fetus 'scalped' in labour? *Lancet* **ii** 94–948

Pardi, G., Tucci, E., Uderzo, A. and Zanini, D. (1974) Fetal electrocardiogram changes in relation to fetal heart rate patterns during labour. *Am J Obstet Gynecol* **118**, 243–50

Patriarco, M. S., Viechnicki, B. M., Hutchinson, T. A., Klasko, S. K. and Yeh, S. Y. (1987) A study of intrauterine fetal resuscitation with terbutaline. *Am J Obstet Gynecol* **157**, 384–7

Pearson, J. E. (1975) 'Induction of labour' in: R. Beard, M. Brudenell, P. Dunn and D. Fairweather (Eds.). *The Managment of Labour. Proceedings of the Third Study Group of the RCOG*, p. 35. London: Royal College of Obstetricians and Gynaecologists

Pello, I. C., Dawes, G. S., Smith, J. and Redman, C. W. G. (1988) Screening of the fetal heart in early labour. *Br J Obstet Gynaecol* **95**, 1128–36

Perkins, R. P. and Papile, L. A. (1985) The very low birth rate infant: incidence and significance of low Apgar scores, 'asphyxia', and morbidity. *Am J Perinatol* **2**, 108–13

Ramin, S. M., Gilstrap, L. C., Leveno, K. J., Burris, J. and Little, B. B. (1989) Umbilical acid base status in the pre term infant. *Obstet Gynecol* **74**, 256–8

Rooth, G. (1973) The time factor in fetal distress. *J Perinat Med* **1**, 7–12

Rosen, K. G., Hokegard, W. H. and Kjellmer, I. (1976) A study of the relationship between the ECG and haemodynamics of the fetal lamb during asphyxia. *Acta Physiol Scand* **98**, 275–84

Rosen, K. G. and Isaksson, O. (1976) Alterations in FHR and ECG correlated to glycogen creatine phosphate and ATP levels during graded hypoxia. *Biol Neonate* **30**, 17–24

Rosen, K. G. and Kjellmer, J. (1975) Change in the fetal heart rate and ECG during hypoxia. *Acta Physiol Scand* **93**, 59–66

Ruth, V. J. and Ravio, K. O. (1988) Perinatal brain damage: predictive value of metabolic acidosis and Apgar score. *BMJ* **297**, 24–7

Schneider, H., Strang, F., Huch, R. *et al.* (1980) Suppression of uterine contractions with fenoterol and its effect of tcPO$_2$ in human term labour. *B J Obstet Gynaecol* **87**, 657–65

Shekerloo, A., Mendez-Bauerl, A. and Freese, U. (1989) Terbutaline for the treatment of acute intrapartum fetal distress. *Am J Obstet Gynecol* **160**, 615–18

Somerset, D. A., Murrills, A. J. and Wheeler, T. (1993) Screening for fetal distress in labour using the umbilical artery blood velocity waveform. *Br J Obstet Gynaecol* **100**, 55–9

Stamm, O., Latscha, U., Janecek, P. *et al.* (1974) Kontinuerliche pH Messung am kindlichen Kopf post partum und sub partu. *Z Geburts Perinatol* **178**, 533–76

Steer, P. J., Eigbe, F., Lissauer, T. J. and Beard, R. W. (1989) Interrelationships among abnormal cardiotocograms in labour, meconium staining of the amniotic fluid, arterial cord blood pH and Apgar scores. *Obstet Gynecol* **74**, 715–21

Sykes, G. S., Malloy, P. M., Johnston, F. *et al.* (1982) Do Apgar scores indicate asphyxia? *Lancet* **ii** 494–6

Thomsen, S. G. and Weber, T. (1984) Fetal transcutaneous carbon dioxide tension during the second stage of labour. *Br J Obstet Gynaecol* **91**, 1103–6

Trudinger, B. J., Giles, W. B. and Cook, C. M. (1985) Flow velocity waveforms in the maternal uteroplacental and umbilical circulations. *Am J Obstet Gynecol* **152**, 155–63

Trudinger, B. J., Cook, C. M., Jones, L. and Giles, W. B. (1986) A comparison of fetal heart rate monitoring and umbilical artery waveforms in the recognition of fetal compromise. *Br J Obstet Gynaecol* **93**, 171–5

Tucker, J. M. and Hauth, J. C. (1990) Intrapartum assessment of fetal wellbeing. *Clin Obstet Gynecol* **33**, 515–53

van Geijn, H. P., Copray, F. J., Donkers, D. K. and Bos, M. H. (1991) Diagnosis and management of intrapartum fetal distress. *Eur J Obstet Gynecol Reprod Biol* **42**, S63–72 van Wijngaarden, W., Sahota, D. S., James, D. K. *et al.* (1996) Improved intrapartum surveillance with PR interval analysis of the fetal ECG — II. A randomised trial showing a reduction in fetal blood sampling. *Am J Obstet Gynecol* **174**, 1295–9

Weber, T. and Nickelsen, C. (1993) in: J. A. D. Spencer and R. H.T. Ward (Eds.). *Intrapartum Fetal Surveillance*, pp. 301–6 London: RCOG Press

Wenstrom, W. D. and Parsons, M. T. (1989) The prevention of meconium aspiration in labour using amnioinfusion. *Obstet Gynecol* **73**, 647–57

Westgate, J., Harris, M., Curnow, J. and Greene, K. R. (1993) Plymouth randomised trial of cardiotocogram only versus ST waveform plus Cardiotocogram for intrapartum monitoring in 2400 cases. *Am J Obstet Gynecol* **169**, 1151–60

Wheble, A. M., Gillmer, M. D. G., Spencer, J. A. D and Sykes, G. S. (1989) Changes in the fetal monitoring practice in the UK: 1977–1984. *Br J Obstet Gynaecol* **96**, 1140–7

Widmark, C., Jansson, T., Lindecrantz, K. and Rosen, K. G. (1991) ECG waveform short term heart rate variability and plasma catecholamine concentrations in response to hypoxia in intrauterine growth retarded guinea pigs. *J Dev Physiol* **15**, 161–8

Wyatt, J. S. and Peebles, D. M. (1993) 'Near infrared spectroscopy and intrapartum fetal surveillance' in: *Intrapartum Fetal Surveillance*, pp. 329–43. London: RCOG Press

Young, B. K., Katz, M. and Wilson, S. J. (1980) Fetal blood and tissue pH with variable deceleration patterns. *Obstet Gynecol* **52**, 170–5

Zuspan, F. P., Quilligan, E. J., Iams, T. D. and van Geijn, H. (1979) Predictors of intrapartum fetal distress: the role of electronic fetal monitoring. *Am J Obstet Gynecol* **35**, 287–91

# 35

# The prevention of preterm birth

*Ronald F. Lamont and Murdoch G. Elder*

With advances in diagnostic fetal ultrasound in the late 1970s and 1980s and the availability of therapeutic termination of pregnancy for fetal malformations, preterm birth has become the major cause of perinatal mortality and morbidity in the developed world (Vilar *et al.* 1994).

The approach to preventing preterm delivery is twofold:

(1) Prevention of the initiation of preterm labour; and

(2) Inhibition of the preterm labour process.

Over 90% of otherwise uncomplicated preterm deliveries occur after 30 weeks' gestation and survival in this group is in excess of 90% (Robertson *et al.* 1992). In contrast, 66% of neonatal deaths occur in pregnancies ending before 29 weeks' gestation (Copper *et al.* 1993). Gestational age provides a better prediction of survival before 29 weeks' gestation, whereas birth weight is a better indicator beyond this time. Morbidity takes on greater importance beyond 30 weeks' gestation, where survival rates are high and obstetricians should not sacrifice any decrease in morbidity with heroic attempts to prolong pregnancy for a minimal increase in survival rate. Conversely, before 30 weeks' gestation, emphasis should be placed on prolonging gestation to improve survival. There is still some doubt as to whether preterm labour is pathological or physiological. Generally, however, the nearer to term this process occurs, the more likely it is to have a large physiological element — the earlier in the gestation this happens, the more likely it is to have a pathological origin.

A number of different approaches and agents have been employed to prevent preterm birth and these are listed in Table 1. They will now be discussed in turn.

## REDUCE RISK FACTORS

Preterm labour is often thought of as a social disease rather than a medical disorder. Over the last 20 years, as society has changed, so have

**Table 1** *Measures to prevent preterm delivery*

*Reduce risk factors, which are:*
 smoking
 multiple pregnancy
 teenage pregnancy
 drug abuse

*Prediction of preterm delivery using:*
 scoring systems:
  risk scoring systems
  cervical scores
 screening tests:
  oncofetal-fibronectin analysis
  bacterial vaginosis

*Prophylactic measures, which include:*
 bed rest
 cervical cerclage
 tocolytics
 antibiotics

*Early diagnosis by:*
 fetal breathing movements
 home monitoring

*Inhibition of preterm labour using:*
 tocolytics
 antibiotics

the risk factors and the emphasis placed on the problem by obstetricians. A review of two leading American peer review journals revealed only nine articles and brief communications for the years 1970 and 1971, but these had risen to 126 by 1990–1991 (Creasy 1993). During this time, the use of assisted conception techniques has made a significant contribution to the problem of early birth in the developed world (Medical Research Council 1990), and it is too early to assess whether reduction in the number of embryos transferred to three or less will reduce the number of higher order births. Other social changes have also contributed to the problem, such as an increase in the teenage birth rate (Anonymous 1991), an increase in maternal age as many working women delay starting their families (Cnattingius *et al.* 1993) and an increase in drug abuse (Cherukuri *et al.* 1988; Chasnoff *et al.* 1989). In this way, despite 20 years of experience of tocolytic agents used to try to prevent preterm birth, the rate of preterm delivery and the morbidity associated with it has not decreased. In the United States, the incidence of preterm birth has increased from 9.4% in 1981 to 10.6% in 1989 (Villar *et al.* 1994).

Some national programmes have been introduced with good effect to try to change society (Papiernik 1984), but three years elapsed before benefit could be observed. In 1978, 40–50% of cases of preterm delivery were thought to be idiopathic and under these circumstances, it is easy to be nihilistic and defeatist. With increasing evidence to implicate infection (McGregor *et al.* 1988; Romero *et al.* 1988; Gibbs *et al.* 1992; Lamont and Fisk 1993) and better efforts to identify the possible causes of preterm labour, the existence of idiopathic preterm labour is in question. In studying 50 women who delivered preterm, despite the use of tocolytics, Lettieri *et al.* (1993) found one or more causes in 96% and two or more in 58% — including faulty placentation (50%), intrauterine infection (38%), immunological factors (30%), cervical incompetence (16%), uterine factors (14%), maternal factors (10%), trauma and surgery (8%) and fetal anomalies (6%).

# PREDICTION OF PRETERM LABOUR

## Scoring systems

### Risk scoring systems

With all the factors associated with preterm labour (Table 2) it should be possible to identify a group of women at risk of preterm delivery using risk scoring systems. Such systems should have a high positive predictive value to warrant some form of intervention and enough sensitivity to affect national outcome measure (e.g. perinatal mortality ad morbidity). The definition of these terms can be seen in Table 3.

A number of risk scoring systems have been suggested, but the number testifies to the failure of each to deliver the appropriate specificity and sensitivity (Newcombe and Chalmers 1981). Most systems rely heavily on past obstetric history and so are inappropriate for nulliparae who constitute 45% of pregnant women. Even if complications of the current pregnancy are included to identify the large number of women who will deliver preterm, there is an unacceptably high false-positive rate. Positive predictive

**Table 2**  *Factors associated with preterm delivery*

*Sociobiological variables:*
  age
  height
  weight
  parity
  socioecomonic group
  nutritional factors
  smoking

*Past obstetric history:*
  therapeutic abortion
  spontaneous abortion
  preterm delivery
  uterine abnormalities
  recurrent urinary tract infection

*Complications of the current pregnancy:*
  antepartum haemorhage
  pregnancy induced hypertension
  multiple pregnancy
  fetal malformation
  polyhydramnios
  oligohydramnios
  abdominal surgery
  inadvertent preterm induction
  infection

**Table 3** *Definitions*

| Term | Definition |
|------|------------|
| Sensitivity | A measure of the ability of a test to detect true cases, and is defined as the number of true-positives as a percentage of the total with the disease |
| Specificity | A measure of the ability of a test to detect disease free individuals and is defined as the number of true-negatives divided by the total without the disease |
| Positive predictive value | The proportion of true cases among all those with a positive test result |
| Negative predictive value | The proportion of negative cases among all those with a negative test result |

values range from 15–30% and sensitivities from 35–60% (Creasy, Gremmer and Liggins 1980; Main and Gabbe 1987).

## Cervical scores

Since substantial changes in the cervix uteri are an essential part of the prelabour and labour process, a number of studies have evaluated the use of cervical scores. Using cervical dilation alone, poor positive predictive values of up to 25% have been obtained (Leveno, Cox and Roark 1986; Stubbs, Van Dorsten and Miller 1986). More recently, reports of cervical scores in multiple pregnancies have been encouraging. Using both length and dilatation (cervical length minus cervical dilatation in centimetres in 154 multiple pregnancies which delivered preterm) the positive predictive value of a cervical score < 0 ranged from 66 to 75%. Only two of the 154 preterm births occurred within a week of a score > 1. As the score became more negative, the interval to preterm delivery became shorter. The positive predictive value increased the earlier in gestation a score < 0 was found (Neilson *et al.* 1988; Newman *et al.* 1991).

## Screening tests

### Oncofetal fibronectin

In 1991, Lockwood and colleagues reported a multicentre study aimed at identifying a biochemical marker (cervicovaginal oncofetal fibronectin) for preterm labour and delivery. Oncofetal fibronectin is an extracellular protein concentrated in amniotic fluid and the extra-

villus trophodecidual interface. The substance is expressed in cervicovaginal secretions during the first 20 weeks of pregnancy, disappears from the secretions after this period and does not normally reappear until spontaneous rupture of the membranes at term. Disregarding the high concentrations of oncofetal fibronectin in vaginal fluid following membrane rupture, any damage of the adhesive oncofetal fibronectin interface between the chorion and the decidua due to mechanical, infective or other aetiologies, may result in the reappearance of the substance in the genital secretions. The use of oncofetal fibronectin appears to have a high sensitivity for detecting subclinical rupture of the membranes (Eriksen *et al.* 1992) and preterm birth, but has a low specificity and high rate of false-positive tests.

Currently, the literature on oncofetal fibronectin is limited. However, in future, published reports are likely to be voluminous as different centres report on the sensitivity, specificity, positive predictive value and negative predictive value of results which evaluate specimens obtained from either the cervix or vagina, in the presence of blood or ruptured (or intact) membranes, the gestational age, levels of fetal fibronectin in the fluid in nanograms per millilitre, the presence or absence of contractions and whether the woman was at low or high risk. The data are shown in Table 4.

For those studies which quoted data, the gestational age at sampling, the gestational age at delivery, the sampling to delivery interval, birth weight, number of contractions and cervical dilatation are shown in Table 5. From the data in Tables 4 and 5, warning of delivery beyond 31 weeks' gestation of an infant weighing

**Table 4** *Presence or absence of oncofetal fibronectin (OFN) as a predictor of preterm delivery*

| Reference | Qualification | Sensitivity | Specificity | Positive predictive value | Negative predictive value |
|---|---|---|---|---|---|
| Lockwood *et al.* (1991) | Cervical or vaginal OFN 50 ng/ml | 81.7 | 82.5 | 83.1 | 81.0 |
| Lockwood *et al.* (1993) | Cervical OFN > 60 ng/ml | 73 | 72 | 25 | 95 |
| Lockwood *et al.* (1993) | Vaginal OFN > 50 ng/ml | 68 | 80 | 30 | 95 |
| Nageotte *et al.* (1994) | Cervical or vaginal OFN > 75 ng/ml (high-risk pregnancies): | | | | |
| | delivery before 37 weeks | 92.6 | 51.7 | 46.3 | 93.9 |
| | delivery before 34 weeks | 92.3 | 59.5 | 28.6 | 97.8 |
| Eriksen *et al.* (1992) | Detection of subclinical membrane rupture with OFN > 50 mg/ml | 98.2 | 26.8 | 87.5 | 75.0 |
| Morrison *et al.* (1993) | Cervicovaginal OFN > 50 ng/ml in women in threatened premature labour | 90 | 72 | 64 | 93 |

**Table 5** *Gestational age and delivery data from three studies which used oncofetal fibronectin as a screening test*

| Parameter measured | Source of data: | | |
|---|---|---|---|
| | *Lockwood* et al. *(1991)* | *Morrison* et al. *(1993)* | *Lockwood* et al. *(1993)* |
| Gestational age at sampling (weeks) | 29.9 | 31.8 | 31.6 |
| Gestational age at delivery (weeks) | 31.3 | 34.3 | 34.4 |
| Sampling – delivery interval (days) | 11 | 21.6 | 24 |
| Birth weight (g) | 1980 | 2199 | 2415 |
| Contractions per hour (*n*) | 10.2 | 12.2 | 32% experienced contractions at 24–36 weeks |
| Cervical dilatation (cm) | 2.6 | — | 18% > 2 cm |

1980–2415 g is unlikely to make a major impact on reducing perinatal mortality and morbidity. Similarly, it might also be argued that when a women is admitted at 30 weeks' gestation, contracting once every six minutes with a cervix dilated more than 2 cm, it does not require a biochemical test to indicate that she is at increased risk of preterm delivery.

It would appear that the measurement of cervicovaginal oncofetal fibronectin levels greater than 50 ng/ml may be a sensitive and specific way to identify those women at subsequent risk of preterm labour and delivery. The use of the test in a high-risk group needs to be assessed to decide whether discrimination is adequate enough for intervention. It may be that, due to the high sensitivity and negative predictive value, the test may prove to be of more value in reassuring women that they are at low risk of preterm delivery if they have, a negative test result.

### Bacterial vaginosis

There is now undeniable evidence that infection is a cause of preterm labour (McGregor *et al.* 1988; Romero *et al.* 1988; Gibbs *et al.* 1992; Lamont and Fisk 1993). This information may be of limited value once a woman is admitted in preterm labour, because by that time there may be irreversible changes in the cervix uteri which renders attempts to inhibit the process unsuccessful. Therefore, it may be more appropriate to use the infected aetiology as a means

of predicting those women at risk of preterm labour and delivery.

Minkoff *et al.* (1984) studied 233 women who were at high risk of preterm delivery using detailed microbiology of high vaginal swabs taken between 14 and 18 weeks' gestation. Those women who were colonised by *Trichomonas vaginalis, Bacteroides* spp. or *Ureaplasma urealyticum* had a statistically increased risk of subsequent preterm labour, preterm delivery and preterm rupture of the membranes.

This degree of microbiological surveillance would be inappropriate as a screening test, because it would be complex and expensive. Some organisms such as anaerobes and *Mycoplasmas* spp. which are commonly found in association with preterm labour and delivery (Lamont *et al.* 1986; Lamont *et al.* 1987; McDonald *et al.* 1991), are also found in association with bacterial vaginosis. In this way, it would seem appropriate to investigate whether the presence of bacterial vaginosis in early pregnancy is a useful indicator of subsequent preterm labour and delivery. Bacterial vaginosis is a polymicrobial condition characterised microbiologically by a marked reduction in lactobacilli with simultaneous increase of up to 1000-fold in other organisms (e.g. anaerobes and *Mycoplasma hominis*). There are also characteristic biochemical imbalances as a result of synergism between these organs, for example:

(1) By increasing the ability of lactobacilli to produce hydrogen peroxide, which is toxic to bacteria; and

(2) By blunting the chemotactic response of polymorphonuclear leucocytes, and by decreasing their killing ability, an environment is created where there are large numbers of potentially pathogenic organisms with very little host response to prevent ascending colonisation of the fetal membranes or decidua (Lamont 1995).

Kurki et al. (1992) found that women with bacterial vaginosis between eight and 17 weeks' gestation had a two- to sixfold increased risk of preterm birth. Hay et al. (1994) found a fivefold increased risk of preterm birth and late miscarriage when bacterial vaginosis was diagnosed by Gram stain on a smear of vaginal secretions taken before 16 weeks' gestation.

Whether bacterial vaginosis is a problem in itself, or whether it is simply a marker for some virulent organism (e.g. *Mycoplasma hominis*), remains unclear. It is also uncertain whether by reversing this imbalance, the subsequent incidence of preterm delivery and late miscarriage can be reduced and this is currently the subject of a multicentre study in the United Kingdom.

In addition, in association with bacterial vaginosis, McGregor et al. (1994) found a 3.3-fold increased risk of preterm birth and a 3.8-fold increased risk of prelabour rupture of the membranes. Extracellular mycolytic enzymes (e.g. as mucinases and sialidases) which allow bacteria to penetrate the cervical mucous plug were also found more often and in higher concentrations in women with bacterial vaginosis. While topical clindamycin cream was found to be effective treatment for bacterial vaginosis and temporarily reduced mucinase and sialidase activity, this did not reduce perinatal morbidity. If given too late in pregnancy, topical treatment may be insufficient to suppress bacterial activation of macrophages in decidua and systemic treatment of bacterial vaginosis may be needed.

Oral metronidazole is an efficient way of treating bacterial vaginosis in pregnancy (McDonald et al. 1994) and when used in women with bacterial vaginosis who had had a previous preterm delivery, resulted in a reduction in the rate of preterm birth (Morales et al. 1994).

## PROPHYLAXIS

### Bed rest

Published studies on the use of bed rest to prevent preterm labour relate mainly to twin pregnancies. Approximately 10% of all preterm deliveries are twin pregnancies and it is estimated that only 50% of twins manage to achieve 36 weeks' gestation. Four randomised studies between 1984 and 1990 examined the use of bed rest in twin pregnancies to prevent preterm delivery. A total of 638 women were hospitalised between 26 and 34 weeks' gestation. None of the trials showed any benefits from bed rest (Hartikainen-Sorri and Jouppila 1984; Crowther et al. 1989; MacLennan et al. 1990; Saunders, Dick and Brown 1995) and, indeed, two showed an increased risk of preterm delivery in hospitalised women (MacLennan et al. 1990; Saunders, Dick and Brown 1995). The majority of women were admitted after 30 weeks' gestation which may be too late to show benefit. Furthermore, there may have been a bias towards admitting women with other complications associated with twins (e.g. antepartum haemorrhage or pregnancy-induced hypertension) which, in themselves, increase the risk of preterm delivery. Alternatively, hospital admission may have resulted in the earlier detection of other complications which indicated earlier delivery. Currently, the weight of evidence would suggest that bed rest is of little or no help in the prevention of preterm birth.

### Cervical cerclage

A belief in cervical incompetence, whether congenital or acquired, is the basis for cervical cerclage. The balance of risk versus benefit of cervical cerclage remains unclear. This uncertainty was studied in the joint Medical Research Council/Royal College of Obstetricians and Gynaecologists multicentre, randomised trial. More than 200 obstetricians from 12 countries submitted 1292 women for randomisation, based upon a doubt as to whether or not cervical cerclage was indicated. The study population carried a high risk of early delivery in the index pregnancy as indicated by an overall preterm delivery rate of 28%. The method of cerclage was not pre-specified.

There was an apparent 4% reduction (from 17 to 13%) of deliveries before 33 weeks' gestation. If real, this would be equivalent to the prevention of one very early preterm delivery for every 25 sutures inserted. The result was only marginally statistically significant and, bearing in mind the confidence intervals, corresponded to the prevention of one very early preterm birth for as few as 12 or as many as 300 cervical sutures inserted.

Overall, the results of this unique study suggest that the operation of cervical cerclage has a beneficial effect, but only in a minority of women. The procedure was associated with an increase in obstetric intervention (e.g. admission to hospital), the use of oral β-agonists, induction of labour and Caesarean section. There was also a twofold increase in risk of having puerperal sepsis (Medical Research Council/Royal College of Obstetricians and Gynaecologist Study Working Party on Cervical Cerclage 1993).

While most cervical cerclage is performed electively, emergency cervical cerclage is rarely used at later gestations. Since the need for such intervention is rare, there are no prospective, randomised, controlled studies and available data come from small and contradictory reports. In a group of 51 cases who underwent emergency cervical cerclage, 19% were nulliparous women with no identifiable risk factors and only 31% of cases might have had identifiable risk factors to make them eligible for cervical cerclage (Wong, Farquaharson and Dansereau 1993).

Contraindications to emergency cervical cerclage include persistent contractions, antepartum haemorrhage, rupture of membranes and chorioamnionitis. Over a 20-year period, the outcome of emergency cervical cerclage in 19 studies comprising 423 women was reviewed. Following emergency cerclage, the incidence of premature rupture of the membranes, chorioamnionitis, preterm delivery and fetal survival was 42%, 29%, 52% and 64%, respectively (Romero et al. 1992).

Two factors were closely associated with adverse outcome following emergency cervical cerclage:

(1) Subclinical chorioamnionitis; and

(2) Greater cervical dilatation.

Amniocentesis has been suggested as a means of detecting subclinical chorioamnionitis (McGregor et al. 1988). In three studies of emergency cervical cerclage where amniocentesis was employed, there was an overall 91% pregnancy loss if the suture was inserted in the presence of undiagnosed subclinical chorioamnionitis (Romero et al. 1992).

## Tocolytic agents

Although there have been isolated reports of success with long-term oral (Edmonds and Letchworth 1982) and parenteral (Lind et al. 1980) administration of β-agonists, there is little evidence that they are useful in the prevention of preterm labour and delivery (Hemminki and Starfield 1978). The only pharmacological prophylactic agent which has been shown to be of any significant use in the prevention of preterm labour is 17α-hydroxyprogesterone administered intramuscularly. In a meta-analysis of six clinical trials, Keirse (1990) found this agent to be effective with an odds ratio of 0.5, although, like many tocolytic agents, the reduction has not been shown to be associated with a reduction in perinatal mortality and morbidity. A different meta-analysis of 15 trials of progestogenic agents used to manage high-risk pregnancy came to a different conclusion. The article appeared in a respected peer review journal, but none of the co-authors were obstetricians and all worked in departments of biomathematical science or health policy and management (Goldstein et al. 1989). They failed to distinguish between the use of progestogens for early miscarriage due to inadequate luteal phase and the main reason for using progestogens for prophylaxis of preterm labour (the maintenance of a quiescent uterus). In addition, they quoted a paper from 1967 in the *Journal of Sexual Research* pertaining to 10 girls who had been exposed to progestogens *in utero* and whose subsequent behaviour was said to exhibit 'tomboyishness'. The credibility of such an meta-analysis should be questioned.

While there is limited evidence that bed rest, cervical cerclage or prophylactic tocolytic therapy are individually of use in the prevention of preterm birth and delivery, it is possible that a combination of these measure may be of help.

In a report which was unashamedly anecdotal, White, Lamont and Letchworth (1989) presented seven women who between them had had 19 midtrimester miscarriages or early preterm deliveries with none of the pregnancies reaching viability. By employing a combination of bed rest, cervical cerclage and tocolytics, all seven women achieved a delivery of a fetus after 36 weeks' gestation with a birth weight of more than 2500 g. It would be impossible to test this management in a randomised, double-blind, placebo-controlled study. The rarity of the condition, the different variables involved, together with the large numbers required to show a difference in perinatal outcome, would render such a study prohibitive.

### Antibiotic prophylaxis

Two randomised, prospective, blind trials have studied the prophylactic use of erythromycin in women with intact membranes who, according to their abnormal genital tract colonisation, were at high risk of preterm labour. Neither study provided any evidence that this antibiotic therapy was effective in women thought to be at risk of preterm labour on the basis of vaginal colonisation (McCormack *et al.* 1987; Eschenback, Nugent and Rao 1991). These studies were reported in 1987 and 1991, before the association between bacterial vaginosis and preterm delivery was recognised (Kurki *et al.* 1992; Hay *et al.* 1994). However, considering the range of organisms found in association with bacterial vaginosis and preterm labour, erythromycin is unlikely to have provided sufficient cover (Lamont *et al.* 1986; Lamont *et al.* 1987).

## EARLY DIAGNOSIS

### Fetal breathing movements

On the basis of contraction alone, 50% of women and 30% of attendants will be wrong in their diagnosis of preterm labour (Anderson and Turnball 1969). On the basis of watery discharge, bloody discharge or abdominal pain, 75% of women were correct in their diagnosis that something was wrong (i.e. they either gave birth or were admitted for more than 48 hours for diagnostic or therapeutic measures). It was concluded, however, that efforts to increase women's awareness of the significance of various symptoms were unlikely to contribute to the early diagnosis of preterm labour (Kragt and Kierse 1990). Moreover, if intervention is delayed until there are progressive cervical changes, attempts to inhibit are more likely to be unsuccessful (Downey and Martin 1983). To overcome this problem of diagnosis, Castle and Turnbull (1983) used the fact that fetal breathing movements normally stop during labour. Using real-time ultrasound, they found that women admitted in preterm labour with fetal breathing movements generally did not progress to established preterm labour and delivery. Conversely, excluding antepartum haemorrhage, when there was absence of fetal breathing movements, there was a high incidence of progressive preterm labour and delivery.

### Home monitoring

The successful use of tocolytic agents requires an early diagnosis of preterm labour, since by the time a woman reaches 4 cm dilatation or spontaneously ruptures her membranes, tocolytics are rarely successful and the risk of infection increases. The first trial on home monitoring depended largely upon patient education and self-palpation as a means of early detection of preterm labour. Even when the approach was extended to include the daily use of instrumental home uterine activity monitoring in high-risk women, the results were controversial.

Many of the studies create difficulties in balancing the relative contribution of electronic detection of uterine contractions with the daily specialised nursing contact. A diagnostic and therapeutic technology assessment panel of the American Medical Association concluded that:

*'it has been shown that the system of home monitoring of uterine activity that includes daily nursing contact, can lower the preterm birth weight in high-risk women ... the relative contribution of the monitored data versus the nursing contact are under question'.*

Only one trial has assessed whether monitoring itself without nursing support is capable of improving early detection of preterm labour. In this trial, in which spontaneous preterm labour was diagnosed in 25% of patients and 24% of controls, the mean cervical dilatation was significantly lower in the monitored group and there were significantly more women in the monitored group with dilatation less than 4 cm (Mou *et al.* 1991).

## INHIBITION OF PRETERM LABOUR

### Tocolytics

In progressive preterm labour, where there are no contraindications to their use, intervention with pharmacological agents remains the current therapy for inhibition of uterine contractions. The risks versus benefits of tocolytic therapy are still being debated, despite 20 years of reported scientific experience. While the recent call for reappraisal has centred on the efficacy and safety of β-adrenergic agonists (Lamont 1993), more information from new and existing tocolytic agents has emerged.

The choice of agents, site of mechanism of action, efficacy, adverse effects and risk:benefit analysis have recently been comprehensively reviewed (Besinger 1994; Schneider 1994). Despite the widespread choice and use of these agents, factors such as gestational age, estimated birth weight, antepartum haemorrhage, pregnancy-induced hypertension, diabetes, intrauterine growth retardation, ruptured membranes, congenital malformations and infections may mitigate against tocolytic intervention in a majority of cases of preterm delivery. Furthermore, while tocolytics may be effective in the short-term inhibition of contractions and, hence, the suppression of labour, this type of use has not been associated with a reduction in perinatal mortality and morbidity (Lamont 1993). This may be due to suboptimal use, or the delay before employing measures, which could significantly improve perinatal mortality and morbidity; for example administration of antepartum glucocorticoids (Crowley, Chambers and Keirse 1990) or arranging *in utero* transfer to a centre with neonatal intensive care facilities (Lamont *et al.* 1983).

Most current tocolytic agents carry risks or undesirable side effects due to their non-selective pharmacological actions on fetomaternal organ systems. Therefore, the benefits of tocolytics for the survival of the fetus should be weighed against the potential fetomaternal adverse effects in each individual case.

### Antibiotics

Five prospective, controlled studies have examined the effectiveness of erythromycin, ampicillin or clindamycin in delaying delivery in women with preterm labour. Consistent with the increasing evidence to implicate infection in aetiology of preterm labour (McGregor *et al.* 1988; Romero *et al.* 1988; Gibbs *et al.* 1992; Lamont and Fisk 1993), four of the studies reported an apparent prolongation of pregnancy with the use of these antibiotics (McGregor *et al.* 1988; Morales *et al.* 1988; Winkler *et al.* 1988; Newton, Dins Moor and Gibbs 1989). In a further study, intravenous clindamycin was compared with a placebo when both were used before 33 weeks' gestation. The mean delay before preterm delivery in the treatment group was 40 days compared to 28 days with the placebo group ($P < 0.05$). Both treatment and placebo were combined with β-mimetics (McGregor, French and Kyung 1991).

## SUMMARY AND CONCLUSION

Excluding malformations, preterm delivery remains the major cause of perinatal mortality and morbidity. The aetiology of preterm labour remains unknown, prediction lacks specificity, prophylaxis is unhelpful, diagnosis is difficult and the benefits and risks of tocolytic therapy are still being debated. The incidence of preterm delivery remains largely unchanged. This is partly due to the increase in the number of women at risk due to factors such as drug abuse, teenage pregnancies, multiple pregnancy or pregnancy in later life. In addition, traditional success has been erroneously measured against the ability to achieve a gestational age beyond 37 weeks' gestation whereas at 24–26 weeks' gestation, success should be measured in terms of each day gained before preterm delivery as each day gained carries a 1% increase in survival rate.

While many studies show success of various treatment modalities in terms of days gained, none can show a significant improvement in perinatal mortality and morbidity. This may be due to the fact that infants with an extremely low birth weight are now considered as part of normal perinatal and neonatal mortality and morbidity statistics. In the recent past, they may have been 'written off' as late miscarriages or nonviable neonatal deaths. We should also consider morbidity as an end-point against which to measure therapeutic regimens, rather than simply mortality.

Currently, most of the efforts of obstetricians to prevent preterm birth are reactive and aimed at inhibiting the process of preterm labour. Unfortunately, all of the currently available tocolytic agents can have unacceptable side effects which limit their use. A better understanding of the mechanisms of term and preterm labour (Challis and Mitchell 1994) may result in the development of new agents to inhibit preterm labour with less dangerous side effects.

With a combination of early and aggressive tocolytics, including multi-agent therapy, it may be possible to combine effective tocolytics with adjuvant therapy to combat the basic pathology responsible for the condition (e.g. a combination of antibiotics and tocolytics for preterm labour associated with infection). It is also attractive to consider that if other measures which identify a woman at risk are used it will allow better screening tests for prediction. Prophylactic measures used either alone or in combination could be employed, together with early detection methods to permit a high-risk group of women to be identified, closely monitored and treated early.

It is also important to remember the concept of susceptibility and exposure which exists in other branches of medicine. A man may smoke heavily for 60 years without developing lung cancer, whereas another exposed only to passive smoking may die from the disease. It is likely that the same balance may exist in preterm labour and delivery. Some women have all the exposure (e.g. twins, antepartum haemorrhage and abnormal genital tract colonisation) without preterm delivery, whereas other women may carry no increased risk factors, but go into labour prematurely in response to nothing more than an increase in fetal movements, which makes the uterus irritable. Similarly, with respect to the role of infection, it is important not to concentrate our attention on the abnormal genital tract flora alone, but look to the host defence mechanisms used to prevent bacterial infiltration of the decidua and upper genital tract.

In this way, with a combined proactive and reactive approach to reducing risk factors, the prediction, and prevention of preterm birth may be improved and the mortality and morbidity with the social emotional and economical consequences may be reduced.

# References

Anderson, A. B. M. and Turnbull, A. C. (1969) Relationship between length of gestation and cervical dilatation, uterine contractility and other factors during pregnancy. *Am J Obstet Gynecol* **105**, 1207–14

Anonymous (1991) Advance report of final natality studies. *Monthly Vital Stat Rep* **40** (Suppl. 8), 40

Besinger, R. D. (1994) 'A systematic review of adverse events documented in the use of currently available treatment of preterm labour' in: M. J. N. C. Keirse (Ed.). New perspectives for the treatment of preterm labour — an international consensus. *Res Clin Forums* **16**, 89–126

Castle, B. M. and Turnbull, A. C. (1983) The presence or absence of fetal breathing movements predicts the outcome of preterm delivery. *Lancet* **ii**, 471–37

Challis, J. R. G. and Mitchell, M. D. (1994) 'Basic mechanism of preterm labour' in: M. J. N. C. Keirse (Eds.). New perspective for the effective treatment of preterm labour — an international consensus. *Res Clin Forums* **16**, 39–58

Chasnoff, I., Griffeth, D., MacGregory, S. *et al.* (1989) Temporal patterns of cocaine use in pregnancy. *J Am Med Assoc* **261**, 1714–24

Cherukuri, R., Minkoff, H., Hansen, R. L. *et al.* (1988) A cohort study of alkaloidal cocaine ('crack') in pregnancy. *Obstet Gynecol* **72**, 147–51

Cnattingius, S., Forman, M. R., Berendes, H., Graubard, B. I. and Isotalo, L. (1993) Effect of age, parity and smoking on pregnancy outcome: a population based study. *Am J Obstet Gynecol* **168**, 16–21

Copper, R. L., Goldenberg, R. L., Creasy, R. K. *et al.* (1993) A multi-center study of preterm birth weight and gestational age — specific neonatal mortality. *Am J Obstet Gynecol* **168**, 78–83

Creasy, R. K. (1993) Preterm birth prevention: where are we? *Am J Obstet Gynecol* **168**, 1223–30

Creasy, R. K., Gremmer, B. A. and Liggins, G. C. (1980) System for predicting preterm birth. *Obstet Gynecol* **55**, 692–5

Crowley, P. Chalmers, I. and Keirse, M. J. N. C. (1990) The effect of corticosteroid administration prior to preterm delivery: an overview of the evidence from controlled trials. *Br J Obstet Gynaecol* **97**, 11–25

Crowther, C. A., Neilson, J. P. Verkuyl, D. A. A. *et al.* (1989) Preterm labour in twin pregnancies: can it be prevented by hospital admission? *Br J Obstet Gynaecol* **96**, 850–3

Downey, L. J. and Martin, A. J. (1983) Ritodrine in the treatment of preterm labour: a study of 213 patients. *Br J Obstet Gynaecol* **90**, 1046–53

Edmonds, D. K. and Letchworth, A. T. (1982) The use of oral prophylactic salbutamol to prevent labour. *Lancet* **i**, 1310–12

Eriksen, N. L., Parisi, V. M., Daoust, S. *et al.* (1992) Fetal fibronectin: a method for detecting the presence of amniotic fluid. *Obstet Gynecol* **80**, 451–4

Eschenback, D. A., Nugent, R. P. and Rao, A. V. (1991) A randomised placebo controlled trial of erythromycin for the treatment of *Ureaplasma urealyticum* to prevent pre-term delivery. *Am J Obstet Gynecol* **164**, 734–42

Gibbs, R. S., Romero, R., Hillier, S. L., Eschenbach, D. A. and Sweet R. L. (1992) A review of premature birth and subclinical infection. *Am J Obstet Gynecol* **166**, 1515–28

Goldstein, P., Berrier, J., Rosen, S., Sacks, H. S. and Chalmers, T. C. (1989) A meta-analysis of randomised controlled trials of progesteronal agents in pregnancy. *Br J Obstet Gynaecol* **96**, 265–74

Hartikainen-Sorri, A. L. and Jouppila, P. (1984) Is routine hospitalisation needed in antenatal care of the twin pregnancy? *Perinat Med* **12**, 31–4

Hay, P. E., Lamont, R. R., Taylor-Robinson, D. *et al.* (1994) Abnormal bacterial colonisation of the genital tract and subsequent preterm delivery and late miscarriage. *BMJ* **308**, 295–8

Hemminki, E. and Starfield, B. (1978) Prevention and treatment of premature labour by drugs: review of controlled clinical trial. *Br J Obstet Gynaecol* **85**, 411–17

Keirse, M. J. N. C. (1990) Progestogen administration in pregnancy may prevent preterm delivery: an overview of the evidence from controlled trials. *Br J Obstet Gynaecol* **97**, 11–25

Kragt, H. and Keirse, M. J. N. C. (1990) How accurate is a woman's diagnosis of threatened preterm delivery? *Br J Obstet Gynaecol* **97**, 317–23

Kurki, T., Sivonen, A., Renkonen, O. V., Savia, E. and Ylikorkala, O. (1992) Bacterial vaginosis in early pregnancy and pregnancy outcome. *Obstet Gynecol* **80**, 173–7

Lamont, R. F. (1993) The contemporary use of β-agonists. *Br J Obstet Gynaecol* **100**, 890–2

Lamont, R. F. (1995) 'Bacterial vaginosis' in: J. W. W. Studd (Ed.). *The Yearbook of the Royal College of Obstetricians and Gynaecologists* 1994, pp. 149–60. Carnforth, Lancashire: Parthenon Publishing Group

Lamont, R. F., Dunlop, P. D. M., Crowley, P., Leven, M. I. and Elder M. G. (1983) Comparative mortality and morbidity of infants transferred *in utero* or postnatally. *J Perinat Med* **11**, 200–3

Lamont, R. F. and Fisk, N. M. (1993) 'The role of infection in the pathogenesis of preterm labour' in: J. W. W. Studd (Ed.). *Progress in Obstetrics and Gynaecology*, Vol. 10, Edinburgh: Churchill Livingstone

Lamont, R. F., Taylor-Robinson, D., Newman, M. *et al.* (1986) Spontaneous early preterm labour associated with abnormal genital bacterial colonisation. *Br J Obstet Gynaecol* **93**, 804–10

Lamont, R. F., Taylor-Robinson, D., Wiggles-

worth, J. S. *et al.* (1987) The role of mycoplasmas, ureaplasmas and chlamydiae in the genital tract of women presenting in spontaneous early preterm labour. *J Med Microbiol* **24**, 253–7

Lettieri, L., Anthony, M., Vintzileos, M. *et al.* (1993) Does 'idiopathic' preterm labor resulting in preterm birth exist? *Am J Obstet Gynecol* **160**, 1480–5

Leveno, J. J., Cox, K. and Roark, M. L. (1986) Cervical dilatation and prematurity revisited. *Obstet Gynecol* **68**, 434–5

Lind, T., Goderey, K. A., Gerrard, J. and Bryson, M. R. (1980) Continuous salbutamol infusion over 17 weeks to pre-empt premature labour. *Lancet* **ii**, 1165–6

Lockwood, C. J., Senyei, A. E, Dische, M. R. *et al.* (1991) Fetal fibronectin in cervical and vaginal secretions as a predictor of preterm delivery. *N Engl J Med* **325**, 669–74

Lockwood, C. J., Wein, R., Lapinski, R. *et al.* (1993) The presence of cervical and vaginal fetal fibronectin predicts preterm delivery in an inner city obstetric population. *Am J Obstet Gynecol* **169**, 798–804

MacLennan, A. H., Green, R. C., O'Shea, R. *et al.* (1990) Routine hospital admission in twin pregnancy between 26 and 30 weeks' gestation. *Lancet* **335**, 267–9

Main, D. M. and Gabbe, S. G. (1987) Risk scoring for preterm labor: where do we go from here? *Am J Obstet Gynecol* **157**, 789–93

McCormack, W. M., Rosner, B., Lee, Y. *et al.* (1987) Effect on birth weight of erythromycin treatment of pregnant women. *Obstet Gynecol* **69**, 202–7

McDonald, H. M., O'Loughlin, J. A., Jolley, P., Vigneswaran, R. and McDonald, P. J. (1991) Vaginal infection and preterm labour. *Br J Obstet Gynaecol* **98**, 427–35

McDonald, H. M., O'Loughlin, J. A., Vigneswaran, R., Jolley, P. T. and McDonald, P. J. (1994) Bacterial vaginosis in pregnancy and efficacy of short course oral metronidazole treatment: a randomised controlled trial. *Obstet Gynecol* **84**, 343–8

McGregor, J. A., French, J. I. and Kyung, S. (1991) Adjunctive clindamycin therapy for preterm labor: results of a double-blind, placebo-controlled trial. *Am J Obstet Gynecol* **165**, 867–75

McGregor, J. A., French, J. I., Lawellin, D., and Todd, J. K. (1988) Preterm birth and infection: pathogenic pssibilities. *Am J Reprod Immunol Microbiol* **16**, 123–32

McGregor, J. A., French, J. I., Jones, W. *et al.* (1994) Bacterial vaginosis is associated with prematurity and vaginal fluid mucinase and sialidase: results of a controlled trial of topical clindamycin cream. *Am J Obstet Gynecol* **170**, 1048–60

McGregor, J. M., French, J. I., Rellier, L. B., Todd, J. K. and Makowski, E. L. (1986) Adjunctive erythromycin treatment for idiopathic preterm labor: results of a randomised double-blinded, placebo-controlled trial. *Am J Obstet Gynecol* **154**, 98–103

Medical Research Council (1990) Working group on children conceived by *in vitro* fertilisation. Births in Great Britain resulting from assisted conception 1978–1987. *BMJ* **300**, 1229–33

Medical Research Council/Royal College of Obstetricians and Gynaecologists Working Party on Cervical Cerclage (1993) Final Report of the MRC/RCOG multicentre randomised trial of cervical cerclage. *Br J Obstet Gynaecol* **100**, 516–23

Minkoff, H., Grunebaum, A. N., Schwarz, R. H. *et al.* (1984) Risk factors for prematurity and premature rupture of the membranes: a prospective study of the vaginal flora in pregnancy. *Am J Obstet Gynecol* **150**, 965–72

Morales, W. J., Angel, J. L., O'Brien, W. F., Knuppel, R. A. and Finazzo, M. A. (1988) A randomized study of antibiotic therapy in idiopathic preterm labor. *Obstet Gynecol* **72**, 829–33

Morales, W. J., Schorr, S. and Albriton, J. (1994) Effect of metronidazole in patients with preterm birth in proceeding pregnancy and bacterial vaginosis: a placebo-controlled, double-blind study. *Am J Obstet Gynecol* **171**, 345–9

Morrison, J. C., Allbert, J. R., McLaughlin, B. N. *et al.* (1993) Oncofetal fibronectin in patients with false labor as a predictor of preterm delivery. *Am J Obstet Gynecol* **168**, 538–42

Mou, S. M., Sunderji, S. G., Gall, S. *et al.* (1991) Multicenter randomized clinical trial of home uterine activity monitoring for detection of preterm labor. *Am J Obstet Gynecol* **165**, 858–66

Nageotte, M. P., Casal, D. and Senyei, A. E. (1994) Fetal fibronectin in patients at increased risk of premature birth. *Am J Obstet Gynecol* **170**, 20–5

Neilson, J. P., Verkuyl, D. A. A., Crowther, C. A. *et al.* (1988) Preterm labor in twin pregnancies: prediction by cervical assessment. *Obstet Gynecol* **72**, 719–23

Newcombe, R. and Chalmers, I. (1981). 'Assessing the risk of preterm labour' in: M. G. Elder and C. H. Hendricks (Eds.). *Preterm Labour,* pp. 47–60. London: Butterworths

Newman, R. B., Godsey, R. K., Ellings, J. M. *et al.* (1991) Quantification of cervical change: relationship to preterm delivery in multifetal gestation. *Am J Obstet Gynecol* **165**, 264–71

Newton, E. R., Dins Moor, M. J. and Gibbs, R. S. (1989) A randomised blinded placebo-controlled trial of antibiotics in idiopathic preterm labor. *Obstet Gynecol* **74**, 562–6

Papiernik, E. (1984) Proposals for a programmed prevention policy of preterm birth. *Clin Obstet Gynecol* **27**, 614–35

Robertson, P. A., Sniderman, S. H., Laros, R. K. Jr *et al.* (1992) Neonatal morbidity according to gestational age and birth weight from five tertiary care centers in the United States, 1983 through 1986. *Am J Obstet Gynecol* **166**, 1629–45

Romero, R., Gonzalez, R., Sepulveda, W. *et al.* (1992) Microbial invasion of the amniotic cavity in patients with suspected cervical incompetence: prevalence and clinical significance. *Am J Obstet Gynecol* **167**, 1086–91

Romero, R., Major, M., Wu, Y. K. *et al.* (1988) Infection in the pathogenesis of preterm labour. *Semin Pathol* **12**, 262–79

Saunders, M. C., Dick, J. S. and Brown, I. M. (1985) The effects of hospital admission for bed rest on the duration of twin pregnancy: a randomised trial. *Lancet* **ii**, 793–5

Schneider, H. (1994) 'Pharmacological intervention in preterm labour' in: M. J. N. C. Keirse (Ed.). New prospectives for the treatment of preterm labour — an international consensus. *Res Clin Forums* **16**, 59–88

Stubbs, T. M., Van Dorsten, P. and Miller, M. C. (1986) The preterm cervix and preterm labor: relative risks, predictive values and change over time. *Am J Obstet Gynecol* **155**, 829–34

Villar, J. Ezcurra, E. J., de la Fuenta, V. G. and Campodonico, L. (1994) 'Preterm delivery syndrome: the unmet need' in: M. J. N. C. Keirse (Ed.). New prospectives for the treatment of preterm labour — an international consensus. *Res Clin Forums* **16**, 9–38

White, B., Lamont, R. F. and Letchworth, A. T. (1989) An approach to the problem of recurrent middle trimester abortion. *J Obstet Gynaecol* **10**, 8–9

Winkler, M., Baumann, L., Ruckhaberle, K. E. and Schiller, E. M. (1988) Erythromycin therapy for subclinical intrauterine infections in threatened preterm delivery — a preliminary report. *J Perinat Med* **159**, 539–43

Wong, G. P., Farquaharson, D. F. and Dansereau, J. (1993) Emergency cervical cerclage: a retrospective view of 51 cases. *Am J Perinatol* **10**, 341–7

# Index